Health Policy and
Advanced Practice Nursing

Kelly A. Goudreau, PhD, RN, ACNS-BC, FAAN, is the Associate Director, Patient Care Services and Nurse Executive at the Kansas City VA Medical Center, Kansas City, Missouri, and associate editor for *Clinical Nurse Specialist: The Journal of Advanced Nursing Practice*. She is also past president of the National Association of Clinical Nurse Specialists (NACNS). She is licensed as a Clinical Nurse Specialist (CNS) in Oregon and is certified by the American Nurses Credentialing Center (ANCC) as a CNS in adult health. Dr. Goudreau has received honors from the Oregon Nurses Association, is a recipient of the Brenda Lyon Leadership Award and the President's Award from NACNS, and is a Fellow of the American Academy of Nursing. She has published more than 30 journal articles and is the coeditor of two books.

Mary C. Smolenski, EdD, MS, FNP, FAANP, is a consultant, registered nurse, and family nurse practitioner with varied experience including graduate education, consulting, the military, primary care, independent practice, and association work with an emphasis on certification and accreditation. She is a retired Air Force reserve colonel and a fellow of the American Association of Nurse Practitioners. Dr. Smolenski served as director of certification services at the ANCC for 11 years. She has served on several nonprofit boards including the American Board of Specialty Nursing Certification and the National Organization of Competency Assurance (now the Institute for Credentialing Excellence [ICE]). Dr. Smolenski has written numerous articles and given presentations on certification, competency, advanced practice nursing, and portfolios both nationally and internationally.

Health Policy and Advanced Practice Nursing

Impact and Implications

SECOND EDITION

Kelly A. Goudreau, PhD, RN, ACNS-BC, FAAN
Mary C. Smolenski, EdD, MS, FNP, FAANP

SPRINGER PUBLISHING COMPANY

Springer Publishing Company, LLC
11 West 42nd Street
New York, NY 10036
www.springerpub.com

Acquisitions Editor: Margaret Zuccarini
Compositor: Newgen KnowledgeWorks

ISBN: 978-0-8261-6944-0
ebook ISBN: 978-0-8261-6945-7
Instructor's PowerPoints ISBN: 978-0-8261-6946-4

Instructor's Materials: Qualified instructors may request supplements by emailing textbook@ springerpub.com

17 18 19 20 / 5 4 3 2 1

The author and the publisher of this Work have made every effort to use sources believed to be reliable to provide information that is accurate and compatible with the standards generally accepted at the time of publication. Because medical science is continually advancing, our knowledge base continues to expand. Therefore, as new information becomes available, changes in procedures become necessary. We recommend that the reader always consult current research and specific institutional policies before performing any clinical procedure. The author and publisher shall not be liable for any special, consequential, or exemplary damages resulting, in whole or in part, from the readers' use of, or reliance on, the information contained in this book. The publisher has no responsibility for the persistence or accuracy of URLs for external or third-party Internet websites referred to in this publication and does not guarantee that any content on such websites is, or will remain, accurate or appropriate.

Library of Congress Cataloging-in-Publication Data
Names: Goudreau, Kelly A., editor. | Smolenski, Mary C. (Mary Catherine), 1950- editor.
Title: Health policy and advanced practice nursing : impact and implications
  / [edited by] Kelly A. Goudreau, Mary C. Smolenski.
Description: Second edition. | New York, NY : Springer Publishing Company,
  LLC, [2018] | Includes bibliographical references and index.
Identifiers: LCCN 2017035507 | ISBN 9780826169440 (pbk.) | ISBN 9780826169457 (ebook) |
  ISBN 9780826169464 (instructor's powerpoints)
Subjects: | MESH: Advanced Practice Nursing | Health Policy | Nurse's Role | United States
Classification: LCC RT89 | NLM WY 128 | DDC 362.17/3—dc23
LC record available at https://lccn.loc.gov/2017035507

Contact us to receive discount rates on bulk purchases.
We can also customize our books to meet your needs.
For more information please contact: sales@springerpub.com

Printed in the United States of America by McNaughton & Gunn.

This book is dedicated to the practitioners and students of nursing who seek to improve the health care environment. It is through your curiosity, perseverance, and advocacy that the world we know will change. We are hopeful that this book will assist you to see what it is, how it will impact your practice, and what may be in the future.

Contents

UNIT III: HEALTH POLICY AND SPECIAL POPULATIONS: IMPLICATIONS

UNIT IV: HEALTH POLICY AND ITS IMPACT ON APRN-DRIVEN QUALITY AND RESEARCH

Contributors

Cynthia Abarado, DNP, RN, APRN, GNP-BC
Retired
University of Texas
MD Anderson Cancer Center
Houston, Texas

Andrea Brassard, PhD, FNP-BC, FAANP
Senior Strategic Policy Adviser
AARP Public Policy Institute
Center to Champion Nursing
  in America
AARP
Washington, DC

Kelly J. Brassil, PhD, RN, AOCNS, ACNS-BC
Director
Nursing Research and Innovation
University of Texas
MD Anderson Cancer Center
Houston, Texas

Linda Brousseau, NP, MN
Nurse Practitioner
Halton Clinical Health Services; and
Doctoral Student and Research
  Trainee
Canadian Centre for Advanced Practice
  Nursing Research
McMaster University
Hamilton, Ontario, Canada

Denise Bryant-Lukosius, PhD, RN
Associate Professor
School of Nursing; and
Co-Director
Canadian Centre for Advanced Practice
  Nursing Research
McMaster University
Hamilton, Ontario, Canada

Garry Brydges, DNP, MBA, ACNP-BC, CRNA
Chief Nurse Anesthetist
Department of Anesthesiology and
  Perioperative Medicine
University of Texas
MD Anderson Cancer Center
Houston, Texas

Nancy Carter, PhD, RN
Assistant Dean and Associate Professor
School of Nursing
Affiliate Faculty, Canadian Centre for
  Advanced Practice Nursing
  Research
McMaster University
Hamilton, Ontario, Canada

Catherine Coates, BA
Senior Advisor
Office of Mental Health
Ministry of Health
Blenheim, New Zealand

Joyce E. Dains, DrPH, JD, RN, FNP-BC, FNAP, FAANP
Associate Professor
Department of Nursing
University of Texas
MD Anderson Cancer Center
Houston, Texas

Kathleen R. Delaney, PhD, PMHNP-BC, FAAN
Professor and Program Director
PMH-NP Program
Rush College of Nursing
Chicago, Illinois

Evelyn Duffy, DNP, AGPCNP-BC, FAANP
Associate Professor
Director of the Adult-Gerontology
    Nurse, Practitioner Program; and
Associate Director of the University
    Center on Aging and Health
Frances Payne Bolton School of Nursing
Case Western University
Cleveland, Ohio

Julia Yuen-Heung To Dutka, EdD
CEO and Senior Advisor to President
CGFNS International, Inc.
Philadelphia, Pennsylvania

Moriah Ellen, PhD
Assistant Professor
Institute of Health Policy, Management,
    and Evaluation at the University of
    Toronto; and
Investigator, McMaster University
Hamilton, Ontario, Canada

Christine C. Filipovich, MSN, RN
Deputy Secretary
Department of Health, Commonwealth
    of Pennsylvania
Harrisburg, Pennsylvania

Kelly A. Goudreau, PhD, RN, ACNS-BC, FAAN
Associate Director
Patient Care Services
VA Kansas City Medical Center
Kansas City, Missouri

James L. Harris, PhD, APRN-BC, MBA, CNL, FAAN
Professor
University of South Alabama
Mobile, Alabama

Susan Hassmiller, PhD, RN, FAAN
Senior Advisor for Nursing
Director, Future of Nursing: *Campaign for Action*
Robert Wood Johnson Foundation
Princeton, New Jersey

Sharon D. Horner, PhD, RN, CNS, FAAN
Associate Dean Research
Dolores V. Sands Chair in Nursing
    Research
University of Texas at Austin
Austin, Texas

Frances Hughes, RN, DNurs, ONZM
Former CEO
International Council of Nurses
Geneva, Switzerland

Susan Kendig, JD, MSN, WHNP-BC, FAANP
Teaching Professor and
    Coordinator
College of Nursing
University of Missouri
St Louis, Missouri

Kelley Kilpatrick, PhD, RN
Associate Professor
CIUSSS EIM-Maisonneuve-Rosemont
    Hospital
Faculty of Nursing, Université de
    Montréal
Affiliate Faculty, Canadian Centre for
    Advanced Practice Nursing
    Research
Montréal, Québec, Canada

Janelle Komorowski, DNP, RN, CNM
Assistant Professor
Frontier Nursing University
Hyden, Kentucky

Elizabeth A. Landin, MSN, MBA, RN, CCRN-K, NE-BC
Associate Chief Nurse
Alaska VA Healthcare System
Department of Veterans Affairs
Anchorage, Alaska

Judy Lentz, RN, MSN
Retired CEO
Hospice and Palliative Nurses Association
Pittsburgh, Pennsylvania

Jennifer M. Manning, DNS, APRN, CNS, CNE
Associate Professor
Louisiana State University Health Sciences Center School of Nursing
New Orleans, Louisiana

Ruth Martin-Misener, PhD, NP
Professor
School of Nursing
Dalhousie University; and
Co-Director
Canadian Centre for Advanced Practice Nursing Research
Halifax, Nova Scotia, Canada

Suzanne Miyamoto, PhD, RN, FAAN
Chief Policy Officer
American Association of Colleges of Nursing
Washington, DC

Liana Orsolini, PhD, RN, ANEF, FAAN
Care Delivery and Advanced Practice System Consultant
Bon Secours Health System
President
Orsolini and Associates
Stafford, Virginia

Tracy Pasek, DNP, RN, CCRN, CCNS
Clinical Nurse Specialist
Children's Hospital of Pittsburgh
University of Pittsburgh
Pittsburgh, Pennsylvania

Elizabeth L. Pestka, MS, PMHCNS-BC, AGN-BC
Clinical Nurse Specialist
Mayo Clinic
Rochester, Minnesota

Melinda Ray, MSN
Executive Director
National Association of Clinical Nurse Specialists
Pittsburgh, Pennsylvania

Susan C. Reinhard, RN, PhD, FAAN
Senior VP
AARP Public Policy Institute
Chief Strategist, Center to Champion Nursing
AARP
Washington, DC

Josette Roussel, RN, MSc, MEd
Senior Nurse Advisor
Policy, Advocacy, and Strategy
Canadian Nurses Association
Ottawa, Ontario, Canada

Madrean M. Schober, PhD, MSN, BGS, ANP, FAANP
President
Schober Global Healthcare Consulting
International Healthcare Consultants
Indianapolis, Indiana

Franklin A. Shaffer, EdD, RN, FAAN, FFNMRcSI
CEO and President
CGFNS International, Inc.
Philadelphia, Pennsylvania

Judith Shamian, RN, PhD, FAAN
Past President of the International Council of Nurses (ICN)
President Emeritus, Immediate Past President, and CEO
Victorian Order of Nurses
Toronto, Ontario, Canada

Maureen Shekleton, PhD, RN, DPNAP, FAAN
Principal
Shekleton, LLC
Chicago, Illinois

Mary C. Smolenski, EdD, MS, FNP, FAANP
Consultant
Lakewood Ranch, Florida

David Stewart, BNRN, MHM
Associate Director
Nursing and Health Policy
International Council of Nurses (ICN)
Saint Francisville, Louisiana

Melissa Stewart, DNP, RN, CPE
Consultant, Author, and International
  Health Literacy Consultant
St. Francisville, Louisiana

Lisa Summers, FACNM. DrPH
Senior Policy Advisor, APRN Issues
Department of Health Policy
American Nurses Association
Washington, DC

Laura J. Thiem, DNP, RN, FNP-BC, Adult PMHCNS-BC, PMHNP-BC, CNE
Clinical Assistant Professor
School of Nursing and Health Studies
University of Missouri—Kansas City
Kansas City, Missouri

Jan Towers, PhD, NP-C, CRNP, FAANP, FAAN
Senior Policy Consultant
American Association of Nurse
  Practitioners
Washington, DC

Christine S. Zambricki, DNAP, CRNA, FAAN
CEO, America's Blood Centers
Former Deputy Executive Director
American Association of Nurse
  Anesthetists
Ann Arbor, Michigan

Karen L. Zanni, RN, PhD, FNP
Research Scientist
TeamHealthNY
New York, New York

Preface

As we develop the second edition of this book, the Patient Protection and Affordable Care Act (PPACA), more commonly known as Obamacare, celebrated its seventh anniversary. It had succeeded in providing millions of Americans with health care coverage who were uninsured and changed the landscape of the health care system. In the midst of this change that put major emphasis on health promotion and prevention as essentials, Advanced Practice Registered Nurses (APRNs) made many strides toward full practice authority and these successes continue. This second edition highlights many of these successes. In spite of successes, the "health" care system, which Dr. Loretta Ford addressed in the Foreword of the first edition, is teetering on the edge of reverting to a "sick" system. This is a perfect time and opportunity for nursing to help move health care from a "curative" culture to a true "culture of health" system. Individuals have tasted the benefits of a health promotion/disease prevention system and embraced its tenets. They are ready for more.

The past few years have kindled in the people of the United States and around the world a desire to become involved and speak up, whatever their views may be. In the United Kingdom, Brexit was a good example. In the United States and worldwide, rallies on January 21, 2017, post–presidential inauguration, spoke to a variety of concerns from health care, women's issues, education, human rights, work issues, and the economy, to name a few. The worldwide universality of this outcry was remarkable, and it continues on a local level. Legislators are being bombarded with phone calls, letters, faxes, emails, and demonstrations at their offices and town halls. Technology has made it easier to have one's voice heard but this desire for change comes from within. People want to be heard and impact policy change. Health care is now also at the forefront of these efforts. When looking at rankings for happiness on a world scale and factors that contribute to this, the countries that score near the top in several polls (Bloomberg and the World Economic Forum) all ensure health care coverage for their populations. The United States ranks 28th in the happiness factor in the 2016 World Economic Forum poll, not even near the top 10. Can it be that healthy people are happy, productive people?

People seem to be ready to take more control of their health care and have a need for knowledge and guidance. The second edition of this book continues to investigate how health policy impacts APRN practice and how, through practice,

APRNs can help improve the lives of their patients/clients. In the first section, efforts such as the J & J Campaign for Nursing's Future and the Consensus Model are brought up to date to show the influence they have had on the nursing practice. The Institute of Medicine (now the National Academy of Medicine) report *The Future of Nursing* pushed for nurses to practice to the full extent of their education and progress toward the defined goals is outlined. A new chapter is presented on independent practice with a case study outlining how state legislative rulings can affect practice. The growing success of the Doctor of Nursing Practice (DNP) programs and graduates is discussed, showing the interest of nurses wanting to be involved and take on more responsibility, including health policy change. A new chapter under special populations provides a review of the evolution and impact of genetics and genetics health policy on APRN practice. A new research chapter titled "Connecting Research, the Research Agenda, and Health Policy" discusses how a research agenda can have a powerful influence on health policy from many perspectives. In Unit IV, organizational perspectives on health policy and APRN practice are updated while in Unit V, global perspectives on APRNs and credentialing are provided by international experts showing how advanced practice nurses are faring worldwide. Finally, the current state of practice for each of the APRN roles is presented.

APRNs have played a role in pushing for full plenary authority as well as contributing to changes to the health care system. Some practice efforts have been more successful than others. An example is well described in the last chapter of the book by Zambricki on Certified Registered Nurse Anesthetists' (CRNAs') efforts to gain full practice authority in the Veterans Affairs (VA) system. As she points out, this is not the time to burn bridges, sit back, or slow down. The same waters may need to be crossed more than once! If the health care system is truly to be a patient-centered system, a culture change needs to happen. If it is to be a patient-choice system, individuals need to be aware of the options open to them, educated about their care including health promotion/prevention and the evidence to support this, and be knowledgeable of the consequences of their choices. Who better to play an integral part in making that happen than APRNs and nurses whose education and roles are grounded in health and well-being, and who better to push for policy changes in the health care system that support patient-centeredness, but APRNs? It is uncertain at this time what changes and deletions may be made to the PPACA with the new Congress or how individual states may deal with these changes. It is also unclear how this will impact APRNs and their practice. All the more important then it is to keep up to date about health policy issues, learn how to interact with lawmakers for positive change for our patients and our practices, and become involved. It is only through a concerted, coordinated effort that as APRNs we can help create a health-oriented culture and address the issues of access, quality, and affordability in our health care system.

Hopefully, this book will help the faculty guide graduate students toward a better understanding of the importance of health policy change and its widespread impact and guide students in taking an active role in these changes. **In addition to the book, we have prepared an instructor's manual of PowerPoint slides. Qualified instructors can obtain a copy of these by emailing textbook@ springerpub.com.** The timing is right, and people are ready for the change. Let's grab the opportunity and make an impact!

Kelly A. Goudreau
Mary C. Smolenski

Acknowledgments

The reality is that this book would not have been possible without the assistance and support of many individuals. We thank our authors who have made each chapter come to fruition and our publishing editors who worked tirelessly to ensure a high-quality product.

I would like to acknowledge the support and patience of my coeditor, Dr. Mary Smolenski. She has been the strength of this edition, and I so very much appreciate her support during some trying times in my personal life.

To my husband, Serge Goudreau, who has been my personal rock during this past year. Thank you does not seem to say enough . . . but thank you.

Health Policy From an Advanced Practice Perspective

CHAPTER 1

Prolific Policy: Implications for Advanced Practice Registered Nurses

Melissa Stewart

Policy can serve as a vehicle for movement or progress in practice. Policy can open doors for opportunity and provide methodology for systematic solidarity in action. Unfortunately, many health care practitioners allow policy to happen around them, but not through them. To truly be an effective advocate, policy must become a tool used to sharpen our practice to meet the needs of our consumers. Tomajan (2012) defined advocacy as "work on the behalf of self and/ or others to raise awareness of a concern and to promote solutions to the issues. Advocacy often requires working through formal, decision-making bodies to achieve desired outcomes."

Milstead (2013) defined policy as "A purposeful, general plan of action, which includes authoritative guidelines, that is developed to respond to a problem. The plan directs human behavior toward specific goals." Policy statements detail values and guidelines to provide precise direction. Actions in the legislative arena at every level—local, state, and federal—directly impact the practice arena, and what occurs in the practice arena in turn impacts legislative action. In order to support the profession and provide for those entrusted to our care, it is essential that Advanced Practice Registered Nurses (APRNs) assume advocacy roles and strengthen their leadership skills in order to become policy leaders. Nursing leaders need a basic platform of understanding, both in advocacy and policy, to combine resources to accomplish identified goals. APRNs must recognize that policy is an integral part of everyday professional nursing practice.

OUR RIGHT TO PROMOTE WELL-BEING

We the people of the United States, in order to form a more perfect union, establish justice, insure domestic tranquility, provide for the common defense, promote the general welfare, and secure the blessings of liberty to ourselves and our posterity, do ordain and establish this Constitution for the United States of America.

The authors of the preamble to the Constitution called for a union of Americans to create optimal conditions for the safety and well-being of America's citizens. This sacred document established a priority to promote welfare among American citizens. Government action toward this directive is derived through policy. Prudent, pragmatic approaches are designed through policy to yield optimal results.

To practitioners, policy often surfaces as regulatory mandates or organizational improvements. Personally and professionally, policy surrounds us daily. From the protection of patient confidentiality to the code used to charge a payer, policy is deeply embedded in our everyday life. The power to influence policy through the political arena is a right of every American. Legislative representatives are servants of the voters, who empower them with their political appointment. The right to vote and contact political figures is often an underutilized resource. Although one may choose to label oneself as not being politically active, one cannot escape the consequences acquiesced to in the political arena.

To many health care professionals, policy is just not appealing enough to hold the providers' attention. The tedious nature of policy is why regulatory changes can sneak in and make chaos out of a once highly functional practice. Legal terms in law, ambiguous terminology in regulations, and robotic language in organizational policy can serve to disengage health care providers. Unfortunately, the perceived pleonasm of policy can deter the health care practitioners, who need to understand and implement the directives in practice. According to Anderson (2011), there are five stages of policy making (Table 1.1).

Stage 1 is policy agenda. In stage 1, the focus is on problems that receive attention of public officials. In policy formulation, stage 2, concentration is on the development of courses of action, acceptable and proposed, for dealing with a public problem. Stage 3 is policy adoption when support for a specific proposal is procured so the policy can be legitimized. Policy implementation is the focus of stage 4; this is where the administrative machinery of government begins to apply the policy. Finally, in stage 5, policy evaluation, policy is evaluated for effectiveness, barriers, and consequences. Table 1.2 compares the five stages of policy making with the nursing process.

Policy is born out of need for communal actions. The need may be identified within an organization to achieve optimal performance from employees, or because of market changes or new legislation passed. Socially, policy is developed to help maintain a civility among populations. Common drivers that influence policy are social and environmental factors, voters, professional organizations, and advocacy groups (Figure 1.1). Irrespective of the reason for the policy, once created, individuals are affected by policy.

TABLE 1.1 Stages of Policy Development

Stage 1 Policy agenda	Assessment
Stage 2 Policy formulation	Diagnosis
Stage 3 Policy adoption	Plan
Stage 4 Policy implementation	Implement
Stage 5 Policy evaluation	Evaluate

TABLE 1.2 Five Stages of Policy Making Compared With the Nursing Process

STAGE 1 POLICY AGENDA	STAGE 2 POLICY FORMULATION	STAGE 3 POLICY ADOPTION	STAGE 4 POLICY IMPLEMENTATION	STAGE 5 POLICY EVALUATION
Those problems that receive the serious attention of public officials	Development of pertinent and acceptable proposed courses of action for dealing with a public problem	Development of support for a specific proposal so a policy can be legitimized or authorized	Application of the policy by the government's administrative machinery	Efforts by the government to determine whether the policy was effective and why or why not

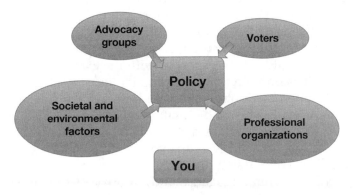

FIGURE 1.1 Drivers of policy.

Social and environmental factors include newsworthy topics such as unemployment, illegal aliens, and the stock market crash. The stock market influences companies' revenue, which in turn impacts employment. The crash of the stock market caused a decrease in capital for companies that translated into layoffs and downsizing. With the loss of employment comes the loss of benefits such as health care benefits. The Affordable Care Act was framed as a way to provide health care coverage for the unemployed and illegal aliens. From bill to law, the Affordable Care Act has ignited political astuteness from political influencers.

It is imperative that health care professionals understand the political process. Health care providers, either (or both?) individually or through professional organizations or advocacy groups, directly influence local, state, and national policy on a regular basis. Professional organizations and advocacy groups through the weight of their votes impact policy. Because the legislative and executive branches of government comprise elected officials, votes and organized groups of voters carry strong lobbying influence when dealing with these two political arms.

Within professional organizations, such as the American Association of Nurse Practitioners [AANP] and the American Nurses Association, member-created resolutions help to push an issue up to the state and national level for organizational support. In the past, a house of delegates would vote on resolutions to help the direction for national organizational boards. The new trend is to have various specialty committees work together to offer expert support. The Institute of Medicine (IOM) often holds roundtables for specific health care issues as a way to provide direction and influence to members, legislators, and other significant parties.

Knowledge of where to introduce proposed policy can determine success or failure. Through the three branches of government, that is, legislative, judicial, and executive, policy is created, implemented, and enforced. The legislative branch, the House of Representatives and the Senate, creates law. The executive branch, which consists of the president federally, at the state level the governor, and at the city level the mayor, implements law. The judicial branch, courts and regulatory agencies, enforces law. To be effective when advocating for law, point of access is critical.

Appropriate point of access for impact is contingent on what a provider is trying to accomplish, because this will determine where personal or professional influence should be introduced. For example, if a bill is in the House, which may limit the practice of the APRN, the practitioner may want to contact legislators and attend committee meetings about the bill. Whereas, if the bill has passed into law and the provider wants to ensure the law is interpreted into practice appropriately, the APRN would want to connect with the executive branch's assigned government entity tasked with implementing the new law. Government entities often tasked with implementing health care laws are the Centers for Medicare and Medicaid Services (CMS) or the State Department of Health and Human Services. Finally, the APRN accesses the judicial arm of government through reporting illegal activity or serving as an expert witness to safeguard intent of the law. Each state's Board of Nursing serves as a judicial arm of government protecting the state's citizens from negligence and/or error of practitioners. Knowing when and where to access can help the health care provider maximize their influential potential (Figure 1.2).

In the process of developing law, a bill has to go through several stages of debate, revision, and voting before it sees the light of day. A proposal from a member of Congress, either from the Senate or the House of Representatives, proposes an idea for a new law or an idea to alter a law that already exists. After the proposal is submitted, it then becomes the proposing official's job to get the proposal written into a bill. Once the bill is created, it must be submitted to one of the two houses of Congress, the Senate or the House of Representatives. The bill is then assigned to a particular committee that deals with the subject of the proposed law. It is the assigned committee's job to debate the value of the law, including its necessity to be passed, and the pros versus the cons. If the bill is favorably passed by the committee, it then goes in front of the entire House or the Senate for debate. It is similar to the debate that occurred within the committee, but now the whole branch of Congress debates the merits and implications of the proposed bill. Once a bill has met with the approval of one of the branches of Congress, it then moves to the other branch to go through the same process. Throughout the journey in Congress, the bill is modified in an effort to be passed by the general consensus. Once the bill is passed by both branches of Congress, it goes to a conference committee to get the modifications added to the original. After the bill has been revised, both houses of Congress vote on it. Finally, the bill is submitted to the president of the United States, who has the power to either put the law into effect or veto it. Even if the president decides to veto the bill, the legislative branch can vote to overrule his decision. If two thirds of the representatives vote to overrule it, the bill becomes a law anyway.

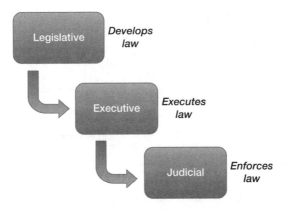

FIGURE 1.2 Point of access for maximum influence.

It is not uncommon, and probably most likely, that organizations and/or lobbyists of special interest groups will try to have as much impact as possible on the early stages of this process, as the idea is being proposed, accepted, and written up as a bill. Getting in on the ground floor of a proposal submission and following it allows for maximum input and to ensure that there is clarity in terminology. It also helps to craft components of the bill with the best interests of the particular group. Most of the initial bills are written by House or Senate staffers, who research elements of the proposal and work on draft after draft until it is ready for committee assignment. The work continues throughout the whole process, because as outlined previously, the bill can be modified, changed, and possibly lose the impact that was originally intended. Knowing where the bill is in the process, what committee it is assigned to and who is on that committee, and contacting legislators and committee members with facts and data to support (or rebuke) the bill are important steps that any APRN can take.

POLICY SHIFT TOWARD ILLNESS PREVENTION

As the 21st century unfolds, a new paradigm in health care begins to emerge with the implementation of the Affordable Care Act. The expansion of health care deliverables, coupled with the movement in health maintenance through prevention services, presents new challenges to address. Redefining providers' scope of practice, adjusting to result-oriented payment structures, and establishing new delivery realms such as transitions in care are just a few of the issues that must be addressed to successfully move forward (CMS, 2011a, 2011b).

The present prevention/wellness movement in health care has always held a presence in our delivery system, especially in the practice of nursing. Nursing theorists such as Florence Nightingale, Dorothea Orem, Betty Neuman, and Nora Pender are just a few who include wellness through prevention as a construct in their theories (Table 1.3). Although healing related to insult or injury has

TABLE 1.3 Nursing Theorists With a Prevention Focus

THEORIST	THEORY
Florence Nightingale	Environmental theory
Dorothea Orem	Self-care deficit
Betty Neuman	Systems theory
Nora Pender	Health promotion model

historically been the crux of health care, the 21st century is focused on personal sustainability through health prevention. With the ever-growing shortage of primary care physicians, frontline access providers are becoming less and less available to the public. In an attempt to address the frontline provider crisis, which has traditionally been a physician, APRNs and in particular Nurse Practitioners (NPs) are assuming this role to meet the public access crisis.

SCOPE OF PRACTICE

Although APRNs are meeting the need of the consumer, they are still limited by reimbursement and collaboration agreements. Even though APRNs are delivering the same level of care in many cases as is rendered by a generalist physician, they are not reimbursed 100% of the treatment billing codes like their physician colleagues. Instead, APRNs are reimbursed at the rate of only 85% of the code allotment. Barnes et al. (2017) noted that APRNs have 20% higher odds of working in an area of practice that is suffering from provider shortages like primary care when they are reimbursed 100% of the physician fee-for-service rate. Payer discrimination between APRNs and physicians only serves to fiscally limit investment in their practices. The harnessing of APRNs through collaboration agreement mandates between APRNs and physicians, further attempts to publicly restrict the independent role of the APRN. Slowly significant policy gains are being made as the AANP publicly identify that 21 states allow APRNs to practice independently to the full extent of their training with unrestricted licensure (AANP, 2016). To maximize the role of APRNs, the legislatively created scope of practice in each state will need to remove these independent practice barriers. The issues of payment and collaborative agreements are regulatory mandates that are hindering the progression of APRNs as they attempt to maximize their practice autonomy. Understanding these issues and having a knowledge of the legislative system can assist in removing the barriers of practice maximization.

RESULT-ORIENTED PAYMENT

Result-oriented reimbursement for health care services was derived from the exponentially rising costs of care with a perception of an ever-decreasing quality of care outcomes. Costs of health care services in the United States continue to soar beyond that of other countries, while U.S. health care consumers continue to experience lower quality in care delivered than that of other industrialized countries (Squires, & Anderson, 2015). It is estimated that by year 2019, health care spending will comprise 20% of the U.S. gross national product (Alonso-Zaldivar, 2010). The United States also pays far more per capita than any other nation when compared with other industrialized nations, almost 50% more than the next closest country, France, in health care expenditures (Squires, & Anderson, 2015). Health care costs in the United States continue to surpass those of other countries even though fewer Americans are covered in comparison to other countries and Americans consume less hospital and physician visits than other industrialized countries (Squires & Anderson, 2015).

According to National Public Radio, the Robert Wood Johnson Foundation, and the Harvard School of Public Health (2012), a survey of U.S. residents with illness found that 73% felt that the cost of health care was a very serious problem and 45% felt that quality was a very serious problem. The survey found that the United States has a below-average life expectancy rate and an above-average infant mortality rate (Organization for Economic Co-Operative Development, 2011). Quality in care continues to be a growing concern in health care; two recent studies have found that approximately one in seven hospitalized patients experiences an adverse event (Landrigan et al., 2010; Office of Inspector General [OIG], 2010), with 44% to 66% of these events found to be preventable. Unfortunately, more often than not, hospital administration may not even be aware that these events have occurred. As noted in the OIG report, only 14% of events that cause harm to patients are captured by hospital tracking systems (OIG, 2012). Downey, Hernandez-Boussard, Banka, and Morton (2012) examined the Agency for Healthcare Research and Quality (AHRQ) patient safety indicators between the years 1988 and 2007 and found little overall change in that time frame. This lack of progress in safety is a poor response to the IOM's publication of the 1999 report, which estimated that almost 100,000 patients die each year from medical errors (IOM, 2000). Another reflection of the quality of care seen in today's health care system can be observed in health care–acquired infections (HAIs), which affect 1.7 million hospitalized patients each year (Klevens et al., 2007), or approximately one in 20 patients. HAIs afflict the U.S. health care system at a cost of $35.7 to $45.0 billion each year (Scott, 2009), resulting in 100,000 deaths and untold disability (Klevens et al., 2007). According to a recent survey, 8% of hospitalized patients report getting an HAI (National Public Radio, Robert Wood Johnson Foundation, & Harvard School of Public Health, 2012). The health care system continues to face many challenges in quality of care coupled with elevating costs, which is evident in the slow progress toward reducing adverse events. In response, the CMS through the Patient Protection and Affordable Care Act (PPACA), along with some private insurance companies, is trying to implement financial incentives that will reward quality care while (at the same time) penalizing care that does not meet quality standards.

Fiscal transparency is a type of health care value-based purchasing incentive (Woodward, 2012). Transparency of measures allows consumers and referrers to make choices between different hospitals and providers based on quality and performance and on cost of services. There are approximately 27 states and the District of Columbia that publicly report HAIs (Frieden, 2010). Provider data on hospital-acquired conditions (HACs), process measures, and patient satisfaction surveys are accessible for public viewing online through Hospital Compare (CMS, n.d.). Beyond referrals and the individual consumer, use of the reporting of quality measures can be a factor in a provider negotiation of insurance contracts and third-party payers. Transparency in value-based purchasing can impact a provider's revenues.

To address the gross disparity between cost and outcomes in care, the PPACA directed the CMS to initiate a value-based purchasing system to financially incentivize quality in health care and lower societal health care costs. At present, in the shift toward outcomes-oriented reimbursement, there are two categories for financial incentives. The first category penalizes payment for the care rendered to an individual patient who acquires an HAC. The second category penalizes or rewards the entire fee for all services and patients who are treated at a facility. The incentive that is selected depends on whether a facility's reimbursement is a payment for individual (line item) services or a bundled payment. Unfortunately, the PPACA provides only a framework for change. A proactive stance in health policy formulation is needed that is based on the best information available.

APRNs must engage in the national redesign and construction of health care under a quality care/wellness delivery paradigm. The literature strongly supports the cost-effectiveness of NPs as well as strong quality in care delivery and outcomes of other APRN roles such as Clinical Nurse Specialists (CNSs; Blackmore et al., 2013; Clavelle, 2012; National Nursing Centers Consortium, n.d.; Schiff, 2012). As the nation moves to redefine health care and apply fiscal incentives, it is a nursing duty to ensure patients receive optimal care for a reasonable fee. It is imperative that advanced practice nurses such as APRNs lead nursing in their political efforts to move health care toward a more patient-centric delivery model.

NEW DELIVERY MODELS

As the nation's health care system revolutionizes its way into a new paradigm of health delivery, policy will need perpetual refurbishment. New health care delivery models such as medical homes and accountable care organizations will require provider and consumer education as well as patience as implementation moves toward maximum impact through new delivery modes. Health care is expanding beyond the traditional care settings and face-to-face delivery model, as noted in the most recent reimbursable phase of health care known as care transitions, which originated from CMS's ninth Scope of Work's (SOW) Care Transitions pilot. CMS's care transitions pilot was framed around Mary Naylor's and Erik Coleman's work in transitioning the patient from an acute level of care to home, where the patient themself or a caregiver delivers personal care. The focus of both Naylor's and Coleman's work is to decrease patient readmissions in chronic care patients by injecting a health care provider's presence into the transitional time frame, which is usually 30 to 45 days postdischarge.

CMS's pilot focused on decreasing the readmission rate of Medicare patients with one or more of five diagnoses—chronic obstructive pulmonary disease, congestive heart failure, myocardial infarction, diabetes, and pneumonia. Both Naylor and Coleman used a coaching model for patient intervention. Naylor's model used an APRN to do home visits, whereas Coleman's model used a registered nurse who did home visits and telephonic coaching. Selected Quality Improvement Organizations (QIOs) were awarded contracts to participate in the care transitions pilot. The QIOs were charged with forging a working relationship with established hospitals for pilot patients. Once recruited, patients were to be enrolled into the QIO's coaching program. Naylor's and Coleman's work helped to inaugurate basic face-to-face and telephonic communication between hired health care providers and patients.

Of the pilot contracts awarded, one QIO found that they were able to make some impact on decreasing readmissions, but not as profound as they wanted. This QIO chose to delve deeper into the communication between patient and provider by implementing the Medagogy model and Understanding Personal Perspectives Instrument© in their coaching program (Stewart, 2012). Then the pilot was able to decrease the enrolled population's inherited 18% readmission rate down to 3% (Griggs, 2011). The marked improvement yielded from their improved patient education efforts and patient engagement led to CMS's acknowledging their work as the nation's most innovative pilot in 2011. Because of the success of the pilot, CMS has created two billing codes that physicians, physician assistants, nurse midwives, CNSs, and NPs can bill under to receive reimbursement for their care transitions work (CMS, 2016). This serves as one example of how nursing, through the work of Naylor, Coleman, and Stewart, made an impact on a policy change at CMS that has improved the bottom line for both patients and providers.

CONCLUSION

Policy making, as it relates to health care during the 21st century, is at an all-time record high. Although it is generally agreed that health care is over-regulated, much of the policy that is sought at this time regards dramatic change in the status quo, to include breaking down traditional provider definitions and creating what would almost appear to be new hybrids of medical professionals. As attempts are made to curtail and control spending, one of the fundamental questions proposed is what constitutes "good" health care, which generates the next question: What role/who is qualified to provide it? A resounding call has been made to use APRNs as primary care providers in the face of the projected shortage of approximately 45,000 primary care physicians expected in the next decade (AARP, 2013; Petterson et al., 2015). Unfortunately, at present, only 16 states allow APRNs to practice autonomously and without oversight. The vast majority of states require limitations to practice, most prominently the requirement that a collaborating practice physician must be contracted in order for any form of health care provision at the APRN level to occur. And despite having data that the quality of care provided by APRNs is commensurate to that of physicians, many managed care organizations do not credential APRNs as primary care providers. This limits the ability to be reimbursed by insurance companies.

It is particularly necessary within the APRN and nursing community at large to acknowledge, embrace, and embark on participating in the political action process so necessary for these times. The intent of the development of laws in the United States was citizen freedom to create and implement action through regulation for the good of all citizens. The process was meant to represent the population of the country and directly address the needs of the citizens.

The initiation and support of legislation are a fundamental right of our birth as Americans; however, it is a laborious process in our whirlwind existence that is unfortunately far too often seen as the responsibility of others. As nurses, we must step up and drive policy—it is in the best interest of all.

REFLECTION QUESTIONS

1. *Who do you see as the present drivers of health care policy change?*
2. *Do you feel those in the position of driver should be there, if not why?*
3. *Can you recall a time when nursing used their political power to advocate for legislative change?*
4. *Have you ever interacted with a level of the political process? If so what level?*
5. *Do you feel Nightingale, Orem, Neuman, and Pender's theories are relevant in today's health care setting? If so why?*
6. *Where do you see nurse's greatest political challenges lie and why?*
7. *Nursing is the largest profession in health care which should lend nursing to have the greatest impact in health care policy. What do you think prevents nursing from using their power to influence health care? How can you change that?*

REFERENCES

Alonso-Zaldivar, R. (2010). Gov't: Spending to rise under health care overhaul. *Associated Press*. Retrieved from http://www.washingtontimes.com/news/2010/sep/9/govt-spending-to-rise-under-health -care-overhaul

American Association of Nurse Practitioners. (2013). Practice/Professional: Medicare update. Retrieved from http://www.aanp.org/practice/reimbursement/68-articles/326-medicare-update

American Association of Nurse Practitioners. (2016). State practice environment. Retrieved from https:// www.aanp.org/legislation-regulation/state-legislation/state-practice-environment

American Association of Retired Persons. (2013). Nurse practitioners: The answer to the doctor shortage? Retrieved from http://blog.aarp.org/2013/03/29/nurse-practitioners-the-answer-to-the-doctor -shortage

Anderson, J. E. (2011). *Public policymaking* (7th ed.). Boston, MA: Wadsworth.

Barnes, H., Maier, C. B., Sarik, D. A., Germack, H. D., Aiken, L. H., & McHugh, M. D. (2017). Effects of regulation and payment policies on nurse practitioners' clinical practices. *Medical Care Research and Review*, 74(4), 431–451. doi:10.1177/1077558716649109

Blackmore, C. C., Edwards, J. W., Searles, C., Wechter, D., Mecklenburg, R., & Kaplan, G. S. (2013). Nurse practitioner-staffed clinic at Virginia Mason improves care and lowers costs for women with benign breast conditions. *Health Affairs*, 32(1), 20–26. doi:10.1377/hlthaff.2012.0006

Centers for Medicare and Medicaid Services. (n.d.). Hospital compare. Retrieved from http://www .hospitalcompare.hhs.gov

Centers for Medicare and Medicaid Services. (2011a). CMS issues final rule for first year of hospital value-based purchasing program. Fact sheets. Retrieved from https://www.cms.gov/Newsroom/ MediaReleaseDatabase/Fact-sheets/2011-Fact-sheets-items/2011-04-29.html

Centers for Medicare and Medicaid Services. (2011b). Medicare program: Hospital inpatient value-based purchasing program. Final rule. *Federal Register*, 76(88), 26490–26547.

Centers for Medicare and Medicaid Services. (2016). Frequently asked questions about billing the Medicare physician fee schedule for transitional care management services. Retrieved from http:// www.cms.gov/Medicare/Medicare-Fee-for-Service-Payment/PhysicianFeeSched/Downloads/ FAQ-TCMS.pdf

Clavelle, J. T. (2012). Implementing Institute of Medicine Future of Nursing recommendations: A model for transforming nurse practitioner privileges. *Journal of Nursing Administration*, 42(9), 404–407. doi:10.1097/NNA.0b013e3182664d1f

Downey, J. R., Hernandez-Boussard, T., Banka, G., & Morton, J. M. (2012). Is patient safety improving? National trends in patient safety indicators: 1998–2007. *Health Services Research, 47*(1, Pt. 2), 414–430. doi:10.1111/j.1475-6773.2011.01361.x

Frieden, T. R. (2010). Maximizing infection prevention in the next decade: Defining the unacceptable. *Infection Control & Hospital Epidemiology, 31*(Suppl. 1), S1–S3. doi:10.1086/656002

Griggs, T. (2011, October). Communication key to patient education. *Louisiana Medical News,* 4–5.

Institute of Medicine. (2000). *To err is human, building a safer health environment.* Washington, DC: National Academy of Science Press.

Klevens, R. M., Edwards, J. R., Richards, C. L., Horan, T. C., Gaynes, R. P., Pollock, D. A., & Cardo, D. M. (2007). Estimating health care-associated infections and deaths in U.S. hospitals, 2002. *Public Health Reports, 122*(2), 160–166. doi:10.1177/003335490712200205

Landrigan, C. P., Parry, G. J., Bones, C. B., Hackbarth, A. D., Goldmann, D. A., & Sharek, P. J. (2010). Temporal trends in rates of patient harm resulting from medical care. *New England Journal of Medicine, 363*(22), 2124–2134. doi:10.1056/NEJMsa1004404

Milstead, J. A. (2013). *Health policy and politics: A nurse's guide* (4th ed.). New York, NY: Jones & Barlett.

National Nursing Centers Consortium. (n.d.). The cost effectiveness of nurse practitioner care. Retrieved from http://www.nncc.us/pdf/Cost-Effectiveness_of_NP_Care.pdf

National Public Radio, Robert Wood Johnson Foundation, & Harvard School of Public Health. (2012, May). Sick in America poll: Chartpack. Retrieved from http://www.rwjf.org/content/dam/farm/reports/surveys_and_polls/2012/rwjf72961

Office of Inspector General. (2010). *Adverse events in hospitals: National incidence among Medicare beneficiaries (OEI-06-09-00090).* Washington, DC: Department of Health and Human Services.

Office of Inspector General. (2012). *Hospital incident reporting systems do not capture most patient harm (OEI-06-09-00091).* Washington, DC: Department of Health and Human Services.

Organization for Economic Co-Operative Development. (2011). *OECD factbook 2011: Economic, environmental and social statistics.* Paris, France: Author.

Schiff, M. (2012). The role of nurse practitioners in meeting increasing demand for primary care. Retrieved from http://www.nga.org/cms/home/nga-center-for-best-practices/center-publications/page-health-publications/col2-content/main-content-list/the-role-of-nurse-practitioners.html

Scott, R. D. (2009). *The direct medical costs of healthcare-associated infection in U.S. hospitals and the benefits of prevention.* Atlanta, GA: Centers for Disease Control and Prevention.

Squires, D., & Anderson, C. (2015). U.S. health care from a global perspective: Spending, use of services, prices, and health in 13 countries. *Issues in International Health Policy.* Retrieved from http://www.commonwealthfund.org/~/media/files/publications/issue-brief/2015/oct/1819_squires_us_hlt_care_global_perspective_oecd_intl_brief_v3.pdf

Stewart, M. (2012). *Practical patient literacy: The Medagogy model.* New York, NY: McGraw-Hill.

Tomajan, K. (2012). Advocating for nurses and nursing. *Online Journal of Issues in Nursing, 17*(1), 4. doi:10.3912/OJIN.Vol17No01Man04

Woodward, N. H. (2012). Seeking transparency: More employers are providing pricing and quality information to help employees make smarter health care purchasing decisions. *HR Magazine, 57*(9), 39–42. Society for Human Resource Management (republished by High Beam Research.)

CHAPTER 2

Turning Health Policy Into Practice: Implications for Advanced Practice Registered Nurses

James L. Harris

Escalating health care costs continue. Approximately 15% of the gross domestic product is spent nationally on health care with projections to increase by 20% on or before 2050 (Congressional Budget Office, 2009). Although there has been rapid growth in biomedical advances and knowledge generation over the past decade, care providers, consumers, and stakeholders remain concerned about the quality, safety, and efficiency of clinical care. Care access coupled with quality and safety concerns is closely aligned with cost containment (Ridenour & Trautman, 2009).

The ongoing debate about health care reform and how to finance escalating costs is an opportunity for Advanced Practice Registered Nurses (APRNs) to engage in policy formation that can shape and influence advanced nursing practice. Health policy that is supported by a business case will further advance APRNs' value in meeting the immediate and future health care needs globally (Grace, 2006).

Policy formation is an overarching process, and the complexities associated with health policy can be even more complex and multidimensional as individuals from various public and private sectors are involved. This complexity requires numerous checks and balances as different strategies are formulated. Making sense of the complexities is straightforward when one considers the domains of process, content, and outcomes. Process provides the context necessary to understand approaches that heighten health policy adoption. Content includes specific elements of the policy that are most likely to have relevance and efficacy. Outcomes provide opportunities for validating efficacy and policy impact(s). Outcomes are further validated as new data are formulated, communicated, used efficiently, and supplemental evidence emerges (Brownson, Chriqui, & Stamatakis, 2009).

Although there are a number of definitions of health policy, the World Health Organization (WHO) broadly defines health policy as actions initiated by governments—local, state, and national—to advance and achieve health care goals of the public (WHO, 2015). It is not a singular process or action, but a series of regulatory and legislative initiatives framed around the goals and pursuit of health. It is the component of health policy that focuses on any health care system, the finances, and provision of health services; a proviso grounded in the U.S. Constitution. The WHO definition is foundational for the more than 222,000 APRNs in practice, and similarly those who engage in policy development and lobbying activities that have practice, education, and research implications.

BACKGROUND

The evolution of advanced practice nursing has been influenced by many factors such as history, advances in care, finances, consumer demands, evolving health care reform legislation, promotion of interprofessional collaboration, innovation, workforce shortages, and regulatory stands to cite a few (Furlong & Smith, 2005; Porter-O'Grady & Malloch, 2015; Spann Communications, 2013). In particular, multiple converging factors are drivers of APRN demand to include: (a) increased demands among an aging American population; (b) enhanced access made possible by Patient Care Action; (c) the Institute of Medicine's (IOM) report calling for less restrictive scope of practice; and (d) leveraging skills, knowledge, and experience in different settings (Clabo et al., 2012; IOM, 2011; Spann Communications, 2013).

What paradoxically seems inevitable is actually a result of multiple years of activity culminating in health policies that will continuously influence APRN practice and affect all populations across the life span (Kronenfeld, 2002). As evidence-based health policies are developed, implemented, and communicated, innovative practices will be universally adopted.

HEALTH POLICY DEVELOPMENT

Numerous authors have written about the various levels, components, and processes associated with health policy development (Block, 2004; Fawcett & Russell, 2001; Hinshaw, 1988). For example, Block (2004) identified six stages of public policy making to include setting the agenda, formulating the policy, adopting the policy, implementing the policy, assessing the policy impact, and modifying the policy as indicated. As health policy is formed, consideration should be given at all levels including health care agencies—state, national, and international interests (Hinshaw & O'Grady, 2011).

So one may pose the question, how do APRNs fit into the processes associated with health policy development? In order to respond to this question, one should first consider four developmental components when developing health policy: (a) policy process—government sets public policy to include formation, implementation, and evaluation; (b) policy reform—changes in programs that may positively or negatively affect practices such as priority reform, financial structures, and the regulatory environment that affect institutions and organizations; (c) policy environment—areas where the process occurs, such as government, public, and/or media; and (d) policy makers—the primary stakeholders and participants within the policy environment. Therefore, APRNs fit into the health policy development through the following actions and activities: (a) policy process—systematically reviewing identified issue(s) and developing dialogue based upon the best available evidence; (b) policy reform—remaining informed and involved in lobbying activities, polls, and meetings; (c) policy environment—remaining visible, articulating position, and disseminating information to stakeholders; and (d) policy makers—demonstrating the value of nurses' contributions to the group and providing credible evidence to support positions. An incremental approach is advisable whereby APRNs can start with current and publicly charged issues that have impacts on health and health services such as community development, social determinants of health, and financing activities. Through purposeful and deliberate action, APRNs will form policy communities that influence the political process while maturing their political competence and strategic foresight (Habegger, 2009; Longest, 1996).

CONCEPTUAL FOUNDATION

The conceptual foundation for this chapter is based on a model of nursing and, specifically, health policy by Fawcett and Russell (2001). Fawcett and Russell's (2001) model "was designed to extend the substantive knowledge of health policy within the discipline of nursing" (p. 108). Ten underlying philosophic assumptions underpin the model, but most notable to this discussion are those specific to public policies, organizational policies, and professional policies. "Public policies are those that are developed by nations, states, cities, and towns. The health policies promulgated by public entities typically have a broad impact on individuals, groups, communities, and health care organizations. Organizational policies are developed by health care institutions, such as hospitals, clinics, and home health agencies to guide practice of a particular institution. Professional policies are standards or guidelines developed by discipline-specific and multidisciplinary associations to provide direction for those individuals and groups who work for or with the associations" (Russell & Fawcett, 2005, p. 320). For the purposes of this chapter, the American Nurses Association (ANA), the National Organization of Nurse Practitioner Faculties (NONPF), the National Association of Clinical Nurse Specialists, and the American Association of Colleges of Nursing are examples of professional policy-making organizations to be used as guides to discussion and related content. Regardless whether it is public, organizational, or professional policies, health care services, personnel, and expenditures are interrelated as related to nursing and health policy.

The model by Russell and Fawcett (2005) consists of four increasingly broad and interacting levels that encompass the concepts of the nursing metaparadigm (human beings, environment, and nursing) posed by Fawcett (2005). The levels are not hierarchical, but are rather increasingly broad as nursing and health policies advance to health care systems. Level 1 emphasizes health policy by focusing on quality relative to the efficacy of nursing practice on the outcomes of individuals, families, groups, and communities. Level 2 focuses on health policy related to quality and cost associated with the effectiveness and efficiency of nursing practice and the health care delivery subsystems created by providers on outcomes of individuals, families, groups, and communities. Level 3 highlights health policy associated with access by focusing on societal demands for equity of access to effective nursing practice, efficient nursing delivery systems, and equity of costs and distribution of care delivery burdens. Level 4 stresses health policy links to quality, cost, and access in relation to social and economic quality and cost-effective services, and health-related resources.

Much dialogue has ensued as to how the model should be used for policy analysis and evaluation. Although there are differing beliefs, the model can be a valuable resource when designing advanced nursing practice learning opportunities and delivering care to individuals, families, groups, and communities. Moreover, the model can also guide policy analysis and evaluation aligned with access, quality, cost, efficiency, and effectiveness. For purposes of this chapter, the utility of the model is applicable to APRN practice evaluation.

APPLICATION OF HEALTH POLICY TO APRNs

APRNs are in pivotal roles to continuously advance nursing practice, education, policy, and the spread of best available evidence. The historical opportunity with health care reform further highlights how APRNs can use policy to leverage widespread social change, especially public policy (Ridenour & Trautman, 2009). This supports the aforementioned conceptual discussion and how the value of health policy priorities shape and influence the welfare of others as organizational policies are developed and implemented.

The impact of APRN practice on health care costs, quality, safety, efficiency, and effectiveness cannot be understated or underestimated. The definitive actions and interventions by APRNs who are linked to individual, family, group, and community needs have never been more profound than today, especially in an era of diminishing resources, manpower, and escalating chronic illnesses. Whether addressing discrepancies in access, prevention and health maintenance, chronic disease management, or workforce education and development, APRNs are a powerful force that influences policy makers and engages numerous stakeholders in advancing health care policy. In an age of information technology and knowledge expansion, APRNs can use advanced knowledge and skill sets of health informatics to engage in comparative analysis of evidentiary interventions and delivery systems that ultimately shape policies in today's constantly changing health care environment.

The myriad of opportunities for APRNs to optimize influence on health care and workforce needs can be more effective when evidence guides actions and there is consistent engagement in policy development. For example, in primary care, APRNs improve access for underserved populations. With the advent of policy reducing the number of medical resident hours, APRNs became an immediate part of the solution (Christmas et al., 2005). The convenience of seeking care has expanded through the use of APRNs in retail clinics and the proliferation of advances in telehealth (Hansen-Turton, Ryan, Miller, Counts, & Nash, 2007; Newhouse et al., 2012). As an integrated workforce, opportunities are abundant for APRNs to advance patient-centered care and drive policy that will allow innovative models of care that bring value to recipients across the life span. However, care environments must be aligned toward improvement, a culture that supports innovation and values evidence, and APRNs functioning at their highest level of knowledge and skill. Otherwise, health policy and APRN practice are marginalized.

As APRNs continue to fill faculty positions in academia, developing the provider workforce for the next decade requires practice, technology and information, policy, and systems leadership competencies to name a few (National Clinical Nurse Specialist [CNS] Competency Task Force, 2010; NONPF, 2007, 2009) and is in support of the IOM (2011) recommendations. For the purposes of this chapter, APRNs must be able to demonstrate the six policy competencies posed by the National Task Force on Quality Nurse Practitioner Education (2012, 2016). For example, two of the six competencies include understanding the specifics for the interdependence of policy and practice, and analyzing the implications of health policy across disciplines. Similarly, the nine Clinical Nurse Specialist core competencies and behaviors associated with the sphere of influence and the nurse characteristics must be demonstrated (National CNS Competency Task Force, 2010). For example, the systems leadership competency (ability to manage, change, and engage others to influence clinical practice and political processes within and across multiple systems) is imperative as health policy is turned into APRN practice (IOM, 2011).

EVALUATION CONCEPTS

Numerous outcomes data are continuously collected in health care systems. Although data collection systems and outcomes management vary between systems, both inform public, organizational, and professional policies. As data are collected and analyzed, approaches to evidence-based care drive policy revision and change. Polit and Beck (2008) support the notion that data stimulate discussions about practice improvement, policy change, validity of evidence-based practices, which groups are at risk for adverse outcomes, and the most pressing priorities. Outcomes measurement linked to quality, cost effectiveness, and value-based care is foundational to advancing APRN practice and complementary policy formation and change.

Although myriad issues and much variation in care exist in the United States, patient, family, and community engagement are increasingly identified as a primary component in achieving a high-quality, affordable health care system (National Quality Forum, 2012). Metrics that align with measuring all provider impacts are fundamental to the overarching goal of meeting needs and moving from single-provider to discipline-specific care delivery (Patient-Centered Primary Care Collaborative, n.d.). The preparation of APRNs allows for individual and group choice in care provision. Care outcomes can subsequently be compared among providers and lead to any policy changes needed to enhance quality, safe, and value-based care (Finkelman & Kenner, 2013). Policy change will be guided by outcomes that benefit consumers and communities. As the number of APRNs increases to meet the escalating care demands, active involvement in policy is imperative for quality. Crafting metrics that amplify efficiency and provide incentives for good care can underpin reimbursement policies that maximize payment for APRN services beyond current rates. Improving workforce data in regard to APRN practice must be included in national databases and will serve as the basis for health care and workforce policy (Newhouse et al., 2012).

The rapid pace of health care change and engagement of the patient at the center of care delivery will continue to require data that will shape policy and generate viable solutions that culminate in evaluating the effectiveness of APRN care delivery. The capacity to use outcomes data and collection systems requires APRNs to be knowledgeable about these and about policy in order to increase the development of effective policies that will shape practice, education, and inquiry in succeeding decades. Being consistent in message, communicating a shared perspective, being visible and innovative, and tailoring activities to identified needs will offer many prospects to evaluate APRN outcomes (Ridenour & Trautman, 2009).

DISCUSSION

"The national landscape surrounding advanced practice nursing roles is undergoing significant change. A perfect storm of forces presents a unique window of opportunity for APRNs to realize their full potential" (Clabo et al., 2012, p. 1). Advances in technology, science, and practice innovation have resulted in people living longer and presenting with multiple care needs. The APRN community and educators are in unique positions to be catalysts for policy development that will shape the preparation of future APRNs who will ultimately function as licensed independent practitioners. Regulation of APRNs varies widely among the 50 states, thus generating mobility barriers that can subsequently limit access to care and the underutilization of skill sets that differentiate advanced and generalist registered nursing practice (Lugo, O'Grady, Hodnicki, & Hanson, 2007; National Council of State Boards of Nursing [NCSBN], 2006; Pearson, 2010). Mobility and access barriers potentiate the creation of roadblocks toward achievement of the nation's goals for safe, efficient, and cost-effective care to all citizens (Lugo et al., 2007; Safriet, 2002). One example of removing such roadblocks is evident from the introduction of H.R.1247, Improving Veterans Access to Quality Care Act of 2015, and S.297, Frontlines to Lifelines Act of 2015 during the 114th Congress. Both acts authorized the Department of Veterans Affairs to allow an APRN the full scope of practice under a set of approved privileges.

Multiple issues and barriers related to education, scope of practice, reimbursement, and prescriptive authority are all embedded in policy and regulatory languages that make it difficult for APRN practice potential and contributions to be realized across the nation. Equally, issues are compounded when collaborative relationships with other regulated disciplines are limited, if not absent. Unquestionably, the issues have significant relevance to advanced nursing practice today and in the future as policies are revised and developed (Hamric, Spross, & Hanson, 2009). This is further rationale for the involvement of APRNs in health policy development that will ultimately impact practice and address the needs of all consumers of care.

For the purposes of this chapter, three issues and potential barriers are further discussed that have significance as public, organizational, and professional policies are developed and implemented. The three issues are (a) education, (b) scope of practice, and (c) reimbursement.

The majority of APRN education is designed and accomplished using a model developed almost a half-century ago where students were involved in siloed clinical learning situations using volunteer preceptors to provide the direct supervision. This education often disregards the growing number of collaborative interprofessional educational opportunities where students learn with and from other disciplines (Culliton & Russell, 2010; Interprofessional Education Collaborative, 2011; IOM, 2011). As Tanner (2012) challenged, "We are approaching a crisis in both the cost of clinical education and the insufficient supply of suitable clinical sites if we continue to use the traditional approach to clinical education" (p. 419). To remedy this situation, changes in educational policy are requisite to success where collaboration between academia and practice across all health professions designs, tests, and implements new models of clinical education. Questions are therefore posed as to whether there should be a specific number of clinical hours for each course, the number of clinical simulation hours used, and how and by whom precepting should occur. Practicing APRNs, educators, interprofessional colleagues, and preceptors can guide this historical journey and craft policy that will contribute to meeting the care needs among various cohorts of consumers in order to meet the impending care demands.

Ongoing challenges remain in overcoming the limits imposed on the sole authority in scope to practice. Several states possess sole authority from state boards of nursing; whereas other states possess joint authority with other professional boards (Hamric et al., 2009). The landmark recommendations by the IOM (2011) are a starting point calling for nurses to practice to the full extent of preparation. This calls for changes and creating opportunities directed at policy involvement that will ultimately result in the best care possible—a timely and responsive patient-centric opportunity.

Although the title, APRN, is a value-based asset, the challenge of equitable reimbursement remains as an impending issue that requires action. Policy makers must continuously be educated about the contribution of APRNs in order to address the debate of equal pay for equal service. The care provided by APRNs cannot be viewed as inferior to that of physicians. But the impending and imposing questions remain—will the education requirement of a doctoral degree for the APRN and recognition of the APRN as a licensed independent practitioner resolve the reimbursement inequity?

Turning health policy into practice has many implications for APRN practice beyond the current decade. The landscape of APRN practice is changing as a result of the rapid pace of impending health needs of the population. The changes imposed by health care reform, cost containment, and mandates for safe and quality care that are patient-centric have become impending requisite actions for active engagement. The time is now for APRNs to become active players in shaping health policy that will guide practice, prove themselves as safe and cost-effective providers to society, and move them forward as professionals who are entrusted as future providers for a healthy America. With the support of Congress and stakeholders, it is possible that all four APRN roles can have the authority to practice to the full extent of their training and expertise.

ETHICAL CONSIDERATIONS

Ethical considerations are moral principles governing behavior with integrity, honesty, and opportunities for advocacy. The ANA *Code of Ethics* provides guidelines available to nurses in practice guiding the conduct of actions in accordance with primary values and standards of the profession (ANA, 2008). The practice of APRNs is central to individual, family, and community needs. According to Kjervik and Brous (2010), APRNs have expanded the standards of care beyond the generalist nursing care. With expanded knowledge and skills, APRNs must understand the obligations and rights associated with advanced practice nursing and roles in advancing health policy that are directed at ethical protection of society. Recognizing that health policy is often driven by the values and biases of policy decision makers or the constituent's influence is a call to action for APRNs to continuously inform and advocate others (Birkland, 2005). Many ethical situations are present daily in practice environments and may not have the same outcomes. Ambiguous areas exist where there is no specific answer. The APRN must function as an advocate for the patient, family, community, and peers. Building consensus among the APRN community can support ethical considerations that must strengthen high-quality, safe, and affordable care.

The nursing and ethical pedagogy for APRNs allows options to utilize knowledge and skills when becoming policy advocates for patients, families, and communities. Evidence-based knowledge is a powerful tool for change and building interprofessional strength that will guide ethical policies and ethical decision making.

As pioneers for change, policy development, and ultimately ethical care, APRNs rely on the knowledge and skills gained through education, practice, and collaboration. As entrusted providers of care, the role of the APRN in ethical policy development-engagement will continue to direct the use of available resources that culminate in quality, safe, and efficient care delivery.

DISCUSSION QUESTIONS

1. *How does policy shape current and future APRN practice?*
2. *Considering the current and impending health care reform mandates, how can a policy framework assist the APRN to become involved in turning health policy into practice?*
3. *What are the impending needs necessary to reform APRN practice, educational preparation, and reimbursement in order to provide quality, safe, and cost-effective care?*
4. *What is the relation of policy formation and implementation to APRN practice in addressing ethical issues?*
5. *What are additional issues/barriers that should be considered in turning health policy into APRN practice?*
6. *Based on information in this chapter, what are two areas of policy change you can identify where legislation could have an impact?*
7. *If you were going to describe the importance of your issue for policy change to potential supporters, what key issues would you stress? How would you describe this to patients?*
8. *Consider the health policy changes discussed in this chapter or those you have described in your analysis and the impact that might occur if these changes are not enacted. In other words, what are the consequences of inaction?*

ANALYSIS, SYNTHESIS, AND CLINICAL APPLICATION

1. *Conduct a focus group of APRNs and educators to gain an understanding of the impact of policy development on future APRN preparation.*
2. *Conduct a focus group of providers and consumers of care to gain an understanding of the impact of APRN practice.*
3. *Interview a policy maker to discuss the advantage(s) of turning health policy into practice for APRNs.*

4. *Interview an elected professional organization member to identify the advantage of APRN involvement in health policy.*
5. *Develop ways to disseminate practices that support policies that guide APRN activities.*
6. *Review the literature and generate a priority list of policy formulation and implementation factors affecting current and future APRN practice.*
7. *Identify ways to expand evidence that will benefit all citizens and differentiate generalist and advanced practice nursing.*
8. *Prepare a letter (pro or con) related to a current bill that supports and advances APRN practice.*

EXERCISES/CONSIDERATIONS

1. *Convey how health policy shapes the meeting of emerging needs of Americans.*
2. *Motivate and educate others to shift priorities in order to guide policy that will shape APRN practice currently and in the future.*
3. *Illustrate the skills, expertise, and dedication of APRNs to meet emerging needs and to strengthen the nation's communities.*
4. *Outline the importance of involving APRNs in developing and implementing health policies and core competencies that result in measurable outcomes.*
5. *Create awareness of policy change, interprofessional learning, and skill development directed at quality, safe, and efficient care delivery.*

REFERENCES

American Nurses Association. (2008). *Code of ethics for nurses with interpretive statements.* Silver Spring, MD: Author.

Birkland, T. A. (2005). *An introduction to the policy process: Theories, concepts and models of public policy making* (2nd ed.). Armonk, NY: M. E. Sharpe.

Block, L. E. (2004). Health policy: What it is and how it works. In C. Harrington & C. L. Estes (Eds.), *Health policy: Crisis and reform in the U.S. health care delivery system* (4th ed., pp. 4–14). Sudbury, MA: Jones & Bartlett.

Brownson, R. C., Chriqui, J. F., & Stamatakis, K. A. (2009). Understanding evidence-based public health policy. *American Journal of Public Health, 99*(9), 1576–1583.

Clabo, L. L., Giddens, J., Jeffries, P., McQuade-Jones, B., Morton, P., & Ryan, S. (2012). A perfect storm: A window of opportunity for revolution in nurse practitioner education. *Journal of Nursing Education, 51,* 539–541.

Christmas, A. B., Reynolds, J., Hodges, S., Franklin, G. A., Miller, F. B., Richardson, J. D., & Rodriguez, J. L. (2005). Physician extenders impact trauma systems. *Journal of Trauma: Injury, Infection & Critical Care, 58,* 917–920.

Congressional Budget Office. (2009, March 1). Cost estimate: Health Insurance Restrictions and Limitations Clarification Act of 2009. Retrieved from https://www.cbo.gov/sites/default/files/111th-congress-2009-2010/costestimate/hr12530.pdf

Culliton, B. J. & Russell, S. (Eds.). (2010). *Who will provide primary care and how will they be trained?* [Conference proceedings]. Durham, NC: Josiah Macy Jr. Foundation.

Fawcett, J. (2005). *Contemporary nursing knowledge: Analysis and evaluation of nursing models and theories* (2nd ed.). Philadelphia, PA: F. A. Davis.

Fawcett, J., & Russell, G. (2001). A conceptual model of nursing and health policy. *Policy, Politics, & Nursing Practice, 2*(2), 108–116.

Finkelman, A., & Kenner, C. (2013). *Professional nursing concepts. Competencies for quality leadership* (2nd ed.). Burlington, MA: Jones & Barlett.

Furlong, E., & Smith, R. (2005). Advanced nursing practice: Policy, education and role development. *Journal of Clinical Nursing, 14*(9), 1059–1066.

Grace, J. A. (2006). New research that illuminates policy issues: Balancing nursing costs and quality of care for patients. *Charting Nursing's Future, 2006*(3), 1–8.

Habegger, B. (2009). Strategic foresight: Anticipation and capacity to act. *CSS Analyses in Security Policy.* Retrieved from http://www.css.ethz.ch/content/dam/ethz/special-interest/gess/cis/center -for-securities-studies/pdfs/CSS-Analyses-52.pdf

Hamric, A. B., Spross, J. A., & Hanson, C. M. (2009). *Advanced practice nursing: An integrated approach* (4th ed.). St. Louis, MO: Elsevier.

Hansen-Turton, T., Ryan, S., Miller, K., Counts, M., & Nash, D. B. (2007). Convenient care clinics: The future of accessible health care. *Disease Management, 10,* 61–73.

Hinshaw, A. S. (1988). Using research to shape policy. *Nursing Outlook, 36*(1), 21–24.

Hinshaw, A. S., & O'Grady, P. A. (Eds.). (2011). *Shaping health policy through nursing research.* New York, NY: Springer Publishing.

Institute of Medicine. (2011). *The future of nursing: Leading change, advancing health.* Washington, DC: National Academies Press.

Interprofessional Education Collaborative. (2011). *Team-building competencies: Building a shared foundation for education and clinical practice* [Conference proceedings]. Durham, NC: Josiah Macy Jr. Foundation.

Kjervik, D., & Brous, E. A. (2010). *Law and ethics in advanced practice nursing.* New York, NY: Springer Publishing.

Kronenfeld, J. J. (2002). *Health care policy: Issues and trends.* Westport, CT: Praeger.

Longest, B. (1996). *Health policymaking in the United States* (4th ed.). Chicago, IL: Health Administration Press.

Lugo, N. R., O'Grady, E., Hodnicki, D., & Hanson, C. (2007). Ranking state NP regulation: Practice environment and consumer healthcare choice. *American Journal of Nurse Practitioners, 11,* 8–24.

National Clinical Nurse Specialist Competency Task Force. (2010). *Clinical nurse specialist core competencies: Executive summary 2006–2008.* Philadelphia, PA: National Association of Clinical Nurse Specialists.

National Council of State Boards of Nursing, Association of Social Work Boards, Federation of State Board of Physical Therapy, Federation of State Medical Boards, National Association of Boards of Pharmacy, & National Board of Certification of Occupational Therapy (Eds.). (2006). *Changes in healthcare professions' scope of practice: Legislative considerations.* Chicago, IL: National Council of State Boards of Nursing.

National Organization of Nurse Practitioner Faculties. (2007, 2009). *The APRN consensus process.* Washington, DC: Author.

National Quality Forum. (2012). *Patient reported outcomes (PROs) in performance measurement* [Draft report for comment]. Washington, DC: Author.

National Task Force on Quality Nurse Practitioner Education. (2012). *Criteria for evaluation of nurse practitioner programs* (4th ed.). Washington, DC: National Organization of Nurse Practitioner Faculties.

National Task Force on Quality Nurse Practioner Education. (2016). *Criteria for evaluation of nurse practitioner programs* (5th ed.). Washington, DC: National Organization of Nurse Practitioner Faculties.

Newhouse, R. P., Weiner, J. P., Stanki-Hutt, J., White, K. M., Johantgen, M., Steinwachs, D., & Bass, E. B. (2012). Policy implications for optimizing advanced practice registered use nationally. *Policy, Politics, & Nursing Practice, 13*(2), 81–89.

Patient-Centered Primary Care Collaborative. (n.d.). History. Retrieved from https://www.pcpcc.org/content/history-0

Pearson, L. J. (2010). The Pearson report. *American Journal for Nurse Practitioners, 14*(2). Retrieved from https://webnponline.wordpress.com/category/american-journal-for-nurse-practitioners

Polit, D. F., & Beck, C. T. (2008). *Nursing research: Generating and assessing evidence for nursing practice.* Philadelphia, PA: Lippincott Williams & Wilkins.

Porter-O'Grady, T., & Malloch, K. (2015). *Quantum leadership: Building better partnerships for sustainable health.* Burlington, MA: Jones & Barlett.

Ridenour, N., & Trautman, D. (2009). A primer for nursing on advancing health reform policy. *Journal of Professional Nursing, 25*(6), 358–362.

Russell, G. E., & Fawcett, J. (2005). The conceptual model for nursing and health policy revisited. *Policy, Politics, & Nursing Practice, 6*(4), 319–326.

Safriet, B. (2002). Closing the gap between can and may in healthcare providers' scope of practice: A primer for policymakers. *Yale Journal of Regulation, 19,* 301–334.

Spann Communications. (2013). Improving patient access to high quality care: How to fully utilize the skills, knowledge, and experience of advanced practice registered nurses. *Charting Nursing's Future, 2013*(20), 1–8.

Tanner, C. A. (2012). Reflections—On leaving the JNE editorship. *Journal of Nursing Education, 51,* 419–420.

World Health Organization. (2015). Health policy. Retrieved from http://www.who.int/topics/health_policy/en

CHAPTER 3

Johnson & Johnson Campaign for Nursing's Future: An Impetus for Change

Mary C. Smolenski

Corporate America has had an impact on nursing, and one company that has helped to change the face of nursing in a positive way is Johnson & Johnson. Johnson & Johnson is an international company developed by three brothers (Robert Wood Johnson, James Wood Johnson, and Edward Mead Johnson) in 1886 and from its beginning has a record of helping communities and populations to solve health care and public health problems. From producing one of the first commercial "First-Aid Kits" and manuals, introducing the first commercially produced sanitary pads—a breakthrough for women's health—and mass-producing dental floss to provide better dental care, to donating products and cash for disaster relief in 1900 starting a long tradition, Johnson & Johnson has been innovative and involved. This company continued to branch out, developing maternity/family planning products, baby products such as baby powder and shampoo, the Band-Aid, various surgical items, and the list goes on and on. The company, started by the three brothers more than 125 years ago, has grown into a worldwide partnership of over 265 companies in more than 60 countries employing approximately 126,500 people. There are products, projects, and efforts in the areas of consumer health, medical devices and diagnostics, and pharmaceuticals touching every facet of health care and the global community and helping to solve problems with a goal of making the world a better place to live in.

The company's credo, written by Robert Wood Johnson in 1943, remains unchanged today and attests to the fact that Johnson & Johnson is committed to and has a responsibility to the doctors, nurses, patients, communities, and world we live in. Johnson & Johnson's progressive and future-oriented set of values began some 70 plus years ago, long before the terminology "corporate social responsibility" came into vogue. The credo outlines Johnson & Johnson's responsibilities to health care providers, recipients of health care, Johnson & Johnson employees, local and worldwide communities, and the Johnson &

Johnson stockholders. A portion of the credo states that we have a responsibility to communities in which we live and work, as well as the world community. We must be good citizens; encourage civic improvement, better health, and education; and maintain property we use, protecting our natural resources and environment.

This dedication and corporate responsibility contribute to, if they are not the reason for, its survival as one of only a handful of companies that has weathered the world's changes over the past 125-year period and one of only two U.S. companies with a triple-A rating.

When James Lenehan, a former vice chairman of Johnson & Johnson, made the rounds on one of his routine executive business reviews in 2001, more than 15 years ago, he was asking one major question: "What's going on in health care and what do we need to focus on?"

One of the recurring comments he received was about the nursing shortage and the impact it might have on health care. Lenehan, whose mother was a nurse, knew well how nurses can and do impact health. Nursing shortages have been a cyclical problem. Numerous factors contributed to the shortage in the early 2000s. The average age of those in the nursing population at the time was the late 40s, and nurse educators were also quickly reaching retirement age. Few young people, typically women, were entering the profession, especially because many more lucrative professions were open to women, unlike decades ago. Men did not typically enter nursing because it was considered a profession for women. Along with the decreased numbers was an increased need for nurses and other caregivers because of the aging population and extended life span. Lenehan asked himself if Johnson & Johnson could make an impact on this problem. The rest is history.

As of this printing, the Johnson & Johnson Campaign for Nursing's Future was initiated more than 15 years ago in February 2002, as a multiyear, $50 million national campaign with its primary goals to enhance the nursing profession's image, to recruit nurses and nursing faculty, and to improve retention in the profession. Johnson & Johnson formed alliances with nursing organizations, schools, hospitals, and other health care organizations already involved in their own efforts to improve nursing's image. Initial efforts also focused on how to increase the number of students entering nursing as a profession at both regional and community levels by helping raise monies for grants and scholarships in nursing. Even nursing camps for elementary and high school students were supported. Now in 2017, the campaign continues to focus on the changing role of the nurse in the new health care environment, the advanced practice role and global expansion.

The "Dare to Care" television commercials launched in 2002, which were aimed at potential new nurses, were born and launched nationwide. Nursing has long been rated/voted the most trusted profession by consumers, and the campaign helped to increase that awareness and get others asking questions. However, over time as awareness increased and efforts around the United States focused more on how to get more individuals to enter the nursing profession, the campaign broadened its view. It was time not only to emphasize that nurses "care" about patients, but also to focus on what nurses "do" for patients (Andrea Higham, senior director, Corporate Equity & Partnerships,

Johnosn & Johnson, personal communication, August 16, 2012). The campaign expanded its reach to develop an appreciation for the acute skills and knowledge base held by nurses in the variety of areas in which they work. It started to look at the technical and diagnostic expertise of nurses along with the many specialties they enter. This broader emphasis also looked at the advanced practice areas open to nurses, once again educating consumers to the variety of roles that nursing professionals are educated for and the level of skills they bring to the health care arena. Primary health care and who would be providing this type of care in the future were a new question that Johnson & Johnson wanted to impact, and Advanced Practice Registered Nurses (APRNs) make a key contribution to the solution.

With the numbers of nurses starting to slowly increase in the early 21st century as a result of the coordinated efforts of many groups, it also became clear that numbers could not continue to increase if there was no one to educate these aspiring "nurses to be," mentor them, provide leadership for them, and find ways to fund their education. Johnson & Johnson reached out and developed multiple partnerships with major nursing organizations to focus more directly on these specific problems.

LOCAL AND REGIONAL SCHOLARSHIP, GRANT, AND FUND-RAISING COMMITMENTS

The Campaign for Nursing's Future, or the campaign as it is called, has had a major goal to raise funds for regional nursing communities. Promise-of-nursing galas were hosted as fundraisers across the country along with other regional events that raised more than $18 million in nursing scholarships and grants, faculty fellowships, and program expansion grants for schools of nursing across the United States to support nursing education. The campaign also partnered with the Foundation of the National Student Nurses Association to award funds in cities and regions where the nursing shortage is most acute. To celebrate National Nurses' week in May 2015 and 2016, Johnson & Johnson donated $1 for every photo shared through their "Donate a Photo" app that month toward nursing scholarships through the Foundation of the National Student Nurses' Association. In addition, the campaign supported a variety of innovative regional programs that promote nursing, including sponsoring nursing camps for elementary and high school students that introduce them to the variety of opportunities available in the nursing profession.

NURSE EDUCATOR INITIATIVES

In September 2007, the Campaign and the American Association of Colleges of Nursing (AACN) launched the Minority Nurse Faculty Scholarship to alleviate the growing shortage of nurse educators and promote diversity through financial and professional support to full-time minority students enrolled in graduate nursing programs who plan to work as nursing faculty upon graduation. This effort focuses on the critical shortage of faculty and supports nurse faculty recruitment and retention.

This program invites applications from students of doctoral and master's programs who will serve as nurse faculty after completing their degree programs. Scholarship recipients are selected by an 11-member review committee with awards in the amount of $18,000 each disbursed in the fall. With the emphasis on moving advanced practice education to the doctoral level and the number of Doctor of Nursing Practice (DNP) programs increasing, this is an important effort to help increase the number of faculty for graduate programs. As of fall 2016, there were 73 minority faculty supported by these scholarships, many of whom are now teaching in APRN programs.

The AACN has administered programs providing more than $40 million in scholarship funding to nursing students since 2007 through a variety of efforts sponsored by the Robert Wood Johnson Foundation, the Jonas Center for Nursing and Veterans Health Care, the Johnson & Johnson Campaign for Nursing's Future, and the California Endowment, as well as through cobranded programs with CertifiedBackground.com, AfterCollege, and Hurst Reviews. The majority of this funding has been awarded to students from diverse ethnic/racial backgrounds and to those with financial need.

NATIONAL LEAGUE FOR NURSING PARTNERSHIP

The National League for Nursing's (NLN) Faculty Leadership and Mentoring Program (2007–2011) is a joint effort between the campaign and the NLN Foundation for Nursing Education designed to use mentoring to enhance leadership skills. From 2007 through 2012, the Johnson & Johnson Campaign provided more than $650,000 in funding to the NLN and the NLN Foundation for Nursing Education. From 2007 through 2011, 20 emerging faculty leaders participated in a mentored 1-year program (five per cohort over four funding cycles) called the Faculty Leadership and Mentoring Program, which was fully supported by Johnson & Johnson. This program aimed to transform the future of nursing education by creating leadership opportunities for nurse educators and building diversity in the nurse educator workforce. Each year, through a highly selective national application process, five early- to mid-career nurse educators were chosen as protégés and matched, according to their interests and experience, with mentors selected from fellows—recognized leaders in nursing education—in the NLN's prestigious Academy of Nursing Education.

In 2012, Johnson & Johnson funding was utilized to partially support the NLN LEAD Program—a component of the NLN Leadership Institute and still continues today. This 1-year program supports nurse faculties who had been rapidly transitioned to administrative roles within associate degree and baccalaureate degree schools of nursing. With NLN mentors, participants focus on strategic planning, building high-performance teams, financial management, and developing a personal career plan to advance in organizational leadership. Built solidly on the NLN core values of caring, integrity, diversity, and excellence, the program calls for promising and talented leaders to develop strong management skills, to advance innovation in curriculum design, and to promote evidence-based nursing education.

Johnson & Johnson has also expanded funding since 2012 to include support for another Leadership Institute Program, the Leadership Development Program for Simulation Educators. This yearlong program is designed for experienced simulation nurse educators who wish to assume a leadership role in simulation within schools of nursing and in affiliated simulation resource centers.

In addition, funding supported the initiation of the Senior Dean Leadership Program, piloted fall 2013 through fall 2014. This program was originally designed for administrators who had been in a dean's role for more than 5 years and aspired to reenergize and reframe their organizational systems for emerging pedagogical and health care outcomes but has now expanded to include the practice arena in addition to education. The program, now called the Executive Leadership in Nursing Education and Practice, is designed for executive leaders in nursing education and practice who have held their positions for more than 5 years and wish to be reenergized, and want to reframe how they think about leadership and themselves as leaders. Participants can become champions for change, harness their authentic leadership, and design and implement strategies to innovate and meet the demands of nursing education and health care.

The campaign's major focus areas have been education, funding, scholarship, and leadership, and numerous partner organizations have benefited from their efforts in addition to AACN and NLN. The campaign has supported the efforts of the American Association of Nurse Practitioners (AANPs— formerly called the American Academy of Nurse Practitioners) to support Nurse Practitioner (NP) scholarships. The American Organization of Nurse Executives (AONE) held national dialog days where AONE nurse executives and industry experts discussed specific issues to help craft AONE Guiding Principles. The Association of Women's Health, Obstetric and Neonatal Nurses (AWHONN) used Johnson & Johnson support for their Emerging Leader Program. The campaign broadens its efforts as the needs of the nursing community change.

IMPACT AND FUTURE OF THE PROGRAM

In 2017, the campaign celebrated 15 years in existence. In 2011, it was cited in a *Health Affairs* article as one of the major initiatives contributing to the increase in the supply of nurses nationwide. Auerbach, Buerhaus, and Staiger (2011) identified a 62% increase in nurses aged 23 to 26 years entering the field between 2002 and 2009, a much higher increase than expected. By 2018, the number of Registered Nurses in the United States is projected to be at 3.2 million according to the Bureau of Labor Statistics, and NPs are listed in the top 10 of the fastest growing occupations in the United States (www.bls.gov/emp/ep_table_103 .htm). However by 2020, there will still be a shortage of 800,000 nurses (rwjf. org). There is still a struggle to keep up with the demand as the aging nurse population continues to retire and the higher median age of the existing workforce persists.

Beverly Malone, PhD, RN, FAAN, chief executive officer of the NLN stated that the Campaign did something for nursing that nursing could not do for itself. Nursing had access to the airwaves and the sensitivity to capture the best parts of nursing and present it in a way that could be understood by all. In the same article, Marla Salmon, RN, ScD, FAAN, professor of nursing and global health at the University of Washington in Seattle, discusses the impact of the program on the value of nurses outside the United States. An effort is under way in the Caribbean to attract young people to nursing and encourage them to stay in their own countries rather than leave for the United States, Britain, or Canada. With the help of the Caribbean nursing leaders and government, an initiative called the Year of the Caribbean Nurse was born. "In many ways, [the Campaign] understood that there was an issue of connecting need, people and resources in ways that have never been done before," Salmon said. "The Campaign set the table for nursing around the world, not just the United States."

Auerbach, Staiger, Meunch, and Buerhaus (2013) published an article about the nursing workforce and the amazing turnaround in the number of nurse graduates. Between 2002 and 2010, the number of graduates went from 74,000 to 157,000, more than double, with many of these being baccalaureate graduates. Nearly 5% of the first-year college students in 2010 claimed nursing as their probable major, the highest level since the 1960s. Initially, there was a surge of 30-somethings returning to the workforce in nursing, attending associate degree programs. This helped to increase nurse graduate numbers. But then the idea of viewing nursing as a career hit the 20-year-olds. If the numbers of nurse graduates entering the workforce stay at the current pace, the shortage may not be felt until around 2025 even considering the numbers of nurses retiring (Auerbach, Buerhaus, & Staiger, 2015). Data from AACN's fall 2014 survey of baccalaureate and graduate nursing programs found enrollment growth across the board, including a 4.2% increase in students in entry-level baccalaureate programs (BSN) and a 10.4% increase in "RN-to-BSN" programs for registered nurses looking to build on their initial education at the associate degree or diploma level (www.aacn.nche.edu/news/articles/2015/enrollment). Although many factors can affect these predictions, they do project a better picture for nursing overall.

Commitment to a career in nursing frequently leads to future education and advancement, a desire to become involved and be more independent in the workplace, all a good sign for the future of advanced practice nursing. Data from AACN enrollments and graduations depicting APRNs from 2005 to 2015 (see Table 12.3; Miyamoto, 2017) show that in master's programs alone the number of APRNs enrolled, except for Clinical Nurse Specialists (CNSs), increased from 2005 to 2015: NPs 2005—20,965 and 2015—68,671, more than tripled; Certified Nurse-Midwives (CNMs) 2005—544 and 2015—1,582 almost tripled; and Certified Registered Nurse Anesthetists (CRNAs) 2005—2,725 and 2015—2,890. CNS enrollments and graduations have continued to decline over the last decade. There were 1,035 CNS graduates in 2005, but only 565 graduates in 2015. This could be due in part to the consensus model and its potential impact on advanced practice authority for CNSs. This model reflects a role (NP, CNS, CNM, or CRNA) and population focus (family, pediatrics, etc.) for legal authority, and the CNS model has generally always been a "specialty or system focus" (rehab, pulmonary, cardiac, etc.), which may decrease the desirability of CNS programs from an advanced practice standpoint. The number of DNP graduates, whether post baccalaureate or post master's, has continued to increase for all APRN roles except CNMs. The number of doctoral NP graduates has almost tripled since 2011, from 630 to 1,836.

The authors state that this phenomenon of large increases in nursing graduates is caused by a confluence of factors (Auerbach et al., 2013). The Johnson & Johnson campaign, initiated in 2002, is identified as a major private sector effort focusing on the nursing shortage affecting these results. The campaign, with its multifaceted, responsive approach to solving the shortage, has made a significant impact on the nursing workforce and ultimately on patient care. The campaign "continues to inform the country about the importance of the nursing profession, promote a positive image of that profession, and entice a new generation of men and women into nursing careers" (p. 1471). The national growing interest and attractiveness of nursing, in conjunction with the recession, increased health care spending and jobs, and a dynamic response from the nursing education system has paved the way for a strong foundation in the nursing workforce for the coming years. Reinforcement will be necessary however and sustainment is not fail-proof, as nursing shortages are cyclical, learning from past history. More important reasons to sustain the growth in the nursing workforce now are the massive aging population and the changes in health care reform seeking to provide health care for all.

Peter Buerhaus noted in an interview in September 2016 for Hospitals and Health Networks, titled the Four Forces That Will Reshape Nursing, that there may not be as much of a nursing shortage now as there is a knowledge shortage in nursing. He points out the fact that the more experienced nurses are retiring and although there are nurses replacing them, they are less experienced. He also points out the need for a higher level of knowledge and education for those entering nursing. This will allow them to be able to navigate the ever-changing health care system, think critically and be able to problem solve and adapt more readily to the ever-changing environment and roles they must play (Larson, 2015). The increase in baccalaureate and graduate degree nurses is a step in the right direction and supports the continued need for Johnson & Johnson's efforts, along with others, in supporting graduate education and faculty development.

The campaign continues to evolve, and Higham says that there is no end date in sight. The impact of the campaign on policies within communities, cities, states, organizations, and probably even on federal policy, is evident when reviewing the more than 15 years of history and the changes over the past decade. The shape and focus of the message are tailored to meet the need. As health care focuses on primary care and community, away from acute hospital settings, Johnson & Johnson has modified its emphasis. As the emphasis on prevention, holistic care, and care coordination grows and the improved care of chronic health conditions becomes more a key focus of health care reform, the nursing model and APRNs are at the forefront of care in helping to make changes and provide quality "health" care. And Johnson & Johnson has helped to lead the way just as their Credo of 1943 says "We are responsible to the communities in which we live and work and the world community as well. We must be good citizens—support good works. . . ."

DISCUSSION QUESTIONS

1. *Johnson & Johnson has had a positive impact on nursing from a corporate perspective. What other companies can you think of that have had similar impact? Can you think of any companies that may have had a negative impact (present or past)?*
2. *Identify individuals past and present, rather than companies, who are having a positive impact on nursing/Nurse Practitioners specifically. On health care?*

ANALYSIS, SYNTHESIS, AND CLINICAL APPLICATION

1. *Promotion of the Baccalaureate in Nursing as entry level nursing has been a goal since the 1960s. As noted in the text from AACN data, there is finally a shift in the majority of BS over ADN graduates. Conduct a debate about the pros and cons of this trend considering current day economics, education, and geopolitical considerations.*
2. *Peter Buerhaus identified four factors affecting the future of nursing. Analyze the factor related to retiring nurses. What is the impact? Look at particular types of nursing. Is it worse for one specialty versus another? Is it possible to slow this rate? How can this level of expertise be utilized even beyond retirement?*
3. *The number of DNP graduates has also increased along with more BS graduates. Select your particular specialty and review the changes that are occurring, or could occur as a result of increased nursing knowledge. What impact has technology had on your specialty? How has education changed for your nursing specialty with regard to faculty, facilities, technologies, etc.?*

ETHICAL CONSIDERATIONS

1. *What, if any, are the ethical considerations of corporate companies (health care products, pharmaceutical, etc.) supporting/endorsing health care workers whether they are nurses, Nurse Practitioners, technicians, physical therapists, other. Again you may want to do a pros and cons list.*

REFERENCES

American Association of Colleges of Nursing. (n.d.). New AACN data confirm enrollment surge in schools of nursing. Retrieved from http://www.aacnnursing.org/Portals/42/Publications/Annual-Reports/AnnualReport15.pdf?ver=2017-08-10-210906-407

Auerbach, D. I., Buerhaus, P. I., & Staiger, D. O. (2011). Registered nurse supply grows faster than projected amid surge in new entrants ages 23-26. *Health Affairs, 30*(12), 2286–2292.

Auerbach, D. I., Buerhaus, P. I., & Staiger, D. O. (2015). Will the RN workforce weather the retirement of the baby boomers? *Medical Care, 53*(10), 850–856.

Auerbach, D. I., Staiger, D. O., Muench, U., & Buerhaus, P. I. (2013). The nursing workforce in an era of health care reform. *The New England Journal of Medicine, 368*(16), 1470–1472.

Johnson & Johnson Credo. (1943). Our credo. Retrieved from http://www.jnj.com/about-jnj/jnj-credo

Larson, L. (2015, September 8). The 4 forces that will reshape nursing: Social and health care changes put pressure on the profession. Retrieved from http://www.hhnmag.com/articles/7522-the-4-forces-that-will-reshape-nursing

Miyamoto, S. (2017, January 6). APRN enrollments and graduations 2005–2015 extracted from AACN enrollments and graduation data, submitted by Susan Miyamoto, AACN.

Nurse.com. (2012, November 12). Still going strong: Johnson & Johnson campaign for nursings future turns 10 [Blog post]. Retrieved from https://www.nurse.com/blog/2012/11/12/still-going-strongjohnson-johnson-campaign-for-nursing%C2%92s-future-turns-10

CHAPTER 4

The IOM Report—*The Future of Nursing*

Liana Orsolini

No one predicted this report would go viral. Since its release, *The Future of Nursing: Leading Change, Advancing Health* has been the most widely read report released by the Institute of Medicine (IOM, 2010) and is associated with a grassroots effort that has spread to all 50 states and Washington, DC, to implement its recommendations. The report's inception came about because the Robert Wood Johnson Foundation (RWJF) partnered with the IOM to study how best to transform the nursing profession to effectively function in a future of health care delivery redesign and be a part of the solution to increasing access to health care for millions more Americans. During the IOM's work, committee members were cognizant that if the Patient Protection and Affordable Care Act, also known as the Affordable Care Act (ACA), became law, up to 30 million more Americans would have access to health care but millions more illegal immigrants would remain without affordable coverage. This report was never meant to aggrandize nursing but rather to significantly increase access to health care and to serve as a blueprint for nursing on how to accomplish this.

BACKGROUND

Let's start with the RWJF. Who are they and why are they so interested in nursing's future? Robert Wood Johnson II of Johnson & Johnson started the foundation in 1972 (RWJF, 2012). The mission of the foundation is to improve public health, and it spends more than $350 million a year on grants to accomplish this (RWJF, 2013). The RWJF views public health as increasing access to and improving the quality of health care improving health, reducing health disparities, stemming the obesity epidemic, increasing prevention effectiveness, reducing the rising cost of health care and creating leaders who are change agents in the community and in the government. When the RWJF realized that the status quo was not sustainable and that sickness prevention would have to be incentivized, they turned to the potential of the nursing workforce for solutions. There are no other health care professional groups that are over 3 million strong, 2.6 million of which are actively working in the health care industry (U.S. Department of Health and Human Services, Health Resources and Services Administration [HRSA], 2010). Nursing was a sleeping giant.

Why did RWJF approach the IOM? Founded in 1970, the IOM is part of the National Academy of Sciences and studies issues around health and health care. The National Academy of Sciences is a bit older than the IOM as it was established under Lincoln's Presidency. The IOM is often sanctioned by Congress, a federal agency such as the National Institutes of Health, or other division within the Department of Health and Human Services (DHHS) to undertake a study with recommendations (National Academy of Medicine [NAM], 2016). Sometimes the IOM is privately funded to hold a study such as *The Future of Nursing* report. The IOM is held to section 15 of the Federal Advisory Committee Act, which means that most of its committee work and process is transparent to the public when a report contains recommendations aimed at a government entity (NAM, 2016). Each IOM committee has stakeholders from many different disciplines as well as content experts. Committee makeup goes through a national public vetting process, and its final reports go through a more structured vetting process with key stakeholders who are not committee members. The IOM is a trusted, non-biased entity that holds their reports to high scientific rigor; they must be evidence based and strive to have consensus-based recommendations. When one wants stakeholders who hold multiple perspectives to take a report seriously, many turn to the IOM. While the IOM changed its name to the National Academy of Medicine in 2015, this chapter refers to the IOM since during the time *The Future of Nursing* was published it was known as the IOM.

RWJF needed a process for *The Future of Nursing* report that would ensure credibility, transparency, an established vetting process to ensure a diversity of stakeholders and that report recommendations were evidence based. While these methods of operation were well in place at the IOM, RWJF needed them to implement some changes to their methods which would not affect the credibility of their process. These changes were unprecedented for the IOM and included allowing RWJF to provide just-in-time research support by an external group of experts, a study director from outside the IOM (Susan Hassmiller, PhD, RN, FAAN, senior advisor for nursing for RWJF), and a communications staff (S. Hassmiller, personal communication, March 9, 2013). The study director's role was to not only serve as a symbolic message that RWJF sanctioned this study, but to also provide crucial continuity between the report recommendations and their implementation through the *Campaign for Action*. The research team implemented needed data analysis to fill gaps the committee members discovered as they poured through evidence. RWJF also funded outside consultations (invited papers) for important topics that committee members discovered few publications about. The communication team blogged and tweeted, helping to keep the public cognizant of the three open public forums on Nursing Education, Care in the Community, and Acute Care held throughout the country, and kept the committee members cognizant about any new evidence that was published in peer-reviewed journals or findings reported by the RWJF research team. They also blogged and tweeted the unveiling of the report, which was met with much fanfare including a mention in *The New York Times* (Chen, 2010). It is important to note that, although social media was applied throughout the IOM process, the core of the process was adhered to, and strict confidentiality of internal discussions and construction of recommendations was strictly confidential at all times.

THE REPORT

The Future of Nursing: Leading Change, Advancing Health committee's charge included reconceptualizing nursing practice with the knowledge that: (a) 78 million baby boomers were rapidly reaching retirement age and a significant number of nurses fit into this category; (b) Americans were living with a higher number of chronic conditions; (c) one third of children were now either overweight or obese; (d) if the ACA passed, up to 30 million more Americans would have access to primary and preventive services, and (e) there was already an acute shortage of primary care practitioners. The committee assumed health care delivery was going to change; they were already seeing a movement away from fee-for-service to accountable care organizations and to other value based models of care where those with chronic conditions were being managed by interprofessional teams who received bundled payments for services. The complexity of care needed for patients was rising while the cost of care was increasing at a proportion far beyond the rate of inflation. Future nurses would have to be prepared for a new way of doing business while nurses in practice would have to be re-tooled with new competencies. While no one could predict when we would completely eliminate the fee-for-service payment structure, many were certain that this was inevitable. A little-known fact of the ACA is that if the Centers for Medicare and Medicaid Innovation (CMMI) collects enough evidence to support a new payment structure, which incentivizes health, through large enough pilot and regional grant funded projects, the Secretary of Health from the DHHS can scale payment reform nationally without the need for legislation (Centers for Medicare and Medicaid Services, 2017a). It is only a matter of time before CMMI collects enough data to support such a move, and there were already 500 hospitals participating in their new bundled payment demonstration project in the early 2000s (Japsen, 2013). The committee was also given the task to expand the ranks of nursing faculty since they knew that thousands of qualified undergraduate and graduate nursing students were turned away each year (and still are as of this writing) due to faculty shortages. The committee was also asked to examine solutions to health care delivery and health professional education in preparation for future changes; in essence they were given the leadership baton for writing an action plan on how to utilize the profession of nursing to get America where it needed to go.

Committee's Vision

The Committee envisions a future system that makes quality care accessible to the diverse populations of the United States, intentionally promotes wellness and disease prevention, reliably improves health outcomes, and provides compassionate care across the lifespan. In this envisioned future, primary care and prevention are central drivers of the health care system. Interprofessional collaboration and coordination are the norm. Payment for health care services rewards value, not volume of services, and quality care is provided at a price that is affordable for both individuals and society. The rate of growth of health expenditures slows. In all these areas, the health care system consistently demonstrates that it is responsive to individuals' needs and desires through the delivery of patient-centered care. (IOM, 2010, p. 2)

Many different stakeholders served on the committee. Donna Shalala, former Secretary of Health for the DHHS under the Clinton administration was the chair while Linda Burnes Bolton, a nurse executive, served as the vice chair. Six members were registered nurses (Liana Orsolini-Hain, Michael Bleich, Jennie Chin Hansen, Rosa Gonzalez-Guarda, Anjli Aurora Hinman, and Linda Burnes Bolton), and 12 came from diverse backgrounds in business, medicine, health policy, consumer advocacy, academia, health care, philanthropy, political science, medical insurance, and economics. This level of diversity increased the credibility and integrity of the report; it was taken more seriously by non-nurses such as physicians because there were physicians on the committee. Lawmakers and the DHHS also took the report seriously. It was a dream team.

The report consists of four key messages, eight major recommendations, and 42 sub-recommendations. It names 31 actors; actors are entities which are directed to carry out the recommendations. Examples of actors named include those from the national level such as Congress, HRSA, the Department of Labor to those at the local level such as frontline nurses and health care organizations. Included in the sub-recommendations are strategies for how the actors are to go about implementing the recommendations. For example, recommendation two, "Expand opportunities for nurses to lead and diffuse collaborative improvement efforts," names the actors: private funders (usually philanthropic organizations), public funders (government), health care organizations (hospitals, clinics, insurance companies), nursing education programs, and nursing associations. The actors are urged to provide more opportunities for nurses to lead when collaborating with others to conduct research and improve the quality of health practice environments. This level of specificity embedded within each of the sub-recommendations makes it a "blueprint" for how to enact these changes.

Key messages of the report:

1. Nurses should practice to the full extent of their education and training.
2. Nurses should achieve higher levels of education and training through an improved education system that promotes seamless academic progression.
3. Nurses should be full partners, with physicians and other health professionals, in redesigning health care in the United States.
4. Effective workforce planning and policy making require better data collection and an improved information infrastructure (IOM, 2010, p. 4).

The first key message is often mistaken to refer solely to Advanced Practice Registered Nurses (APRNs). *All* nurses should practice to the full extent of their education and training. It is shocking, however, how few states allow APRNs to practice independently of a physician, whether it is in running a nurse-managed clinic, assessing patients, prescribing medications or delivering anesthesia and treatments for chronic pain. Since the report was released in October of 2010 a total of 28 states and the District of Columbia have laws that allow Nurse Practitioners (NPs) to practice and prescribe independently from a physician. This is an increase from 16 states in 2010 (National Council of State Boards of Nursing [NCSBN], 2016). Certified Registered Nurse Anesthetists (CRNAs) can both practice and prescribe independently in 26 states and in the District of Columbia, Clinical Nurse-Midwives (CNMs) can both practice and prescribe independently in 17 states and the District of Columbia, and Clinical Nurse

Specialists can do so in 20 states and the District of Columbia (NCSBN, 2016). (NOTE: These numbers may vary depending on the source and definition of "independent" practice authority.) The committee saw the value of the care millions of nurses could deliver if only allowed to work at their full capacity. This would likely exponentially increase access to health care and hopefully, significantly reduce health disparities. This key message could lead to achieving a little more social justice for those without access to a primary care. provider. This would be a difficult key message for others to accept, and sure enough it became the most controversial key message, pulling along with it recommendation one, "Remove scope-of-practice barriers." Nurses and supportive stakeholders would have to battle professional territorialism and fear.

The second key message, "Nurses should achieve higher levels of education and training through an improved education system that promotes seamless academic progression," calls for a better educated nursing workforce but stops short of demanding that the baccalaureate degree be the entry level into nursing practice. This key message disappointed many academic nurses since they had been advocating for the baccalaureate in nursing (BSN) degree as the entry requirement for nurses to sit for their state board licensing exam since at least the mid-1960s (Orsolini-Hain & Waters, 2009). Why didn't this landmark report call for the BSN as entry level into practice? It seemed the perfect opportunity, especially after the Carnegie Foundation for the Advancement of Teaching's national nursing education study, "Educating Nurses: A Call for Radical Transformation," not only called for the BSN as entry into practice but also recommended that all nurses get a master's degree within 10 years of initial licensure (Benner, Sutphen, Leonard, & Day, 2010).

The evidence the IOM had available at the time of this report was mixed. While some studies showed a difference in outcomes for nurses with at least a BSN degree (Aiken, Clarke, Cheung, Sloane, & Silber, 2003; Estabrooks, Midodzi, Cummings, Ricker, & Giovannetti, 2005; Tourangeau et al., 2006), others did not (Sales et al., 2008) and instead linked outcomes with level of experience (Blegen, Vaughn, & Goode, 2001). So if the evidence was mixed and the IOM did not have enough research findings to support such a key message or recommendation why did the report call for a better educated nursing workforce? There were several reasons for this. Of the 900,000 nurses reaching retirement age, a significant number of them were nursing educators. One of two main reasons nursing programs have been turning away thousands of qualified students each year from nursing schools is due to shortages of faculty. All knew we were heading toward a retirement cliff in nursing, but especially so with nursing faculty. Aging and retiring nursing faculty desperately needed to be replaced. Most nursing faculty have a master's degree if they are teaching at the community college level, and community colleges educate 50% to 60% of our undergraduate nursing workforce. At least 50% of faculty in BSN programs have a PhD or other doctoral level degree and most faculty who teach in graduate programs have a doctoral level degree since they conduct clinical nursing and other research. Some committee members were wondering if we could even replace the number of nursing researchers needed to continue the level of National Institutes of Health–funded nursing research. To replace the number of retiring nurses seemed a daunting task with the worsening nursing faculty shortage; in addition, more APRNs were needed to provide access to care for at least up to 30 million more Americans after the ACA passed. Although the master's degree has been the required entry point into advanced practice registered nursing for many years, now there is a strong national movement to require the Doctorate of Nursing Practice (DNP; American Association of Colleges of Nursing [AACN], 2004), which would require even more faculty who could teach at the doctoral level. We would also need to retool the current nursing workforce for the inevitable changes in health care delivery, which would require more continuing education. Lastly, due to the rising complexity of patients and the rising need for chronic care management, we would need a better educated nursing workforce with higher level competencies to deliver more preventive and population health services.

The third key message, "Nurses should be full partners, with physicians and other health professionals, in redesigning health care in the United States," was the second most controversial statement in the report. This key message ties into the second recommendation, which states, "Expand opportunities for nurses to lead and diffuse collaborative improvement efforts." When an IOM report states that nurses should "lead," many physicians get very nervous. The American Medical Association was anxious about this key message and recommendation and publicly stated so at the meeting convened in Washington, DC, to unveil the report at a public forum in 2010. The only way Virginia's action coalition could get buy-in legislation to remove barriers to practice for its APRNs was to capitulate to the idea that physicians would always lead the patient-care team and that physicians could now "collaborate" with six Nurse Practitioners instead of four (HB 346, 2012).

With a growing national movement toward interprofessional health education and practice, the IOM's Global Forum on Innovations in Health Professional Education sponsored Lloyd Michener, MD, Director, Duke Center for Community Research in North Carolina, at their meeting in November 2012, who showcased how medical homes using Nurse Practitioners and other health professionals collaborate in interprofessional teams (Michener, 2012). They used a patient centered approach: The health professional who could best help the patient's problem became the designated "leader" for that patient in that situation. Dr. Michener stated, " 'Lead' isn't quite the right term, as it suggests that individuals are either leading or following, as opposed to a sense of shared, coordinated leadership with clear roles, well-coordinated around the needs of the patient(s). If the primary need is for social services, the 'lead' is likely a social worker; if mental health, might be a psychologist" (L. Michener, personal communication, November 4, 2012). Leadership was fluid and contextual. When professional egos don't get in the way, this approach can work well. In addition, Duke University recently partnered with Johnson & Johnson to offer a nurse leadership fellowship program to teach leadership competencies to APRNs necessary to successfully lead nurse-managed health clinics and to "act on behalf of patients to address needs within the larger health care system" (Duke University School of Nursing, n.d.). How can nurses and how should nurses lead on a national level so they can make a significant impact to improve the health of the nation? The obvious answer is to not wait to be asked to lead; just lead. Examples of this on a national scale are evident in three areas: (a) the sweeping movement in the Action Coalitions, (b) the proliferation of nurse managed health clinics (NMHCs), and (c) the Million Hearts Initiative.

In 2010, the RWJF, the country's largest philanthropy devoted to health, joined the AARP Foundation and AARP, the nation's largest consumer organization, to create The Future of Nursing: *Campaign for Action* to improve America's health through nursing. The Campaign is coordinated through the Center to Champion Nursing in America, also an initiative of the AARP Foundation, AARP, and RWJF (campaignforaction .org/about/our-story).The *Campaign for Action* is discussed in detail in another chapter. This national phenomenon in nursing is creating a new national awareness in leaders among several stakeholder groups about nurses' goals to do what needs to be done to make a dent in improving access to health care and to improve health for millions more people living in America. The Action Coalition movement has reached the awareness of politicians on the Hill and in the White House and leaders in the administration, such as in the DHSS. There are nurses throughout the Hill and in the administration who work in health policy who are very interested in the potential of the nursing workforce to help implement the ACA and to make implementation of the ACA sustainable. For example, Marilyn Tavenner was only the second nurse ever to lead the CMS. Mary Wakefield, a PhD-prepared registered nurse was the administrator of HRSA, an agency which is key to developing the health professional workforce, and under the Obama administration served as the acting deputy secretary of the DHHS. They both understand the potential of nurses who act to the full extent of their education and training.

NHMCs are proliferating, are run by APRNs and are staffed by a variety of health professional practitioners who work together in teams. They provide primary care and preventive services to communities traditionally underserved who remain vulnerable to chronic illness. They are usually associated with an institution such as a college, university, department or school of nursing, Federally Qualified Health Center (FQHC), nonprofit foundation, or some other group (National Nursing Centers Consortium [NNCC], 2016). FQHCs are community-based centers that provide Comprehensive Primary Care services to populations that have traditionally had significantly less health care than average Americans (HRSA, 2013).

In 2010, when the IOM released *The Future of Nursing* report, there were at least 200 NHMCs in 37 states with an estimated two million patient encounters per year (Kovner & Walani, 2010). About 60% of these patients were either uninsured or had Medicaid. According to Jamie Ware, the Policy Director of NNCC as of October 2012, there were about 500 nurse-managed primary care clinics, preventive care clinics, birthing centers, and school-based health centers across the country that NNCC could track (J. Ware, personal communication, November 1, 2012). It is difficult to track all these centers because they use different funding sources. See Exhibit 4.1 for services provided by nurse-managed health clinics.

The Million Hearts Initiative, which is discussed in more detail in another chapter, is a CMS and Centers for Disease Control and Prevention (CDC)–led national effort to prevent 1 million heart attacks and strokes (refer to https://million hearts.hhs.gov/data-reports/data.html for up-to-date progress; a final report will be available by 2019 [https://millionhearts.hhs.gov/files/MH-meaningful-progress.pdf]). APRNs led by national nurse leaders are taking the challenge of lowering blood pressure in hypertensive patients without asking permission to join their interdisciplinary peers. Instead, APRNs are asking their interdisciplinary peers to join them in efforts to improve the health of the nation and are even being asked to lead in this effort due to this initiative. Most health professionals are beginning to realize that they need to work together instead of in separate

SERVICES PROVIDED BY NURSE MANAGED HEALTH CLINICS	EXHIBIT 4.1

1. Promotion and maintenance of health
2. Prevention of illness and disability
3. Basic care during acute and chronic phases of illness
4. Guidance and counseling of individuals and families
5. Referral to other health care providers and community resources when appropriate
6. Nurse-midwifery services

Source: HRSA (2012).

silos to make a difference in eliminating health disparities and to significantly improve health, which is the ultimate goal of increasing access to health care.

The fourth key message of the IOM *Future of Nursing* report, "Effective workforce planning and policy making require better data collection and an improved information infrastructure," reflects the lack of ability of the report committee to predict how many and which types of nurses we need to prepare for the future, and in which geographical areas shortages exist. The committee did not know where APRNs practice geographically and what types of practices they were working in. At the time of the report's formation, the committee did not know how quickly health service delivery redesign was going to occur, or even if the ACA was going to pass, or if it did pass, whether President Obama would be reelected for a second term in office. The committee did not know how quickly CMS would be able to eliminate a fee-for-service system that provides incentives for volume of care for a system of value-based health care delivery incentives that would provide hospitals monetary rewards to keep their beds empty by incentivizing health. If this happened the committee speculated that hospitals would surely turn into big intensive care units with operating rooms and an emergency room. Hospitals would require fewer beds and regions would require more community-based clinics with expanded ambulatory roles for registered nurses. Telehealth would expand because care teams would be able to see more patients virtually at home. These changes would require academic institutions to change the way they educate the health professional workforce. Health care professionals would have to learn new competencies for caring for people in their own environments versus in the hospital. Additionally new competencies would be needed to work in interprofessional and transdisciplinary teams. Examples of interprofessional colleagues are registered nurses, APRNs, registered dieticians, physical therapists, pharmacists and physicians, and examples of transdisciplinary colleagues include certified nurse assistants, health coaches, and community workers. There were too many variables and uncertainty for the IOM report committee to list the number and types of registered nurses Americans needed for the future.

In addition to the four key messages *The Future of Nursing* report has eight recommendations (see Exhibit 4.2). The first recommendation, "Remove scope-of-practice barriers," is necessary in order for nurses to practice to the full extent of their education and training. As stated earlier in this chapter, the Center to Champion Nursing in America through its Action Coalitions, is working toward

| RECOMMENDATIONS OF THE REPORT | EXHIBIT 4.2 |

1. Remove scope-of-practice barriers.
2. Expand opportunities for nurses to lead and diffuse collaborative improvements efforts.
3. Implement nurse residency programs.
4. Increase the proportion of nurses with a baccalaureate degree to 80% by 2020.
5. Double the number of nurses with a doctorate by 2020.
6. Ensure that nurses engage in lifelong learning.
7. Prepare and enable nurses to lead change to advance health.
8. Build an infrastructure for the collection and analysis of interprofessional health care workforce data.

Source: IOM (2010, pp. 9–15).

increasing the independence of all APRNs through state legislation. Refer to the AARP initiatives chapter for more detail. While the Action Coalitions work to remove scope-of-practice barriers at the state level, the Federal Trade Commission (FTC) is working to prevent physician-run monopolies that squeeze out APRNs from the federal level. Directed by the Senate Commerce Committee, the FTC reviews all state practice laws and regulations to see if any of these preclude nurses from working to the full extent of their education and training. They are asking several state legislatures such as those in Texas, Louisiana, and other states to remove "unduly restrictive regulations . . . to amend them to allow advanced practice registered nurses to provide care to patients in all circumstances in which they are qualified to do so" (FTC, 2013). Sub-recommendations in the report also asked CMS to change regulations to permit more direct reimbursement to APRNs for services rendered independently of a physician. For example, the Physician Fee Rule was revised in 2012 to include stronger language to enable CRNAs to get direct Medicare reimbursement for chronic pain management to include related care such as all the diagnostic and interventional measures for monitoring, placement of medication, and treatment (CMS, 2017b). Health policy scholars in CMS and throughout DHHS realize that removing these practice restrictions is likely to reduce the cost of health care.

The second recommendation, "Expand opportunities for nurses to lead and diffuse collaborative improvement efforts," was not only a call for a variety of organizations to invite registered nurses to lead in redesigning and improving health practice environments, but it was also a call to these nurses to seek out these types of leadership rolls. There are few nurses and fewer nurse leaders in health policy arenas. These areas are hard to break into mid-career because many high level positions in the Administration require that one start from a low-paying position in order to get hired into an agency. Many mid-career nurses cannot afford to remain in a low level position until they have worked their way up into a position of higher influence. It is the same for elected officials who are nurses; it usually takes many years of local and regional public service before being elected to be a state or federal legislator. While there are many physicians in leadership in public health arenas and there are many physicians and lawyers in Congress and in the Administration, there are few nurses whose voices are heard. Conversely, while most hospitals and employers of registered nurses have a chief nursing officer, there are few nurses on their boards. In 2011 the percentage of registered nurses on hospital boards was only 6% while 20% were physicians (Hassmiller & Combes, 2012). Even more dismal, the percentage of nurses on boards of non-profit hospitals was a mere 2% in 2010 (Totten, 2010). To help insure a higher number of registered nurses in boardrooms, leadership training should include competencies needed to serve on governing boards. In addition, more health policy leadership strategies such as offering dual degrees for APRNs are needed. Many schools of medicine offer a medical doctor *and* master's in public health dual-degree program. APRNs can also minor in health care or public health administration. More nurses need to work in the administration in agencies such as CMS, the Agency for Healthcare Research and Quality (AHRQ), Institutes at the National Institutes of Health besides National Institute of Nursing Research, and in the Immediate Office of the Secretary of Health in DHHS.

Recommendation three states that we should "implement nurse residency programs." Nurse residency programs are also known as transition-to-practice programs and include transition to new practice areas, not solely to new nursing practice. For example, a nurse who wishes to move to intensive care from medical surgical hospital practice should have a transition-to-practice residency. New graduate registered nurses should have transition-to-practice programs that last longer than an orientation of new employee's program. Nurses entering advanced practice should have a transition-to-practice program. NCSBN conducted a study of patient health outcomes linked to transition-to-practice programs for new graduate nurses across 105 hospitals in three states (NCSBN, 2013). They found that hospitals using established transition programs experienced higher retention rates, fewer medical errors, higher nurse competency levels, fewer negative safety practices and greater nursing satisfaction (Spector et al., 2015). Funding for these residencies may be perceived as a challenge by employers of registered nurses and APRNs. Increased retention of nurses will likely pay for these programs because orienting even experienced nurses takes thousands of dollars in these care environments, which must be compliant with much regulation.

Recommendation four, "Increase the proportion of nurses with a baccalaureate degree to 80% by 2020," and five, "Double the number of nurses with a doctorate by 2020," tie in with the second key message that nurses should "achieve higher levels of education." The report speaks extensively about making it seamless for nurses to continue with their education whether they are continuing students or have been in practice for years. Seamless refers to processes in place that go beyond the ease of good articulation agreements between community college and university nursing programs. Seamless means without barriers or roadblocks (Orsolini-Hain & Waters, 2009). Many studies have shown that deterrents to returning to school for a more advanced degree in nursing are redundant curricula, needing to be on site too often during working hours, lack of flexibility with courses and many others (Kovner, Brewer, Katigbak, Djukic, & Fatehi, 2012; Orsolini-Hain, 2008). In order to achieve recommendation four, 778,879 nurses or about a third of the workforce would need to earn a BSN by 2020; and for recommendation five, 21,000 more nurses would need to earn a doctoral level degree (Kovner et al., 2012). Although this seemed unlikely when nursing schools continue to turn away thousands of qualified applicants yearly in both undergraduate and graduate programs due to faculty and/or clinical site shortages, over

21,000 nurses had earned a doctoral degree in nursing by 2014, likely due to the explosion of DNP programs, thereby achieving recommendation five (*Campaign for Action*, 2016). The AACN's survey data show that nursing schools turned away 64,067 qualified applicants from baccalaureate and graduate nursing programs in 2016, with lack of faculty being one of the reasons. The data show a national nurse faculty vacancy rate of 7.9%. Most of the vacancies (92.8%) were faculty positions requiring or preferring a doctoral degree (AACN, 2017). The DNP has become more attractive to nurses than a PhD in nursing such that as of 2011 there were double the enrollments in DNP programs as in research focused doctorates (AACN, 2012). This demand for DNP programs has encouraged their growth. As of April the number of DNP programs grew from 20 to 292 as of 2014 while the number of research focused doctoral programs grew from 103 to only 126 as of 2012 (AACN, 2012, 2016).

Recommendations four and five are critical to facilitate nursing's success in interdisciplinary health professional practices of the future. The paradigm of nursing blindly following physicians' orders is becoming prehistoric as accountability and engagement in higher levels of frontline leadership require a more active role in the health care team. Better educated nurses will be taken more seriously and are likely to acquire more credibility as they increase interactions with other health professionals whose entry into their practice requires graduate degrees. If an advanced practice registered nursing program does not require interprofessional health education learning experiences then it is not preparing its students for future practice. All health professionals, even APRNs and not solely physicians, are being called to practice together. Emerging evidence shows that it is more effective to practice together than alone, especially to reduce blood pressure in complex patients (CDC, 2012). Even if allowed to practice independently, APRNs work with physicians and psychiatrists, social workers, pharmacists, physical therapists, and a myriad of others in care teams.

Recommendation six, "Ensure that nurses engage in lifelong learning," speaks to staying currently competent to give safe and culturally appropriate care in a changing environment and in changing health care delivery systems. It is not enough to get a more advanced degree in nursing; one must continually strive to stay up to date with emerging evidence, for improvement of skills for chronic care management, and for effective population preventive health measures. Care is becoming more complex as we are urged by legislatures, the administration, employers and health insurers to lower health care costs while improving care safety and effectiveness. The Institute for Healthcare Improvement (IHI), a non-profit organization which believes everyone should receive the best health care possible developed the Triple Aim framework. The three aims are to (1) improve the quality of care, which should increase patient satisfaction; (2) improve the health of populations; and (3) reduce the cost of health care (IHI, 2013). These aims must be achieved simultaneously by everyone in the business of health care for this approach to make a difference. We can no longer afford *not* to operate by the triple aim framework. For access to health care and access to health for all in America to be sustainable we must reduce the expenditures of health care down from 17% of the gross national product, which is projected to rise to even higher levels (CMS, 2012).

One of the best ways to ensure that all nurses engage in life-long learning is for employers of nurses to form strong collaborative partnerships. These partnerships can bring academia and health care organizations together to combine strengths to provide residency programs, continuing education to retool the current workforce, seamless education pathways leading to more advanced degrees, and process improvements. These partnerships can work together to transition interprofessional education of health professionals into new ways of doing interprofessional practices. The literature on models of these new collaboratives is expanding. These collaboratives have the potential to help nursing faculty stay current in the nursing field as they can lead to joint appointments and exposure to health care organizations' quality and safety committees. Conversely, these collaboratives can strengthen undergraduate and graduate nursing curricula since health care organization leaders can be exposed to nursing program curriculum committees and serve on nursing program advisory boards. Perhaps we will begin to see nursing educators serving on health care boards.

Recommendation seven, "Prepare and enable nurses to lead change to advance health," ties to keynote message three, "Nurses should be full partners, with physicians and other health professionals, in redesigning health care in the United States," and with the title of the report itself *Leading Change, Advancing Health*. In order to implement this recommendation nurses need to be leaders at the national level and not solely at regional and local levels. Nurses need to think beyond their own practice environments and start to care about the health of communities and populations. Nurses have to care about social justice and feel the need to reduce health disparities by reducing or eliminating social determinants that reduce health. These social determinants include poverty, social structures lack of resources to improve health literacy, substance abuse, tobacco use, unsafe physical living environments, social environments that encourage racial discrimination, reduced or no physical access to health preventive and primary care services, and a myriad of others leading to health inequities (CDC, 2014). Nurses have to start caring beyond their single-patient encounters and work on what really matters for improving health if they are seriously determined to improve the health of this nation.

Advanced practice registered nursing students can prepare for leadership roles by taking as many courses in leadership, health policy, health administration and economics as possible while in school. APRNs can lead by joining their national organizations and by getting involved. Most advanced practice nursing organizations are headquartered or have an office in or near Washington, DC, which gives them access to legislators and to agencies in DHHS such as Medicare and Medicaid. It is critical that APRNs stay abreast of Medicare and Medicaid regulations because future proposed rules and legislation may eliminate direct reimbursement or limit independent practice. Limiting direct reimbursement to APRNs and limiting their scope of practice will certainly decrease access to care, especially to the already disenfranchised. Some advanced practice organizations were working on getting state insurance exchanges mandated by the ACA to recognize nurse-led health clinics as "essential community providers," which allows direct reimbursement by Medicare and Medicaid insurance contractors (NNCC, 2016). APRNs can engage in lifelong learning by taking executive leadership courses and training through their professional and other organizations. They can step up to the plate and run a clinic or medical center and even run for public office.

The eighth recommendation states, "Build an infrastructure for the collection and analysis of interprofessional health care workforce data." We could not have leveraged $200 million in graduate nursing education monies had we not shown a shortage in primary care providers in the United States. We need this data and it needs to be uniform across states. The National Forum of State Nursing Workforce Centers has developed three minimum datasets that each state should collect as frequently as is affordable in order to continue monitoring the makeup of the nursing workforce. The three datasets include nurse supply, nurse demand, and level of nurse education (The National Forum of State Nursing Workforce Centers, 2016). This national effort to standardize states' collection of data about the nursing workforce is especially important since HRSA is no longer able to fund conducting the National Sample Survey of Nursing in the near future that they have been previously conducting every four years since 1977. Although it is unlikely Congress will appropriate money for the ACA's mandated National Health Care Workforce Commission, IOM recommendations are still calling for it. The IOM's recent report, *Geographic Adjustment in Medicare Payment Phase II: Implications for Access, Quality, and Efficiency*, calls for the Workforce Commission as one of six recommendations in order to propose evidence-based actionable items regarding professional health workforce distribution and supply, and to allow APRNs to practice to the full extent of their education and training (IOM, 2012).

DIVERSITY AND THE IOM REPORT

Many nurses criticized the IOM *Future of Nursing* report because they perceived that it did not do enough to increase the diversity of the nursing workforce. If one reads *The Future of Nursing* report cover to cover the reader will notice that increasing the diversity in the nursing workforce is a thread throughout its chapters. The report calls for bringing and educating more people from diverse ethnic backgrounds, including men, into the profession of nursing. Nurses should racially, ethnically, by gender and other categories of diversity reflect the population in the United States; all nurses must have or gain the competency of providing culturally competent care and that concern over diversity must be integrated into all levels of nursing practice. Diversity is so integral to the *Campaign for Action* in order to fully implement *The Future of Nursing* recommendations that the Campaign unveiled its Diversity Steering Committee to work on implementing a national diversity action plan and is giving technical assistance to state Action Coalitions on diversity strategies. See Exhibit 4.3 for the mission of the Diversity Steering Committee.

Members on the Diversity Steering Committee represent the following national nursing organizations: National Black Nurses Association, National Association of Hispanic Nurses, American Assembly for Men in Nursing, Asian American/Pacific Islander Nurses Association, Philippine Nurses Association, and National Alaska Native American Indian Nurses Association. Why was diversity in nursing such a concern to the IOM Future of Nursing committee and continues to be a concern to the *Campaign for Action*? By 2042 the US Census Bureau predicts that minority groups will make up 54% of our population (U.S. Census Bureau, 2012). By 2042 while the non-Hispanic White population will be the largest single group, no single ethnic group will be the majority. Contrast this to the racial makeup of nurses in 2008, which remained predominantly White and female (HRSA, 2010). While about 85% of registered nurses in the United States are White, only 5.5% are Asian, 5.4%

MISSION OF THE *CAMPAIGN FOR ACTION* DIVERSITY STEERING	EXHIBIT 4.3

The Future of Nursing: *Campaign for Action*'s Diversity Steering Committee works to ensure that all Americans, regardless of race, religion, creed, ethnicity, gender, sexual orientation, or any aspect of identity will have access to high-quality, patient-centered care in a health care system where nurses contribute as essential partners in achieving success

Source: Campaign for Action (n.d.).

are Black, 3.6% are Hispanic, and Alaska Native and American Native Indian are combined at less than 1%. It is widely believed that a more diverse nursing workforce will give more culturally competent care. An executive summary published by the Commonwealth Fund reports that this racial discordance in professional health care has serious consequences. The degree of continued racial disparities in health care is the fruit of this gross mismatch of mostly white practitioners to non-white patients and populations. It is naïve to think that the color of skin is solely the issue. Since many white health professionals come from a background that facilitated them to go to medical or nursing school they likely lead mostly middle- to upper-middle-class lives. They do not have the kind of cultural insight that comes with living in poverty, where life is completely different than being white and middle class in America. White, middle-class health professionals constantly make assumptions about their racially and ethnically non-white patients such as that they can afford to fill their prescriptions, that they have access to transportation, and that they can afford to buy non-subsidized fruits and vegetables. Several studies link racial concordance with better patient satisfaction and better health outcomes (Cooper & Powe, 2004).

ASSESSING THE PROGRESS

The NAM convened a team to assess the progress of the IOM *Future of Nursing* report (NAM, 2015). While some progress was acknowledged with achieving the report's recommendations, the report brief called for more work to achieve higher levels of nursing education, more skillful teamwork, care coordination and prevention training. See Exhibit 4.4 for the list of recommendations. In addition, the progress report calls for making diversity a campaign priority. The progress assessment stated that nursing is having a "wide-ranging impact" on increasing our population's access to patient-centered and affordable health care. While *The Future of Nursing* created the tipping point in bringing nursing communities across the United States together to work together to achieve the recommendations, the profession is still facing significant challenges in removing scope-of-practice barriers. The progress report recommends that nursing "build common ground around scope of practice and other issues in policy and practice." It recommended that the *Campaign for Action* broaden its stakeholders and work on these issues, which serve as a prevention from nursing contributing its full potential to the health of populations.

RECOMMENDATIONS OF THE ASSESSING PROGRESS ON THE IOM *FUTURE OF NURSING REPORT*	**EXHIBIT 4.4**

Removing Barriers to Practice and Care

1. Build common ground around scope of practice and other issues in policy and practice.

Achieving Higher Levels of Education

2. Continue pathways toward increasing the percentage of nurses with a baccalaureate degree.
3. Create and fund transition-to-practice residency programs.
4. Promote nurses' pursuit of doctoral degrees.
5. Promote nurses' interprofessional and lifelong learning.

Promoting Diversity

6. Make diversity in the nursing workforce a priority.

Collaborating and Leading in Care Delivery and Redesign

7. Expand efforts and opportunities for interprofessional collaboration and leadership development for nurses.
8. Promote the involvement of nurses in the redesign of care delivery and payment systems.
9. Communicate with a wider and more diverse audience to gain broad support for campaign objectives.

Improving Workforce Data Infrastructure

10. Improve workforce data collection.

Source: National Academy of Medicine (2015).

CONCLUSION

The Future of Nursing report has put a strong spotlight onto the nursing profession. This report is essentially challenging the profession of nursing to commit to mobilize for changes that will make a difference in people's health and in the quality of their lives. Wouldn't it be more meaningful for nurses if interventions could make lasting health changes in patients' lives rather than solely relief from a single acute illness event? Nurses must take to heart the rest of the American Nurses Association (ANA) definition of nursing, which is to advocate for the health of families, communities, and populations (ANA, 2010). The IOM's *Future of Nursing* report is not only telling nurses they are capable of increasing the health of Americans but also telling them that they must care enough to return to school and to lead in these efforts.

DISCUSSION QUESTIONS

1. *How has increased interprofessional practice among APRNs and other practitioners resulted in improved health outcomes for patients, families, and communities?*

2. *How can health coaches and community workers affect the practice of APRNs?*
3. *Is a transition to practice residency really necessary for APRNs, especially since research shows good health outcomes of APRNs who never had such a residency?*
4. *Are there any practice barriers in your state and if so what are they and what does this mean for your practice?*
5. *Why might an APRN choose to earn a PhD over a DNP?*

ANALYSIS, SYNTHESIS, AND CLINICAL APPLICATION

1. *Interview leaders in your state or district's Action Coalition and analyze the extent to which your state has implemented any or all of the eight recommendations of* The Future of Nursing *report.*
2. *Interview an APRN who works in a NHMC about his or her practice in relation to the eight recommendations of* The Future of Nursing *report. Ask about concerns over the health of the community and ideas to promote the health of the community.*
3. *Find an APRN who is racially/ethnically neither White nor female and ask this person what (if any) the barriers were to becoming an APRN. Ask how diversity enhances their nursing practice.*
4. *What are several ways you can enhance your cultural competencies? Why does this matter?*

EXERCISES/CONSIDERATIONS

1. *APRNs will have to learn ways of increasing interprofessional practice, especially if their state allows independent practice.*
2. *APRNs will increasingly be asked to extend their practices by engaging in trans-disciplinary teams, such as including community health workers.*
3. *APRNs will increasingly work with registered nurses in increasingly complex care environments in the ambulatory setting.*
4. *APRNs will increasingly use telehealth to manage patients with chronic illness, engage in "hospital at home" programs, provide consultation, determine if patients are appropriate for transfer, and improve access to palliative care consultations and services.*
5. *APRNs will increase their engagement in population/preventive health measures.*

REFERENCES

Aiken, L. H., Clarke, S. P., Cheung, R. B., Sloane, D. M., & Silber, J. H. (2003). Educational levels of hospital nurses and surgical patient mortality. *Journal of the American Medical Association, 290*(12), 1617–1623.

American Association of Colleges of Nursing. (2004). AACN position statement on the practice doctorate in nursing. Retrieved from http://www.aacnnursing.org/News-Information/Position-Statements-White-Papers/Practice-Doctorate

American Association of Colleges of Nursing. (2012). Retrieved from http://www.aacn.nche.edu/membership/members-only/presentations/2012/12doctoral/Potempa-Doc-Programs.pdf

American Association of Colleges of Nursing. (2016). DNP fact sheet. Retrieved from http://www.aacnnursing.org/News-Information/Fact-Sheets/DNP-Fact-Sheet

American Association of Colleges of Nursing. (2017). Nursing faculty shortage fact sheet. Retrieved from http://www.aacnnursing.org/Portals/42/News/Factsheets/Faculty-Shortage-Factsheet-2017.pdf?ver=2017-07-11-103742-167

American Nurses Association. (2010). *Nursing's social policy statement: The essence of the profession* (3rd ed.). Silver Spring, MD: Author.

Benner, P., Sutphen, M., Leonard, V., & Day, L. (2010). *Educating nurses: A call for radical transformation.* San Francisco, CA: Jossey-Bass.

Blegen, M. A., Vaughn, T. E., & Goode, C. J. (2001). Nurse experience and education: Effect on quality of care. *Journal of NursingAdministration, 31*(1), 33–39.

Campaign for Action. (n.d.). Diversity steering committee: Mission. Retrieved from https://campaign foraction.org/about/diversity-steering-committee

Campaign for Action. (2016). Welcome to the future of nursing: *Campaign for Action* dashboard. Retrieved from http://campaignforaction.org/wp-content/uploads/2016/04/Campaign-Dashboard-5-19 -16.pdf

Centers for Disease Control and Prevention. (2012). Task force recommends team-based care for improving blood pressure control. Retrieved from http://www.cdc.gov/media/releases/2012/p0515_ bp_control.html

Centers for Disease Control and Prevention. (2014). NCHHSTP social determinants of health. Retrieved from http://www.cdc.gov/socialdeterminants/Definitions.html

Centers for Medicare and Medicaid Services. (2012). National health expenditures projections 2010–2012. Retrieved from https://www.cms.gov/Research-Statistics-Data-and-Systems/Statistics-Trends -and-Reports/NationalHealthExpendData/Downloads/Proj2012.pdf

Centers for Medicare and Medicaid Services. (2017a). About the CMS Innovation Center. Retrieved from http://innovation.cms.gov/about/index.html

Centers for Medicare and Medicaid Services. (2017b). Physician fee schedule. Retrieved from http:// www.cms.gov/Medicare/Medicare-Fee-for-Service-Payment/PhysicianFeeSched/index .html?redirect=/PhysicianFeeSched

Chen, P. W. (2010, November 18). Nurses' role in the future of health care. *New York Times.* Retrieved from http://www.nytimes.com/2010/11/18/health/views/18chen.html?_r=0

Cooper, L. A., & Powe, N. R. (2004). Disparities in patient experiences, health care processes, and outcomes: The role of patient-provider racial, ethnic, and language concordance. Retrieved from http://www.commonwealthfund.org/programs/minority/cooper_raceconcordance_753.pdf

Duke University School of Nursing. (n.d.). Nursing and health care leadership major. Retrieved from https://nursing.duke.edu/academics/programs/msn/nursing-and-health-care-leadership -major?gclid=Cj0KCQjwub7NBRDJARIsAP7wlT9WMCGV_6wSv15WQ2QwjVMvEUApLFojL2b aJChIQ6s1_zM9dUO3MHcaAu_4EALw_wcB

Estabrooks, C. A., Midodzi, W. K., Cummings, G. C., Ricker, K. L., & Giovannetti, P. (2005). The impact of hospital nursing characteristics on 30-day mortality. *Nursing Research, 54*(2), 74–84.

Federal Trade Commission. (2013). Retrieved from http://www.ftc.gov

Hassmiller, S., & Combes, J. (2012). Nurse leaders in the boardroom: A fitting choice. *Journal of Healthcare Management, 57*(1), 8–11.

HB 346. (2012). Retrieved from http://lis.virginia.gov/cgi-bin/legp604.exe?ses=121&typ=bil&val =HB346

Institute for Healthcare Improvement. (2013). IHI triple aim initiative. Retrieved from http://www.ihi .org/offerings/Initiatives/TripleAim/Pages/default.aspx

Institute of Medicine. (2010). The future of nursing: Leading change, advancing health. Retrieved from https://www.nap.edu/read/12956/chapter/1

Institute of Medicine. (2012). Geographic adjustment in Medicare Payment Phase II: Implications for access, quality, and efficiency. Retrieved from https://www.nationalacademies.org/hmd/~/ media/Files/Report%20Files/2012/Geographic-Adjustment-Phase-II/geoadjustment_phaseII_ RB.pdf

Japsen, B. (2013). Though Obamacare pays less, providers flock to 'bundled' Medicare payments. *Forbes.* Retrieved from http://www.forbes.com/sites/brucejapsen/2013/02/01/though-obamacare-pays -less-medical-providers-flock-to-bundled-medicare-payments

Kovner, C. T., Brewer, C., Katigbak, C., Djukic, M., & Fatehi, F. (2012). Charting the course for nurses' achievement of higher education levels. *Journal of Professional Nursing, 28*(6), 333–343.

Kovner, C., & Walani, S. (2010). Nurse managed health centers (NMHCs). Retrieved from https:// campaignforaction.org/resource/nurse-managed-health-centers-nmhcs

Michener, L. (November, 2012). *Durham and Duke: A story of one community's journey towards health and what it has meant for practice and training*. Presented at the Institute of Medicine Global Forum on Innovation in Health Professional Education, Washington, DC.

National Academy of Medicine. (2015). Assessing progress on the IOM report the future of nursing. Retrieved from http://www.nationalacademies.org/hmd/Reports/2015/Assessing-Progress-on-the-IOM-Report-The-Future-of-Nursing.aspx

National Academy of Medicine. (2016). About the National Academy of Medicine. Retrieved from https://nam.edu/about-the-nam

National Council of State Boards of Nursing. (2013). Transition to practice. Retrieved from https://www.ncsbn.org/transition-to-practice.htm

National Council of State Boards of Nursing. (2016). CNP independent practice map. Retrieved from https://www.ncsbn.org/5407.htm

National Forum of State Nursing Workforce Centers. (2016). Nursing minimum dataset surveys. Retrieved from https://nfsnwc.wpengine.com/minimum-datasets

National Nursing Centers Consortium. (2016). Retrieved from http://www.nncc.us

Orsolini-Hain, L. (2008). An interpretive phenomenological study on the influences on associate degree prepared nurses to return to school to earn a higher degree in nursing. Retrieved from ProQuest Dissertations and Theses database (UNI No. 3324576).

Orsolini-Hain, L., & Waters, V. (2009). Education evolution: A historical perspective of associate degree nursing. *Journal of Nursing Education, 48*(5), 266–271.

Robert Wood Johnson Foundation. (2012). The billion dollar hei$t. Retrieved from http://www.rwjf.org/en/library/research/2012/05/the-billion-dollar-heist.html

Robert Wood Johnson Foundation. (2013). Grant's explorer. Retrieved from http://www.rwjf.org/en/grants.html#q/maptype/grants

Sales, A., Sharp, N., Li, Y. F., Lowy, E., Greiner, G., Liu, C. F., . . . Needleman, J. (2008). The association between nursing factors and patient mortality in the Veterans Health Administration: The view from the nursing unit level. *Medical Care, 46*(9), 938–945.

Spector, N., Blegen, M., Silvestre, J., Barnsteiner, J., Lynn, M., Ulrich, B., . . . Alexander, M. (2015). *Journal of Nursing Regulation, 5*(4), 24–38. Retrieved from https://www.ncsbn.org/Spector_Transition_to_Practice_Study_in_Hospital_Settings.pdf

Totten, M. K. (2010, May/June). Nurses on healthcare boards: A smart and logical move to make. *Healthcare Executive Magazine*, 84–87.

Tourangeau, A. E., Doran, D. M., McGillis-Hall, L., O'Brian-Pallus, L., Pringles, D., Tu, J. V., & Cranley, L. A. (2006). Impact of hospital nursing care on 30-day mortality for acute medical patients. *Journal of Advanced Nursing, 57*(1), 32–44.

U.S. Census Bureau. (2012). U.S. Census Bureau projections show a slower growing, older, more diverse nation a half century from now. Retrieved from http://www.census.gov/newsroom/releases/archives/population/cb12-243.html

U.S. Department of Health and Human Services, Health Resources and Services Administration. (2010). The registered nurse population: Initial findings from the 2008 National Sample Survey of Registered Nurses. Retrieved from https://bhw.hrsa.gov/sites/default/files/bhw/nchwa/rnsurveyfinal.pdf

U.S. Department of Health and Human Services, Health Resources and Services Administration. (2012). Affordable Care Act nurse managed health clinics: Frequently asked questions. Retrieved from https://www.hrsa.gov/grants/healthprofessions/acafaq.pdf

U.S. Department of Health and Human Services, Health Resources and Services Administration. (2013). What is a health center? Retrieved from http://bphc.hrsa.gov/about/what-is-a-health-center/index.html

Updates on the Implications for Practice: *The Consensus Model for APRN Regulation*

Kelly A. Goudreau

The Consensus Model for APRN Regulation: Licensure, Accreditation, Certification, and Education (APRN Consensus Work Group & National Council of State Boards of Nursing APRN Advisory Committee, 2008) is a historic document that will have implications for practice for all four of the identified Advanced Practice Registered Nurse (APRN) roles (Clinical Nurse Specialist [CNS], Nurse Practitioner [NP], Certified Nurse-Midwife [CNM], and Certified Registered Nurse Anesthetist [CRNA]) for many years to come. Even today, the effects of the statements made in that document continue to be felt across the four roles in numerous ways and in all states as the states begin or continue to adopt the principles in the 2008 vision for the future. Other chapters in this text define the specific implications of the document. This chapter provides a brief history of how the document was created, explores how things have changed since the first edition of this book, indicates how it is being applied today to APRN practice, evaluates the outcomes of the document to date, and identifies how and why APRNs continue to need to be engaged in the discussions relative to the implementation of the *Consensus Model*.

BRIEF HISTORICAL BACKGROUND

The landscape of advanced practice nursing has been a confusing patchwork quilt of differing definitions for scope of practice, expectations of autonomy, prescriptive authority, and educational preparation. Before the *Consensus Model* (2008), and still today, each state has to work with its legislative body to affirm the existence of APRNs and define the functionality of each of the roles. The *Consensus Model* (2008) was created through a difficult and sometimes laborious process that took approximately 4 years of discussion between 23 nursing organizations and the National Council of State Boards of Nursing (NCSBN). Representatives came and went from the various organizations, but the document and its outcomes became the paramount outcome desired by all. That outcome was the singular voice for all advanced practice nursing having full practice authority across the United States.

The chaos related to regulation of advanced practice nursing has been recognized for a long time. As roles were added in the 1980s (NP) and the clear delineation between nursing practice and medical practice became blurred, there was increasing resistance from medical practitioners in a variety of states. That resistance took the form of negotiated limits on the function and autonomy of nurses in advanced roles. Those limits were different in each state and therefore there were multiple models for regulation of APRNs. In an effort to bring some order to the national chaos that was advanced practice regulation and to standardize the expectations for each of the roles, the NCSBN adopted a position paper on the licensure of advanced practice nursing in 1993 that included model language for legislation and a template for state-level administrative rules (Stanley, 2009). Unfortunately, the work done in the position paper had little effect, and the confusion and chaos in state-by-state rules and regulation of APRNs continued. Areas of concern were lack of uniformity in how an APRN was defined, inability to cross state lines and provide care of a consistent nature, and lack of a clear definition of a specialty or subspecialty and how one was educated to provide specialized care. Each state was doing what it could to try to make the APRN language work in concert with the legislative understanding of the roles and how they could impact quality, safety, and access to care for constituents, but it became a confusing jumble that did not allow nurses to move freely across state lines when necessary.

In 2004, in a continuing effort to more clearly define the advanced practice role and provide guidance to the state member constituents the NCSBN APRN Advisory Panel—essentially a special interest group of the NCSBN focused on APRN regulatory issues nationally—began work a draft APRN vision paper. This document was being created simultaneously with another document that was being written by the APRN Consensus Work Group that had been convened in response to concerns from the American Nurses Association (ANA), the National Organization of Nurse Practitioner Faculties (NONPF), and the American Association of Colleges of Nursing (AACN). The APRN Consensus Work Group had been working on a document since 2004 in parallel to the NCSBN but was unaware of the work that was being done by NCSBN APRN Advisory Panel.

The NCSBN APRN Advisory Panel completed a draft of their paper and disseminated it in 2006 to a broad audience including multiple nursing organizations that were engaged in the APRN Consensus Work Group process. The response was immediate and not favorable. Although created in a parallel process, there were significant differences from the document that was nearing completion in the APRN Consensus Work Group.

Rather than continue on parallel pathways, it was determined that APRNs would be better served by a consensus among the various organizations. In order to achieve that consensus, there needed to be significant dialogue to explore the similarities and differences between the NCSBN draft document and the APRN Consensus Work Group draft document. In order to do that work, seven representatives were selected from each of the two groups, the NCSBN APRN Panel, and the APRN Consensus Work Group. The initial goal of the group was to discuss how best to ensure that the content was at least complimentary and not contradictory if two documents were to be maintained. After initial discussions and returning to the two other groups with the discussion content, the final decision, however, was that there could not be differing documents in an already chaotic environment. There needed to be consistency in the recommendations in order to guide the work of states as they wrestled with how best to categorize and ensure ongoing access to APRNs. This smaller group of 14 became known as the APRN Joint Dialogue Group and began meeting in early 2007.

The work of the APRN Joint Dialogue Group progressed for a year. The group took on a specific aim of "doing no harm" to any APRN group in order to better the lot of another, and also determined that the group must listen to each concern voiced and determine a collective and consensus response. In that year each area of the two papers was examined and openly discussed in regard to implications, and a decision was made to combine the documents and come forward with a single consensus paper that could guide the regulation of APRN practice across the country. The final document, the *Consensus Model for APRN Regulation; Licensure, Accreditation, Certification, and Education* (APRN Consensus Work Group & National Council of State Boards of Nursing APRN Advisory Committee, 2008) was released to nursing and regulatory organizations in July 2008.

The *Consensus Model*, as it has come to be known, has generated much discussion among the four APRN roles as the implications of the statements in it have been dissected and analyzed in the effort to implement the recommendations. The document was also used in part as an element of the document created by the Institute of Medicine (IOM) on *The Future of Nursing: Leading Change, Advancing Health* (2010), further validating its impact on the APRN roles.

APPLICATION TO APRN PRACTICE

Since the release of the *Consensus Model* in 2008, there has been much work accomplished in each of the four areas of licensure, accreditation, certification, and education (LACE). A separate workgroup (LACE) was created from the Joint Dialogue Workgroup that is continuing the work of the transition and monitoring the progress toward full implementation of the APRN Consensus document.

The work of reducing the chaos and standardizing the expectations for APRNs across the United States is well under way now in 2016. The stated goal of full implementation of the model by 2015 has passed, however, and yet there continues to be a significant amount of work still left to complete. All of the organizations that represent the four areas of LACE continue to have work to do. The work includes considerations in licensure, accreditation processes for educational programs, certification, and changes to the core educational process for each of the four roles involved as well as the increasingly important continuation of the communication between the groups that represent the four elements of LACE. Each of the roles has been impacted differently, but the goal is that no change in one group will negatively impact another. An analysis of the impact to each of the areas reveals much about the intrinsic philosophic approach taken in the foundation of each of the roles.

Licensure

The nature of the comprehensive change this agreement is generating is clearly evident when one looks at the issues arising from the proposed changes in licensure across the country. The APRN *Consensus Model* was intended to provide standardization of LACE in nursing. Licensure is only one of those elements that is not fully controlled by nursing. Developing the laws that become the licensure regulations in each state is an outcome of the political process in that state. As such, the rules are different in each and every state. It is a monumental undertaking to change the laws governing nursing in each state. The APRN *Consensus Model* calls for some consistent rules to apply to all four of the advanced practice roles.

These requirements may seem simple on the surface, but when attempting to implement them consistently across the nation for four advanced practice roles, the issues become complex. Difficulty arises when the state board of nursing in each state must open the state practice act in order to have the language modified to meet the previously stated requirements. Opening the state practice act allows for any interested stakeholder to voice concerns with one or more sections of the existing law and any proposed changes. Great opposition has been raised by physician groups in particular in relation to prescriptive authority and the maintenance of supervised/collaborative practice agreements in many states. Another issue is the one surrounding licensure of existing APRNs when no prior recognition for them existed under the old rules or regulations. Many issues are arising for those individuals who may have been carrying the name of one or more of the groups of APRNs without the appropriate education or certification to match. This issue is, unfortunately, most recognized for the CNS group. Per the *Consensus Model* language it is imperative that the SBN be actively engaged in the process of licensure of APRNs in their state (see Box 5.1).

The NCSBN continues to be actively engaged in the discussion. From the outset of the Joint Dialogue Group, the NCSBN began to develop tools that are

---

FOUNDATIONAL REQUIREMENTS FOR LICENSURE   **BOX 5.1**

Boards of nursing will:

1. License APRNs in the categories of CRNA, Certified Nurse-Midwife, CNS or NP within a specific population focus
2. Be solely responsible for licensing APRN
3. Only license graduates of accredited graduate programs that prepare graduates with the APRN core, role, and population competencies
4. Require successful completion of a national certification examination that assesses APRN core, role, and population competencies for APRN licensure
5. Not issue a temporary license
6. Only license an APRN when education and certification are congruent
7. License APRNs as independent practitioners with no regulatory requirements for collaboration, direction, or supervision
8. Allow for mutual recognition of advanced practice registered nursing through the APRN Compact
9. Have at least one APRN representative position on the board and utilize an APRN advisory committee that includes representatives of all four APRN roles
10. Institute a grandfathering clause that will exempt those APRNs already practicing in the state from new eligibility requirements.

APRN, Advanced Practice Registered Nurse; CNS, Clinical Nurse Specialist; CRNA, Certified Registered Nurse Anesthetist; NP, Nurse Practitioner.

Source: APRN Consensus Work Group & National Council of State Boards of Nursing APRN Advisory Committee (2008, pp. 14–15).

being used by nurses with an interest in the current discussion related to where their state is presently as measured against the *Consensus Model* language. The tools can also inform the nurses whether or not their state or neighboring states are proposing changes to the laws and subsequently the rules and regulations surrounding licensure of APRNs. Look at the NCSBN web page located at www. ncsbn.org/5397.htm for a synopsis of all states and territories and where they are in reaching the goal of compliance with the *Consensus Model.*

Although the licensure is moving toward full practice authority in many states, there continues to be some resistance across the nation. The health branch of the Veterans Affairs (VA), the Veterans Health Administration (VHA), recently moved to authorize full practice authority for all APRNs employed in its multiple medical centers and community-based outpatient clinics (CBOCs). At the time of the writing of this chapter, the issue had not been fully resolved. Per regulatory requirement, the VHA needed to print its intent in the Federal Register so that the public and any stakeholders could provide their feedback to the proposal of full practice authority for APRNs employed by the VA. The response was over- whelming. More comments were received on this one issue than any other in the history of the Federal Register. Comments came from both sides of the issue (for and against) with an alarming number of negative comments coming from the National Association of Anesthetists. Each comment needs to be considered in the issue, and it is taking time to process through all comments. All will be seri- ously considered when looking at the current language being proposed as the VHA moves to fully implement full practice authority for APRNs.

Accreditation

The APRN *Consensus Model* outlined expectations for the accrediting bodies as well as licensure, certification, and education entities. The goal again was to achieve con- sistency in the processes used to accredit educational programs that prepare APRNs. Those changes were defined as shown in Box 5.2.

ACCREDITORS WILL	BOX 5.2

1. Be responsible for evaluating APRN education programs including graduate- degree-granting and postgraduate certificate programs
2. Through their established accreditation standards and process, assess APRN education programs in light of the APRN core, role core, and population core competencies
3. Assess developing APRN education programs and tracks by reviewing them using established accreditation standards and granting pre-approval, pre-accreditation, or accreditation prior to student enrollment
4. Include an APRN on the visiting team when an APRN program/track is being reviewed
5. Monitor APRN educational programs throughout the accreditation period by reviewing them using established accreditation standards and processes

APRN, Advanced Practice Registered Nurse.

Source: APRN Consensus Work Group & National Council of State Boards of Nursing APRN Advisory Committee (2008, p. 15).

The accrediting bodies, including the Accreditation Commission for Education in Nursing, Inc. (ACEN), the Commission on Collegiate Nursing Education (CCNE), the Accreditation Commission for Midwifery Education (ACME), and the Council on Accreditation of Nurse Anesthesia Educational Programs (COA), have all undergone some changes as a result of the implementation of the *Consensus Model*. The major changes have occurred as a reflection of the requirement that APRN programs be evaluated in relation to the role and population foci. This is no longer new territory for many of the accrediting agencies, and the transitions appear to have been fairly smooth.

Two of the accrediting agencies had never considered pre-accreditation review of programs. Both the ACEN and the CCNE needed to shift their perspectives and realign their accreditation standards to meet this requirement. The pre-accreditation process was in use by the ACME and COA before the Joint Dialogue discussions. The intent of pre-accreditation processes is to ensure that educational programs in the role meet the outcome standards and expectations prior to final accreditation. By looking at a pre-accreditation process, the educational preparation for all classes of graduates (including the previously exempt first class of students) would be able to be fully accredited upon graduation. This standardization was called for during the LACE discussions and is intended to provide counsel, strength, and consistency to both the CNS and NP educational programs in addition to the nurse anesthetist and midwifery programs.

For the two agencies newly doing pre-accreditation visits, the inclusion of an APRN on the team when programs are being evaluated continues to be a work in process. At present, there may be an NP on the team, or a CNS, and they are then responsible for reviewing both the NP and CNS tracks when they themselves may not be as knowledgeable as they could be for the alternative role. For the CNM and CRNA programs, there is no question that there will be an appropriate APRN on the team as the program review is specific to the role. This is an area that continues to need refinement as the full implementation of the APRN *Consensus Model* gets closer.

All of the accrediting agencies for higher education programs are overseen by the U.S. Department of Education (2017) through a process of review and evaluation of the standards set by each of the accrediting agencies. Per the Department of Education website, "The goal of accreditation is to ensure that education provided by institutions of higher education meet acceptable levels of quality" (www2.ed.gov/admins/finaid/accred/accreditation.html#Overview). The Department of Education relies on review of all educational accrediting agencies by the National Advisory Committee on Institutional Quality and Integrity (NACIQI), a politically appointed board of 18 individuals who are nominated in equal numbers by each party. The members are identified by peers and reviewed for political appointment to the committee. Criteria for selection include expertise in educational matters and a proclivity for integrity and objectivity. All four of the nursing accrediting bodies have been reviewed by the NACIQI and are approved to accredit nursing programs in higher education. In order to maintain their ability to accredit programs, they must meet or exceed the standards articulated by the Department of Education and reviewed by the NACIQI.

Certification

CRNAs and CNMs already determined many years ago that they needed certification as an entry to practice element before the APRN *Consensus Model* discussions and subsequent to its implementation. CRNAs and CNMs developed certification as an adjunct to their educational process and an outgrowth of the professional expectations for competency-based assessments of skill. NPs, too, were using certification as an entry to practice assessment of competency prior to practice in most states. CNSs however were not. Until the discussions at the Joint Dialogue Group table, the CNS leadership had maintained the perception that certification was a mark of excellence rather than an element to assess competence for entry to practice. Therefore, most, if not all, CNS certification examinations had a requirement for 2 to 3 years of practice as an element of eligibility to sit for the examination. This major paradigm shift has created great difficulty in the transition period for the CNSs. The conceptual framework for CNSs was based on some core elements of competency that span all of the specialty foci, but each CNS was flexible enough to move fluidly within and between populations based on the specialty content of their practice. For example, a CNS who specialized in diabetes or pulmonary could move between populations in acute, community, or age brackets. Their specialty was foremost in their practice. Within a regulatory model, however, which calls for standardization in order to protect the public, there is little tolerance of unique perspectives, regardless of the need. CNSs have had to reframe their entire construct of certification and ultimately of the core educational framework.

A further issue is emerging as the APRN *Consensus Model* implementation evolves and practice environments become more and more in need of providers. As the physician shortage increases in primary care, hospitalist care, and frontline specialty foci, the practice areas are increasing their use of APRNs in specialty areas for which they may not have received training. The certification framework within the APRN *Consensus Model* allows for some flexibility in that the core elements of the role and population are what need to be the focus for surrogate licensure. The intent of the model was to allow not only for the regulation of the core foundations but also for expansion of the specialty as an unregulated element (in licensure terms) but overseen by the professional organizations that focus on that specialty. The intent was that the focus of the CNS group on certification being the mark of excellence would still stand within the specialty areas developed by each individual APRN. Unfortunately, certification examinations are costly to create and difficult to maintain as psychometrically sound if there are relatively few individuals taking the tests. This is creating a situation where many APRNs are functioning in specialty roles without certification to support the quality of their practice.

In order to meet the intent of the APRN *Consensus Model* certification examinations to be a proxy for licensure at the advanced practice level, all four of the roles needed to look at the certification examinations they were offering and refine them to meet the criteria of the new model. Specifically, the primary change for the roles has been to align in the format of role and population foci. As mentioned previously, CNSs did not focus on a single population as described in the *Consensus Model*. The population foci in the model include six primary groupings: Adult-Gerontology, Pediatrics, Gender Specific, Psychiatric, Family/Individual Across the Life Span, and Neonatal.

CNSs moved across these population foci depending on their specialty focus. Primary certification for CNSs has been in the specialty role, so moving to a population foci has meant a complete shift in how the CNS certification examinations are written. The NPs have also had to shift somewhat. Although the population foci fit much better with the NP perspective, there has been some drift as CNSs have been nonexistent in many areas; yet, the specialty need has continued, so they too moved into a specialty focus in many instances. The realignment of both the NP and the CNS examinations has been a disruptive innovation for both groups. The CNMs can fit into multiple categories as well, which has opened up their perspective on caring for individual women and their partners through young, middle, and old adulthood as well as the neonate. Nurse anesthetists have, like CNSs, moved fluidly across the populations due to their specialty approach to care. The examinations have shifted since the first writing of this chapter, and it is noted they will continue to shift and change as the roles are more clearly defined or as the needs of society dictate.

Education

Again, the need for change has varied among the four APRN roles, and the APRN *Consensus Model* language has impacted one or two more than the others. Primary elements of the needs in education are outlined in Figure 5.1 as defined in the APRN *Consensus Model*.

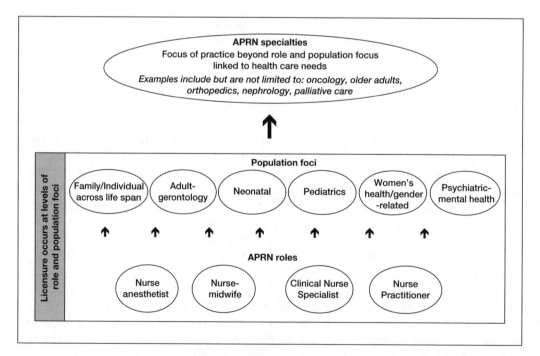

FIGURE 5.1 APRN Regulatory Model.

APRN, Advanced Practice Registered Nurse.

Source: APRN Consensus Work Group & National Council of State Boards of Nursing APRN Advisory Committee (2008, p. 10).

Additionally, there were changes to the curriculum expectations for the four roles. Some of the changes experienced by the CRNAs, CNMs, and CNSs have been the inclusion of three separate courses on pathophysiology, physical and health assessment, and pharmacology, commonly referred to as the "three Ps." The course content may have been present for all three of the roles in the curriculum but not necessarily pulled out in three separate and distinct courses as defined in the *Essentials of Master's Education for Advanced Practice Nursing* (AACN, 2011). The NP programs had pulled these courses into separate credits since the implementation of the NONPF agreement on core competencies and outcome expectations in the "Task Force Criteria" document first published in 1990 and updated most recently in 2014. An update to the 2014 criteria was sent out in the summer of 2016 for public comment and was released in early 2017.

The CNM and CRNA curriculum has been established for a very long time and is based on demonstrated competency in tasks and skills and repetitive application of same. The CNS, however, has seen many changes in licensure (simple recognition as an APRN role in some states), accreditation (incorporation of the core competency documents into accreditation standards is still pending), certification (transition from recognition of expert specialty focus to entry to practice population-focused examinations), and education (establishment of core competencies through a consensus process and refocusing to a population rather than specialty) (Goudreau, 2009; National Association of Clinical Nurse Specialists, 2012). All of these are significant paradigm shifts for any role but ones that will pay dividends in the end.

The changes have been substantial for all four of the roles. Some of the roles have had the backbone and infrastructure in place for most of the needed implementation (CRNA and CNM), some have had old battles to fight in state

---

FOUNDATIONAL REQUIREMENTS FOR EDUCATION   BOX 5.3

APRN education programs/tracks leading to APRN licensure, including graduate-degree-granting and postgraduate certificate programs will:

1. Follow established educational standards and ensure attainment of the APRN core, role core, and population core competencies.
2. Be accredited by a nursing accrediting organization that is recognized by the U.S. Department of Education (USDE) and/or the Council for Higher Education Accreditation (CHEA)
3. Be preapproved, preaccredited, or accredited before the acceptance of students, including all developing APRN education programs and tracks
4. Ensure that graduates of the program are eligible for national certification and state licensure
5. Ensure that official documentation (e.g., transcript) specifies the role and population focus of the graduate

APRN, Advanced Practice Registered Nurse.

Source: APRN Consensus Work Group & National Council of State Boards of Nursing APRN Advisory Committee (2008, p. 16).

legislatures regarding independent practice and prescriptive authority (NP), and some have had to build again essentially from the ground up in defining consistent curriculum expectations and outcomes (CNS), but the changes are occurring.

EVALUATION OF THE *CONSENSUS MODEL*

The evaluation of the *Consensus Model* will take many years. The work was done over a period of 4 years and took much discussion, collaboration, and assessment of the principle of doing no harm to any of the four advanced practice roles. It also took a lot of dialogue to determine the definition of APRN versus nurses who practice at an advanced level. When looking at the discussions in the remainder of this text, this definition may seem arbitrary and lacking in substance, but it is the definition of terminology that will help to clearly define the boundaries of APRN practice. When the next generation of APRNs look back on the work done in the early 2000s, will they look at it with an appreciation of the work done or disdain for the barriers that were put in place for APRN practice? It is hard to tell at this point. The IOM identified the anticipated barriers in their 2010 document, and unfortunately many of them have come to be recognized even in 2016.

Those barriers include:

1. The resistance of organized medicine to support expanded APRN scope of practice
2. The resistance of state legislators to introduce bills that expand scope of practice for APRNs
3. Restrictive credentialing and privileging practices within health care institutions
4. A lack of public awareness and recognition of the education, training, and clinical abilities of APRNs
5. A lack of standardized education, licensure, and certification requirements for APRNs from state to state (IOM, 2010; Kleinpell et al., 2014)

There are not only many gains for the APRN roles but also many losses of the values of the past and the intent of the roles when they were first created. All things must evolve. This is the evolution or the revolution of APRN practice in the 21st century in the United States. This initiative has already reached other countries and has impacted the consideration of outcomes of APRN definitions and practice in those countries. It has already been used as an exemplar of what not to do or will clearly define the pitfalls that need to be avoided and is assisting other countries as they consider their journey on the APRN path. Only time will tell if that will mean consistency in APRN practice internationally as the roles are examined and applied within multiple health care organizations.

THE *CONSENSUS MODEL* AS HEALTH POLICY

The *Consensus Model for APRN Regulation* is the epitome of health policy that has already had a direct impact on the practice of APRNs across the United States. It will also influence the outcomes of similar discussions around the world as other countries consider their need for expansion of the APRN role. The role of the leaders in APRN practice in the United States was significant and took 4 years to bring to consensus. The implementation process continues to use the consensus process and attempts to hold all parties accountable to not harming any other stakeholder in the process of their evolution as a segment of the nursing profession. The APRN *Consensus Model* document has already provided guidance for the development of health policies specific to the recognition and implementation of the APRN role in each and every state in the union and in the VHA, a national health care system.

Although the work of the APRN consensus leaders is complete at this time, many of them have continued the journey as the words are being taken and put to task in new practice acts that are being created in each state. It truly is up to the APRNs in each state, region, or county to speak up as to their specific needs that can support the patients they see and the access to health care in their community. Only by speaking with a singular voice about the impact of APRN care can the legislators hear about the impact and possibilities of APRN practice.

Now it is your turn to work on the issues. Raise your voice and address your legislator(s). Let them know if the current legislation surrounding APRN practice is insufficient. Tell them what you need in order to practice to the full scope of your license as defined in the IOM's report on *The Future of Nursing: Leading Change, Advancing Health* (IOM, 2010). Identify health policies that need to be generated as a result of this landmark consensus document and work for a brighter future for all APRNs and your patients.

CONCLUSION

The *Consensus Model* was a work of collaboration, integration, focused energy, and a will to define clearly for now and the future what an APRN is and should be able to do. The consensus around the elements of regulation was landmark and groundbreaking. To have more than 40 nursing organizations agree in principle to elements that provide the foundation for LACE of APRNs across the country took tremendous work from all involved. The key element of not wanting to do any harm to any of the four groups was upheld by all and continues to be upheld as the document and the ripples it has created impact the practice of APRNs nationwide. The right to self-determination of the roles was also upheld and respected, and the members around the discussion table stopped and listened to the needs of each group as issues of concern were raised. It was not a perfect process and although there are many issues that have been raised for a variety of the roles, it was at least a place to start. The foundational document has created much more discussion than it took to create it as the details have been worked out and new processes put into place. The recognition of the four roles and provision of definitions for each has set an expectation and a standard that will be discussed and perhaps emulated internationally.

It is the sincere hope of this author that the work that was done will stand the test of time and will endure, so that changes can be made at all levels of policy across the United States and now internationally as an exemplar of APRN regulation. Only through sweeping changes such as proposed in the *Consensus Model* can there be clear understanding of the importance, role, and implications for APRNs everywhere. On to the future.

DISCUSSION QUESTIONS

1. *Based on the information in this chapter, list at least two areas of policy change you can identify where legislation could have an impact.*
2. *If you were going to describe the importance of your issue for policy change to potential supporters, what key issues would you stress? How would you describe this to your patients?*
3. *Consider the health policy changes discussed in this chapter or those you have described in your analysis and consider the impact that might occur if these changes are NOT enacted. In other words, what are the consequences of not taking action?*
4. *Identify one change in your state that has already occurred or is in process as a result of the APRN Consensus Model implementation.*
5. *Discuss how the APRN Consensus Model has impacted your role as an APRN. Has it been positive? Negative? Has the APRN Consensus Model created or removed barriers for your APRN role?*
6. *Identify how the APRN Consensus Model has changed certification of APRNs in your role or population focus.*
7. *Identify how the APRN Consensus Model has changed your educational program. Have there been curriculum changes that have occurred over the past 2 years? Five years? How has that change impacted your education specifically?*

ANALYSIS, SYNTHESIS, AND CLINICAL APPLICATION

1. *Go to the website for your state legislature and/or your state board of nursing and look for legislation that is being proposed. Determine if the legislative change being proposed is in relation to the changes required by the APRN Consensus Model. If related to the APRN Consensus Model, plan to attend the hearings in the committee where the legislation was created or is being heard. Identify how your voice should be heard on the issue and prepare written testimony for presentation to the committee for their consideration.*
2. *Is there a rule or regulation that simply does not make sense in your state? Examples could include the inability of APRNs to sign state orders for life-sustaining treatment, death certificates, or ordering of physical therapy for patients who need it. Does the rule or regulation impact your practice directly? Consider approaching a legislator to educate the person about the situation and propose new legislation that would address the issue.*

EXERCISES/CONSIDERATIONS

1. *In your analysis of the regulations and rules for APRN practice in your state, do you see any specific barriers that will impact your practice or may have already impacted your practice? Describe the steps that would need to be taken in order to rectify this situation.*
2. *As you prepare for one of the four roles of APRN practice, how do you see your practice interface with the other three roles? How will full practice authority impact your ability or need to interact with the other three roles?*
3. *How will full practice authority impact your interaction with other disciplines?*

REFERENCES

American Association of Colleges of Nursing. (2011). *Essentials of master's education for advanced practice nursing.* Washington, DC: Author.

APRN Consensus Work Group & National Council of State Boards of Nursing APRN Advisory Committee. (2008). *Consensus model for APRN regulation: Licensure, accreditation, certification & education.* Retrieved from https://www.ncsbn.org/aprn-consensus.htm

Goudreau, K. A. (2009). What clinical nurse specialists need to know about the Consensus Model for advanced practice registered nurse regulation. *Clinical Nurse Specialist, 23*(2), 50–51.

Institute of Medicine. (2010). *The future of nursing: Leading change, advancing health.* Washington, DC: National Academies Press. Retrieved from http://www.nap.edu/catalog/12956.html

Kleinpell, R., Scanlon, A., Hibbert, D., DeKeyser, F., East, L., Fraser, D., . . . Beauschesne, M. (2014). Addressing issues impacting advanced nursing practice worldwide. *Online Journal of Issues in Nursing, 19*(2). Retrieved from http://www.nursingworld.org/mainmenucategories/anamarket place/anaperiodicals/ojin/tableofcontents/vol-19-2014/no2-may-2014/advanced-nursing -practice-worldwide.html

National Association of Clinical Nurse Specialists. (2012). *Statement on the APRN Consensus Model implementation.* Retrieved from http://www.nacns.org/docs/NACNSConsensusModel.pdf

Stanley, J. M. (2009). Reaching consensus on a regulatory model: What does this mean for APRNs? *Journal for Nurse Practitioners, 5*(2), 99–104.

U.S. Department of Education. (2017). Accreditation in the United States. Retrieved from http://www2 .ed.gov/admins/finaid/accred/accreditation_pg13.html

CHAPTER 6

Effective State-Level APRN Leadership in Health Policy

Christine C. Filipovich

Becoming an effective advocate requires experiences in the real world where policy is made. This chapter provides information and suggestions to prepare the reader for effective interaction with policy and decision makers. The content is intended to help the Advanced Practice Registered Nurse (APRN) to be a knowledgeable and effective advocate in his or her own state, where much policy affecting health care, nursing, and advanced practice nursing originates.

Legislation, regulation, and court rulings related to health care service delivery and reimbursement are types of government "policy" that directly impact nurses and nursing practice. The focus of this chapter is on how an APRN can identify issues of health policy and then work with the legislature and agencies under the jurisdiction of the governor to advance the practice of nursing at the state level.

HEALTH POLICY AND PUBLIC POLICY DEFINED

Broadly speaking, health policy is a course of action that influences health care decisions (World Health Organization, n.d.). Public policy refers to policy that is generated by governmental agencies and enacted through legislation. Public policy is made on behalf of the citizens and is influenced by factors such as economics, social issues, research, and technology. Health policy influences decisions about the health of a society. Similar to public policy, health policy is also influenced by factors such as health status of the citizens, research, and economics. Health policy can be developed and implemented:

- On an institutional level to address workplace issues, such as in hospitals to establish limitations on the number of patients an RN can care for

- To shape nursing practice through professional organization policies by established standards of care or a code of ethics
- To promote healthy communities through community, regional, or national policies (e.g., improving air quality or implementing health screening processes; New Jersey Collaborating Center for Nursing Workforce Development, 2003)

THE APRN IS AN EXPERT

Registered nurses prepared at the advanced practice level, by definition, possess knowledge and skill for expert practice in a specialized field of nursing. As most professionals, APRNs are lifelong learners because advances in science, technology, and theoretical foundations of nursing practice require continuous learning in order to remain professionally competent.

Most undergraduate and graduate nursing education programs include learning experiences that expose students to some aspects of legal and regulatory matters affecting nursing, such as the state's licensing law and regulations. However, neither formal education programs nor years of clinical practice are likely to equip the APRN for effective policy advocacy. This expertise comes from experience and real-time exposure to the policy-making process.

Nurses are widely respected in their communities, and public polls rank nurses near or at the top of the most admired and trusted professions. This public trust positions the nursing profession to be a powerful influence in health policy matters. There are many gains within reach of nurses who capitalize on the public's respect. APRNs are especially well positioned to insert the nursing profession into policy discussions and to lead the way for nurses to effectively advocate for themselves.

The APRN has expert knowledge of the health care delivery system and advanced clinical nursing skills. In addition, the APRN has well-developed critical thinking skills and both knowledge and experience in applying change theory and principles to effectively lead system transformation. Historically, education of Clinical Nurse Specialists (CNSs) has emphasized preparation to be a change agent. More recently, the Doctor of Nursing Practice (DNP) has incorporated aspects of both change management and systems level analysis into preparation for all four of the APRN roles.

Through leadership and influence, APRNs impact policy making and policy decisions within an agency or health system. Thus, the APRN has an excellent foundation for effectively impacting and influencing health policy and policy decisions in a broader scope. Health policy within the scope of state government and the implications of the APRN to influence that policy are discussed.

APRN POLICY/ADVOCACY COMPETENCIES

Practice competencies published by national organizations representing APRNs outline the role expectations and activities of APRNs in policy advocacy. Each of the four roles of CNS, Certified Nurse Practitioner (CNP), Certified Nurse-Midwife (CNM), and Certified Registered Nurse Anesthetist (CRNA) has defined competencies within its core documents for educational preparation for the role.

CNSs are expected to evaluate the impact of legislative and regulatory policies as they apply to nursing practice and patient or population outcomes. CNSs also are expected to advocate for the CNS/APRN role and for positive legislative response to issues affecting nursing practice (National CNS Core Competency Task Force, 2010). Nurse Practitioners are expected to participate in health policy activities at the local, state, national, and international levels (American Association of Nurse Practitioners, 2013). CNMs are expected to know issues and trends in health care health policy and systems, to evaluate women's health policy issues within a variety of jurisdictions (local to federal), and to demonstrate the ability to develop remedies to promote health improvement for women and newborns (American College of Nurse-Midwives, 2011).

Until 2008, public health nurses were considered to be a part of the CNS role, but their professional organization made the decision to exclude components of the evolving definition of APRN. For that reason, they are no longer considered to be APRNs but do provide advanced nursing care. Although not currently considered APRNs, public health nurses are also expected to demonstrate expertise in understanding and interpreting health policy, as defined by the Quad Council's 2011 competencies intended to guide public health nursing education and practice at all levels. The Quad Council of Public Health Nursing Organizations is comprised of the Association of Community Health Nurse Educators (ACHNE), the Association of State and Territorial Directors of Nursing (ASTDN), the American Public Health Association Public Health Nursing Section (APHA) and the American Nurses Association's Congress on Nursing Practice and Economics (ANA). They made the decision to not include core educational elements from the APRN Consensus Work Group & the National Council of State Boards of Nursing APRN Advisory Committee (2008) and so determined that the public health and community health nurses would no longer be considered APRNs.

According to the American Association of Colleges of Nursing (AACN), APRNs who earn a DNP degree are educationally prepared to assume a leadership role in the development of health policy, and DNP graduates have the capacity to engage proactively in the development and implementation of health policy at all levels, including institutional, local, state, regional, federal, and international (AACN, 2006).

The APRN leadership role in health policy may take many forms and may be carried out by the individual APRN or by groups of individuals who work together to accomplish a common goal. Leadership in any form requires current knowledge of the issues that affect nursing and health care as well as how policy decisions pertaining to those issues are made. Federal legislation, such as the Affordable Care Act, is enacted in large measure at the state level and often the effects are directly evident in clinical care at the bedside. For example, the increased focus on quality measures and value-based payment models creates the perfect environment for APRN leaders to demonstrate the value of APRN care. In fact, it demands that APRNs lay claim to their essential role in promoting wellness and improving chronic disease management. By designing, conducting, and publishing research pertinent to emerging national issues, APRNs create the foundation for advocating for their critical role in current health care delivery systems and promoting effective future models of care. When APRNs can demonstrate the value of their work in terms of cost savings and improved patient outcomes, policy makers listen. Finding an open door to the arenas where policy is made and, once inside, proving to be an effective advocate will lead to influence.

INTERACTING WITH POLICY MAKERS AND POLICY-MAKING BODIES

Nursing's concerns are related to all three branches of government: the administration, the legislature, and the courts. The infrastructure of policy making in each state revolves around government bodies—the legislature, agencies, and regulatory boards—that are unique to each state. For example, a governor's decision to expand Medicaid is a legislative matter with potential for significant impact at the agency level where Medicaid programs are administered, and perhaps also impacting scope-of-practice decisions by the APRN licensing board. Through state-level advocacy, APRNs can raise the awareness of both government officials and the public about the role that APRNs play in expanding access to care for Medicaid recipients.

Two foundational steps toward effective advocacy are identifying the key policy leaders at the state level and gaining a clear understanding of the detailed processes through which state legislation and regulations are made. This includes knowing who sets the policy agenda, who determines policy goals and alternatives, who formulates policy, and who implements and evaluates policy.

In the governor's office, the governor, lieutenant governor, attorney general, and secretary of state all have roles that influence nursing. In the legislature, the licensing committees take the lead in matters affecting professional licensure, but other committees such as health and consumer safety blaze the trail for nurses and nursing issues. For example, public discussion of a proposal to authorize unlicensed, minimally trained health aids to provide services to elderly residents in their homes may be initiated in a legislative committee responsible for consumer safety.

Each state in the United States passes its own laws regulating APRNs based on the health care environment within that state. Hence the reason that rules and regulations governing the practice of the APRN vary in each state.

Legislatures differ from state to state. Two key differences among states are (a) some legislatures are full time and others are part time and (b) the frequency with which the state legislature meets to conduct business varies. Some state legislatures are similar to Congress in that an elected seat in the legislature is considered a full-time job and the legislatures meet in year-round session. California, New York, Michigan, and Pennsylvania top the list of states considered to have a "full time" legislature, while the smaller, more rural states—Montana, New Hampshire, North Dakota, South Dakota, Utah, and Wyoming—have "citizen legislatures" made up of elected representatives who have full-time occupations in addition to being legislators (National Conference of State Legislatures, 2017).

Perhaps the policy-making government agency most familiar to nurses is the state nurse licensing board. The term "state board of nursing" will be used to refer to the state entity responsible for nurse licensing. The name of the nurse licensing board varies among states, however, as does the composition of the state board and the position of the board within the regulatory structure of the state. For example, the Pennsylvania State Board of Nursing is one of many licensing boards within the Pennsylvania Department of State's Bureau of Professional and Occupational Affairs. The North Carolina Board of Nursing is independent and self-supporting, not part of another state government agency. In some states, the nurse practice act dictates the composition of the board by specifying a certain number of board seats to be filled by individuals with certain qualifications. For example, the Illinois nursing law establishes four board seats for APRNs representing CNS, CNP, CNM, and CRNA practice.

To effectively impact state governance of the nursing profession, all APRNs must understand the role of the state board and know both the state nursing law (known as the nurse practice act or similar name) and rules and regulations promulgated by the board to carry out the act. It is also important to clearly understand the composition of the board and the process through which individuals gain seats on the board. Appointment to a licensing board is usually made by the governor. Often, endorsement by professional associations and other influential bodies is necessary for success in being selected by the governor for such an appointment.

In addition to knowing the composition of the board, it is very helpful to know the individual board members' alliances with special interest groups. In some states, these relationships are permitted, while in other states, a clear connection to an affected group of licensees or other interest group precludes eligibility to sit on the board. If these alliances are known, it may impact the decisions made by an individual and subsequently the board. This can have a significant impact on the rules and regulations that then affect all members of the nursing profession in that state.

State "sunshine laws" provide for open meetings that allow members of the public to be present at board meetings. Attending and observing state board meetings is an excellent and easily available way to learn the functions, scope, and limits of regulatory agencies. Remember that there are a lot of "behind the scenes" discussions that you are not privy to that will influence the decisions made at the board meetings. See if you can sit with someone who is a long-term attendee who may be able and/or willing to mentor you or a lobbyist who has a vested interest in the outcomes of a particular decision. Their insights will be invaluable to you as you learn the processes.

Licensing boards typically make regulations and amend them in collaboration with stakeholder groups; however, boards vary with respect to how they interact with and communicate with their licensees and leaders who represent the licensees. Some state boards actively and routinely seek input from licensees when matters come before the board that affect or have the potential to impact their practice. The interaction may be informal, with representatives of the licensees serving as subject matter experts with whom the board consults. The board may hold public hearings to more formally gather information and perspectives from an array of interested parties. In addition, an interested stakeholder or group may request to be placed on the board's meeting agenda to address the board in public session.

WHO SPEAKS FOR APRNs?

Every APRN should know the representatives of the nursing profession speaking as advanced practice nursing experts to the state board, to legislators, and to state agencies. In addition to knowing who those representatives are, it is important to know the topics they are discussing and the positions they are advancing. Those who have the ear of the decision makers may be promoting policy decisions that are not in the best interest of APRNs or advanced nursing practice. Never assume that a nurse or nursing organization will understand and advocate for the best interests of APRNs unless APRNs have contributed to the development of the underlying position.

An effective working relationship with legislators and state regulatory boards is critical for organizations that represent nurses. Often, the state nurses' association is the representative of nursing interests most recognized and consulted by state legislators and regulators. Although there may be many voices speaking for APRNs presenting varied positions on a given issue, in general, the state nurses' association is usually viewed as a key leader for carrying nursing's positions forward.

Agencies such as state health departments may have a designated office of policy or policy director responsible for developing major policy positions for the department, consistent with the governor's goals and objectives. The policy office or director ensures that policies and initiatives supported by the governor are implemented within the agency and, conversely, that the agency's positions and views are communicated to the governor's office for consideration in policy decision making.

Communications with stakeholders are an important function of the agency's policy office or director, and that interaction typically takes place through contact with lobbyists representing the stakeholder groups. Bringing stakeholders into discussion of proposed legislation that the agency is negotiating with the legislature is a common strategy for garnering support for positions and proposals that satisfy the stakeholders' interests as well as the intent of legislators and agency leaders.

ADVOCACY STRATEGY TOOLS AND RESOURCES

Governments exist to protect the welfare of the public. Advocacy efforts with government officials and agencies should be built on this premise. It is strategically important to know the governor's priorities and priority initiatives and, if possible, to demonstrate how these priorities can be achieved or positively affected by the proposal or position being presented or recommended.

Many APRNs are very good at applying their advanced analytical skills to understanding a policy issue and then using their clinical reasoning to formulate a solution. However, the influence of statewide politics and political positioning must be taken into consideration in order to be strategically effective. Detailed personal knowledge of a policy problem or issue and a logical solution are a good start but will not necessarily lead to effective policy change. The knowledge and expertise of APRNs as individuals, combined with the knowledge and expertise of others who know the political landscape and how to navigate it, will likely be more effective.

In many cases, strategic alliances with other stakeholders are necessary for positioning a proposal or issue so that it will get attention and action. This requires building and maintaining collegial relationships with groups both within and outside of nursing. This does not necessarily include just those groups that share priorities and perspectives supportive of nursing or APRNs. In the course of daily practice, APRNs are likely to interact with leaders of organizations such as the state medical society, the hospital association, the long-term care association, and other groups that have interest and influence in state health care matters. Cultivating those individual relationships is beneficial for both the information exchange and sharing of perspectives on policy issues that can result. APRNs and practitioners of disciplines outside nursing who interact positively as colleagues in clinical settings are likely to engage comfortably in conversation about policy issues, even if they espouse differing views. Even though APRNs and other practitioners, such as physicians, often have conflicting positions with regard to policy matters pertaining to scope of practice, they can easily coalesce around other current policy issues that have direct, high impact on health care delivery, for example, gun violence. It is equally important to know the reasons driving antagonists to oppose your position. Knowing the basis of adversarial positions is a key factor in successful negotiation of more compatible working relationships.

By working with state leaders in disciplines other than nursing to learn about their priorities and activities, nurses and nursing groups can identify potential allies and adversaries who may pursue policy initiatives that impact APRNs and APRN practice. It is important to recognize opportunities to informally or formally support them. Participation in other organizations' activities provides the opportunity to develop acquaintances that promote collegial relationships and greater familiarity with how and why others take the positions that they do.

Both active involvement in the groups that represent APRNs' interests at the state level and development of one's own skills are important for effective advocacy. APRNs who belong to these organizations support effective policy leadership by their individual contributions and leadership within these organizations. Individuals' skills develop over time and are built on exposure to and experience in a variety of policy arenas.

The ability to write and speak clearly and concisely in a style that can be understood by the public and legislators is critical for effective advocacy. Understanding the frame of reference of the intended audience and presenting information in terms that have meaning within that frame of reference will increase the effectiveness of communications. APRNs can develop skill in preparing issue briefing papers that outline a problem or concern in a manner that reaches beyond the clinical patient care world and makes the matter meaningful to the public, the legislator, or the regulator.

APRNs clearly understand the critical value of data. Facts and figures presented in an easily understood manner can make it easier to garner support for a policy position. Telling an audience what "should" happen and why from the perspective of the health care provider or patient is often more effective when accompanied by undeniable, unemotional statements of fact about how supporting an issue or position will result in better outcomes, that is, lives saved, public spending reduced or eliminated, costs to the citizens or to the government minimized. Citations from the law or literature are important components of an effective advocacy presentation. A position supported by precedent set in law or a citation from the law will have impact with policy decision makers and will contribute to evidence-based decision making. As an APRN faced with trying to influence policy makers, be prepared with your clear, rational, and well thought out discussion of the facts in the situation that should sway the decision in the direction you feel it needs to go.

In addition to effective communications, relationships are also a valuable tool. Creating and maintaining relationships with those who make policy and influence decision making is an important strategy for nurses as individuals and for nursing groups collectively. By introducing themselves to elected representatives who serve in the state legislature and becoming acquainted, APRNs can establish an identity as an expert resource among the representative's constituents. Ongoing communication with elected representatives and/or their staff, based on issues of mutual concern or about matters that fall within the APRN's scope of expertise, will help that relationship develop. The APRN who has specialized expertise in chronic illness, for example, or violence prevention can be a valuable source of information as an unpaid consultant for his or her legislator when proposed legislation or policy decisions relating to those topics are developing or are presented.

Nursing knowledge is intellectual capital that APRNs should feel comfortable sharing. For example, a perinatal CNS can talk to a legislator about the importance of funding preterm birth prevention programs based on the authority of his or her own experience and knowledge. While speaking to an audience of policy makers who are not health professionals, the nurse is likely to be the person in the room most qualified to address topics pertaining to the delivery of health care.

Negotiating skills and understanding how negotiation works in the political and policy environment are also important. Understanding who has the power to set policy and to make policy decisions is critical. Understanding who is in the decision-making role and their scope of authority and appealing to the right agency or the right office or person within the agency also will prevent time wasting that undermines efforts to influence change. Knowing and working with other stakeholders to gain strength from shared positioning are an important part of negotiation.

Along with negotiation, patience is more than just a virtue—it is essential for effective advocacy. The APRN who has a mindset based on clinical reasoning and is accustomed to making rapid, decisive actions in response to a need for change may find a high level of frustration with the plodding nature of negotiation and the perceived expectation to "give away" some pieces of a policy proposal in order to gain support for other remaining pieces of it. The essence is acquiring one small gain each time the issue is brought forward to the legislative process and not taking an "all or nothing" stance.

Policy initiatives that require legislation are often subject to extensive and complex negotiation. These are most effectively managed by professional lobbyists whose daily work enables them to have depth and breadth of knowledge of the players and the power structure. The opportunity to do advocacy work in collaboration with a lobbyist contributes to the APRNs knowledge of the bigger picture, the views held by policy leaders in the world outside of health care who are making decisions that affect nursing and patient care.

Timing is crucial. Those who work in policy day in and day out have the best knowledge about when the state political climate and broader policy direction are amenable to a policy proposal and knowing when a proposal, no matter how well conceived and planned, will not succeed and why. APRNs and other nursing leaders must collaborate with individuals and groups who are connected, sensitive, and can speak the language and negotiate the complexities of state government on their behalf. Even though a policy proposal may be perfectly sound, thoroughly supported with logic, and good for the public, there may be political reasons that will make it impossible to move forward. Policy is based on both politics and rational, evidence-based logic. Knowing the legislature's priorities is crucial to effective advocacy. For example, when a legislative priority focuses on a state's bedside nursing capacity (Joint State Government Commission, 2015), there is an opportunity to address broader issues pertaining to the adequacy of the nursing workforce and appropriate education for professional practice.

In addition to working with personnel who have expertise in government relations to lead and advise APRN policy initiatives, individuals who want to develop expertise can access other resources. Most states' statutes are accessible for free online, offering the actual text of existing laws. Licensing boards' laws, such as the state nurse practice act and the administrative rules/regulations promulgated by the board may be accessed by the board's web pages. Likewise, a state agency's web pages may offer access to the specific statutes and regulations that establish the agency's duties, responsibilities, and programs. When legislators develop a statute, committee conference notes are documented. These conference notes reflect discussion about the wording, text, staff thoughts, and decisions made as the law was drafted. They are available to the public and offer valuable insight and understanding about the intended meaning of the statutory language.

Information about current policy initiatives of interest to APRNs is likely to be available through the state professional organizations that are sponsoring them. Access to some information may be offered only to the organization's members. When activity is occurring in the legislature on bills that the professional organization has sponsored or supported, the organization may provide regular updates for members and/or for the public via the website.

Professional organizations also provide specific materials for individuals' advocacy efforts. Examples include the National Association of Clinical Nurse Specialists' (NACNS) "Starter Kit for Impacting Change at the Government Level: How to Work with Your State Legislators and Regulators"; materials developed by the Oregon Nurses Association that address reimbursement for Nurse Practitioners; the Pennsylvania State Nurses Association's advocacy training titled "Advocacy 101: Advocating for Your Future"; and a study of the economic impact of greater utilization of APRNs publicized in May 2012, by The Texas Coalition of Nurses in Advanced Practice (CNAP). By taking advantage of these resources, you become a better advocate for your discipline and the health care provided in your state.

TEACH/MENTOR/MODEL

Leadership in policy issues is a critical role for advanced nursing leaders globally. Noting that nursing and therefore nursing leadership are shaped dramatically by the impact of politics and policy, a Royal College of Nursing study concluded that effective nursing leadership currently is a vehicle through which *both* nursing practice and health policy can be influenced and shaped (Antrobus & Kitson, 1999). The APRN is in a position to serve as a teacher, mentor, and role model for colleagues, students, staff, and other health care workers. Just as nursing practice expertise evolves over time through continuous search for new knowledge and opportunities, expertise in policy leadership can develop for the APRN who seeks these opportunities either as an individual or as a member of a professional organization. Modeling this role for other APRNs new to practice and supporting their development of skills in this area is critical for nursing's advancement in the health care marketplace.

CONCLUSION

This chapter has presented information to stimulate more thinking about how APRNs can assume a position to lead health care policy efforts. The current significant focus on transparency in government, legislative, and regulatory affairs offers a wealth of opportunity for those who want to learn more. State government is highly visible through the Internet, with proposed rule making, regulations, and other policies available on the government's website. A motivated APRN constituency can become a powerful force in exerting control of APRN practice at the state level. Competent professional practice includes knowledge and competence in policy and advocacy to benefit nursing practice and health care. APRNs should be leaders who seek and accept every opportunity for visibility, for advocacy, and for taking ownership of their own professional practice.

DISCUSSION QUESTIONS

1. *Based on the information in this chapter, list at least two areas of policy change you can identify where legislation could have an impact.*
2. *If you were going to describe the importance of your issue for policy change to potential supporters, what key issues would you stress? How would you describe this to your patients?*
3. *Consider the health policy changes discussed in this chapter or those you have described in your analysis and consider the impact that might occur if these changes are NOT enacted. In other words what are the consequences of inaction.*

ANALYSIS, SYNTHESIS, AND CLINICAL APPLICATION

1. *What do newspaper and/or university public opinion polls indicate about the public's perceptions of nursing. On what basis does the public form these opinions?*
2. *Who are the nurses in your state legislature and what are their educational and clinical backgrounds?*
3. *What are the sources of rules in your state regarding APRN reimbursement (state law or regulations? Agency policies or policy interpretation?)*
4. *What organizations outside nursing share a stake in policy matters that concern APRNs? How do they stand to benefit from being involved in and/or influencing policy decisions that affect nursing practice or nursing education?*

EXERCISES/CONSIDERATIONS

1. *Identify the current state governor's priorities and learn about the initiatives the governor is supporting.*
2. *Meet with the lobbyist for the state nurses association. Discuss the lobbyist's view of the most influential leaders driving the health care agenda in the state and their priorities.*

3. *Identify at least one board or advisory panel convened by state government (a state agency other than the state licensing board) that makes decisions affecting your practice. Investigate how appointments to that board/advisory panel are made and whether or not nurses serve on it.*
4. *Identify the agency in your state that administers the state's Medicaid program. Learn how decisions are made regarding provider reimbursement for APRNs.*

ETHICAL CONSIDERATIONS

1. *APRN is an umbrella designation for four separate groups. How should APRN leaders reconcile policy positions that are beneficial to some of the four but harmful to others when all four groups have agreed to advocate as one APRN voice?*
2. *When and how should APRNs in clinical practice empower their patients to become engaged in advocating for health policy matters that affect patient care, access to care or clinical services that the patients themselves need?*

REFERENCES

American Association of Colleges of Nursing. (2006). The essentials of doctoral education for advanced nursing practice. Retrieved from http://www.aacnnursing.org/Portals/42/Publications/DNPEssentials.pdf

American Association of Nurse Practitioners. (2013). Standards of practice for nurse practitioners. Retrieved from http://www.aanp.org/images/documents/publications/standardsofpractice.pdf

American College of Nurse-Midwives. (2011). The practice doctorate in midwifery. Retrieved from http://www.midwife.org/ACNM/files/ACNMLibraryData/UPLOADFILENAME/000000000260/Practice%20Doctorate%20in%20Midwifery%20Sept%202011.pdf

Antrobus, S., & Kitson, A. (1999). Nursing leadership: Influencing and shaping health policy and nursing practice. *Journal of Advanced Nursing, 29,* 746–753. doi:10.1046/j.1365-2648.1999.00945.x

APRN Consensus Work Group & the National Council of State Boards of Nursing APRN Advisory Committee. (2008). Consensus model for APRN regulation: Licensure, accreditation, certification & education. Retrieved from https://www.ncsbn.org/aprn-consensus.htm

Joint State Government Commission. (2015). Professional bedside nursing in Pennsylvania: A staff study. Retrieved from http://jsg.legis.state.pa.us/resources/documents/ftp/publications/2015-413-HR920FINALREPORT6.30.15.pdf

National CNS Core Competency Task Force. (2010). Clinical nurse specialist core competencies: Executive summary 2006–2008. Retrieved from http://www.nacns.org/wp-content/uploads/2017/01/CNSCoreCompetenciesBroch.pdf

National Conference of State Legislatures. (2017). Full and part time legislatures. Retrieved from http://www.ncsl.org/legislatures-elections/legislatures/full-and-part-time-legislatures.aspx

New Jersey Collaborating Center for Nursing Workforce Development. (2003). Nursing in public and health policy. Retrieved from http://www.njccn.org/category/njccn

World Health Organization. (n.d.). Health policy. Retrieved from http://www.who.int/topics/health_policy/en

CHAPTER 7

State Implementation of the APRN *Consensus Model*: Progress to Date

Kelly A. Goudreau

When the *Consensus Model for APRN Regulation: Licensure, Accreditation, Certification, and Education* (APRN Joint Dialogue Group, 2008) was endorsed and became a part of nursing history, the profession of nursing took a significant step toward consistency. Specifically, consistency in how Advanced Practice Registered Nurses (APRNs) are educationally prepared, certified, and recognized by their state for purposes of practice. The National Council of State Boards of Nursing (NCSBN), along with a wide variety of nursing organizations, had a role to play in the crafting of the document and continues to play an important role in the implementation of the APRN Joint Dialogue Group (2008) document nationwide. Although the NCSBN is a nonregulatory body composed of a member group of all state and territorial boards of nursing and does not hold regulatory sway over the various state boards of nursing (SBON), it does carry influence and indirectly impacts the direction that the various states move in regard to regulation of all nursing, including APRNs. The APRN *Consensus Model*, as it came to be known, has been implemented to varying degrees in each state and movement toward achieving full regulatory recognition for the APRN roles is well under way. Although the 2015 deadline articulated in the document has come and gone, great progress has been made and continues to be made each year.

The purpose of this chapter is to identify the current state of implementation within various states, note what movement states have made or are in the process of making at the time of the writing of this document, and discuss policy principles and concepts as applied to the full implementation of the *Consensus Model*.

BACKGROUND

The APRN *Consensus Model* was created through a sometimes-difficult process whereby nursing representatives from each of the APRN roles and representatives from the NCSBN came together to discuss and define specific terms and

expectations for the process and the outcome of full regulatory practice authority. The final outcome was expected to be increased access to APRNs and a
demonstrable positive outcome to health care of multiple populations. In order
to achieve this monumental task, there needed to be an open and transparent
dialogue between the NCSBN, the member SBON, the accreditation teams for
educational programs, the educational preparation expectations, and the certification processes.

Not the least of these was a consensus on what to call the advanced practice
roles so that there could be consistency and understanding of the expectations
for practice. The term APRN was chosen as the term that would apply to all
four of the roles identified as advanced practice. This umbrella term included
the Certified Nurse Practitioner (CNP), Certified Registered Nurse Anesthetist
(CRNA), Certified Registered Nurse-Midwife (CRNM), and Clinical Nurse
Specialist (CNS). The intent was that the term APRN would be a restricted and
ultimately statutorily protected term that could not be used by any nurse other
than those with specific advanced training and education.

Based on the educational preparation that was agreed to in the APRN
Consensus Model (2008), all APRNs must have educational preparation to prescribe, can and should practice autonomously, and can manage individual
patients in defined populations. APRNs must be nationally certified after graduate education at the master's or doctoral level. The certification examination
was seen as a proxy for a second licensure examination and is recognized by the
NCSBN and the member states as such. It is notable that there was a significant
discussion in the Joint Dialogue group regarding how to define APRN as compared to nurses with advanced degrees in education, informatics, community
health, or policy. These degrees were recognized as advanced preparation but not
as advanced practice. The difference may seem simply a statement of semantics,
but the fundamental difference was the practice component in direct care with
patients. This had, and continues to have, significant implications for the individual states as they look to regulate those who have a master's degree or doctoral-
level preparation in areas other than the four designated roles.

Although a guiding principle in the Joint Dialogue Group was specifically
to "do no harm" to any of the four roles, there were some significant issues that
arose in the discussions. As a result there needed to be an ongoing body that
would address the issues as they arose and ensure that the four roles (and others
if they arose) would have clear expectations and could articulate the issues to the
other members of the team. This group became known as the LACE group and
was representative of the licensure, accreditation, certification, and education
group.

APRN *CONSENSUS MODEL* VERSUS STATE
PROCESSES OF LAW

Before the implementation of the APRN *Consensus Model* (APRN Joint Dialogue
Group, 2008), there were as many variations in the licensure of APRNs as there
were states/territories licensing APRNs. The APRN *Consensus Model* is not a
legal or regulatory document. It is simply a collective agreement by the four
elements of regulation as described by Styles, Schumann, Bickner, and White
(2008) and serves as an organizing document that helps define terms, state

relationships, and provides guiding principles for institutional implementation. Regulatory bodies, such as the SBON have to use the political process state by state to adopt changes to the nurse practice act and be able to implement rules that will allow for full practice authority and the full realization of the *Consensus Model* (Cahill, Alexander, & Gross, 2014). States are strongly encouraged to use the language developed and adopted by the NCSBN through the Joint Dialogue Group to implement changes in their state that conform to the *Consensus Model* (APRN Joint Dialogue Group, 2008). To that end, the NCSBN created a mirror document to the APRN *Consensus Model*, which puts the terminology of the model into regulatory terms and could be used as an exemplar for how to structure state regulations and subsequent rule making. The model act and rules are available through the NCSBN website (available at www.ncsbn .org/739.htm), and state representatives are encouraged to freely download and distribute these tools for use in evaluating and modifying existing state nurse practice acts (NCSBN, n.d.).

NCSBN (2012) also provides visual prompts in the form of color-coded maps that regularly update the public and APRNs in each state regarding state-based legislative changes and how close they are to meeting the requirements of the APRN *Consensus Model* (available at www.ncsbn.org/5397.htm).

Finally, the NCSBN (2015) has provided model language for implementation of an APRN compact licensure process so that APRNs can practice across state lines in states that are part of the APRN compact. This is perceived to move more closely to the nationalization of APRN licensure and reduce barriers as nurses implement new technologies such as telehealth initiatives, which are predicted to increase access to health care providers in the future (NCSBN, 2014b).

A CONCEPTUAL MODEL FOR EVALUATION OF PROGRESS TO DATE

In order to fully understand the process and its implementation to date, we need to consider the change in terms of a frame of reference or conceptual framework. Hardee, Irani, MacInnis, and Hamilton (2012) describe a conceptual framework that links the development and implementation of health policy to health systems and evaluation of intended health outcomes. This conceptual framework presents a sound comparative reference for the APRN *Consensus Model* (APRN Joint Dialogue Group, 2008) and evaluation of the progress to date.

CONCEPTUAL FRAMEWORK

There are five key elements in the conceptual framework on health care outcomes linked to health policy as described by Hardee et al. (2012): (a) An enabling environment, (b) health-related policy development, (c) program and policy implementation, (d) healthy systems and health outcomes, and finally (e) policy monitoring and program evaluation. These elements are complex and intertwine to create either an opportunity or barriers to full health policy implementation. The context of the *Consensus Model* (Joint Dialogue Group, 2008) will be discussed using the *Linking Health Policy with Health Systems and Health Outcomes* (Hardee et al., 2012) conceptual framework.

Enabling Environment

Hardee et al. (2012) describe the enabling environment as being an overarching concept composed of governance. Governance includes concepts such as political stability, rule of law/regulation, government effectiveness, control of corruption, and accountability and voice. Additionally, an enabling environment also includes the political/sociocultural/economic environment. The authors describe this as including political context, cultural and gender context/factors, and economic context factors. The environment at the time of the development of the *Consensus Model* was fully enabled and primed by a number of things including the election of a new president who was strongly in favor of increased access to care and insurance for all, and the development of research and evaluation of health care that showed that patients were not engaged in their own care, the quality of care was lacking, and cost was higher than it should be (Berwick, Nolan, & Whittington, 2008). Finally, a desire within nursing itself to sort out some of the complexities of regulation was making itself known and the Institute of Medicine (2011) released their seminal work on *The Future of Nursing: Leading Change, Advancing Health*. The time was ripe for the development and implementation of the *Consensus Model*.

The supportive environment had a great deal to do with a perceived crisis in health care with reports of declining numbers of physicians, increasing costs of care, and decreasing quality of care. This triumvirate of elements meant that the door was open to an alternative to physicians that could provide high-quality care at a lower cost and was supported by the Patient Protection and Affordable Care Act (PPACA, 2010) initiative. Only through the blending and merging of these key factors could the discussions occur and the *Consensus Model* be created.

Finally, the nursing community saw the need to move toward creation of a document that would serve the needs of nursing to more clearly define the key elements of advanced practice roles, clarify the needs for regulation, specialization, educational foundations, and protection of the public welfare. Driven by the American Nurses Association (ANA) and the NCSBN, the Joint Dialogue Group came together with the specific purpose of bringing very divergent concepts to advanced practice into alignment and consensus on core concepts and principles around the roles.

Health-Related Policy Development

Systems improvements were needed within nursing in order to position the discipline for the coming changes in health care. Problems were emerging in the context of licensure for APRNs. The NCSBN was pushing to regulate the APRNs in order to meet the mandate of the individual states' needs for protection of the public. The confusion at the state level led to an NCSBN committee being created that looked into the process and proposed a regulatory model for APRNs. The concern of the group was how to define advanced practice nursing and then license the many areas of advanced practice in a unified model that could be adopted and adapted by individual states. The subspecialization of many APRNs was making it very difficult to clearly define the boundaries of care and regulate this population of nurses. As an example, and to bring this issue into focus, the

NCSBN was figuratively asking "should the nurse practitioner who specializes in the right great toe be licensed for just that practice?" The question may seem ridiculous when looking back, but the reality was that it was that concept that regulators were wrestling with as they tried to determine the best course of action to uphold their societal mandate: protecting the public. At the same time, the ANA had convened a group that was looking at the same issue and was struggling to complete its work in a timely manner as this group too wrestled with the best way to define the practice of APRNs. By finally identifying that the two groups were doing parallel work and there was a need to bring the two streams of consciousness together into a single statement by the nursing community forward momentum was achieved. Klein (2014) wrote that:

> The [APRN] *Consensus Model* is an exemplar of social construction impacting specific target populations. Social construction is an explanatory theory used to identify and consciously build a group through policy design. Policy design selects a target population who will receive benefits in exchange for some perceived burdens. The group, in this case APRNs, develops and implicitly endorses stated goals to be achieved, tools intended to change behavior, rules for inclusion or exclusion, a rationale for the policy change, and an implementation structure. The success of social construction depends upon the ability of its assumptions to be legitimized in authoritative policy. (p. 324)

The work of both teams came together in the form of the Joint Dialogue Group. The 4 years of work on both sides were examined in detail, clearly understood in terms of intent and meaning, merged, fine-tuned, and agreed on by the members of both teams. The subsequent document prepared by the dual team was endorsed by more than 40 professional nursing groups. The document demonstrated multisectorial collaboration and defined a regulatory framework for the states to begin implementation of full practice authority for all APRNs within their state. The initial work, an authoritative policy of the expected systems change, had been completed. Now it was up to the states, the professional organizations, the certifying bodies, and the educators to make the policy a reality.

Program and Policy Implementation

Once the policy was created and endorsed as substantively meeting the needs of the discipline of nursing advanced practice, it needed to be enacted. Initial implementation of the APRN *Consensus Model* was slower than expected (ANA, 2009). Although the document was being created, the team members were going back to their respective organizations and informing their teams of the pending changes. There was a tremendous amount of work to be done if the implementation was to be successfully carried out by the anticipated date. The date of the intended implementation deadline was set 7 years into the future because the changes would take time to accomplish. That date, the year 2015, was intended to allow time for the many changes that needed to occur in order to align the licensure, accreditation, certification, and educational components of the regulatory model.

As of the writing of this chapter, the model has still not been fully implemented nationwide, but strong movement toward full implementation has occurred. As of August 22, 2016, there were 16 states/territories that met the expectations of the APRN *Consensus Model* to the extent that they were identified as having 100% compliance (NCSBN, 2012). Eleven more states/territories were identified as having between 75% and 96% compliance (NCSBN, 2012). With the majority of states/territories more than half way to being fully in alignment with the model, it is simply a matter of time and continued education of the remaining SBON before the remaining states move in the direction of full practice authority for APRNs.

Some barriers to the implementation have been noted, however, and are not easily overcome. The American Medical Association (AMA) stands strongly against the independent and full practice authority for APRNs (AMA, 2016). The relationship and power dynamic between nursing and medicine has been in play for many years but is making itself known in the implementation of full practice authority for APRNs in the Department of Veterans Affairs, Veterans Health Administration (VHA). The VHA has proposed to implement federal supremacy and allow APRNs employed within the system to function to the full capacity of their education and training regardless of state rules and regulations (VHA, 2016). This proposal, which is substantially the enactment of the APRN *Consensus Model*, has met with significant resistance from the AMA particularly focused on CRNAs and to a lesser extent CNPs.

Healthy Systems and Health Outcomes

The next element in the *Linking Health Policy with Health Systems and Health Outcomes* (Hardee et al., 2012) conceptual framework is assessing the impact of the policy on the health of the system and the outcomes of care resulting from the policy implementation. As the full implementation of the policy as outlined in the APRN *Consensus Model* has not yet occurred across all states and organizations, it is difficult to determine what the outcomes will be for health systems and health outcomes. An analysis of the literature on health outcomes identified a number of articles touting the outcomes of care of APRNs over many years (Newhouse et al., 2011; Selway, 2011; Waszynski, Murakami, & Lewis, 2000). The work has not yet been conducted, however, to evaluate the outcomes of care within the context of full practice authority and advanced practice nursing roles. As full practice authority is realized, it is hoped that many positive outcomes will result in terms of access (Livanos, 2016) and other measures of positive health care for all. This work, however, is far from complete and so remains to be evaluated over time.

Policy Monitoring and Program Evaluation

The final component of the conceptual model refers to ongoing policy monitoring in order to sustain the changes created by the policy enactment and to evaluate the policy for needed revisions and refinements. Again, as the full implementation of the policy has not been realized as of yet, it is nearly impossible to monitor and evaluate the program outcomes. It is evident that the expectations for the APRN *Consensus Model* are vast and all-encompassing, and hopes are high that the infusion of fully enabled APRNs will increase access to high-quality, efficient, and effective health care for the majority of individuals in the United States. The focus of the work of the LACE consortium has been on the implementation and the monitoring of the implementation of the *Consensus Model*. The work being done by that group has not, however, been focused on the evaluation of the program/policy implementation and the outcomes of care. Perhaps the group should now set its sights and focus on the evaluation of the policy and the intended effects as full practice authority is realized in wider and wider circles.

INDIVIDUAL STATE PROGRESS TO DATE

The wider and wider circles noted previously are visible on the NCSBN web page, which denotes progress to date with the implementation of full practice authority (www.ncsbn.org/5397.htm). As identified earlier in the chapter, progress is being made but it is slow to come. Reasons for the length of time to date are primarily the process that must be used in a state-by-state approach. The laws must be changed in order for APRNs to have full practice authority. Those changes have been incremental and slow to come (Kaplan, Brown, Andrilla, & Hart, 2006; Keeling, 2007; Klein, 2012; Madler, Kalanek, & Rising, 2012). That means that each state must craft a bill that details the needs and then must move that bill through the legislative process. In some instances, it can take up to three legislative sessions to have the bill passed. Also, as the bill moves through the legislative process, it can be changed from the original intent and may be modified by pleas from lobbyists for a variety of organizations. This process can have harmful effects on the original bill and could change it to such an extent that it no longer provides the same level of autonomy as was intended in the APRN *Consensus Model*.

The NCSBN has clearly stated its support for the *Consensus Model* by including that support in its stated strategic initiatives for 2014 to 2016:

> With the advent of the Affordable Care Act and other initiatives to improve the health of the nation, NCSBN encourages state and federal legislation that promotes and complies with the recommendations in the *Consensus Model for APRN Regulation*. This model contains education, accreditation, licensure and certification requirements for all four categories of APRNs in the U.S. These national standards will increase mobility for APRNs, increase access to care, help fill gaps in areas that need health care providers, and assure the public that every APRN has met the same standards and is competent and safe to practice. Given the evidence provided by numerous studies on the safety of APRNs and the growing need for their services, NCSBN supports legislation that encourages independent practice and prescriptive authority of these practitioners. (NCSBN, 2014a, p.11)

Many states are making significant progress toward the full implementation of the *Consensus Model* since the document was first published. A few have clearly articulated the journey in the literature (Madler, Kalanek, & Rising, 2014; Nutty, 2015; Senner, 2014; Weise, 2015). The ANA supports the movement (Brassard, 2014), and some professional organizations have supported the document in their literature as well (National Association of Clinical Nurse Specialists, 2012).

With the recent decision by the Veterans Affairs, VHA (Livanos, 2016; Summers, 2016) to move toward full practice authority, it will likely not be long before states move to align with the federal government. It is hoped that the VHA will fully assess the outcomes of care provided by the APRNs within its organization and will be able to support the premise that the full practice authority for APRNs will mean increased access to care for millions of veterans.

The alignment of APRNs within the VHA to full practice authority will hopefully push the momentum forward for those states that have hesitated to move forward or have not had a clear imperative to do so. The enactment of the federal supremacy in this instance, although rarely used, will perhaps be an enticement to the states to continue to pursue licensure freedoms and practice expectations that will ultimately meet the need of the American people for inexpensive access to quality health care.

CONCLUSION

When determining whether a policy implementation has been successful, it is important to assess five key elements to determine if health care outcomes can be linked to health policy (Hardee et al., 2012). These five key elements include: (a) An enabling environment, (b) health-related policy development, (c) program and policy implementation, (d) healthy systems and health outcomes, and finally (e) policy monitoring and program evaluation. When looking at the *APRN Consensus Model* implementation, only two have fully been implemented at this point in time. The policy itself, although proposed and moved forward in 2008, has not been fully implemented yet, which places it firmly in the category of still being rolled out. Only when fully implemented can the assessments of effectiveness be determined. The implementation of the policy in pockets nationwide could be considered pilot programs for purposes of evaluation of health outcomes. The difficulty is that the manner in which the policy has been implemented is fragmented and disparate among the various states due to regulatory issues in the full implementation and adjustments made by individual state legislatures. These variations will prove somewhat problematic when evaluation is attempted between the various states and their versions of full practice authority.

The greatest hope of seeing positive health outcomes from a consistent application of the policy comes from the current steps being undertaken by the VHA. It is hoped that the full practice authority implementation will be effective and will be administered in a consistent manner nationwide. Recent discussions and presentations at the national VHA joint nurse executive/chief of staff meeting held in Leesburg, Virginia, would indicate that there may be some discontent among the medical providers even within the Veterans Affairs system. Time will tell as the policy is rolled out across the very large VHA facilities.

Only when fully implemented can the policy be monitored and the programs spawned by the policy be evaluated. The policy has come a long way in its implementation but still has many years to go before its effectiveness can be fully evaluated and validated. In the interim, this social policy experiment will go on and the real-life implications to both the quality and quantity of care available to the American people will be felt. It is my sincere hope that the policy will be fully implemented and the value and worth of the APRN can be fully appreciated in all aspects of care. The change is coming, even if incrementally, and it is having an impact on APRN issues internationally (Nardi & Diallo, 2014). The present initiative has been moving forward steadily. Only time will tell the full story as it unfolds.

It is imperative though to keep in mind the need to evaluate the outcomes of care as linked to the full practice authority initiative. Only through tough, thoughtful, and complete evaluation of the outcomes of care can the APRN roles be seen as fully contributory to the health and well-being of people nationally and internationally. The story continues to unfold and will be an important aspect of how nursing, and in particular advanced practice nursing, develops in the future.

DISCUSSION QUESTIONS

1. *Identify several ways to evaluate successful outcomes in APRN state law change related to recommendations in the* Consensus Model.
   a) *Patient based*
   b) *System based*
   c) *Policy based*
2. *Using your state as an example, name four key non-nursing stakeholders who could form a coalition with APRNs interested in changing state law to enhance the APRN scope of practice. Why would their help be useful and what would be their focus of interest in APRN practice?*

ANALYSIS, SYNTHESIS, AND CLINICAL APPLICATION

1. *Your state legislator is on a committee that will vote on removing mandatory supervision of CRNAs by physicians. Write a one-page summary (Talking Points) with scholarly citations to provide your legislator information on why he or she should support this change.*
2. *Attend a SBON meeting or committee meeting which has at least one agenda item related to APRN practice. Write a summary of the issue with the supporting and opposing views expressed, and provide your conclusion of support or opposition.*

EXERCISES/CONSIDERATIONS

1. *Propose a model for grandfathering APRNs who practice in your state and are not eligible for national certification as proposed by the* Consensus Model *(APRN Joint Dialogue Group, 2008).*
2. *Your state law allows CNSs to be credentialed and privileged as APRNs in a hospital setting. You have just been hired as a CNS in the cardiology intensive care unit. Physicians, nurses, and physicians' assistants primarily staff the unit, and the medical staff has no familiarity with CNS practice and scope. Write a three- to four-page document that could be used to obtain privileges utilizing CNS core competencies (National Association of Clinical Nurse Specialists) and other appropriate documents.*

REFERENCES

American Medical Association. (2016, May). *Statement on VA proposed rule on advanced practice nurses.* Chicago, IL: Author. Retrieved from https://www.ama-assn.org/ama-statement-va-proposed-rule-advanced-practice-nurses

American Nurses Association. (2009). APRN Consensus Model toolkit. Retrieved from http://nursingworld.org/EspeciallyForYou/AdvancedPracticeNurses/Consensus-Model-Toolkit.aspx

APRN Joint Dialogue Group. (2008, July 7). *Consensus model for APRN regulation: Licensure, accreditation, certification, and education.* Retrieved from https://www.ncsbn.org/Consensus_Model_for_APRN_Regulation_July_2008.pdf

Berwick, D. M., Nolan, T. W., & Whittington, J. (2008). The triple aim: Care, health, and cost. *Health Affairs, 27*(3), 759–769.

Brassard, A. (2014). Calling all nurses: State legislation needed to implement the APRN Consensus Model. *The American Nurse, 46*(1), 9.

Cahill, M., Alexander, M., & Gross, L. (2014). The 2014 NCSBN consensus report on APRN regulation. *Journal of Nursing Regulation, 4*(4), 5–12.

Hardee, K., Irani, L., MacInnis, R., & Hamilton, M. (2012). *Linking health policy with health systems and health outcomes: A conceptual framework.* Washington, DC: Futures Group, Health Policy Project.

Institute of Medicine. (2011). *The future of nursing: Leading change, advancing health.* Washington, DC: National Academies Press.

Kaplan, L., Brown, M. A., Andrilla, H., & Hart, L. G. (2006). Barriers to autonomous practice. *The Nurse Practitioner, 31*(1), 57–63.

Keeling, A. (2007). *Nursing and the privilege of prescription, 1893–2000.* Columbus: The Ohio State University Press.

Klein, T. (2014). State implementation of the APRN consensus model. In K. A. Goudreau & M. C. Smolenski (Eds.), *Health policy and advanced practice nursing: Impact and implications* (pp. 323–336). New York, NY: Springer Publishing.

Klein, T. A. (2012). Implementing autonomous clinical nurse specialist prescriptive authority: A competency-based transition model. *Clinical Nurse Specialist, 26*(5), 254–262.

Livanos, N. (2016). Increasing avenues to care: Department of Veterans Affairs makes move to grant APRNs full practice authority. *Journal of Nursing Regulation, 7*(3), 58–62.

Madler, B., Kalanek, C., & Rising, C. (2012). An incremental regulatory approach to implementing the APRN Consensus Model. *Journal of Nursing Regulation, 3*(2), 11–15.

Madler, B., Kalanek, C., & Rising, C. (2014). Gaining independent prescriptive practice: One state's experience in adoption of the APRN Consensus Model. *Policy, Politics, & Nursing Practice, 15*(3–4), 111–118. doi:10.1177/1527154414562299

Nardi, D. A., & Diallo, R. (2014). Global trends and issues in APN practice: Engage in the change. *Journal of Professional Nursing, 30*(3), 228–232.

National Association of Clinical Nurse Specialists. (2012). National Association of Clinical Nurse Specialists' statement on the APRN Consensus Model implementation. Retrieved from http://www.nacns.org/docs/NACNSConsensusModel.pdf

National Council of State Boards of Nursing. (n.d.). APRN Consensus Model toolkit. Retrieved from https://www.ncsbn.org/739.htm

National Council of State Boards of Nursing. (2012). Model act and rules. Retrieved from https://www.ncsbn.org/2012_APRN_Model_and_Rules.pdf

National Council of State Boards of Nursing. (2014a). Public policy agenda: 2014–2016. Retrieved from https://www.ncsbn.org/PublicPolicyAgenda-2014-2016.pdf

National Council of State Boards of Nursing. (2014b). State based licensure and telehealth. Retrieved from https://www.ncsbn.org/federal.htm

National Council of State Boards of Nursing. (2015). Advanced practice registered nurse compact. Retrieved from https://www.ncsbn.org/APRN_Compact_Final_050415.pdf

Newhouse, R., Stanik-Hutt, J., White, K., Johantgen, M., Bass, E., Zangaro, G., . . . Weiner, J. (2011). Advanced practice nurse outcomes 1990–2008: A systematic review. *Nursing Economics, 29*(5). Retrieved from http://www.nursingeconomics.net/ce/2013/article3001021.pdf

Nutty, A. (2015). Alaska APRN Consensus Model bill introduced. *Alaska Nurse, 66*(2), 12.

Patient Protection and Affordable Care Act. (2010). Retrieved from https://www.healthcare.gov/glossary/patient-protection-and-affordable-care-act

Selway, J. S. (2011). New systematic review on APRN outcomes. *Journal for Nurse Practitioners, 7*(9), 710–714.

Senner, P. (2014). Continuing education: APRN Consensus Model. *The Alaska Nurse, 65*(2), 13.

Styles, M. M., Schumann, M. J., Bickford, C. J., & White, K. (Eds.). (2008). *Specializing and credentialing in nursing revisited: Understanding the issues, advancing the profession.* Silver Spring, MD: American Nurses Association.

Summers, L. (2016). Update: Transition to full practice authority for APRNs. *The American Nurse, 48*(3), 11.

Veterans Health Administration. (2016). *AP44—Proposed rule—Advanced practice registered nurses.* Retrieved from https://www.regulations.gov/document?D=VA-2016-VHA-0011-0001

Waszynski, C. M., Murakami, W., & Lewis, M. (2000). Community care management: Advanced practice nurses as care managers. *Care Management Journals, 2*(3), 148–152.

Weise, T. (2015). Alaska APRN alliance defines trajectory, requests participation. *The Alaska Nurse, 66*(6), 6.

Implications of Health Care Reform and Finance on APRN Practice

CHAPTER 8

The Patient Protection Affordable Care Act (PPACA)

Jan Towers

Improving and updating the health care system in the United States have been on the agenda of legislators, regulators, and other policy makers as well as health care providers for decades. Beginning with unsuccessful national health insurance proposals of Theodore Roosevelt and later with Franklin Roosevelt's more successful social reforms, it has been continuously on the agenda of both Republicans and Democrats in the White House and Congress, as well as many state legislatures, to the present day.

The initiation of the Medicare and Medicaid programs in 1965 was arguably the most significant step taken to assure the elderly and underserved of access to and payment for health care. As early as 1945 President Truman proposed the formation of these programs that were signed into law 20 years later by Lyndon Johnson. Although many attempts to improve upon these programs were initiated through the years, it was not until 2003 that the next piece of legislation to improve access to health care was signed into law. That was when the Medicare Modernization Act (MMA) that sought to improve outpatient care and payment for medications to eligible Medicare recipients was passed and signed by President George W. Bush.

In the intervening years, the need for health care reform was recognized by a variety of presidents and legislators. President Richard Nixon in the early and mid 1970s, proposed legislation (Comprehensive Health Manpower Act and the Nurse Training Act) that initiated, among other things, federal funding for Nurse Practitioner education and was passed and signed into law. At that time, he also proposed a "National Health Strategy" that included a fee-for-service or health maintenance organization (HMO) coverage for all citizens through their employer or special government programs. Likewise, President Gerald Ford signed into law the first health care privacy act, and President Jimmy Carter, in anticipation of the implementation of national health insurance, consolidated various health care administration entities into what was first known as the

Health Care Financing Administration (HCFA) and more recently as the Centers for Medicare and Medicaid (CMS).

Most of the health care reform proposals, however, were controversial. Both President Reagan and President Clinton encountered setbacks in proposals that slowed the progression of health care reform for close to 20 years. A bill was passed during the Reagan administration (the Medicare Catastrophic Coverage Act of 1988) that included catastrophic medical care coverage and prescription drug benefits that was subsequently repealed in the George H. W. Bush administration. Later, in the 1990s, although the Health Insurance Portability and Accountability Act that provided patients with privacy and insurance protection benefits was passed, a major health care reform bill providing for universal health care coverage to all Americans proposed by President Clinton disintegrated before votes could be taken because there was so much controversy over its provisions. Then in 2003, legislation that included drug benefits and preventive care benefits was passed under George W. Bush.

During this time, Nurse Practitioners did become federally authorized providers first in the Federal Employees Health Insurance Program, then in rural and long-term care settings, and finally in the Medicare program at large.

THE ACT

With the advent of the Obama administration, another attempt to initiate and pass health care reform legislation was undertaken. Bills were introduced in both the House and the Senate that would revise many costly and cumbersome provisions in Medicare and Medicaid law, provide increased access to health care by the nation's large uninsured population and establish insurance processes to enhance access, protect patients, stimulate increases in the primary care workforce, and implement the provision of primary care services including health promotion and disease prevention. Creating legislation that would lead to cost-effective care and bend the spiraling cost curve for health care soon became a contentious and convoluted process. As the contentiousness increased, mainly along party lines, the ability to reach agreement in the House and Senate decreased. Added to the confusion was the death of one of the lead senators in the Democratic-led proposal for this legislation, which initially included provisions for a publicly funded universal health care program. In the end, a somewhat watered-down proposal was passed and signed into law. The bill was called the Patient Protection and Affordable Care Act (PPACA) of 2010 (Office of Legislative Council, 2010).

Provisions in the act were constructed so that they were not required to be implemented immediately. Instead, their implementation would be phased in over several years, in order to allow time for insurance carriers, providers, hospitals, and government agencies including state governments to prepare for the new or revised provisions included in the legislation.

Patient protection provisions such as banning preexisting condition clauses in insurance contracts that prevent patients from obtaining later coverage for those conditions began immediately after passage of the bill in 2010. Those provisions were immediately implemented for children and 6 months later for adults. Similar approaches were taken regarding provisions that limited the practice of setting caps on coverage that would subsequently prohibit patients from obtaining needed health care services.

Provisions that protected patient choice of provider and payment nondiscrimination toward providers were to be implemented as the new requirements were implemented. These provisions protect the right of patients to keep or choose the health care provider they desire to see and prohibit health care insurers from providing new insurance to patients to discriminate against a class of providers such as Nurse Practitioners. Other provisions, such as increasing Medicare payment for medical care including prescriptions to close gaps (commonly referred to as the doughnut hole) created by the 2003 MMA payment schemes were designed to gradually go into effect over a 10-year period. The 2003 "doughnut hole" legislation provided payment for prescriptions of Medicare patients up to a certain level, then the patient was responsible for payment beyond that level until costs reached what was considered to be catastrophic, at which time payment would again be initiated for prescription costs that exceeded that threshold (Before the 2003 legislation, Medicare did not cover prescriptions for medications). The PPACA provision continued to pay for prescriptions as legislated in 2003 and gradually raised the first-level threshold until it met the second or "catastrophic level" by the year 2010, thus eliminating the "doughnut hole" for payment for prescriptions initiated in 2003.

Other provisions such as the implementation of universal coverage and Medicaid expansion were delayed to allow regulations to be developed and methodologies for implementation put in place. These delayed provisions were the most controversial pieces of the legislation and led to drastic attempts by its opponents to remove the provisions. Initially, the House of Representatives voted to repeal the entire bill. However, the Senate rejected that proposal and the president had announced that such a piece of legislation would be vetoed by his office. This was followed by attempts to challenge the constitutionality of the legislation in the courts and further attempts to repeal or block appropriations for some of the provisions in the statute.

As the challenges moved through the courts, implementation of many of the provisions moved forward according to the required schedule set in the legislation. It was not until the spring of 2012 that the Supreme Court agreed to hear the case against the constitutionality of the new legislation. The questions the Court considered included whether the Supreme Court could actually hear the case prior to implementation of the legislation; whether the universal coverage mandate was constitutional; whether expansion of Medicaid (basically a state controlled entity) was constitutional, and whether pieces of the proposed legislation could be determined unconstitutional without declaring the entire bill unconstitutional (severability).

The conclusion was that the Court determined they could hear the bill, despite the fact that not all parts had been implemented; that the universal health provision was constitutional; and that the federal government could not require the states to implement the expanded Medicaid coverage in the bill (567 U.S., 2012 Opinion of Roberts, C. J. Supreme Court of the United States). The rest of the statute remained untouched. Although the road had been opened for implementation of the new legislation, opponents of the legislation determined that they would keep this bill from being implemented by blocking implementation through other means. The House (with a Republican majority) has voted twice to repeal the entire new statute, but the measure was not taken up in the Senate where there was a Democratic majority. Likewise, measures were successfully introduced to repeal sections of the bill in the House; again these were not addressed by the Senate, thus stopping their progress. In addition, steps were taken in appropriations legislation to block the funding of many of the measures within the statute that require funding in order to implement them. Although expansion of Medicaid suffered some setbacks, depending on whether the states opted to cover the additional populations/groups authorized federally to receive Medicaid, the steps to initiate all of the provisions of the bill continued to move forward. As of this reading, updated information is maintained at the following websites: www.whitehouse.gov/healthreform or www.CMS.gov. *Note: This may change as the transition to the new administration proceeds.*

NURSE PRACTITIONERS AND THE PPACA

Through the years, beginning in the late 1980s, Nurse Practitioners made progress with every reform bill that was passed. The PPACA was no exception. In the well-known presence of the need for primary care providers, Nurse Practitioners were identified as a significant part of the resolution of the health care crisis. At the time this legislation was passed, there were greater than 155,000 Nurse Practitioners. More than 88% of them were prepared as primary care providers and approximately 70% were practicing in primary care settings (American Association of Nurse Practitioners [AANP], 2013). Currently there are more than 220,000 Nurse Practitioners, with greater than 83% prepared as primary care Nurse Practitioners, 87% of whom are practicing in primary care (AANP, 2015).

For the first time, legislation was predominantly provider neutral and "clinicians," rather than "physicians," were identified as providers throughout the statute. This included Advanced Practice Registered Nurses (APRNs). Although the PPACA addresses all clinicians, APRNs providing primary care services were most affected by this legislation.

In the area of strengthening the health care workforce, Title VIII funding for the graduate nurse education (GNE) workforce that includes appropriations for APRN education programs and traineeships, faculty loan repayment, and grants to nurse managed clinics was reauthorized. In addition, payment to nurse managed clinics and fellowships for family nurse practitioners in Federally Qualified Health Centers was authorized, though not immediately funded. What was immediately funded was a GNE demonstration that provided funding for clinical preparation through a competitive bidding process to five APRN programs to increase the number of APRN graduates prepared to practice in community-based primary care. The participants were Rush University, Chicago, Illinois; Duke University, Durham, North Carolina; Hospitals of the University of Pennsylvania, Philadelphia, Pennsylvania (consortia); Memorial Medical Center, Houston, Texas (consortia); and Scottsdale Medical Center, Scottsdale, Arizona (consortia).

Other significant programs within this legislation afforded opportunities for APRNs to obtain funding or participate in innovative programs focusing on the delivery of primary care services. A CMS-Centers for Medicare and Medicaid Innovation (CMMI) was created to allow CMS to experiment and implement programs more efficiently than currently allowed. Prior to its development, successful demonstrations had to be reapproved by Congress if the programs were to be continued. Of particular importance to Nurse Practitioners is that CMMI innovations were not limited to physicians and hospitals. Although the first rounds of the funding cycle were dedicated to large established practices, later funding cycles included more innovative projects that incorporated APRNs and allowed for smaller practices to compete.

Among the most prominent innovations included in this legislation was the formation of insurance exchanges/marketplaces for individuals not covered by existing government or third-party insurance programs, the formation of a Medicare primary care accountable care organization (ACO) pilot called Shared Savings, an emphasis placed on the utilization of medical home standards in a variety of government payment innovations, the development of a medical home for homebound patients, the development of programs that reimburse for transitional care of patients being discharged from hospitals and funding for the coordination of complex patient care. As the rules for implementation of these programs developed, APRNs were recognized as eligible providers within applicable programs.

INSURANCE EXCHANGES AND MEDICAL HOMES

Currently, the regulations for the development of insurance exchanges allow APRNs to become providers within the systems being developed. However, because there is no mandate, APRNs have needed to be vigilant within their states, becoming involved in the development and implementation of these programs. This means they had and continue to need to be at the table, acquainted with the state's insurance commissioners, involved in associated task forces and committees, and involved with the insurance carriers associated with the programs. Likewise it was and continues to be important for APRNs to be vigilant, as state regulations are developed, to be sure that practices are recognized as medical homes within those regulations and regulations for other state-controlled programs affecting health care. Currently Nurse Practitioner practices are recognized by Medical Home certifiers and may receive recognition from the recognized national certification programs. The principles of the Medical Home Practice have been the centerpiece for Nurse Practitioner practice from the beginning: wholistic patient centered care, with an emphasis on access, quality, and safety (AANP, 2012).

ACCOUNTABLE CARE ORGANIZATIONS

In this legislation, Nurse Practitioners are recognized as ACO providers. However, last-minute changes in the Shared Savings provision for Medicare patients have determined for that program that the only eligible beneficiaries will be patients of primary care physicians. Although Nurse Practitioners may be participants in a Shared Savings ACO, their patients must be seen at least once by a physician in a funding measurement year. Changes continue to be needed in the statute that will allow patients of Nurse Practitioners to be beneficiaries in this program. Although this provision dis-incentivizes APRNs in the Shared Savings program, it does not, however, prevent them from becoming members of other ACOs or forming ACOs of their own.

The Shared Savings program is a pilot Medicare primary care ACO, designed for primary care practices within the Medicare system. Practices will participate in shared savings activities, which include the performance of a predetermined set of quality indicators and reported cost savings by practices with one physician who performs primary care services to Medicare patients. The statute is in place as of this writing; however it still requires a change to allow patients of APRNs to become identified beneficiaries in the program.

TRANSITIONAL CARE AND CARE COORDINATION AND MEDICAID EXPANSION

As in other areas, studies have already demonstrated that APRNs are particularly skilled in implementing transitional care and coordinating care for patients both in public and commercial insurance plans. Transitional care speaks to the care of patients postdischarge (usually 30 days) from hospitals and other health care institutions usually at home and in primary care practices. Care coordination refers to the activities all professional nurses have been prepared to provide, which involves the maintenance of patient-centered continuity of care; communication among health care providers, families, other community resources, and the patient that provides for and maintains the health and welfare of patients in our communities. The goal of both transitional care and care coordination is to sustain maximal functioning outside the health care institution and keep the patients from being admitted or readmitted with the same problem. Involvement in the development of these programs at the community level and involvement with the reimbursement planning at the policy level are musts for APRNs. Likewise, the expansion of Medicaid coverage has necessitated the continued authorization of APRNs as full participants in the health care systems, to address the needs of increased numbers of patients requiring primary care services.

HEALTH PROMOTION/DISEASE PREVENTION

The legislation has continued to emphasize the importance of health promotion and disease prevention through the expansion of payment for health promotion, disease prevention services, and the development of programs that APRNs are particularly prepared to deliver. It will be important for APRNs to continue to seek out opportunities to utilize this authorization in the provision of the care on which APRN education is built.

OBSTACLES/BARRIERS

One of the unfortunate aspects of the passage of legislation such as this has been the opposition of some power brokers in the country's health care system. Of particular significance to APRNs is organized medicine's opposition to changes in the care models that are being authorized. This has created particular challenges to APRNs, who have the potential to increase the quantity and quality of health care services to both public and private patients throughout the country. It has been and will continue to be up to APRNs to seize the appropriate moments to demonstrate their worth and expertise in meeting the health care needs of the nation, and to continue to use their influence to make changes in the country's health care system that will improve the health and welfare of its citizens.

Likewise, the presence of other statutory barriers to practice that are grounded in obsolete laws will continue to interfere with the ability of APRNs to fully implement the opportunities provided in this legislation until they are changed. The need for all APRNs to function at their full scope of preparation and for obsolete barriers related to physician oversight and Medicare Conditions of Participation to be removed continues to exist at this writing.

Significant improvements in the status of APRNs have been achieved with the recent passage of the Medicare Access and CHIP Reauthorization (MACRA) Act of 2015 legislation that is moving Medicare billing away from quantity-based fee-for-service reimbursement to value-based patient-centered payment for care called the Quality Payment Program (QPP; qpp.cms.gov). In this recently passed legislation Nurse Practitioners, clinical specialists, and nurse anesthetists will be authorized along with physicians to participate in a new value-based system that will emphasize quality and cost-effectiveness of care to their patients. In addition, Nurse Practitioners are recognized in the medical home requirements for chronic care management as providers, managers, and owners of primary care medical homes in this legislation.

As we move into the 115th congressional session with a new president and the renewed efforts of parts of Congress to repeal the PPACA once again, the status of this now implemented legislation is up in the air. It will be important for APRNs to be vigilant and proactive in helping to maintain high-quality, cost-effective care for their patients in the coming months and years as the national health care system is debated once again.

CONCLUSION

As with all legislation, the statutory provisions in this legislation have their limitations, but similar to health care reform legislation in the past, they have provided significantly increased opportunities for APRNs to practice to the full extent of their education and licensure. It will be important for APRNs to continue to take advantage of the opportunities provided in the PPACA and its subsequent iterations by seizing the moment to demonstrate their worth and expertise in meeting the health care needs of the nation and to continue to use their influence to make changes in the country's health care system that will improve the health and welfare of its citizens.

DISCUSSION QUESTIONS

1. *What do you think an APRN should/can do to assist with the implementation of the PPACA?*
2. *How should the PPACA affect your patient's health?*
3. *Identify two provisions of the PPACA that would help the patients of APRNs.*
4. *Identify two provisions of the current PPACA that would help APRNs in their practices. Give examples.*
5. *Identify any changes that could occur in the provisions of the PPACA during a new administration and discuss how they could affect the APRN role in primary care.*

REFERENCES

American Association of Nurse Practitioners. (2012). *Survey results national data base*. Austin, TX: Author.

American Association of Nurse Practitioners. (2013). *Nurse practitioners in primary care*. Austin, TX: Author. Retrieved from http://www.aanp.org/publications/position-statements-papers

Centers for Medicare and Medicaid Services. (2013). *Tracing the history of CMS programs*. Retrieved from https://www.cms.gov/About-CMS/Agency-Information/History/Downloads/President CMSMilestones.pdf

Office of Legislative Council. (2010). Patient Protection and Affordable Care Act (as Amended Through May 1, 2010, Including Patient Protection and Affordable Care Act Health Related Portions of the Health Care and Education Reconciliation Act of 2010). Washington, DC: U.S. Government Printing Office.

567 U.S. (2012). Opinion of Roberts, C.J. Supreme Court of the United States Nos. 11-393, 11-398, and 11-400. National federation of Independent Business, et al., Petitioners vs. Kathleen Sebelius, Secretary of Health and Human Services, et al., Department of Health and Human Services, Department of Health and Human Services, et al., Petitioners vs. Florida et al. Petitioners, Florida et al. vs Department of Health and Human Services et al. On Writs of Certiorari To The United States Court of Appeals for the Eleventh Circuit. Retrieved from https://www.supremecourt.gov/docket/PPAACA.aspx

CHAPTER 9

AARP Initiatives

Andrea Brassard and Susan C. Reinhard

WHAT IS AARP?

Established in 1958, and formerly known as the American Association of Retired Persons, AARP is now the official name of the nation's leading membership organization for people aged 50 years and older. AARP is a nonprofit, nonpartisan membership organization with a membership of more than 37 million people. It is dedicated to enhancing the quality of life for all, nationally and globally, and leading positive social change by providing information, advocacy, and service to its members and the public. AARP's founder, Dr. Ethel Percy Andrus, was a high school principal in Los Angeles when she retired at the age of 60 to take care of her mother. Her mother recovered and Dr. Andrus volunteered with the California Retired Teachers Association and led its committee for retired teachers' welfare. On learning that many retired educators had no health insurance and inadequate pensions, Dr. Andrus testified before the California legislature. Her efforts resulted in the formation of the National Retired Teachers Association in 1947 to advocate for educators throughout the United States. She developed benefits and programs, such as group health insurance for older people and a discount mail order pharmacy service. These programs were so popular that thousands of people asked the association to open its membership to noneducators and, in 1958, AARP was founded. In 1999, its name was changed to the four-letter acronym AARP because the membership is open to people of age 50 years and older, with almost half of the current membership continuing to work. The National Retired Teachers Association continues as a division of AARP.

As a nonprofit, nonpartisan organization, AARP does not endorse candidates for public office or make contributions to either political campaigns or candidates. The AARP Foundation is an affiliated charity that provides security, protection, and empowerment to older people in need with support from thousands of volunteers, donors, and sponsors. AARP has staffed offices in all 50 states, the District of Columbia, Puerto Rico, and the U.S. Virgin Islands.

Located within AARP is the prestigious Public Policy Institute (PPI), staffed by approximately 60 researchers and issue experts who inform public debate on critical issues. PPI conducts policy research and analysis, and convenes leading policy experts for discussion of national, international, and state policy issues. PPI's research and analysis informs AARP's national policy efforts aimed at improving economic security, health care and quality of life, and advocacy work by AARP state offices. These research findings are shared throughout the national policy-making community, such as other researchers, advocacy organizations, legislative and executive branch officials, and the media.

CENTER TO CHAMPION NURSING IN AMERICA

Launched in December 2007, the Center to Champion Nursing in America (CCNA) is a joint initiative of the Robert Wood Johnson Foundation (RWJF), AARP, and the AARP Foundation. CCNA's chief strategist is Dr. Susan Reinhard, who is the senior vice president of AARP's PPI. CCNA's vision is that all Americans have access to a highly skilled nurse when and where they need one.

In its first 2 years, CCNA focused primarily on building nursing education capacity through state teams and three national invitation-only summits. The first summit was held in June 2008. Eighteen state teams of diverse stakeholders such as representatives from nursing education, employers, state nursing work-force centers, government agencies, and AARP state offices developed action plans to increase nursing education enrollment in their states. In preparation for the summit, RWJF, CCNA, and the U.S. Department of Labor, Employment, and Training Administration commissioned a white paper, "Blowing Open the Bottleneck: Designing New Approaches to Increase Nurse Education Capacity" (www.rwjf.org/content/rwjf/en/research-publications/find-rwjf-research/2008/05/blowing-open-the-bottleneck.html). Four approaches to effective solutions were outlined as follows: (a) create strategic partnerships to align and leverage stakeholder resources; (b) increase nurse faculty capacity and diversity; (c) redesign nurse education—for example, use simulation technology, redesign clinical education, and create dedicated educational units; and (d) capitalize on the role played by the government and accrediting organizations in nurse education.

CCNA's initial goals were to (a) strengthen our nation's educational pathways to prepare the nursing workforce of the future; (b) increase the number and diversity of nurses entering and remaining in the profession; (c) remove barriers that limit nurses' ability to provide the health care consumers need; and (d) enhance the influence of nurses in high levels of health care, policy, business, and community decision making. In December 2008, CCNA founded the Champion Nursing Coalition, whose member organizations such as Aetna, Families USA, and Verizon represent the voices of consumers, purchasers, and providers of health care. The Champion Nursing Coalition is raising awareness of the roles of nurses in increasing access to primary care, transitional care, and chronic care management in a reformed health care delivery system. CCNA also convened the Champion Nursing Council, an advisory group made up of national nursing organizations.

In 2009, 12 additional state teams were added to the CCNA education transformation project to increase education capacity in the states. The 30 multistakeholder teams included representatives from multiple AARP state offices. CCNA provided advocacy training and communications support to stakeholders to help them communicate more effectively with policy makers and private-sector leaders. Several AARP state offices contacted CCNA advocacy staff about the scope-of-practice limitations for Advanced Practice Registered Nurses (APRNs) in their states. In response to this advocacy work, the AARP policy book was amended with input from CCNA to increase access to APRN practice and care.

AARP POLICY BOOK REVISION

In the spring of 2010, the health chapter in the AARP policy book was amended to include all four APRN categories in its "Professional Schools and Licensing" section and in the policy book glossary shown in Box 9.1. The new language called for states to "amend current nursing and, where applicable, medical licensing laws to allow nurses, APRNs and allied health professionals to perform duties for which they have been educated, and certified. . . ." An additional bullet was added that "current state nurse practice acts and accompanying rules should be interpreted and/or amended where necessary to allow APRNs to fully and independently practice as defined by their education and certification" (AARP, 2013).

CCNA FOCUS EVOLVES TO IMPLEMENT THE RECOMMENDATIONS OF THE INSTITUTE OF MEDICINE REPORT

In October 2010, the Institute of Medicine (IOM) released *The Future of Nursing: Leading Change, Advancing Health*, a thorough examination of how nurses' roles, responsibilities, and education should change to meet the needs of an aging, increasingly diverse population, and to respond to a complex, evolving health care system. The four key messages and eight major recommendations (see Boxes 9.2 and 9.3) in the report focus on the critical intersection between the health needs of patients across the life span and the readiness of the nursing workforce. These recommendations are intended to support efforts to improve health care for all Americans by enhancing nurses' contributions to the delivery of care.

CAMPAIGN FOR ACTION

The Future of Nursing: *Campaign for Action* is a national initiative to guide implementation of the recommendations in *The Future of Nursing: Leading Change, Advancing Health*, a landmark IOM (2011) report. The Campaign envisions a

---

GLOSSARY	BOX 9.1

Advanced Practice Registered Nurses (APRNs):

> Nurses who receive advanced clinical preparation (generally a master's degree and/or post-master's certificate, although the Doctor of Nursing Practice degree is increasingly being granted). Specific titles and credentials vary by state approval processes, formal recognition, and scope of practice as well as by board certification. APRNs fall into four broad categories: Nurse Practitioner, Clinical Nurse Specialist, Nurse Anesthetist, and Nurse-Midwife.

KEY MESSAGES	BOX 9.2

- Nurses should practice to the full extent of their education and training.
- Nurses should achieve higher levels of education and training through an improved education system that promotes seamless academic progression.
- Nurses should be full partners, with physicians and other health care professionals, in redesigning health care in the United States.
- Effective workforce planning and policy making require better data collection and an improved information infrastructure.

REPORT RECOMMENDATIONS	BOX 9.3

1. Remove scope-of-practice barriers.
2. Expand opportunities for nurses to lead and diffuse collaborative improvement efforts.
3. Implement nurse residency programs.
4. Increase the proportion of nurses with a baccalaureate degree to 80% by 2020.
5. Double the number of nurses with a doctorate by 2020.
6. Ensure that nurses engage in life-long learning.
7. Prepare and enable nurses to lead change to advance health.
8. Build an infrastructure for the collection and analysis of interprofessional health care workforce data.

health care system where all Americans have access to high-quality care, with nurses contributing to the full extent of their capabilities.

The Campaign includes 50 states' plus Washington, DC, action coalitions and a wide range of health care providers, consumer advocates, policy makers, and business, academic, and philanthropic leaders. Many of the action coalitions evolved from CCNA's education transformation state teams.

The *Campaign for Action* is working to implement all eight recommendations of *The Future of Nursing: Leading Change, Advancing Health.* Any work performed by CCNA staff that relates to advocacy or lobbying is funded by AARP, because RWJF grant funds cannot be used to fund lobbying or political campaign activities. CCNA tracks legislative and regulatory activity pertaining to all eight recommendations. Advocacy efforts in areas such as advancing nursing education are funded by AARP. To date, of the eight recommendations, advocacy work has largely focused on removing scope-of-practice barriers for APRNs at both the federal and state levels.

RECOMMENDATION NO. 1: REMOVE SCOPE-OF-PRACTICE BARRIERS

To fully realize nurses' potential contribution to a patient- and family-centered, seamless, transformed health care system, the *Campaign for Action* is leading efforts to modernize outdated policies (public and private), change state and federal laws and regulations, and remove cultural and organizational barriers.

The *Campaign for Action* is implementing a learning collaborative to help states achieve success; engaging national stakeholder partners in state, federal, and private sector efforts; and engaging stakeholders to ensure inclusion of nurses practicing in all sectors.

As described previously, advocacy work around Recommendation No. 1 is funded through AARP's portion of the *Campaign for Action*. AARP has a consumer focus—the goal is to increase access to care by removing barriers to APRN practice. CCNA's placement within the PPI of AARP provides an opportunity to offer research and analysis to inform the consumer-focused health policy advocacy agenda of AARP.

AARP WEST VIRGINIA MODERNIZES APRN LAW

The West Virginia state office of AARP made removal of the required restrictive collaborative agreement between APRNs and physicians its top legislative priority. West Virginia AARP framed the issue around increasing access to care. Increasing access to APRN practice and care helps West Virginians statewide and is especially important to residents in rural and underserved parts of the state—as well as to the state's 300,000 family caregivers who are responsible for the safety and well-being of their older parents, spouses, and other loved ones.

West Virginia AARP staff and volunteers advocated for the successful 2016 West Virginia legislation that removed the restrictive collaborative agreement for APRNs after 3 years. The law also expands the prescription formulary for APRNs and permits APRNs to sign documents previously signed only by physicians. It also retires old statutes restricting the individual practices of nurse midwives and certified nurse anesthetists to bring them under the one designation of APRN.

The tireless, consolidated effort was led by the West Virginia Nurses Association and AARP and supported by the Future of Nursing West Virginia, West Virginia Board of Nurse Examiners, Healthy Kids and Families Coalition, West Virginians for Affordable Healthcare, Citizens Action Group, Heritage Foundation, Federal Trade Commission, and other organizations, as well as delegates and senators who championed the bill on its journey.

The Future of Nursing West Virginia Coalition Practice Team developed information fact sheets and trained nurse policy advocates in each West Virginia senatorial district on the key issues. They presented the issues and stories to AARP volunteers and participated in strategy sessions with the AARP and nursing lobbyists throughout the legislative session.

The biggest beneficiaries of this legislation are the 170,000 new Medicaid recipients who acquired health care for the first time through Medicaid expansion and had no access to adequate primary care resources until now. Before passing this legislation, West Virginia APRN practices were closing because of an unavailability of physicians to sign collaborative agreements. Now nurses are free to open practices again in this state where 50 of the 55 counties are considered undeserved health care areas.

states.aarp.org/wva6-healing-powers
campaignforaction.org/wv-aprn-bill-signed-law

AARP'S PPI PUBLICATIONS

AARP has published two papers that align with the first recommendation of *The Future of Nursing: Leading Change, Advancing Health*. The first of these papers is titled "Removing Barriers to Advanced Practice Registered Nurse Care: Hospital Privileges" (Brassard & Smolenski, 2011). This article discusses barriers to hospital privileges and expands on the IOM report recommendations that APRNs be eligible for hospital clinical privileges, admitting privileges, and hospital medical staff membership and also be permitted to perform hospital admission assessments—documenting medical histories and performing physical examinations.

The second paper that aligns with the IOM report is "Removing Barriers to Advanced Practice Registered Nurse Care: Home Health and Hospice Services" (Brassard, 2012). This chapter expands on the IOM report recommendations that APRNs be allowed to certify patients for Medicare payment of home health and hospice services and shows how removing the barrier to this would benefit consumers, physicians, and the health care system. Allowing APRNs to certify home health and hospice services can potentially decrease costs, expedite treatment by eliminating the need for physician sign-off, and allow patient-centered health care teams to practice more efficiently.

GRADUATE NURSE EDUCATION DEMONSTRATION PROGRAM

True to the CCNA vision to ensure that Americans have the highly skilled nurses needed to provide affordable, quality health care, now and in the future, AARP continues to advocate for state and national funding for nursing education. AARP advocates for funding to advance education progression in nursing and to increase the supply of RNs, APRNs, and nursing faculty.

AARP advocated for the Graduate Nurse Education (GNE) Demonstration Program, which is an important part of the 2010 Affordable Care Act (ACA). ACA set aside $200 million over 4 years to test the idea of providing Medicare funding for GNE to fund hospitals and collaborating colleges of nursing to educate more APRNs. Selected hospitals are partnering with accredited schools of nursing and non-hospital community-based care settings to expand clinical education within and beyond the hospital setting. Consumers, nurses, and health care groups issued a collective cheer when the selected institutions—the Hospital of the University of Pennsylvania, Duke University Hospital, Scottsdale Healthcare Medical Center, Rush University Medical Center, and Memorial Hermann-Texas Medical Center Hospital—were announced in July 2012 (Quinn, Reinhard, Thornhill, & Reinecke, 2015).

Preliminary findings include expanded access to clinical training sites—especially in community-based clinics, which are ideal for educating APRNs and other primary care providers. Models of care in demonstration partner sites include preventive care, transitional care, and primary care. An evaluation report is due to Congress by October 2017 and could prompt Medicare to change its current nursing education payment policies and create a permanent funding stream to boost graduate nursing education nationwide.

CARE ACT

As previously described, CCNA is a strategic initiative within AARP's PPI. Another PPI strategic initiative aims to improve the capacity of nurses to meet the needs of family caregivers. According to a groundbreaking study by the AARP PPI and the United Hospital Fund titled *Home Alone: Family Caregivers Providing Complex Chronic Care* (Reinhard, Levine, & Samis, 2012), most family caregivers perform complex medical/nursing tasks with very little guidance. Family caregivers are providing much more complex care than what many had thought, with little or no training or home visits. Understandably, family caregivers performing medical/nursing tasks were most likely to report feeling stressed and worried about making a mistake. More than half reported feeling down, depressed, or hopeless in the last two weeks, and more than a third reported fair or poor health. These negative impacts increased with the number of the care recipients' chronic conditions (Reinhard, Levine, & Samis, 2012).

Family caregivers reported receiving little formal training in medical/nursing tasks such as managing medications, performing wound care, or operating medical equipment, despite patients' frequent hospitalizations. When nurses in selected hospitals, nursing homes, and home care agencies were surveyed about how well they trained family caregivers, most were very positive. Family caregivers of patients who had been discharged from the same settings did not agree (Levine, Halper, Rutberg, & Gould, 2013). "Staff may have indeed given family caregivers . . . information, but not in a way that those family caregivers understood and could use" (Levine et al., 2013, p. 20).

In response to the *Home Alone* report, AARP developed model legislation to help family caregivers get the recognition, information, and instruction they need to perform the complex medical/nursing tasks that they are often expected to perform. The Caregiver Advise, Record, Enable (CARE) Act requires hospitals to ask patients to designate a caregiver, to notify the caregiver before discharge, and to educate the caregiver in medical/nursing tasks they are expected to perform (AARP, 2015). Educating caregivers on medical/nursing tasks includes providing training and the opportunity for return demonstration of procedures. Thirty-three states and territories had enacted the CARE Act as of October 2016.

Implementing the CARE Act in hospital settings is just getting started. The AARP PPI is conducting a national scan of implementation efforts to uncover promising practices and potential barriers. For example, APRNs in hospital settings have needed to advocate for institutional policy changes to allow caregivers to perform procedures such as insulin administration or tracheostomy suctioning to their hospitalized loved one (S. McMillan, personal communication, June 7, 2016).

As our health care system continues to evolve, APRNs can look to AARP for ongoing research and policy initiatives that are relevant to APRN practice and care.

DISCUSSION QUESTIONS

1. *Review the two AARP PPI publications that refer to Recommendation No. 1 of the IOM report. What legislative or regulatory changes are needed to remove these policy barriers?*
2. *If you were going to describe the importance of hospital privileges and/or home health certification for policy change to potential supporters, what key issues would you stress? How would you describe this to your patients?*
3. *To date, federal legislation has not been enacted to allow APRNs to certify home health services. What have been the consequences of federal inaction?*

ANALYSIS, SYNTHESIS, AND CLINICAL APPLICATION

1. *What other barriers to APRN practice and care impact consumers? Would federal or state or institutional policy changes be needed?*
2. *How does the GNE Demonstration Program impact your school's current or future APRN programs?*
3. *Has the CARE Act been enacted in your state? If it has been enacted, how does this legislation impact your current RN or future APRN practice? If it has not been enacted, what can you do to promote it?*
4. *Should the CARE Act be extended to home health and rehabilitation settings? What are the consequences when patients are discharged from these settings without caregiver training on medical/nursing tasks?*

EXERCISES/CONSIDERATIONS

1. *APRNs can partner with AARP to increase consumers' access to care.*
2. *APRNs can look to AARP for policy initiatives that are relevant to APRN practice and care.*

REFERENCES

American Association of Retired Persons. (2013). *The policy book: AARP Public Policies, 2013–2014* (Chapter 7, p. 145). Washington, DC: Author.

American Association of Retired Persons. (2015). New state law to help family caregivers. Retrieved from http://www.aarp.org/politics-society/advocacy/caregiving-advocacy/info-2014/aarp-creates -modelstate-bill.html

Brassard, A. (2012, July). Removing barriers to advanced practice registered nurse care: Home health and hospice services. *AARP Public Policy Institute, Insight on the Issues 66*. Retrieved from http://www .aarp.org/health/medicare-insurance/info-07-2012/removing-barriers-to-advanced-practice -registered-nurse-care-home-health-hospice-AARP-ppi-health.html

Brassard, A., & Smolenski, M. (2011, September). Removing barriers to advanced practice registered nurse care: Hospital privileges. *AARP Public Policy Institute, Insight on the Issues 55*. Retrieved from http://www.aarp.org/health/doctors-hospitals/info-10-2011/Removing-Barriers-to-Advanced -Practice-Registered-Nurse-Care-Hospital-Privileges.html

Institute of Medicine. (2011). *The future of nursing: Leading change, advancing health.* Washington, DC: National Academies Press.

Levine, C., Halper, D. E., Rutberg, J. C., & Gould, D. A. (2013). Engaging family caregivers as partners in transition. Retrieved from http://www.uhfnyc.org/publications/880905

Quinn, W., Reinhard, S., Thornhill, L., & Reinecke, P. (2015, June). Improving access to high-quality care: Medicare program for graduate nurse education. *AARP Public Policy Institute, Insight on the Issues 103*. Retrieved from http://www.aarp.org/content/dam/aarp/ppi/2015/improving -access-to-high-quality-care-revised.pdf

Reinhard, S., Levine, C., & Samis, S. (2012). *Home alone: Family caregivers providing complex chronic care.* A report of the AARP Public Policy Institute and the United Hospital Fund. Retrieved from http://www.aarp.org/content/dam/aarp/research/public_policy_institute/health/home-alone -family-caregivers-providing-complex-chronic-care-rev-AARP-ppi-health.pdf

CHAPTER 10

Million Hearts®

Liana Orsolini and Mary C. Smolenski

The Institute of Medicine's (IOM) *The Future of Nursing: Leading Change, Advancing Health* report's seventh recommendation calls everyone to "prepare and enable nurses to lead change to advance health" (2010, p. 43), and the American Nurses Association Social Policy Statement's definition of nursing includes advocating for ". . . the care of individuals, families, communities and populations" (2010, p. 10). Both documents call for nurses to improve the health of communities and populations; an imperative nursing has mostly ignored until recently. Advanced Practice Registered Nurses (APRNs) have opportunities to improve the health of communities and populations through public–private partnerships and involvement with federal programs.

Federal efforts to improve health are certainly not new but have gathered momentum with the start of the U.S. Department of Health and Human Services' (USDHHS) launch of Healthy People in 2000 (National Center for Health Statistics [NCHS], 2001). Unlike Healthy People 2020 (USDHHS, Office of Disease Prevention and Health Promotion, 2016), which covers a myriad of health topics from access to health services to improving the visual health of the nation, Million Hearts aims to prevent 1 million heart attacks and strokes by 2017 (USDHHS, 2016c; HealthyPeople 2020). Because Million Hearts has prevented more than half a million heart attacks and strokes it will continue for at least another 5 years (Centers for Medicare and Medicaid Services [CMS], 2017b).

The DHHS launched Million Hearts in 2011. This initiative not only works to align existing efforts but is creating new programs to improve heart health and to help Americans live longer, more productive lives. The Centers for Disease Control and Prevention (CDC) and CMS, colead Million Hearts and are working alongside other federal agencies and private- and public-sector organizations to institutionalize effective cardiovascular disease (CVD) prevention strategies within communities. Community strategies include targeting smoking and artificial trans fat and sodium consumption, while clinical strategies include targeting appropriate aspirin use, blood pressure control, cholesterol control, and smoking cessation (ABCS). Clinical strategies also include improving health information technology (HIT) and innovative care models to meet national goals. Federal agencies involved in Million Hearts include the Administration for Community Living, National Institutes of Health (NIH), the Agency for Healthcare Research and Quality, the Food and Drug Administration, the Health Resources and Services Administration (HRSA), the Substance Abuse and Mental Health Services Administration, the Office of the National Coordinator, and the Veterans Administration. Among the many private-sector partners are the American Heart Association (AHA)/ American Stroke Association, American Academy of Nursing (AAN), American Association of Nurse Practitioners (AANP), American Association of Colleges of Nursing, American Nurses Association, Association of Public Health Nurses, Preventive Cardiovascular Nurses Association and a nurse managed clinic, Lewis and Clark Family Health Clinic. Dr. Janet Wright, an accomplished cardiologist who served as senior vice president for science and quality at the American College of Cardiology, is the executive director of Million Hearts. Under her leadership, many national nursing organizations have been asked and are still being asked to partner with Million Hearts. According to Dr. Wright, if this initiative is to be successful it has to take a comprehensive interprofessional and transdisciplinary effort across multiple types of stakeholder organizations (J. Wright, personal communication, May 9, 2013).

The private sector initiatives include a variety of efforts. All official partners are listed on www.millionhearts.hhs.gov/partners-progress/partners.html and feature a variety of different community efforts to prevent heart attacks and strokes. The AAN published a policy brief/call-to-action for all nurses to get heart healthy in *Nursing Outlook* and presented a policy dialogue at the 2016 Academy Annual Policy conference (AAN, 2016). The subgroup also published, "The Million Hearts initiative: Guidelines and best practices," in *The Nurse Practitioner* (Melnyk et al., 2016). Their Million Hearts subcommittee has collected data on the heart health of nurses across the nation and the effects of their health (or lack of it) in their nursing practice.

Why should APRNs be interested in Million Hearts? Heart disease causes one in every three deaths or 800,000 deaths per year in the United States, which costs about $110 billion each year for coronary disease alone in treatment costs and loss of productivity (CDC, 2015b; Mozaffarian et al., 2016). While 81 million Americans are affected by some form of CVD (Lloyd-Jones et al., 2010), this number is expected to increase as 70.7% of the U.S. population age older than 20 years are either overweight or obese (CDC, 2017b) and one in every three children is overweight or obese (AHA, 2014). Strokes are also a leading killer, taking 130,000 American lives each year (Kochanek, Xu, Murphy, Miniño, & Kung, 2011). If one adds up *all* the deaths each year from heart attacks, strokes, and related vascular diseases, we are confronted with the staggering costs of about $1 billion a day or $1 out of every $6 spent on direct medical costs (CDC, 2011b), which is predicted to exceed $275 billion in lost productivity by 2030 (CDC, 2015a). Although the CDC (2011a) began the National Heart Disease and Stroke Prevention Program in 1998, which is now in all 50 states and the District of Columbia, heart disease and stroke continue to increase. A likely cause of CVD is that one in every three, or 75 million, Americans has high blood pressure and 20% of these, or about 14 million people, do not know they have it and only about half of those with high blood pressure have it controlled (CDC, 2017a). Self-reported hypertension rose by almost 10% from 2005 to 2009, and the data continue to show racial and geographic disparities (CDC, 2013b). In addition, another 30% of Americans have prehypertension (CDC, 2016b). When documenting the extent of the problem of CVD prevention and the lack of evidence-based treatment patients receive, Frieden and Berwick (2011) draw our attention to the chasm between clinical guidelines and practice:

> Currently, less than half of people with ischemic heart disease take daily aspirin or another antiplatelet agent; less than half with hypertension have it adequately controlled; only a third with hyperlipidemia have adequate treatment; and less than a quarter of smokers who try to quit get counseling or medications.

Clearly, CVD in the United States is not well managed, and this should have the attention of APRNs if nursing is to lead in advancing the health of the nation. APRNs care for significant amounts of the U.S. population (ANA, 2011) and have an enormous capacity to bring blood pressure and other controllable risk factors under control. Data from the AANP's sample survey completed in the spring of 2016 indicate that 83.4% of the over 222,000 Nurse Practitioners (NPs) are prepared in primary care. Just over one out of three (35.4%) patients seen by NPs is a Medicare patient, and one in five is on Medicaid. Many of their patients are between the ages of 66 years and 85 years. A majority of these patients present with multisystem disease. Of the 7.7% prepared as acute care NPs, 20% of their practice focuses on cardiology (AANP, 2016). Over 97% of NPs prescribe medications, and of all the prescriptions written, three of the top four drugs prescribed are antihypertensives, diabetic drugs, and dyslipidemias, making up 63.5% of all the drugs they prescribe (AANP, 2012). NP managed clinics have shown excellent outcomes for managing high blood pressure (Wright, Romboli, DiTulio, Wogen, & Belletti, 2011). Furthermore, nurse-managed health clinics are proliferating (J. M. Ware, personal communication, October 1, 2012) and are operating in at least 37 states, with an estimated 2 million patient encounters per year, mostly for Medicaid recipients and for the uninsured (Kovner & Walani, 2010). More NPs work in rural areas and other remote areas than any other primary care practitioner (Fauteux, 2012). Dr. McMenamin (2013), a senior policy analyst for the American Nurses Association, analyzed Medicare data and discovered that APRNs served more than 30% of Medicare fee-for-service beneficiaries across the United States. Through nurse-managed health clinics, APRNs and NPs can lead the nation in improving blood pressure control and other controllable risk factors that contribute to heart attack and stroke. Table 10.1 shows what all health professionals were asked to do by taking the Million Hearts Pledge.

Although prevention of illness and injury is a desirable proposition, it is difficult to sustain because success usually means the absence of a condition. Results are intangible and may take months or even years to realize. Patients often give up on strategies and methods because results seem slow, unreachable, or out of sight. Most effects and benefits of prevention have been shown in retrospective or highly controlled longitudinal studies. In a world where people are conditioned to expect instant feedback and immediate results, prevention efforts need to create incentives for both practitioners and patients alike. Integrating population health measures into primary care is a natural strategy for APRNs who have been leading the way in this arena for many years (Health Affairs, 2013). NPs

TABLE 10.1 By Taking the Pledge, as a Health Care Provider, You Commit To

TREAT high blood pressure and cholesterol in your patients.
TREAT appropriate patients with aspirin.
ESTABLISH and **DISCUSS** with patients their specific goals for treatment and the most effective ways that they can help control their risk factors for heart disease and stroke.
COACH your patients to develop heart-healthy habits, such as regular exercise and a diet rich in fresh fruits and vegetables, and stress reduction techniques. Provide tools to show their progress and access to team members to help them succeed.
ASK your patients about their smoking status and provide cessation support and medication when appropriate.
ASK about barriers to medication adherence and help find solutions.
USE health information technology, such as electronic health records and decision support tools, to improve the delivery of care and control of the **ABCS.**

ABCS, appropriate aspirin use, blood pressure control, cholesterol control, and smoking cessation.

and other APRNs are a natural fit to "lead change and advance health" through Million Hearts. The Patient Protection and Affordable Care Act (PPACA) created this opportunity by mandating prevention and quality care.

The PPACA's Title III, Improving the Quality and Efficiency of Healthcare, Part II, National Strategy to Improve Health Care, mandates the first National Quality Strategy (NQS; USDHHS, 2016b). The three aims of the NQS are:

- Better Care: Improve the overall quality, by making health care more patient-centered, reliable, accessible, and safe.
- Healthy People/Healthy Communities: Improve the health of the U.S. population by supporting proven interventions to address behavioral, social and, environmental determinants of health in addition to delivering higher quality care.
- Affordable Care: Reduce the cost of quality health care for individuals, families, employers, and government (USDHH, 2016a).

Million Hearts meets the NQS's goal to "promote the most effective prevention and treatment practices for the leading causes of mortality, starting with cardiovascular disease" (USDHHS, 2012a). At the beginning of Million Hearts there were two main goals:

- Better prevention efforts by "empowering Americans to make healthy choices such as preventing tobacco use and reducing sodium and trans fat consumption"
- Better treatment by, "improving care for people who do need treatment by encouraging a targeted focus on the ABCS," which includes the ABCS of aspirin as appropriate for people at risk, blood pressure control, cholesterol management and smoking cessation (CDC, 2011c)

As Million Hearts matured, these were expanded by adding the aims of improving access to effective and quality care, activating the public to lead healthy lifestyles, and improving medication adherence (Million Hearts, 2016).

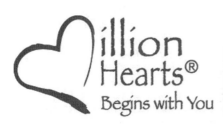

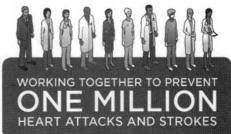

WORKING TOGETHER TO PREVENT
ONE MILLION
HEART ATTACKS AND STROKES

1 of every **3**
deaths is caused by heart disease and stroke

Health care costs for heart attack and stroke:
$312.6 BILLION

Leading cause of **PREVENTABLE DEATH** in people 40–65 years of age

2 MILLION+
heart attacks and strokes each year

To prevent 1 million heart attacks and strokes, health care professionals and public health workers should do what we know works:

FOCUS ON THE ABCS

Aspirin when appropriate
Blood pressure control
Cholesterol management
Smoking cessation

USE HEALTH IT

Use **electronic** health records and other health IT to identify patients who need support to improve their ABCS and then track their progress over time.

USE **TEAM-BASED** CARE

Use clinical innovations, including:
♥ Use everyone who interacts with patients to the top of their skills and license
♥ Self-measured blood pressure monitoring with clinical support
♥ Reward and recognize excellence in the ABCS

By doing what we know works, health care professionals, health care systems, and public health organizations can help prevent 1,000,000 heart attacks and strokes and meet these goals by 2017:

47% to **70%**
increase in aspirin use for secondary prevention

46% to **70%**
increase in blood pressure control

33% to **70%**
increase in cholesterol management

23% to **70%**
increase in help for those who want to quit smoking

20%
reduction in sodium consumption

50%
reduction in trans fat consumption

* For more information on effectiveness of team-based care, visit:
www.thecommunityguide.org/cvd/teambasedcare.html

www.cdc.gov/media/dpk/2013/dpk_13_in_2013.html
www.millionhearts.hhs.gov

CS234777E

CDC

**U.S. Department of
Health and Human Services**
Centers for Disease
Control and Prevention

FIGURE 10.1 Million Hearts infographic.
Source: Million Hearts (2016).

Strategies for prevention efforts aimed to improve the health of American lifestyles by preventing tobacco use and reducing sodium and trans fat consumption rely on community engagement efforts. Let's begin by examining tobacco use in the United States.

Although tobacco use declined shortly after the 1998 Master Settlement Agreement that eliminated the use of advertising directed toward underage youth, the United States is currently quickly losing ground (USDHHS, 2012b). Tragically, nearly one in four high school seniors smoke and most of these become adult smokers (USDHHS, 2012b). The success of big tobacco in the United States is evidenced by the figures that more than 600,000 middle-school students and 3 million high school students smoke cigarettes. These numbers are expected to increase because every day more than 1,200 people die because of smoking and at least two youth or young adults take their place. This means 2,400 young people begin smoking each day (USDHHS, 2012b). Certainly school nurses/practitioners and school-based health centers are key players in the prevention of tobacco product use and smoking cessation in children and youth. As of 2008, there were 73,697 registered nurses working as school nurses and nearly 2,000 school-based health centers (HRSA, n.d., 2010). School-based health centers routinely provide tobacco prevention services (Strozer, Juszczak, & Ammerman, 2010). In a study of 35 high schools, limited school nurse intervention using the 5As model (see Table 10.2) resulted in successful short-term abstinence in adolescent boys (Pbert et al., 2011). More research needs to be conducted to determine if a longer intervention period would lead to sustained abstinence among all genders.

The incidence of tobacco use in adults in the United States remains problematic. The CDC (2016a) estimates that 40 million people or about 17% of adults over 18 smoke cigarettes and that cigarette smoking accounts for over 480,000 deaths each year in the United States. Sadly, 70% of smokers wish to quit yet continue smoking (CDC, 2013a). The CDC is using the PPACA's Prevention and Public Health Fund to finance its newest campaign against smoking. Most television viewers familiar with the CDC's "Tips from Former Smokers" campaign recognize Terrie, a middle-aged woman with a disfigured face and stoma, who tells her story of smoking, which she started at age 13 years. The CDC television ads where Terrie and other former smokers tells their stories can be reviewed at: www.cdc.gov/tobacco/campaign/tips/resources/videos/terrie-videos.html #terrie-2. *Note: Terrie Hall died on September 16, 2013, aged 53 years.*

These ads caused the call volume to the CDC's 1-800-QUIT-NOW number to double, and visits to the campaign website (www.cdc.gov/tips) increased more than fivefold (CDC, 2013a). Every APRN should follow the Clinical Practice Guidelines for Treating Tobacco Use and Dependence updated in 2008 by the USDHHS Public Health Service (USDHHS, 2008). These guidelines list evidence-based ways to facilitate successful tobacco use cessation in population-specific patients both willing and unwilling to quit at the time of visit with their health care practitioner. In an evidence review of over 8,000 articles from 1975, the 2008 updated guidelines stress that combined counseling and medication is more effective than either alone. It is also noteworthy that the evidence to screen all adult patients and especially pregnant women for tobacco use at every visit to a primary care provider is an A level recommendation by the U.S. Preventive Services Task Force (UPSTF, 2015). Diet is another focus area for community prevention efforts of Million Hearts.

TABLE 10.2 5As and 5Rs

5As	
Ask about tobacco use	Identify and document tobacco use status of every patient at every visit.
Advise to quit	In a clear, strong, and personalized manner, urge every tobacco user to quit.
Assess	For a current tobacco user, is he or she willing to make a quit attempt at this time? For the ex-tobacco user, how recently did he or she quit and are there any challenges to remaining abstinent?
Assist	For the patient willing to make a quit attempt, offer medication and provide or refer for counseling or additional behavioral treatment to help the patient quit. For patients unwilling to quit at this time, provide motivational interventions designed to increase future quit attempts. For the recent quitter and anyone with remaining challenges, provide relapse prevention
Arrange	All those receiving the previous As should receive follow-up.
5Rs	
Relevance	Encourage the patient to indicate why quitting is personally relevant, being as specific as possible. Motivational information has the greatest impact if it is relevant to a patient's disease status or risk, family or social situation (e.g., having children in the home), health concerns, age, gender, and other important patient characteristics (e.g., prior quitting experience, personal barriers to cessation).
Risks	The clinician should ask the patient to identify potential negative consequences of tobacco use. The clinician may suggest and highlight those that seem most relevant to the patient. The clinician should emphasize that smoking low-tar/low-nicotine cigarettes or use of other forms of tobacco (e.g., smokeless tobacco, cigars, and pipes) will not eliminate these risks. Examples of risks are: • *Acute risks*: Shortness of breath, exacerbation of asthma or bronchitis, increased risk of respiratory infections, harm to pregnancy, impotence, infertility. • *Long-term risks*: Heart attacks and strokes, lung and other cancers (e.g., larynx, oral cavity, pharynx, esophagus, pancreas, stomach, kidney, bladder, cervix, and acute myelocytic leukemia), chronic obstructive pulmonary diseases (chronic bronchitis and emphysema), osteoporosis, long-term disability, and need for extended care. • *Environmental risks*: Increased risk of lung cancer and heart disease in spouses; increased risk of low birth weight, sudden infant death syndrome (SIDS), asthma, middle ear disease, and respiratory infections in children of smokers.
Rewards	The clinician should ask the patient to identify potential benefits of stopping tobacco use. The clinician may suggest and highlight those that seem most relevant to the patient. Examples of rewards follow: • Improved health • Food tasting better • Improved sense of smell • Saving money • Feeling better about yourself • Home, car, clothing, breath smelling better • Setting a good example for children and decreasing the likelihood that they will smoke

(continued)

TABLE 10.2 5As and 5Rs (*continued*)

5Rs	
	• Having healthier babies and children • Feeling better physically • Performing better in physical activities • Improved appearance, including reduced wrinkling/aging of skin and whiter teeth
Roadblocks	The clinician should ask the patient to identify barriers or impediments to quitting and provide treatment (problem-solving counseling, medication) that could address barriers. Typical barriers might include: • Withdrawal symptoms • Fear of failure • Weight gain • Lack of support • Depression • Enjoyment of tobacco • Being around other tobacco users • Limited knowledge of effective treatment options
Repetition	The motivational intervention should be repeated every time an unmotivated patient visits the clinic setting. Tobacco users who have failed in previous quit attempts should be told that most people make repeated quit attempts before they are successful and that you will continue to raise their tobacco use with them.

Source: Agency for Healthcare Research and Quality (2008).

About hypertension, too much sodium intake increases the risk of developing high blood pressure (CDC, 2012b), and 90% of Americans eat more sodium than is recommended. Although the U.S. Dietary Guidelines recommend ingesting less than 2.3 g of sodium/day, Americans ingest an average of 3.3 g/day. Moreover, those at risk for CVD such as African Americans, anyone older than 50 years, those with high blood pressure, diabetes, or chronic kidney disease should ingest no more than 1,500 mg of sodium per day (U.S. Department of Agriculture and USDHHS, 2010). Although the IOM (2013) recommends further research on the effects of sodium on patient outcomes in population subgroups, there is much evidence to link a high sodium intake with CVD. Most consumers are not aware that high amounts of sodium in the American diet come from surprising sources such as cottage cheese, raw chicken and pork injected with a sodium solution, bread, soup, and salsa. There are many resources APRNs can use to educate their patients about lowering their salt intake and salt intake's relationship to blood pressure. The NIH has a user-friendly guide for the public on how to lower blood pressure by reducing salt consumption (https://www.nhlbi.nih.gov/health/health-topics/topics/dash; www.nhlbi.nih.gov/health/resources/heart/hbp-dash-introduction-html). The site has easy-to-read instructions on how to read food labels for sodium, sample eating plans, and recipes for heart health. The Preventive Cardiovascular Nurse Association (PCNA) has many downloadable resources as well as tools for health care providers at http://pcna.net/clinical-tools/education-for-your-patients. In addition to limiting salt intake or sodium, Americans must also limit their intake of trans fats.

The amount of publicity linking ingestion of trans fats to coronary heart disease has led to a marked decrease in their consumption and the reformulation

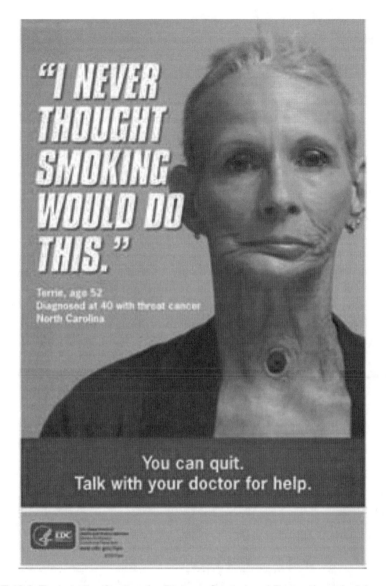

FIGURE 10.2 Terrie in the Centers for Disease Control and Prevention television ads for
Tips From Former Smokers® campaign.

Source: Picture reprinted with permission from the Department of Health and Human Services, Centers
for Disease Control and Prevention, Office on Smoking and Health. https://www.cdc.gov/tobacco/campaign/tips/resources

of many foods to greatly decrease amounts of trans fat or eliminate them (CDC, 2012d). Despite this progress, Americans continue to consume 1.3 g of artificial trans fat or partially hydrogenated oils per day. Few realize that although an ingredient label states that there is 0 trans fat, manufacturers are allowed to add less than 0.5 g and remain within the law. As no trans fat is a good trans fat, patients should be told to avoid all products containing partially hydrogenated oils such as frozen pizza, microwave popcorn, ready-to-use-frostings, margarine, pies, cookies, coffee creamers, and fried foods. Many prepackaged foods and preprepared and fried foods still contain high amounts of trans fats. APRNs can encourage patients to read every label and cook for themselves as much as possible. Certainly a nutritionist should be part of the interprofessional team and should be available as a patient resource. Once an APRN determines that a patient needs treatment to prevent heart attacks and strokes, efforts are placed on the ABCS.

A is for appropriate aspirin use. Appropriate aspirin use has been widely studied. The U.S. Preventive Service Task Force (USPSTF), a nongovernmental panel of interprofessional clinical experts and scientists, conducts evidence reviews on a large variety of primary care preventive health services and then publishes its recommendations. These recommendations are weighed according to the level of evidence. For instance, an A or B recommendation means there is high (A) or moderate (B) certainty that the preventive service should be offered to a targeted population, and a while a C recommendation means that the service should be used more selectively as the benefit is small (USPSTF, 2012). As of September 23, 2010, the PPACA has mandated that new insurance plans must cover all A and B preventive services recommended by the USPSTF at no cost sharing (Health Affairs, 2010). See Table 10.3 for the USPSF's recommendations for the use of aspirin to prevent CVD and colorectal cancer.

The CDC analyzed data from the National Ambulatory Medical Care Survey and from the National Hospital Ambulatory Medical Care Survey representing a total of 198,042 patient visits among adults aged older than 18 years in order to "estimate the prevalence of physician-prescribed aspirin and other antiplatelet medications" (George, Tong, Sonnenfeld, & Hong, 2012). Although prescribing increased from 32.8% in 2003 to 46.9% by 2008, this analysis concluded that prevalence of prescribing aspirin or other appropriate antiplatelet medications remains low for those in which prevention is recommended because

TABLE 10.3 USPSTF Recommendations for Appropriate Aspirin Use

• The USPSTF recommends initiating low-dose aspirin use for the primary prevention of CVD and colorectal cancer (CRC) in adults aged 50 to 59 years who have a 10% or greater 10-year CVD risk, are not at an increased risk for bleeding, have a life expectancy of at least 10 years, and are willing to take low-dose aspirin daily for at least 10 years.
Grade: B recommendation
• The decision to initiate low-dose aspirin use for the primary prevention of CVD and CRC in adults aged 60 to 69 years who have a 10% or greater 10-year CVD risk should be an individual one. People who are not at an increased risk for bleeding, have a life expectancy of at least 10 years, and are willing to take low-dose aspirin daily for at least 10 years are more likely to benefit. People who place a higher value on the potential benefits than the potential harms may choose to initiate low-dose aspirin.
Grade: C recommendation
• The current evidence is insufficient to assess the balance of benefits and harms of initiating aspirin use for the primary prevention of CVD and CRC in adults younger than 50 years.
Grade: I recommendation
• The current evidence is insufficient to assess the balance of benefits and harms of initiating aspirin use for the primary prevention of CVD and CRC in adults aged 70 years or older.
Grade: D recommendation

CVD, cardiovascular disease; USPSTF, U.S. Preventive Service Task Force.

Source: Adapted with permission of USPSTF (2016).

of the presence of either ischemic vascular disease or risk factors. Despite knowing which patients were already on an aspirin regimen and thus did not need their physician to prescribe it, or aspirin use was contraindicated, the authors determined that a higher percentage of patients should be on aspirin prevention therapy. Appropriate aspirin therapy for the secondary prevention of CVD is an integral part of the Million Hearts Initiative (Parekh, Galloway, Hong, & Wright, 2013). If APRNs followed the UPSTF guidelines, the gap in appropriate aspirin use could surely be narrowed.

B is for blood pressure control. Blood pressure control is challenging, as evidenced by the millions of Americans that live with uncontrolled hypertension. The NIH's National Heart, Lung, and Blood Institute (NHLBI) published the eighth report of the Joint National Committee on Prevention, Detection, Evaluation, and Treatment of High Blood Pressure (JNC 8) in 2014 (James et al., 2014). The first step in effectively controlling hypertension is assessing for it correctly. The standard of care for in-office blood pressure measurement is to take the average of two readings 5 minutes apart with appropriate cuff size while the patient is sitting in a chair with both legs flat on the floor. An abnormal reading should be confirmed in the contralateral arm. Home blood pressure monitoring should be strongly encouraged for those with known to have or who are at high risk for hypertension. Although the USPSTF currently supports ambulatory blood pressure measurement as the gold standard for diagnosing hypertension, there is growing evidence to support home blood pressure monitoring over ambulatory blood pressure monitoring because patients' readings are closer to the readings taken by 24-hour ambulatory monitors, which eliminates falsely elevated readings from white coat syndrome (Pickering et al., 2008). With the plethora of technologically savvy health devices, there are blood pressure cuffs that plug into iphones, ipads, and other smart devices, which collect blood pressure data and then transmit the data to clinicians. As many of these devices have not been validated for accuracy, it is necessary to educate patients about checking for device validation and U.S. Food and Drug Administration (FDA) approval. Electronic health records can record the data and send an alert to the patient's clinician when the blood pressure becomes out of target range. Leslie L. Davis PhD, RN, ANP-BC published a useful tutorial for clinicians to use to implement home blood pressure monitoring for their patients (Davis, 2011). Dr. Davis is active in supporting Million Hearts and is a clinical assistant professor at the University of North Carolina at Chapel Hill in the School of Medicine, Division of Cardiology. Accurate and consistent blood pressure monitoring is necessary for diagnosing and controlling hypertension.

Million Hearts was founded on and continues to adhere to the JNC 7 guidelines as the new JNC 8 recommendations do not explicitly push healthy diets, weight control, or exercise. These therapeutic lifestyle modifications benefit those with hypertension and are recommended in the 2013 Lifestyles Work Group (Eckel et al., 2014). Therapeutic lifestyle modifications include weight loss, the Dietary Approaches to Stop Hypertension (DASH) eating plan, regular exercise, limited alcohol intake, and cessation of use of tobacco products. Heartening for both care practitioners and patients alike is that weight loss as little as 10 lbs. (4.5 kg) can reduce blood pressure significantly. The DASH diet includes eating many fruits and vegetables, choosing low-fat varieties of dairy products, choosing low cholesterol protein sources, reducing overall fat intake to include reduced saturated fats and elimination of trans fat, and reducing sodium intake. The overall

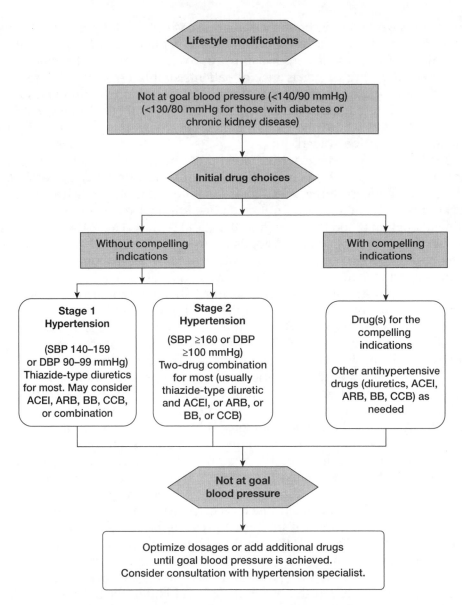

FIGURE 10.3 The JNC 7 Algorithm for Treating Hypertension.

Source: National Heart, Lung, and Blood Institute (2004).

diet should be rich in calcium and potassium. In addition, everyone should engage in an aerobic physical activity for at least 30 minutes on most days.

Noteworthy in the JNC 8 recommendations is that all patients with hypertension need to be on medication management while they implement lifestyle modifications. Most people with hypertension require more than one drug to bring their hypertension under adequate control, and no recommendation initiates medication regimen(s) with a beta blocker. Some clinicians may begin therapy using a thiazide diuretic alone or in combination with other classes of agents, especially if the patient is an African American, has diabetes, is obese, and/or has other cardiovascular chronic diseases. The JNC 8 includes goals and modifications of treatment for hypertension that vary for different categories of clinical complexity including race. The advantage of using multidrug therapy is achieving greater blood pressure reduction at lower doses with fewer side effects. The consideration to prescribe multiple medications should be balanced with the patient's ability to pay for multiple medications and to adhere to taking multiple drugs, especially if they are needed to be taken more than once or twice a day. However, experiencing fewer side effects will likely increase adherence. Moreover, noteworthy for adherence considerations is that older diuretics and older beta blockers dampen erectile function whereas many newer drugs do not (Manolis, & Doumas, 2012). Some patients may be hesitant to speak about erectile dysfunction to their clinician, so it behooves the clinician to consider erectile dysfunction when assessing causes of low medication adherence. Following the NIH NHBLI guidelines for follow-up and monitoring of hypertensive patients is essential.

C is for cholesterol management. The American College of Cardiology in conjunction with the AHA updated guidelines for the treatment of blood cholesterol to reduce CVD risk (Stone et al., 2014). These guidelines stress that reducing atherosclerotic cardiovascular disease (ASCVD) risk in those most likely to benefit from this risk reduction is critical. Aside from a group of New York Heart Association (NYHA) class II–IV heart failure patients not receiving hemodialysis, extensive and consistent evidence supports the use of statins for high-risk primary prevention and all secondary prevention. The guidelines stress that although statins play a key role in risk reduction, lifestyle changes remain essential. Although statins decrease ASCVD risk, they are not without their side effects. Side effects such as myopathy or the perceived risk of side effects have led to high levels of statin nonadherence (Harrison et al., 2013). As statins do increase the risk of myopathy and kidney disease, patients should be educated to report side effects as soon as possible (Yongbin et al., 2016).

The S is for smoking cessation, which is already covered in this chapter. While smoking cessation is critical for primary and secondary prevention of CVD, it is also necessary to assess if the patient is using smokeless tobacco products. Nicotine, whether inhaled or absorbed through the mouth, causes vasoconstriction of blood vessels and rises in blood pressure. According to the CDC, in 2014, 3.4% of adults used smokeless tobacco. Six percent of high school students used smokeless tobacco products as of 2015 (CDC, 2016c). These numbers are likely to increase because tobacco companies are spending hundreds of millions of dollars promoting smokeless tobacco products.

Health information technology (HIT) is an integral pillar of Million Hearts. HIT includes the use of patient registries to identify gaps in CVD prevention, use of multiple methods to track the progress of patients being treated for hypertension or hyperlipidemia, point-of-care risk assessment tools built into electronic health records (EHRs) to assist clinicians in identifying those at higher risk for disease or undiagnosed for hypertension, clinical decision support mechanisms through EHR systems to assist clinicians to deliver patient-specific care the first time and every time that the patient gets examined, and electronic reminders for consumers that assist them to develop and stick to new, healthier habits that may include medication adherence (J. O'Brien, PharmD, MPH, personal communication, March 3, 2011). For more information on Million Hearts and HIT visit www.millionhearts.hhs.gov/tools-protocols/tools/health-IT.html. It is critical to find patients with undiagnosed hypertension, and this is a key part of the HIT portfolio. More information about this can be found at millionhearts.hhs.gov/tools -protocols/hiding-plain-sight/index.html. A number of applications, or apps, for smart devices have also been developed as a result of private and public partner engagement in Million Hearts. The winner of the 2012 Million Hearts Risk Check Challenge, sponsored by the Office of the National Coordinator, is the Marshfield Clinic Research Foundation in Wisconsin. Their Heart Health mobile app is available in the Apple App Store or as a web-based version (www.hearthealth mobile.com) and is designed to reach those who may not know that they are at risk for coronary heart disease. The app conducts a quick health risk assessment within an engaging user interface, motivates users to pursue learning their blood pressure and cholesterol values, and directs them to pharmacies in their communities which offer affordable and convenient blood pressure and cholesterol screenings. Other app finalists whose apps remain available include HeartHealthMobile also by Marshfield Clinic Research Foundation (www.hearthealthmobile.com), and PharmaSmart Blood Pressure Tracker (www.pharma-smart.com). The Million Hearts website also has three app-like interfaces under the tool section to help consumers track and manage their heart health, determine 10-year risk of having a heart attack or dying from coronary heart disease, and learn the state of one's heart and about heart healthy behaviors (millionhearts.hhs.gov/resources/tools .html). These and other innovations are increasing the reach of Million Hearts.

A pleasant surprise of Million Hearts has been its unintended consequences. This initiative's effort has had an important positive impact on interagency collaboration within the DHHS, has resulted in the creation of many new private-public partnerships, especially for national nursing organizations, and has led to evidence discovery for interprofessional practice for the common goal of preventing and decreasing the harms of CVD. The Community Preventive Services Task Force does evidence-based reviews about interventions to promote public health and safety. Their members are appointed by the director of the CDC. In an analysis of 80 studies, team-based care was significantly superior for lowering both systolic and diastolic pressure and improved outcomes for a greater proportion of patients with diabetes and hyperlipidemia than physicians practicing solo (CDC, 2012a). Teams consisted of a primary care provider and another health professional such as a nurse, pharmacist, social worker, dietician, and/ or community health worker. Teams with the greatest proportion of successful blood pressure control were those in which the team members could change medications independently or with the approval of the primary care provider. Team member behaviors extended the work of the primary care provider by ". . . providing support and sharing responsibility for hypertension care, such as medication management, patient follow-up, and helping the patient adhere to their blood pressure control plan, including monitoring blood pressure routinely, taking medications as prescribed, reducing sodium in the diet, and increasing physical activity (CDC, 2012c). It is no coincidence that team-based care is a central pillar of Million Hearts.

Another unintended consequence of Million Hearts is that it is changing the paradigm of practice among the health professions. As discussed, there is a national "tipping point" push for interprofessional and transdisciplinary (includes direct care workers and others without advanced degrees) practice which involves the use of team specific competencies (Frenk et al., 2010; Interprofessional Education Collaborative Expert Panel, 2011). This team approach to practice, which breaks institutionalized silos between the health professions, is creating higher quality care. Furthermore, through participation in Million Hearts, these interprofessional teams and new public/private partnerships are creating more aggressive outreach to identify and begin early intervention of high blood pressure. Another paradigm change is the concept that "It takes a village to prevent and manage hypertension." Dentists, as well as optometrists and pharmacists, are taking blood pressures as a routine part of their intake process. Although the patient has always been the common element across providers of care, Million Hearts provides a more focused strategy and emphasizes the need for everyone to pay attention to the whole patient, whether they are having their eyes examined, getting their teeth cleaned, or having their medications evaluated at a regular checkup. Patients with high blood pressures or prehypertension are referred to their primary care clinician for follow-up. As the PPACA's reach and level of implementation widen, population health become a greater focus of health professionals who were previously focused solely on their patients. There is great optimism that these unintended consequences and many other strategies help meet the Million Hearts aim.

Million Hearts set both intervention target goals for clinical systems and target goals for the population as a whole to be reached by the end of 2016. Table 10.4 shows baseline data from 2011 as well as the target goals.

To reach target goals, Million Hearts has worked with public and private partners to align and embed the ABCS into major quality reporting initiatives, including the Physician Quality Reporting System (PQRS). This reporting system provides Medicare bonus payments or payment reduction for all eligible providers depending on their level of performance and patient outcomes. All APRNs were eligible to report PQRS measures (CMS, 2015). Moreover, beginning in 2013 eligible health professionals who did not report quality measures lost incentive payments and received less Medicare Part B reimbursement in a fee-for-service

TABLE 10.4 Million Hearts®: Status and Targets for the ABCS

INTERVENTION	BASELINE (2011)	DECEMBER 2016 TARGET FOR THE POPULATION AS A WHOLE	INTERVENTION TARGET FOR CLINICAL SYSTEMS OF CARE (%)
Aspirin, for those at high risk	47%	65%	70
Blood pressure control	46%	65%	70
Cholesterol management	33%	65%	70
Smoking cessation	23%	65%	70
Smoking prevalence	19%	17%	
Sodium intake (average)	3.5 g/d	20% reduction	
Artificial trans fat consumption (average)	1% of calories/day	50% reduction	

ABCS, appropriate aspirin use, blood pressure control, cholesterol control, and smoking cessation.

Sources: Baseline: http://www.cdc.gov/mmwr/preview/mmwrhtml/mm6036a4.htm?s_cid=mm6036a4_w 2017 goals of MH: http://millionhearts.hhs.gov/Docs/MH_Fact_Sheet.pdf

Clinical target goals: http://www.cdc.gov/about/grand-rounds/archives/2012/pdfs/GR_MH_ALL_FINAL_Feb28.pdf

system (CMS, 2015, 2017a). Table 10.5 shows which PQRS measures align with which part of the ABCS. Another reporting strategy is that all community health centers funded by HRSA had to report their progress on the ABCS to track and improve their performance.

The new Medicare Access and CHIP Reauthorization Act of 2015 (MACRA), which rolled out in 2017, incentivizes the ABCS of Million Hearts to a whole new level with a Merit-Based Incentive Payment System (MIPS) and Advanced Alternative Payment Models (APMs). MACRA consolidates PQRS, the Value Modifier Program, and Medicare incentives to use the electronic health record incentives under MIPS (Caresync, 2016). Although Medicare

TABLE 10.5 PQRS Measures That Support the ABCS

ABCS	DOMAIN	MEASURES	2012 PHYSICIAN QUALITY REPORTING SYSTEM (PQRS)
A	Aspirin use	The percentage of patients aged 18 years and older with the ischemic vascular disease will have documented use of aspirin or other antithrombotic therapy	#204
B	Blood pressure screening	The percentage of patients aged 18 years and older who are screened for high BP and have a documented follow-up plan based on current BP readings	#317
	Blood pressure control	The percentage of patients aged between 18 years and 85 years who have a diagnosis of HTN and whose BP was adequately controlled (<140/90) during the measurement year	#236
C	Cholesterol Screening and Control	The percentage of patients aged between 20 and 79 years whose risk factors have been assessed and a fasting low-density lipoprotein (LDL) test performed, and their fasting LDL is at or below the recommended LDL goal after risk stratification	#316
	Cholesterol Control – Diabetes	The percentage of patients aged between 18 and 75 years with diabetes mellitus who had their most recent LDL-C level in control	#2
	Cholesterol Control – Ischemic Vascular Disease	The percentage of patients aged 18 years and older with the ischemic vascular disease who received at least one lipid profile within 12 months and who had their most recent LDL-C under control (<100 mg/dL)	#241
S	Smoking cessation	The percentage of patients aged 18 years and older who are screened for tobacco use one or more times within 24 months and received cessation counseling intervention(s) if identified as a tobacco user	#226

ABCS, appropriate aspirin use, blood pressure control, cholesterol control, and smoking cessation; BP, blood pressure; HTN, hypertension; LDL-C, low density lipoprotein cholesterol.

Source: Million Hearts® (2012).

LEARNING SCENARIO #1

Mrs. S, an African American obese female has an appointment with you for a yearly physical that is mandated by her employer, a public metro agency where she works as a bus driver. You read on the electronic medical record that last year she weighed 275 pounds and that her height is 5'5". She was borderline hypertensive and was encouraged to engage in lifestyle modifications. There is a history of adult onset diabetes and hypertension on her mother's side of the family and history of heart disease on her father's side of the family. You assess her on this visit and find that her resting blood pressure (average taken 5 minutes apart) is 150/95, pulse 85, and fasting blood sugar is 110. Her fasting cholesterol remains high, with total cholesterol 275 mg/dL, LDL 180 mg/dL, high-density lipoproteins (HDL) 30 mg/dL, and triglycerides 350 mg/dL. She reports that she drinks alcohol occasionally and is down to smoking one pack of cigarettes a day. She has no idea how many mg of sodium she consumes every day. She notices that she is getting more short of breath going up the stairs in her home.

1. Does Mrs. S need primary or secondary prevention measures to prevent heart attack and stroke?
2. What other physical and psychosocial information do you need to collect to come up with an appropriate treatment plan for Mrs. S?
3. How would you individualize the ABCS for Mrs. S?
4. Are there any referrals you would like to make and if so what are they?
5. How will you follow up with Mrs. S?

Activities

1. Role play this scenario with one student playing Mrs. S and another student playing the APRN.
2. Write a sample office visit history and physical and treatment narrative.

Practice the components of motivational interviewing using Mrs. S as the patient.

LEARNING SCENARIO #2

You work in a primary care practice medical home for a health system with a Medicare Shared Savings Accountable Care Organization. You just had a practice meeting about what MACRA mean for your practice's reimbursement.

1. What quality and reimbursement levels do you bring to the meeting to support clinicians' investment in Million Hearts?
2. What ways can the entire medical home team work together to ensure patients understand how to avoid a heart attack or stroke and adhere to evidence-based preventive measures?
3. How would you go about finding out what percentage of your patients had their blood pressure under control?
4. What other metrics about your performance regarding Million Hearts would you want to find out ?

estimates 700,000 providers will be held accountable to MIPS, nurse midwives are exempt as well as any provider generating less than $10,000 in Medicare Part B reimbursement and those who have less than 100 Medicare beneficiaries. In addition, any provider determined by Medicare to be significantly participating in an APM is exempt from MIPS. The AANP has resources on MACRA on their web page (https://www.aanp.org/legislation-regulation/federal-legislation/macra-s-quality-payment-program#macra-resources), as does the American Academy of Family Physicians (www.aafp.org/practice-management/payment/medicare-payment.html).

In conclusion, APRNs can lead in improving the health of the nation by simply stepping up what they do well, and that is blood pressure control and other means to prevent CVD and its complications. There are so many opportunities for nurses to partner with the federal government and become a significant part of implementing the PPACA in the area of population health than ever before through participation in the Million Hearts Initiative. Federal agencies, as well as the White House, have taken notice of the role APRNs can have in providing high-value primary care with integration of preventive services. For more information about Million Hearts and to access CVD risk assessment tools and a variety of clinical decision support tools (i.e., evidence-based protocols, action guides, and other tools and information) visit millionhearts.hhs.gov. Million Hearts is a trademark of the USDHHS.

REFERENCES

Agency for Healthcare Research and Quality. (2008). Treating tobacco use and dependence. Retrieved from https://www.ahrq.gov/sites/default/files/wysiwyg/professionals/clinicians-providers/guidelines-recommendations/tobacco/clinicians/references/quickref/tobaqrg.pdf

American Academy of Nurses. (2016). Call to action: Nursing action necessary to prevent one million heart attacks and strokes by 2017. *Nursing Outlook, 64*(2), 197–199.

American Association of Nurse Practitioners. (2012). 2012 AANP National NP sample survey. Report on prescribing. Retrieved from https://www.aanp.org/membership/153-research/public-research-accordion/1409-aanp-national-np-sample-survey-p

American Association of Nurse Practitioners. (2016). 2016 AANP National NP sample survey. Retrieved from https://www.aanp.org/membership/153-research/public-research-accordion/1409-aanp-national-np-sample-survey-p

American Heart Association. (2014). Overweight in children. Retrieved from http://www.heart.org/HEARTORG/GettingHealthy/Overweight-in-Children_UCM_304054_Article.jsp

American Nurses Association. (2011). Advanced practice nursing: A new age in healthcare. Retrieved from http://www.nursingworld.org/FunctionalMenuCategories/MediaResources/MediaBackgrounders/APRN-A-New-Age-in-Health-Care.pdf

Caresync. (2016). Game changer: Preparing for success with MACRA. Retrieved from http://learn.caresync.com/white-paper-macra/?GA_network=g&GA_device=c&GA_campaign=625287781&GA_adgroup=33790221681&GA_target=&GA_placement=&GA_creative=116042842761&GA_extension=&GA_keyword=macra&GA_loc_physical_ms=9008238&GA_landingpage=http://learn.caresync.com/white-paper-macra/&gclid=Cj0KEQjwhbzABRDHw_i4q6fXoLIBEiQANZKGW-U-Qb3CsAy9Nm5B1c8sHhCBsf_s8Rsh_ea6NzMVbSYaAoWR8P8HAQ

Centers for Disease Control and Prevention. (2011a). CDC National Heart Disease and Stroke Prevention Program: Staff orientation guide. Retrieved from http://www.cdc.gov/dhdsp/programs/spha/docs/orientation_manual.pdf

Centers for Disease Control and Prevention. (2011b). Most Americans with high blood pressure and high cholesterol at unnecessary risk for heart attack and stroke. Retrieved from http://www.cdc.gov/media/releases/2011/p0201_vitalsigns.html

Centers for Disease Control and Prevention. (2011c). New Million Hearts tools announced by partners. Retrieved from http://millionhearts.hhs.gov/docs/MH_Partners_Press_Release_11-3-2011.pdf

Centers for Disease Control and Prevention. (2012a). Cardiovascular disease: Team-based care to improve blood pressure control: Task force finding and rationale statement. Retrieved from https://www.thecommunityguide.org/findings/cardiovascular-disease-team-based-care-improve-blood-pressure-control

Centers for Disease Control and Prevention. (2012b). CDC vital signs. Where's the sodium? There's too much in many common foods. Retrieved from http://www.cdc.gov/vitalsigns/Sodium/index.html

Centers for Disease Control and Prevention. (2012c). Task force recommends team-based care for improving blood pressure control. Retrieved from http://www.cdc.gov/media/releases/2012/p0515_bp_control.html

Centers for Disease Control and Prevention. (2012d). Trans fat: The facts. Retrieved from http://www.cdc.gov/nutrition/downloads/trans_fat_final.pdf

Centers for Disease Control and Prevention. (2013a). Education campaign returns with powerful stories to help Americans quit smoking. Retrieved from http://www.cdc.gov/media/releases/2013/p0328_TIPS_campaign.html

Centers for Disease Control and Prevention. (2013b). Self-reported hypertension and use of antihypertensive medication among adults—United States, 2005–2009. *Morbidity and Mortality Weekly Report, 62*(13), 237–244. Retrieved from http://www.cdc.gov/mmwr/preview/mmwrhtml/mm6213a2.htm?s_cid=mm6213a2_e

Centers for Disease Control and Prevention. (2015a). Heart disease and stroke cost America nearly $1 billion a day in medical costs, lost productivity. Retrieved from http://www.cdcfoundation.org/pr/2015/heart-disease-and-stroke-cost-america-nearly-1-billion-day-medical-costs-lost-productivity

Centers for Disease Control and Prevention. (2015b). Heart disease fact sheet. Retrieved from https://www.cdc.gov/dhdsp/data_statistics/fact_sheets/fs_heart_disease.htm

Centers for Disease Control and Prevention. (2016a). Current cigarette smoking among adults in the United States. Retrieved from http://www.cdc.gov/tobacco/data_statistics/fact_sheets/adult_data/cig_smoking/index.htm

Centers for Disease Control and Prevention. (2016b). High blood pressure facts. Retrieved from http://www.cdc.gov/bloodpressure/facts.htm

Centers for Disease Control and Prevention. (2016c). Smokeless tobacco use in the United States. Retrieved from https://www.cdc.gov/tobacco/data_statistics/fact_sheets/smokeless/use_us/index.htm

Centers for Disease Control and Prevention. (2017a). High blood pressure. Retrieved from http://www.cdc.gov/bloodpressure

Centers for Disease Control and Prevention. (2017b). Obesity and overweight. Retrieved from http://www.cdc.gov/nchs/fastats/obesity-overweight.htm

Centers for Medicare and Medicaid Services. (2015). Physician Quality Reporting System (PQRS): List of eligible professionals. Retrieved from http://www.cms.gov/Medicare/Quality-Initiatives-Patient-Assessment-Instruments/PQRS/Downloads/PQRS_List-of-EligibleProfessionals_022813.pdf

Centers for Medicare and Medicaid Services. (2017a). Spotlight. Retrieved from http://www.cms.gov/Medicare/Quality-Initiatives-Patient-Assessment-Instruments/PQRS/Spotlight.html

Centers for Medicare and Medicaid Services. (2017b). 2016 CMS Quality Conference news & announcements. Retrieved from http://qioprogram.org/qionews/articles/2016-cms-quality-conference-news-announcements

Davis, L. (2011). How to implement home BP monitoring. *The Clinical Advisor.* Retrieved from http://www.clinicaladvisor.com/how-to-implement-home-bp-monitoring/article/206808/1

Eckel, R., Jakicic, J. M., Ard, J. D., de Jesus, J. M., Houston Miller, N., Hubbard, V. S., . . . Yanovski, S. Z. (2014). 2013 AHA/ACC guideline on lifestyle management to reduce cardiovascular risk: A report of the American College of Cardiology/American Heart Association Task Force on practice guidelines. *Circulation, 129*(25, Suppl. 2), S76–S99. doi:10.1161/01.cir.0000437740.48606.d1

Fauteux, N. (2012). Implementing the Future of Nursing Report–part III: Issue 18 of the Charting Nursing's Future series shows how nurses are solving some of primary care's most pressing challenges. Retrieved from http://www.rwjf.org/en/library/research/2012/07/cnf-implementing-the-future-of-nursing-report-part-three.html

Frenk, J., Chen, L., Bhutta, Z. A., Cohen, J., Crisp, N., & Evans, T., . . . Zurayk, H. (2010). Health professionals for a new century: Transforming education to strengthen health systems in an interdependent world. *The Lancet, 376*(9756), 1923–1958.

Frieden, T. R., & Berwick, D. M. (2011). The "Million Hearts" initiative—Preventing heart attacks and strokes. *New England Journal of Medicine, 365,* e27. Retrieved from http://www.nejm.org/doi/full/10.1056/NEJMp1110421

George, M. G., Tong, X., Sonnenfeld, N., & Hong, Y. (2012). Recommended use of aspirin and other antiplatelet medications among adults—National Ambulatory Medical Care Survey and National Hospital Ambulatory Medical Care Survey, United States, 2005–2008. *Morbidity and Mortality Weekly Report Supplements, 61*(2), 11–18. Retrieved from http://www.cdc.gov/mmwr/preview/mmwrhtml/su6102a3.htm

Harrison, T. N., Derose, S. F., Cheetham, T. C., Chiu, V., Vansomphone, S. S., Green, K., . . . Reynolds, K. (2013). Primary nonadherence to statin therapy: Patients' perceptions. *American Journal of Managed Care, 19*(4), e133–e139.

Health Affairs. (2010). Health policy briefs: Preventive services without cost sharing. *Health Affairs.* Retrieved from http://www.healthaffairs.org/healthpolicybriefs/brief.php?brief_id=37

Health Affairs. (2013). Health policy brief: Nurse practitioners and primary care. *Health Affairs.* Retrieved from http://healthaffairs.org/healthpolicybriefs/brief_pdfs/healthpolicybrief_92.pdf

Health Resources and Services Administration. (n.d.). School-based health centers. Retrieved from http://www.hrsa.gov/ourstories/schoolhealthcenters

Health Resources and Services Administration. (2010). The registered nurse population: Findings from the 2008 National Sample Survey of Registered Nurses. Retrieved from https://bhw.hrsa.gov/sites/default/files/bhw/nchwa/rnsurveyfinal.pdf

HealthyPeople 2020. (n.d.). Heart disease and stroke. Retrieved from http://www.healthypeople.gov/2020/topicsobjectives2020/overview.aspx?topicid=21#two

Institute of Medicine. (2010). *The future of nursing: Leading change, advancing health.* Washington, DC: National Academies Press. Retrieved from http://www.nationalacademies.org/Reports/2010/The-Future-of-Nursing-Leading-Change-Advancing-Health.aspx

Institute of Medicine. (2013). *Sodium intake in populations: Assessment of evidence.* Washington, DC: National Academies Press. Retrieved from https://www.nap.edu/catalog/18311/sodium-intake-in-populations-assessment-of-evidence

Interprofessional Education Collaborative Expert Panel. (2011). Core competencies for interprofessional collaborative practice: Report of an expert panel. Washington, DC: Interprofessional Education Collaborative. Retrieved from https://www.aamc.org/download/186750/data/core_competencies.pdf

James, P., Oparil, S., Carter, B., Cushman, W., Cennison-Himmelfarb, C., Handler, J., . . . Ortiz, E. (2014). 2014 evidence-based guideline for the management of high blood pressure in adults: A report from the panel members appointed to the Eighth Joint National Committee (JNC 8). *Journal of the American Medical Association, 311*(5), 507–520. Retrieved from http://jamanetwork.com/journals/jama/fullarticle/1791497

Kochanek, K. D., Xu, J. Q., Murphy, S. L., Miniño, A. M., & Kung, H. C. (2011). Deaths: Final data for 2009. *National Vital Statistics Reports, 60*(3). Retrieved from http://www.cdc.gov/nchs/data/nvsr/nvsr60/nvsr60_03.pdf

Kovner, C., & Walani, S. (2010). Nurse managed health centers. *Robert Wood Johnson Foundation Research Brief.* Retrieved from https://campaignforaction.org/wp-content/uploads/2016/04/Research-Brief-Nurse-Managed-Health-Centers.pdf

Lloyd-Jones, D., Adams, R. J., Brown, T. M., Carnethon, M., Dai, S., De Simone, G., . . . Wylie-Rosett, J. (2010). Heart disease and stroke statistics—2010 update: A report from the American Heart Association. *Circulation, 121*(7), e46–e215. doi:10.1161/CIRCULATIONAHA.109.192667

Manolis, A., & Doumas, M. (2012). Antihypertensive treatment and sexual dysfunction. *Current Hypertension Reports, 14*(4), 285–292.

McMenamin, P. (2013). In 2011 in every state thousands of medicare F-F-S beneficiaries were treated by an APRN. *American Nurses Association Nurse Space.* Retrieved from http://www.ananursespace.org/BlogsMain/BlogViewer/?BlogKey=9632c2fa-6fc3-4a1b-93ad-343cd90058f1&ssopc=1

Melnyk, B., Orsolini, L., Gawlik, K., Braun, L., Chyun, D., Conn, V., . . . Olin, A. (2016). The Million Hearts initiative: Guidelines and best practices. *The Nurse Practitioner, 41*(2), 46–53.

Million Hearts®. (2012). Opportunities for engagement in Million Hearts. Retrieved from https://dph.georgia.gov/sites/dph.georgia.gov/files/3.%20Million_Hearts_Opportunities_for_Engagement.pdf

Million Hearts®. (2016). About Million Hearts®. Retrieved from https://millionhearts.hhs.gov/about-million-hearts/index.html

Mozaffarian, D., Benjamin, E., Go, A., Arnett, D., Blaha, M. Cushman, M., . . . Turner, M. (2016). Heart disease and stroke statistics—2016 update: A report from the American Heart Association. *Circulation, 133*, 447–454. doi:10.1161/CIR.0000000000000350

National Center for Health Statistics. (2001). *Healthy People 2000 final review*. Hyattsville, MD: Public Health Service. Retrieved from http://www.cdc.gov/nchs/data/hp2000/hp2k01.pdf

National Heart, Lung, and Blood Institute. (2004). The seventh report of the Joint National Committee on prevention, detection, evaluation, and treatment of high blood pressure. Retrieved from http://www.nhlbi.nih.gov/guidelines/hypertension/jnc7full.pdf

Parekh, A. K., Galloway, J. M., Hong, Y., & Wright, J. S. (2013). Aspirin in the secondary prevention of cardiovascular disease. *New England Journal of Medicine, 368*(3), 204–205.

Pbert, L., Druker, S., DiFranza, J. R., Gorak, D., Reed, G., Magner, R., . . . Osganian, S. (2011). Effectiveness of a school nurse-delivered smoking-cessation intervention for adolescents. *Pediatrics, 128*(5), 926–936.

Pickering, T. G., Houston Miller, N., Ogedegbe, G., Krakoff, L. R., Artinian, N. T., & Goff, D. (2008). Call to action on use and reimbursement for home blood pressure monitoring: A joint scientific statement from the American Heart Association, American Society of Hypertension, and Preventive Cardiovascular Nurses Association. *Hypertension, 52*, 10–29. Retrieved from http://hyper.aha journals.org/content/52/1/10.full.pdf+html

Stone, N., Robinson, J., Lichtenstein, A., Merz, N., Blum, C., Eckel, R., . . . Wilson, P. (2014). 2013 ACC/AHA guideline on the treatment of blood cholesterol to reduce atherosclerotic cardiovascular risk in adults: A report of the American College of Cardiology/American Heart Association Task Force on practice guidelines. *Circulation, 129*(25, Suppl. 2), S1–S45. doi:10.1161/01.cir.0000437738.63853.7a

Strozer, J., Juszczak, L., & Ammerman, A. (2010). School-based health centers: National Census 2007–2008. Retrieved from http://www.sbh4all.org/wp-content/uploads/2015/06/NASBHC-2007-08-Census-Report-Final.pdf

U.S. Department of Agriculture and U.S. Department of Health and Human Services. (2010). Dietary guidelines for Americans 2010. Retrieved from http://health.gov/dietaryguidelines/dga2010/dietaryguidelines2010.pdf

U.S. Department of Health and Human Services. (2012a). Attachment to the Annual Progress Report to Congress national strategy for quality improvement in healthcare: Agency-specific quality strategic plans. Retrieved from http://www.ahrq.gov/workingforquality/nqs/nqsplans .pdf

U.S. Department of Health and Human Services. (2012b). *Preventing tobacco use among youth and young adults: A report of the surgeon general*. Atlanta, GA: U.S. Department of Health and Human Services, Centers for Disease Control and Prevention, National Center for Chronic Disease Prevention and Health Promotion, Office on Smoking and Health. Retrieved from http://www.surgeongeneral .gov/library/reports/preventing-youth-tobacco-use/full-report.pdf

U.S. Department of Health and Human Services. (2016a). About the National Quality Strategy. Retrieved from http://www.ahrq.gov/workingforquality/about.htm

U.S. Department of Health and Human Services. (2016b). About the Affordable Care Act. Retrieved from https://www.hhs.gov/healthcare/about-the-aca/index.html

U.S. Department of Health and Human Services. (2016c). The Million Hearts initiative. Retrieved from http://millionhearts.hhs.gov/index.html

U.S. Department of Health and Human Services, Office of Disease Prevention and Health Promotion. (2016). Healthy people 2020. Retrieved from www.healthypeople.gov

U.S. Department of Health and Human Services Public Health Service. (2008). Clinical practice guideline: Treating tobacco use and dependence 2008 update. Retrieved from https://www.ahrq.gov/sites/default/files/wysiwyg/professionals/clinicians-providers/guidelines-recommendations/tobacco/clinicians/update/treating_tobacco_use08.pdf

U.S. Preventive Service Task Force. (2012). Grade definitions. Retrieved from http://www.uspreventive servicestaskforce.org/uspstf/grades.htm

U.S. Preventive Service Task Force. (2015). Tobacco smoking cessation in adults, including pregnant women: Behavioral and pharmacotherapy interventions. Retrieved from https://www.uspreventiveservicestaskforce.org/Page/Document/UpdateSummaryFinal/tobacco-use-in-adults-and-pregnant-women-counseling-and-interventions1

U.S. Preventive Service Task Force. (2016). Aspirin use to prevent of cardiovascular disease and colorectal cancer: Preventive medicine. Retrieved from https://www.uspreventiveservices taskforce.org/Page/Document/UpdateSummaryFinal/aspirin-to-prevent-cardiovascular -disease-and-cancer?ds=1&s=aspirin

Wright, W. L., Romboli, J. E., DiTulio, M. A., Wogen, J., & Belletti, D. A. (2011). Hypertension treatment and control within an independent nurse practitioner setting. *American Journal of Managed Care, 17*(1), 58–65. Retrieved from http://www.ajmc.com/publications/issue/2011/2011-1-vol17-n1/AJMC_2011jan_Wright_58to65/3

Yongbin, L., Cheng, Z., Zhao, Y., Chang, X., Chan, C., Bai, Y., & Cheng, N. (2016). Efficacy and safety of long-term treatment with statins for coronary heart disease: A Bayesian network meta-analysis. *Atherosclerosis, 254,* 215–227. doi:10.1016/j.atherosclerosis.2016.10.025

CHAPTER 11

Value-Based Purchasing and Its Impact on Advanced Practice Nursing

Elizabeth A. Landin

A pivotal strategy to improve the quality of health care while lowering costs in the United States is value-based purchasing (VBP). VBP, referring to a comprehensive set of performance-based payment strategies, links performance on quality measures to provider reimbursement rather than reimbursement from a fee-for-service/volume-based system. Although originally implemented by Medicare for inpatient care only, VBP now includes providers of outpatient care enabling purchasers of health care to hold providers accountable. Additionally, the quality-performance measures apply to all patients, not just those on Medicare.

The Centers for Medicare and Medicaid Services (CMS) has developed a quality strategy that focuses on improving care by using incentives, using new payment models that tie payment to value, changing how care is given through better teamwork, improving coordination across health care settings, creating more awareness about population health, and putting health care information to work. The CMS website lists the quality strategy goals as making care safer by reducing harm to patients, helping patients to be involved in their care, promoting coordination of care and effective communication, promoting effective treatment and/or prevention of chronic disease, assisting communities in remaining healthy, and making care affordable. To meet these goals, the CMS quality strategy builds on four foundational principles: (a) eliminating racial and ethnic disparities; (b) strengthening data systems and infrastructure; (c) enabling innovations at a local level; and (d) fostering learning organizations. These goals and principles guide the aim of the value-based programs by providing better care for patients at a lower cost (CMS, 2016).

Currently, CMS has nine existing or planned value-based programs (discussed later in this chapter) resulting from four different legislations passed: in 2008, Medicare Improvements for Patients and Providers Act (MIPPA); in 2010, the Affordable Care Act (ACA); in 2014, Protecting Access to Medicare Act (PAMA);

and in 2015, the Medicare Access and CHIP Reauthorization Act of 2015 (MACRA; CMS, 2016). Five that have started are: the End-Stage Renal Disease Quality Incentive Program (ESRD QIP); the Hospital-Acquired Condition Reduction Program (HACRP); the Hospital Readmissions Reduction Program (HRR); the Hospital Value-Based Purchasing (HVBP) Program; the Home Health Value-Based Purchasing (HHVBP) Program; and the Value Modifier (VM) or Physician Value-Based Modifier (PVBM). Still to come are: in 2018, the Skilled Nursing Facility Value-Based Purchasing (SNFVBP) Program and in 2019, the Alternative Payment Models (APMs) and the Merit-Based Incentive Payment System (MIPS; CMS, 2016). As health care reform progresses, Advanced Practice Registered Nurses (APRNs) must become thoroughly familiar with VBP and its role in their practice.

BRIEF HISTORICAL BACKGROUND

In the 1990s, the increases in the American health insurance benefit demands and the increase in health care costs in conjunction with the compounded projection of Medicare costs amplified the burden on the federal budget. At that time fee-for-service reimbursement was volume-based, thus producing fragmentation, inefficiency, waste of resources, ineffective processes, and a decreased focus on quality (Aroh, Colella, Douglas, & Eddings, 2015). In 1994, the Institute of Medicine (IOM) issued a report titled *America's Health in Transition: Protecting and Improving Quality*. This report confirmed a need to direct attention to the quality of health care in America and improve on it (IOM, 1994). Thus, the IOM recommended a three-phase tactic. In the first phase, the lack of quality in health care delivery was documented. In the second phase, occurring from 1999 to 2001, several reports were issued by the Committee on the Quality of Health Care in America and the IOM. This included the IOM report, *To Err Is Human: Building a Safer Health Care System* in 1999 and in 2001 *Crossing the Quality Chasm: a New Health System for the 21st Century* (Marjoua & Bozic, 2012). The *Quality Chasm* report outlined a health care system, which was the objective of the third phase. To change the health care delivery system from the disease management medical model to a focus on health maintenance and disease prevention that will advance chronic disease outcomes and population health, CMS began investigating pay-for-performance (P4P; Aroh et al., 2015).

Four criteria must be met to use quality measures and data reporting and pay-for-performance. First, the measurement strategy must be grounded on a robust footing of research that demonstrates that the process addressed by the measure leads to improved clinical outcomes when performed correctly. Second, the strategy must correctly capture if evidence-based care has been given. Third, the measure should address a process adjacent to the desired outcome with relatively few prevailing processes. Finally, there should be no unintentional or minimal adverse consequences (Chassin, Loeb, Schmaltz, & Wachter, 2010). These four criteria are used to guide accountability measures and ensuring evidence-based practice as the quality of care and patient outcomes continue to advance—these are the drivers for VBP. CMS and The Joint Commission (TJC) work together to systematize these measures to lessen the occurrence of duplicate reporting while realizing that these measures need to be constantly changing to synchronize with developing science.

In 2003, the Social Security Act for CMS was mandated by the legislature to inaugurate a VBP reimbursement program. In October 2012, the VBP Program was introduced as part of health care reform under the Patient Protection and Affordable Care Act (PPACA), also called the ACA, which was launched in 2010 (Berwick & Hackbarth, 2012; Henkel & Maryland, 2015). Under VBP, CMS rewards hospitals based on the quality of care, use of and compliance with best clinical practices, and patient satisfaction with care during a hospital stay (CMS, 2015). This translates to payment for patient outcomes and satisfaction but not how many patients a given person cared for.

APPLICATION TO APRN PRACTICE

As previously stated, VBP connects performance on quality measures and costs to provider reimbursement. Simply put, the value is a connotation of both cost and quality. The VBP initiative assesses the patient experience and includes evidence-based practice. VBP is a program that continues to evolve every fiscal year with changes in measurement, indicators, and reimbursements, and APRNs need to be familiar with the VBP programs and the changes as they occur. According to the National Business Coalition on Health (2011), there are four elements to producing a framework for effective VBP. The first element consists of standardized performance measurement that should be accomplished by health plans, hospitals, physician groups, and individual health care practitioners. This standardized information should be converted into information that purchasers, payers, and consumers can access, enabling them to make an informed decision for payments and provider selection. Element two is transparency and regular and timely public reporting. Transparency should be evidence in informing consumers of health care costs in advance of standard procedures or visits—emergent issues cannot always be predicted. The third element is a successful payment innovation such as the CMS programs. Element four consists of an informed consumer choice through consumer education.

Types of VBP. According to a research report conducted by RAND Health, there are three broad types of VBP: pay-for-performance, accountable care organization, and bundled payments (Damberg et al., 2014). Pay-for-performance is a reimbursement system in which providers are either rewarded or penalized based on meeting benchmarks for quality and/or efficiency measures. Accountable care organizations are composed of providers and hospitals who coordinate care and "agree to be held accountable for the overall cost and quality of care for an assigned population of patients" (Damberg et al., 2014, p. 6). In bundled payments, financial and quality performance responsibility regulate the expected costs for a bundle of related health care services or a clinically defined episode. Table 11.1 gives an overview of the three types of VBP as well as incentives and risks associated with these types.

CMS VBP programs. Although all of the CMS's value-based programs are moving our nation's hospitals and providers toward payment for quality rather than quantity, there are specific programs identified, each similar in appearance but with different measures. This section briefly discusses each program. It should be noted that while VBP and the scoring system were designed to maximize patient outcomes, they do not direct how hospitals should achieve these outcomes. This gives facilities and providers the flexibility to implement changes to increase the value of services delivered to their patients. Additionally, the

TABLE 11.1 VBP Types

VBP TYPE	SUMMARY OVERVIEW	INCENTIVE	RISK
Pay-for-performance	• Works by establishing, measuring, and reporting clinical quality benchmarks. • Focus is on quality.	• Rewards providers for reaching clinical quality aims. • Allows smaller practices to align provider payment with value to avoid large capital expenditures such as clinical integration and information technology (IT).	• Viewed as a still rewarding provider for volume rather than value without necessarily reducing services.
Accountable care organization	• Includes shared risk, global capitation, and provider-sponsored health plans. • Involves set prices or budgets where the provider agrees to assume accountability.	• Stakeholders are motivated to work together to reduce costs by placing an emphasis on disease prevention and health maintenance. • Gives incentives for improving care and increased market penetration.	• If targeted costs are exceeded (cost variation), liability for a portion of the cost of care falls on the provider.
Bundled payments	• These are like fixed-price contracts where a budget is provided to cover estimated costs associated with all patient care for an episode, condition, or procedure. • Objective is to maximize the value for the patient per episode.	• Performance incentives are related to quality, patient experience, and cost efficiency. • Rewards provider for providing less costly episodes of care. • May have an added incentive to prevent unnecessary procedures. • Allows provider flexibility to decide which services are offered to achieve the desired outcome.	• The largest risk occurs when the episode of care or condition exceeds the negotiated cost of service. • These are like fee-for-service, which can increase the potential for payment as episode or procedures for a given patient increase.

VBP, value-based purchasing.

Source: Adapted from Henkel and Maryland (2015) and Damberg et al. (2014).

facilities can increase the amounts of incentive payment received by identifying which measures impact performance scores the most. More information on these programs, including the formulas to calculate the adjustment factors and payment adjustment amounts, can be found on the CMS website (www.cms.gov).

ESRD QIP. As part of the MIPPA, the ESRD program was implemented in 2012. In 2016, the fourth year for this program, there were eight clinical and five reporting measures; by 2018, the clinical measures will increase to 11 with a continuation of the five reporting measures for a total of 16 measures (CMS, 2016). The goal of this program is to promote high-quality services in outpatient dialysis facilities that treat patients with the end-stage renal disease. The program will link a portion of the treatment payment directly to the facility's ESRD quality care performance measures. If the facility does not meet or exceed certain performance standards, the facility will receive reduced payments. For 2016, clinical measures

TABLE 11.2 Reimbursement Domains and Measurement

Hospital Value-Based Program	2017 (%)	2018 (%)
Clinical care (in 2017: Outcomes—25% and Process—5%)	30	25
Patient and caregiver-centered experience of care/care coordination	25	25
Safety	20	25
Efficiency and cost reduction	25	25

included maintaining a patient's hemoglobin greater than 12 g/dL, availability and outcome of different dialysis types, tracking bloodstream infections, keeping track of hemodialysis outpatients, and monitoring for hypercalcemia. Reporting measures include mineral metabolism and anemia management.

HVBP. Although VBP is a Medicare program, for hospitals under the HVBP, which began in 2012 under the ACA, the quality performance measures include all hospital patients of participating facilities no matter what type of insurance the patient has. The only facilities not affected by the CMS reimbursement shift now are psychiatric, rehabilitation, long-term care, children's cancer, critical access, and U.S. territory hospitals. Although participation is not required, eligible hospitals that do not participate will have no way of recovering the diagnosis-related group (DRG) reimbursement reductions and so may suffer significant annual financial losses (Aroh et al., 2015). Incentive payments made by Medicare are based on how well the hospital performs on given measures within specific domains and the amount of performance improvement from a baseline period. Table 11.2 gives the domains and the weighted percentages for 2017 and 2018; these scores may change each fiscal year (CMS, 2015).

Scoring within each domain is dependent on program measures such as fibrinolytic therapy following a myocardial infarction, influenza immunizations, antibiotics administration for surgical patients, and mortality rates for acute myocardial infarction's, heart failure, and pneumonia. To calculate a hospital's total performance score (TPS), a hospital's achievement or improvement points for each measure are combined, and the hospital's TPS is the greater of the two. The final score will determine whether the facility receives an incentive. More information on scoring for hospitals can be found at www.CMS.gov.

HRR. Another program introduced in 2012 and implemented under the ACA, the HRR program focuses on prevention of hospital readmission within 30 days after discharge. Readmission within 30 days applies to readmissions that meet certain measures and includes readmission to any hospital, not just where the original hospitalization occurred. However certain planned readmissions, such as a scheduled surgery, are not included. In 2016, hospital measures are based on readmission rates for patients with acute myocardial infarction, heart failure, pneumonia, chronic obstructive pulmonary disease, total hip and/or total knee replacement, and coronary artery bypass graft surgery. A few strategies for hospitals to lower the rates of readmissions are improving coordination of care, communication, discharge planning, and education. Two other strategies are ensuring discharge patients have follow-ups and using electronic medical records to share information and thereby improve continuity of care.

HACRP. Implemented in 2014 under the ACA, by providing incentives, this program encourages hospitals to improve patient safety and decrease the number of hospital-acquired conditions. According to the CMS, HACRP saves Medicare approximately $350 million every year—the savings are gained by reducing payments to the hospitals with the worst calculated Total HAC Score which is based on two domains (CMS, 2016).

Domain 1 consists of patient safety indicators at either the provider level or area level. As of 2016, there are 19 provider-level indicators, which include death rates in a low mortality DRG, postoperative respiratory failure rate, and transfusion reaction counts. The seven area-level indicators, as of 2016, include indicators such as retained surgical items, postoperative wound dehiscence rates, and transfusion reaction rates. More information on patient safety indicators can be found on the Agency for Healthcare Research and Quality website (http://qualityindicators.ahrq.gov/Modules/psi_overview.aspx). Domain 2 consists of health care–associated infection measures, including central line-associated bloodstream infections (CLABSI), catheter-associated urinary tract infection (CAUTI), surgical site infections (SSIs), methicillin-resistant *Staphylococcus aureus* (MRSA) bacteremia, and Clostridium difficile infection (CDI; QualityNet, n.d.).

VM or PVBM. Created in 2015 as part of the ACA, this program determines the amount of Medicare physician payment based on performance on specific quality and cost measures; it rewards quality performance and lower costs. This program is being implemented in phases. In 2016, physicians in groups of 10 or more eligible professionals will have their payments adjusted based on their performance in 2014. In 2017, the payment adjustments will apply to physician solo practitioners and physicians and groups of two or more eligible practitioners based on the 2015 performance. In 2018, CMS will make adjusted payments based on 2016 performance to physician solo practitioners and physicians in groups of two or more eligible practitioners. In 2018, eligible practitioners will include Nurse Practitioners, physician assistants, Clinical Nurse Specialists, and Certified Registered Nurse Anesthetists who are solo practitioners or are in groups of two or more eligible practitioners. Measures used in the VM program are based on both quality and cost.

Quality measures in the VM program consist of three outcome measures that are calculated from Medicare fee-for-service claims. There are two composite measures of ambulatory care-sensitive condition hospital admissions, one for acute conditions and one for chronic conditions. The third measure is hospital readmissions within 30 days for any cause. Cost measures include six areas of performance such as total per capita costs for patients with specific conditions: diabetes, coronary artery disease, chronic obstructive pulmonary disease, or heart failure. The last two cost measures are total per capita costs for all beneficiaries and Medicare Spending per Beneficiary. More information can be found on the CMS website (CMS, 2016).

HHVBP Program. Not yet a program, HHVBP program began on January 1, 2016, under the ACA. The HHVBP program was implemented in all Medicare-certified home health agencies (HHAs) in nine randomly selected states representing geographic areas of the nation: Arizona, Florida, Iowa, Maryland, Massachusetts, Nebraska, North Carolina, Tennessee, and Washington. HHAs in these states are required to compete on the value in the HHVBP program where payment adjustments are tied to quality performance. Under the program, different quality measures are evaluated to calculate a TPS for the HHVBP program. For an agency to receive a score on a measure, it must have a minimum of 20 home health episodes of care for that measure. Payments will not be adjusted until the HHA generates scores on five or more measures.

SNFVBP. Under the PAMA, the SNFVBP will begin in 2019. Measures under this program will include a 30-day all-cause readmission measure and a 30-day potentially preventable readmission measure. The 30-day all-cause readmission measure will estimate the rate of unexpected readmissions within 30 days for people with fee-for-service Medicare who were patients at a prospective payment system, critical access or psychiatric hospital for any cause or condition. The 30-day potentially preventable readmission measure will estimate the standardized risk rate of unexpected, potentially preventable readmission within 30 days for people with fee-for-service Medicare who were inpatient at a prospective payment system, critical access or psychiatric hospital.

Advanced APM and MIPS. As part of the Quality Payment Program and under the Medicare Access and CHIP Reauthorization Act of 2015, both will begin in 2019. However, providers will need to start collecting performance data between January 1 and October 2 of 2017. The Quality Payment Program will replace the sustainable growth rate formula, which potentially left clinicians with probable payment decreases for 13 years. Applicable to providers who participate in Medicare Part B, the clinician may choose between the Advanced APM or MIPS. By choosing to participate in the advanced APM, clinicians participating in Medicare Part B may earn incentive payments for participation. If choosing MIPS, clinicians will continue to participate in the traditional Medicare Part B in which earnings may include a performance-based payment adjustment.

Participation in the Quality Payment Program will apply to any physician, physician assistant, Nurse Practitioner, Clinical Nurse Specialist, or Certified Registered Nurse Anesthetist who bills Medicare for more than $30,000 per year and provides care for more than 100 Medicare patients per year. It is important to note that if 2017 is the provider's first year to participate in Medicare, that provider is not eligible for the MIPS track of the Quality Payment Program. Under MIPS, payment adjustments are based on evidence-based and practice-specific quality data: a quality that replaces the Physician Quality Reporting System (PQRS); improvement activities; and advancing care information that replaces the Medicare Electronic Health Record (EHR) Incentive Program. In 2018, the cost will replace the Value-Based Modifier. Further information and updates can be found on the Quality Payment Program website (qpp.cms.gov).

CONCLUSION

To promote quality outcomes health care providers must remain well informed of quality initiatives through continuous education. With an increasing emphasis on quality, promoting quality outcomes is a priority. Additionally, to succeed cultural transformation is crucial as traditional performance improvement projects will no longer serve the evolving health paradigm. APRNs can lead this transformation through collaboration, coaching/mentoring, direct patient care, research, ethics, and leadership. To achieve success in improving patient safety and outcomes, leaders must focus on interprofessional, team-based collaboration to effectively lead all involved to system and process improvements in the delivery of care.

APRNs should align themselves with VBP by CMS guidelines. By implementing quality improvements or evidence- and value-based practices, the APRN can influence future changes to value-based health care. APRNs should also take professional accountability to become knowledgeable about the ACA and VBP, not just the program that applies to the APRN's practice but about all programs, and discuss these with other providers, colleagues, and patients. Finally, APRNs must also become involved in policy making to remove barriers for all nurses and to allow APRNs to practice at their highest level of education, skill, and competency.

DISCUSSION QUESTIONS

1. *Based on the information in this chapter, list at least two areas of policy change you can identify where legislation could have an impact and explain what type of change is needed.*
2. *If you were going to describe the importance of your issue for policy change to potential supporters, what key points would you stress? How would you describe them to your patients?*

ANALYSIS, SYNTHESIS, AND CLINICAL APPLICATION

1. *What has the nursing discipline been doing about health policy?*
2. *What can APRNs do to help make these changes on a local level? Hospital level? State level? National level? International level?*
3. *Who are the key players/organizations/entities from a nursing practice perspective? Legislative perspective?*
4. *What does the future hold for providers? For patients? For organizations?*
5. *What are the hurdles yet to cross?*
6. *How does health policy impact my practice? For example:*
   - *Who can I see or care for?*
   - *What kind of care can I provide?*
   - *What do I get paid?*
   - *Where and how restricted is my practice?*
   - *How can I make things better for my patients and myself?*
   - *What things need to change?*

EXERCISES/CONSIDERATIONS

1. *Using Table 11.1 and considering your area of specialty, determine which value-based program(s) you could utilize. What are the barriers to your practice?*

ETHICAL CONSIDERATIONS

1. *Consider the health policy changes discussed in this chapter or those you have described in your analysis and consider the impact that might result if these changes are NOT enacted. In other words, what are the consequences of inaction? Consider how inaction may affect patient care.*

For More Information

Quality Payment Program: qpp.cms.gov

CMS Value-Based Programs: www.cms.gov/Medicare/Quality-Initiatives-Patient-Assessment-Instru ments/Value-Based-Programs/Value-Based-Programs.html

Agency for Healthcare Research and Quality. (1997, November). Theory and reality of value-based purchasing: Lessons from the pioneer. Retrieved from http://www.ahrq.gov/professionals/ quality-patient-safety/quality-resources/tools/meyer/index.html

REFERENCES

Aroh, D., Colella, J., Douglas, C., & Eddings, A. (2015). An example of translating value-based purchasing into value-based care. *Urologic Nursing, 35*(2), 61–74.

Berwick, D. M., & Hackbarth, A. D. (2012). Eliminating waste in US health care. *Journal of the American Medical Association, 307*(14), 1513–1516.

Centers for Medicare and Medicaid Services. (2015). Hospital value-based purchasing. Retrieved from https://www.cms.gov/Outreach-and-Education/Medicare-Learning-Network-MLN/ MLNProducts/downloads/Hospital_VBPurchasing_Fact_Sheet_ICN907664.pdf

Centers for Medicare and Medicaid Services. (2016). What are the value-based programs? Retrieved from https://www.cms.gov/Medicare/Quality-Initiatives-Patient-Assessment-Instruments/Value -Based-Programs/Value-Based-Programs.html

Chassin, M. R., Loeb, J. M., Schmaltz, S. P., & Wachter, R. M. (2010). Accountability measures—Using measurement to promote quality improvement. *New England Journal of Medicine, 363*(7), 683–688. doi:10.1056/NEJMsb1002320

Damberg, C. L., Sorbero, M. E., Lovejoy, S. L., Martsolf, G., Raaen, L., & Mandel, D. (2014). Meauring success in health care value-based purchasing programs: Findings from an environmental scan, literature review, and expert panel discussions. *Rand Health Quarterly, 4*(3), 9. Retrieved from http:// www.rand.org/pubs/research_reports/RR306.html

Henkel, R. J., & Maryland, P. A. (2015). The risks and rewards of value-based reimbursement. *Frontiers of Health Services Management, 32*(2), 3–16.

Institute of Medicine. (1994). *America's health in transition: Protecting and improving quality.* Washington, DC: National Academies Press.

Marjoua, Y., & Bozic, K. J. (2012). Brief history of quality movement in US healthcare. *Current Reviews in Musculoskeletal Medicine, 5*(4), 265–273. doi:10.1007/s12178-012-9137-8

National Business Coalition on Health. (2011). Value-based purchasing: A definition. Retrieved from http://w.nbch.org/Value-based-Purchasing-A-Definition

QualityNet. (n.d.). Overview: Hospital-Acquired Condition (HAC) Reduction Program. Retrieved from https://www.qualitynet.org/dcs/ContentServer?c=Page&pagename=QnetPublic%2FPage%2FQ netTier2&cid=1228774189166

Funding of APRN Education and Residency Programs

Suzanne Miyamoto

A HISTORICAL PERSPECTIVE

The political roots for nursing education funding can be traced back to the administration of President John Adams when the Public Health Service (PHS) was created in 1798 (Kalisch & Kalisch, 1982). To this day, nurses are a vital part of the PHS and the use of health care professionals to provide public services spans the centuries as well as the investment by the federal government. In 1902, the U.S. PHS was established and eventually the Division of Nursing (Kalisch & Kalisch, 1982), currently housed within the U.S. Department of Health and Human Services (HHS), Health Resources and Services Administration (HRSA) and recently renamed the Division of Nursing and Public Health.

However, the nation's attention to the importance of nurses became increasingly evident during World War I. Nurses who were a part of the PHS were deployed to military camps and asked to care for the civilian populations around the camps by teaching proper sanitation, treating children, and investigating communicable diseases (Kalisch & Kalisch, 1982). The care these nurses provided during wartime demonstrated the critical importance of public health nursing.

> In general, the public health expenditures of the 1920s proved that public health nursing could be a purchasable commodity: the public health nursing programs, which had grown up in the first quarter of the 20th century, had helped to lower the mortality rate, to increase life expectancy and reduce significantly the morbidity rate from tuberculosis, typhoid fever, smallpox, malaria, and most infant diseases. (Kalisch & Kalisch, 1982, p. 170)

The Great Depression, the next chapter in U.S. history, caused federal funding for PHSs to be slashed. In 1933, the New Deal allowed the federal government to invest in programs that were cut during the Great Depression, which included nursing. Congress established the Federal Emergency Relief Administration and the Civil Works Administration, which significantly invested in nursing (Kalisch & Kalisch, 1982). It was during this era that the federal government provided postgraduate training for public health nurses. Yet, one of the most notable federal investments for nursing education policy came in the 1940s. The United States had entered World War II and again, the call for nursing care had intensified.

During this time, the PHS funded a national nursing survey and allocated dollars to support nursing programs for the imminent increase in students. This work was conducted by the Nursing Council for National Defense that was created by the nation's nursing leaders (Kalisch & Kalisch, 1982). A total of $1.2 million was allocated for basic training and administered by the Public Health Nursing section of the Division of States Relation of the PHS. This marked the first federal investment in nursing education. But it was the creation of the U.S. Cadet Nurse Corps in 1943 that established more comprehensive funding for nursing education (Kalisch & Kalisch, 1982).

Nurses were being drafted to serve in the military and this in turn led to a shortage of nurses in civilian hospitals, marking the first American nursing shortage. Given this demand for nurses in both the military and civilian sectors, proposals were offered to shorten nursing education programs. However, they were strongly opposed by nursing leaders as they feared a "massive collapse of the already meager educational standards" (Kalisch & Kalisch, 1982, p. 173). The initial objections were quickly overshadowed by the great need for nurses. In 1943, the U.S. Cadet Nurse Corps was introduced by Congresswoman Frances Payne Bolton (R-OH) and signed into law by President Roosevelt on June 15 of that year. Nursing students entering this 24- or 30-month program received free tuition, a monthly stipend, and uniforms. To oversee the corps, the PHS Surgeon General created the Division of Nursing Education (DNE). The U.S. Cadet Nurse Corps was the "largest experiment in federally subsidized education in the history of the United States up to that time" (Kalisch & Kalisch, 1982, p. 174).

The U.S. Cadet Nurse Corps was a major success, but the importance of this program as well as the DNE ended after the war. Congress viewed this particular federal investment as part of the war effort and phased out both programs. The result made a drastic impact on nursing school enrollments, and the nation's hospitals experienced severe nursing shortages (Kalisch & Kalisch, 1982). Moreover, the effects created a shortage of nursing faculty, and many nursing leaders were concerned over the academic standards.

Ninety-seven percent of nursing education was hospital-based programs (Kalisch & Kalisch, 1982). The profession needed to investigate its trajectory. In 1948, the Carnegie Corporation and the Russell Sage Foundation sponsored the report *Nursing for the Future* (Kalisch & Kalisch, 1982). The recommendations included one that has withstood decades: nursing programs should be housed in colleges and universities and subpar programs should be closed. In 1948, the American Medical Association concurred with this recommendation through its Committee on Nursing Problems that investigated patient care standards and stressed the importance of nursing education at the baccalaureate level (Kalisch & Kalisch, 1982).

Although no major funding streams from Congress were appropriated for nursing education during this time, support on Capitol Hill was gaining momentum. As Kalisch and Kalisch (1982) note, "their [nursing legislation] recurring appearance before each session of Congress indicated that they had acquired a permanent base of support" (p. 180). The only federal support for nursing from 1948 to 1956 was through the National Mental Health Act of 1946 that provided funding for psychiatric nursing education (Kalisch & Kalisch, 1982). The next major congressional action to support nursing education (beyond mental health nursing) was through the Health Amendments Act of 1956. In its first year, this legislation authorized $2 million in traineeships for approximately 3,800 nurses pursuing a career in education or administration (Kalisch & Kalisch, 1982). However, nursing leaders knew the piecemeal approach to funding nursing education would not be sufficient. The demand had surfaced for consistent federal funding for nursing education.

CONGRESSIONAL ACTION TO ESTABLISH CONSISTENT FUNDING FOR NURSING EDUCATION

The United States faced its second significant nursing shortage in the late 1950s and early 1960s as the nation's hospitals reported high RN vacancy rates (Buerhaus, Staiger, & Auerbach, 2009). In 1961, the reported vacancy rate soared to 23.2% (Yett, 1975) much higher than the documented rates in the late 1990s and early 2000s. The shortage was driven by expanding positions for nurses in the hospital setting. As Kalisch and Kalisch (1982) noted:

> In the 1940s, hospitals had about one professional nurse for every fifteen beds and one practical nurse, or other auxiliary, for every ten beds. By the 1960s, one professional nurse was required for every five beds and one auxiliary for every three beds. Health care was given to a greater variety of people, and the primary focus of care had shifted from the home to the institution. (p. 186)

The nursing shortage impacted quality nursing care. Without the supervision of licensed RNs, nonprofessional personnel were providing direct patient care, resulting in dangerous errors (Yett, 1966). The impact of the nursing shortage on patient care was quickly rising to the national agenda. Its effects were highlighted in medical, nursing, and public health journals, in magazines and public newspapers (Yett, 1966). As cited by Yett, "Gradually, and inevitably, an awareness of this situation has become a part of what John Kenneth Galbraith so aptly has described as our 'conventional wisdom'" (p. 190). The RN vacancy rate was on the rise from 5% in the 1940s to 10% to 15% in the 1950s and eventually 20% in the 1960s (Yett, 1966). It was at this time in history that hospitals lobbied Congress to enact legislation that would fund nursing education and help address the demand for nurses (Buerhaus et al., 2009).

In 1963, the Surgeon General released the report *Toward Quality in Nursing, Needs and Goals* (Congressional Research Service [CRS], 2005). This report signified the need for comprehensive legislation for nursing workforce development. It recommended that the supply of practicing RNs be increased to 850,000 by 1970, a growth of 55%. It also recommended that nursing school graduates increase by 75% to meet this goal and more specifically noted that nurses with graduate degrees should increase by 194%, baccalaureate prepared nurses by 100%, and licensed practical nurses by 50% (Kalisch & Kalisch, 1982).

The Nurse Training Act (NTA) of 1964 (P.L. 88–581) established Title VIII of the Public Health Service Act (PHSA), which is known today as the Nursing

Workforce Development programs. While the legislation authorized a total of $238 million for five programs over 5 years, when it was signed into law by President Johnson on September 4, 1964, it received $9.92 million in its first year (Kalisch & Kalisch, 1982). "On signing the act, President Johnson observed that the Nurse Training Act of 1964 was the most significant nursing legislation in the history of the country" (Kalisch & Kalisch, 1982, p. 188). Further, "he believed that it would enable the nation to attract more qualified young people to this 'great and noble calling'" (Kalisch & Kalisch, 1977, p. 855).

The five programs included nursing student loans, professional nurse traineeships, construction grants, project grants, and formula grants to diploma schools (Scott, 1967; see Table 12.1).

To administer the new authorities, the Division of Nursing created the Nursing Education and Training Branch (Kalisch & Kalisch, 1982). The programs made a significant impact. Between the years 1964 and 1967, the Nursing Student Loan program supported over 32,000 nursing students (Scott, 1967). The Professional Nurse Traineeship program was expanded to include long-term and short-term traineeships for graduate nurses seeking a clinical specialty track, and from 1964 to 1967 a total of 17,000 RNs were supported (Scott, 1967).

The other Title VIII programs focused more on the didactical and the "brick and mortar" of nursing education. Scott (1967) noted that the construction grants were established to help address the overcrowding in the nation's nursing schools and the obsolete buildings. Sixty-two schools were funded to renovate their buildings between 1964 and 1967, which resulted in 2,600 more students enrolled (Scott, 1967). In addition, nine new nursing schools were developed due to the construction grants. The project grants that were created by the NTA awarded 116 schools federal dollars and benefited 33,000 students (Scott, 1967). The grant money was used for projects such as investing in multimedia to enhance education and teaching students in the community, away from the hospital setting. The final program created through the NTA went to support a total of 414 diploma programs given the high costs incurred by the hospitals in administering them (Scott, 1967).

TABLE 12.1 Title VIII Programs and Authorization Level

PROGRAMS	AUTHORIZATION	PURPOSE
Nursing student loans	$85 million	Those who received the awards agreed to work 5 years after graduation and would be forgiven half of their loan.
Professional nurse traineeship	$50 million	Continuation of existing professional nurse traineeship programs.
Construction grants	$90 million	Construction and improvement of nursing facilities. $55 million for diploma and associate degree programs. $35 million for baccalaureate programs.
Project grants	$17 million	Improvements to teaching methodologies and other special projects.
Formula grants to diploma schools	$41 million	Improvements to hospital based nursing programs such as the quality of instruction.

Source: Kalisch and Kalisch (1982) and Scott (1967).

Nursing experts of the 1960s noted that the NTA would significantly help alleviate the nursing shortage. However, others felt the original projections made in 1963 to increase the profession to 850,000 practicing nurses were not achievable. Yett's (1966) analysis of the NTA and the Surgeon General's report revealed a discrepancy of 170,000 nurses. According to the Surgeon General's Consultant Group on Nursing, who wrote the 1963 report,

> a feasible goal for 1970 is to increase the supply of professional nurses in practice to about 680,000 and that to meet this goal schools of nursing must produce 53,000 graduates a year by 1969 (including 13,000 baccalaureate, and an additional 3,000 at the master's level). (U.S. Public Health Service, 1963 as cited in Yett, 1966)

Adding to the shortfall, Kalisch and Kalisch described in their 1977 unpublished study for the Division of Nursing that "It soon became obvious that unless the shortage of classroom and other training space in hospital schools of nursing and junior college nursing programs was corrected, it would stand in the way of the nation's goal of having 680,000 nurses in active practice by 1970" (p. 834).

When the NTA was up for reauthorization in 1969, a committee was established to evaluate the five authorities. They found them to be effective in addressing the national nursing shortage through investments in nursing education but noted the NTA should be expanded to address planning, recruitment, and research (Kalisch & Kalisch, 1982). Congressional hearings were held on the NTA and other legislation supporting health professionals to determine how to act on the recommendations of the various committees. The Health Manpower Act of 1968 reauthorized the NTA. The reauthorization weakened the accreditation standards (the original bill required accreditation by the National League for Nursing, which, at the time only accredited baccalaureate programs, weakening federal support for diploma programs) due in large part to the associate degree lobby, but it did increase the number of scholarship provisions (Kalisch & Kalisch, 1982).

In the 1970s and 1980s, the Title VIII programs saw a number of amendments and reauthorizations. The NTA of 1971 (P.S. 92–158) and 1975 (P.L. 94–63), for the first time, provided grants for all types of nursing education programs (Kalisch & Kalisch, 1977). Known as capitation grants, they were "based on the well-established need to maintain the quality of education in schools of nursing by establishing a firm core of financial support" (Kalisch & Kalisch, 1977, p. 1135). Capitation grants provided formula grants based on enrollment rates in schools of nursing (American Association of Colleges of Nursing [AACN], 2008a). Schools were awarded the grants if they could demonstrate enrollment growth over the previous year and could use the funds to hire faculty, recruit students, enhance clinical laboratories, expand school of nursing buildings, or for other learning equipment (AACN, 2008a). For collegiate schools of nursing, Congress provided "$400 for each full-time baccalaureate student enrolled in the last two years of a nursing program, and approximately $275 for each student enrolled in an associate degree or diploma program" (AACN, 2008a, para. 3). Capitation grants received significant funding support from Congress and in fiscal years (FYs) 1977 and 1978 the program was appropriated $55 million (AACN, 2008b).

The capitation grant program proved to be a powerful source of funding for the nation's nursing schools. However, politics played a significant role in its eventual elimination. The program was endorsed by the liberal Congress, but not the conservative Nixon Administration. While President Nixon signed the NTA into law in 1971, continual debates between the Administration and Congress over the appropriate funding levels for nursing education led President Nixon to veto a number of bills that would have created higher levels of support (Kalisch & Kalisch, 1982). In 1972 and 1973, Congress passed continual resolutions (appropriations bills funded at the previous year's level), but President Nixon impounded $73 million nursing appropriations that were later recovered through a federal court case (Kalisch & Kalisch, 1982). Funding for nursing education continued to be a target. In 1974, President Nixon's budget request slashed the $160 million appropriated to Title VIII in 1973 to $49 million (Kalisch & Kalisch, 1982). Although Congress was able to secure funding for Title VIII above the president's request and $139 million was finally appropriated for the NTA programs in FY 1974 (Division of Nursing, personal communication, May 2008), nursing would continue to fight for necessary federal support.

The Ford administration also made cuts to nursing education funding. President Ford vetoed the NTA of 1974, claiming it was too expensive (Kalisch & Kalisch, 1982). Additionally, the Administration felt that the nurse scholarship and loan programs were unnecessary as nursing students were eligible for other federal loans (Kalisch & Kalisch, 1982). The NTA of 1975 attempted to find a middle ground with the Administration. It decreased federal funding for the Title VIII programs but extended their authorization through FY 1978. However, the most notable difference of the NTA of 1975 was the creation of the Advanced Nurse Training program. This legislation provided funding for the expansion of master's and doctoral nursing education programs, most notably those for Advanced Practice Registered Nurses (APRNs). President Ford vetoed this bill, but Congress was able to override his veto (Kalisch & Kalisch, 1982).

The nursing community fought with their congressional champions to keep the legislation intact and funded. When President Carter took office, he viewed the programs similarly to his predecessors, Presidents Nixon and Ford. He believed that nursing students could obtain funding from other federal programs, the NTA had helped address the nursing shortage, and the funding levels were too excessive (Kalisch & Kalisch, 1982). In President Carter's fiscal year 1978 budget, he provided no funding for nurse training "and foreboded the probable end of the Division of Nursing had his administration continued" (Kalisch & Kalisch, 1977, p. 1225). Congress did pass an extension to the NTA in 1978, but it was pocket-vetoed on November 11, 1978, by President Carter (Kalisch & Kalisch, 1982). This move ignited outrage from the nursing community.

The following year, a new version of the legislation was drafted. It required a national study to be conducted by the Institute of Medicine (IOM—now, National Academy of Medicine) to determine if the federal government should continue to provide institutional support, if there was an actual nursing shortage, if the government should subsidize all of a nursing student's loan, and how Congress should address the unequal distribution of nurses and the increase in nursing specialization (CRS, 2005). The NTA of 1979 was signed into law by President Carter on September 29 of that year given the provision of the study (Kalisch & Kalisch, 1982). The IOM report, *Nursing and Nursing Education: Policies and Private Actions*, found that federal support for the "overall supply of nurses was not needed, but that generalist education programs should continue to help sustain the nursing supply" (CRS, 2005, p. CRS-2). The results of the report caused further cuts to the Title VIII programs and eliminated the construction grants, capitation grants, and scholarships at schools of nursing. Laws passed in 1981 and 1982 repealed most of the programs that were created in the 1960s and 1970s (CRS, 2005).

CURRENT FEDERAL FUNDING FOR APRNS

As noted through arguments mentioned previously by various political leaders, the reality is that nursing students, including APRN students, as well as all other health professions or college students can receive federal financial support from varying sources, particularly those that are funded by the U.S. Department of Education. Pell grants, Public Service Loan Forgiveness, Graduate Assistance in Areas of National Need, and Stafford Loans, are to name only a few (AACN, 2016b). Others are included in the U.S. Department of Labor that focuses more on technical needs and demand areas. This chapter continues to focus on dedicated funding for nurses or programs focused on health professionals. Like other health disciplines, particularly medicine and Graduate Medical Education, dedicated funding is critical to workforce training and sustainability. With that said, despite the political battles the Title VIII Nursing Workforce Development programs faced over the years, they still represent the largest dedicated source of federal funding for nursing education (Nursing Community, 2016). They also continue to support APRNs through consistent funding.

To date, the Title VIII programs have seven authorities: (a) Advanced Education Nursing (AEN) grants (Sec. 811); (b) Nursing Workforce Diversity (Sec. 821); (c) Nursing Education, Practice, Quality, and Retention (Sec. 831); (d) Nursing Student Loan program (Sec. 835); (e) Nurse Loan Repayment and Scholarship program (Sec. 846)—Renamed NURSE Corps; (f) Nurse Faculty Loan Program (Sec. 846A); and (g) Comprehensive Geriatric Education Grants (Sec. 855). Each of these programs has the potential to support APRNs. However, one major program within Title VIII focuses on APRN training, the AEN grants.

AEN grants (Sec. 811 of the PHSA) are modeled after the traineeship programs that were originally created in the 1960s and 1970s. There are three distinct programs authorized under this section. First, they provide schools of nursing, academic health centers, and other nonprofit entities funding to improve the education and practice of Nurse Practitioners (NPs), Certified Nurse-Midwives (CNMs), Certified Registered Nurse Anesthetists (CRNAs), Clinical Nurse Specialists (CNSs), nurse educators, nurse administrators, public health nurses, and other nurses pursuing AEN (P.L. 107–205).

Second, they provide full or partial traineeship support for graduate nursing students to help with the expense of tuition, books, program fees, and other reasonable living expenses (P.L. 107–205). This program is known as the Advanced Education Nursing Traineeships (AENT). Finally, the AEN section of Title VIII also funds the Nurse Anesthetist Traineeship (NAT), which provides the same type of support as the AENT to students in nurse anesthetist programs. As seen in Table 12.2, funding for the AEN programs represents a substantial portion of Title VIII funding. The average percent of funding allocated for the program over the last decade and a half is approximately 36%. The increase in funding seen after 2002 can be attributed to the enactment of the Nurse Reinvestment

TABLE 12.2   Percent of AEN Funding Compared to Total Title VIII Dollars

FISCAL YEAR	TOTAL TITLE VIII FUNDING (IN MILLIONS)	FUNDING FOR AEN (IN MILLIONS)	AEN OF TITLE VIII FUNDING (%)
2002	$92.74	$60.04	64.7
2003	$112.76	$50.17	44.5
2004	$141.92	$58.65	41.3
2005	$150.67	$58.17	38.6
2006	$149.68	$57.06	38.1
2007	$149.68	$57.06	38.1
2008	$156.05	$61.88	39.7
2009	$171.03	$64.44	37.7
2010	$243.87	$64.44	26.4
2011	$242.39	$64.05	26.4
2012	$231.01	$63.93	27.7
2013	$217.50	$59.94	27.6
2014	$223.84	$61.58	27.5
2015	$231.62	$63.58	27.5
2016	$229.47	$64.58	28.1

AEN, Advanced Education Nursing.

Source: American Association of Colleges of Nursing (2016a).

Act of 2002 in which a number of new programs were added to Title VIII, which impacted future allocations.

In 2010, the Patient Protection and Affordable Care Act (P.L. 111–148) was signed into law and the subsequent appropriations cycles increased funding levels, but later, due to political battles between a Republican Congress and the Obama administration the funding fell. These cuts were to all nondefense discretionary programs as a result of negotiations around the debt ceiling or the fiscal cliff in 2011. A number of laws were passed, the Budget Control Act of 2011 (P.L. 112–125) and the American Taxpayer Relief Act of 2012 (P.L. 112–240), that included seques-tration, across-the-board cuts to discretionary spending in fiscal years 2013 and 2014, which negatively impacted Title VIII (AACN, 2012b). Continued debates on how to control national funding resulted in continuing resolutions and smaller across-the-board cuts, somewhat stabilizing federal funding.

Two additional sources of federal support for APRN education and train-ing are funded through the National Health Service Corps (NHSC) and the U.S. PHS. The NHSC was created through the Emergency Health Personnel Act (P.L. 91–623) in 1970 (Politzer et al., 2000). The intent of the legislation was to cre-ate a program that would direct commissioned officers and civil service per-sonnel to national health professional shortage areas (HPSAs). The health care professionals were to provide primary care to those in rural and underserved areas. The goal was to ensure that after the health care professional finished a tour, he or she would find the work to be rewarding and would choose to stay and practice in the community (Redman, 1973, as cited in Politzer et al.). The first cohort of 20 commissioned officers began in 1972 and included two nurses. As the importance of this effort grew, the federal government established a scholarship and loan repayment program within the NHSC.

Based on each school year, the scholarship program provides financial support if health professional students agree to serve in a NHSC-approved site that is located in a HPSA. For each full or partial school year that is reimbursed, the program requires a minimum of a 2-year commitment (NHSC, 2016a). The NHSC scholarship program supports NPs and CNMs.

The loan repayment program offers three options for primary care providers. The NHSC loan repayment program is offered to primary care providers who seek to work in an approved NHSC site. The Students to Service Loan Repayment program provides loan repayment to medical students in their fourth year. Finally, the state loan repayment program is a "federally-funded grant program to states and territories that provides cost-sharing grants to assist them in operating their own state educational loan repayment programs for primary care providers working in health professional shortage areas (HPSAs) within their state" (HRSA, 2016b, para. 1). Currently, the NHSC loan repayment program funds primary care NPs, CNMs, and psychiatric CNSs.

As noted, the U.S. PHS began in 1798 under the Adams Administration and was designated as one of the nation's seven uniformed services. Nearly a century later, in 1889, the Commissioned Corps was officially established. But it was in 1944 that the PHSA authorized nurses and other health professionals into the commissioned corps (Debisette, Martinelli, Couig, & Braun, 2010). In 1949, when the PHS was restructured, the chief nurse officer position was created with the rank of Assistant Surgeon General (Rear Admiral; Debisette et al., 2010). To a nurse in the U.S. PHS, like in the Army, Navy, and Air Force, loan repayment options are available.

THE PATIENT PROTECTION AND AFFORDABLE CARE ACT: INVESTING IN APRN EDUCATION

Beginning in 2008, the health care community was deeply engaged and excited by the potential for health care reform. Discussion regarding massive and overarching changes to increase health care access, reduce expenditures, and improve quality resonated inside and outside the capital beltway. The nursing community was no exception. It would be through this legislative vehicle that they could achieve substantial and even monumental provisions that would invest in nursing education and practice with the ultimate goal of helping to meet the nation's changing patient care needs.

One of the first coordinated efforts by the nursing community was the reauthorization of the Title VIII Nursing Workforce Development programs. On January 24, 2008, Senator Barbara Mikulski (D-MD), a longtime nursing champion, contacted nursing leaders and requested they develop a single document that detailed the priorities for a stand-alone Title VIII reauthorization bill (Nursing Community, 2008). Headed by AACN, a Title VIII

Reauthorization task force was created to develop the consensus document that Senator Mikulski's office had requested. The nursing organizations around the table had a short deadline of 3 weeks to agree on a set of priorities and set them to paper. By the end of the first week, nursing organizations participating had to submit priorities and recommendations for the reauthorization. During the second week, the task force voted on which of the presented recommendations would be appropriate for a Title VIII reauthorization. The final week was spent drafting the recommendations and their accompanying rationale.

The document included one overarching principle, increase funding for Title VIII—all other principles were contingent on increased funding levels, and four guiding principles: (a) increase support for nurse faculty education, (b) strengthen specific resources for the education of APRNs and advanced education nursing, (c) increase efforts to develop and retain a diverse and professional nursing workforce for the transforming health care delivery system, and (d) increase efforts of HRSA and the Division of Nursing to release timely and more comprehensive data on the nursing workforce (Nursing Community, 2008).

This document was signed by 37 national nursing organizations such as the AACN, American Nurses Association, and major APRN organizations like the American Academy of Nurse Practitioners (AANP), the American College of Nurse Practitioners (ACNP; AANP and ACNP have now merged to become the American Association of Nurse Practitioners), the National Organization of Nurse Practitioner Faculties (NONPF), the American Association of Nurse Anesthetists (AANA), the American College of Nurse-Midwives (ACNM), and the National Association of Clinical Nurse Specialists (NACNS). It was presented to Senator Mikulski's office and while a stand-alone bill to reauthorize Title VIII was not introduced, the document was used as a tool by the senator and the nursing community in preparing the Title VIII provisions that were included in the Patient Protection and Affordable Care Act or ACA (P.L. 111–148).

Near the end of May 2009, 29 national nursing organizations, led by AACN, came together and agreed on a set of statutory language changes to Title VIII. Two significant changes were important to future APRN education funding. First, the AEN grant program included a clause under Section 296j(f) (2) that stated, "The Secretary may not obligate more than 10% of the traineeships under subsection (a) of this section for individuals in doctorate degree programs" ("Title VIII Reauthorization," 2009, p. 3). Education for APRNs and those seeking advanced education in nursing was changing. The doctorate of nursing practice (DNP) was gaining momentum across the country, and the data clearly indicated a need for more nurse faculty with doctoral degrees ("Title VIII Reauthorization," 2009). This clause severely limited the nation's nursing schools from supporting those who were enrolled in DNP or PhD programs. Second, under the AEN grant program, the definition of authorized midwifery programs was included to remain current with the changes in midwifery education. These provision changes were eventually included in the ACA.

In relation to the Title VIII AEN program, the Affordable Care Act also led to the development of the Prevention and Public Health Fund (Sec. 4002). The fund, administered by HHS, provided support for programs authorized by the PHSA that focused on public health, wellness, and prevention (P.L. 111–148). It was through this fund that HRSA had the authority to create the Advanced Nursing

Education Expansion (ANEE) grant program in 2010. According to HRSA's 2010 funding opportunity announcement,

> The program's two purposes are (1) to increase the number of students enrolled full time in accredited primary care Nurse Practitioner and Nurse Midwifery programs and (2) to accelerate the graduation of part time students in such programs by encouraging full time enrollment. (p. 1)

In the rationale, HRSA noted

> The need for primary care continues to grow because of expanded health care coverage for the un-insured and under-insured provided by the Affordable Care Act. The ANEE program will help meet this need by increasing the supply of primary care nurse practitioners and nurse-midwives. (p. 1)

The total amount of funding was $30 million over a 5-year period and 26 grants were made to schools of nursing across the country (InsideGov, n.d.). While the program was not funded again through the Prevention and Public Health Fund, the noteworthy investment and recognition by the federal government of the important role NPs and CNMs play in providing primary care was substantial.

However, one of the most significant investments made to APRN education through the passage of the ACA was the Graduate Nurse Education (GNE) Demonstration (Sec. 5509). This program amended Title XVIII of the Social Security Act (SSA) to provide up to five hospitals with reimbursement for the clinical training of APRNs (P.L. 111–148). The road to achieve this important provision for APRN education was long, and it demanded the attention of critical nursing champions and a strong coalition of health care expertise. Table 12.3 shows the growth in numbers of enrollments and graduates in all types of DNP programs from 2005 to 2015.

THE ROAD TO THE GNE DEMONSTRATION

To understand the development of the GNE demonstration, a historical base must be laid for mandatory APRN education funding. Mandatory funding for nursing education and attempts to secure mandatory funding for APRN education are long embedded in nursing's history. In fact, mandatory funding for nursing education dates back to the creation of Medicare through Title XVIII of the SSA (Theis & Harper, 2004). Graduate Medical Education (GME) essentially reimburses hospitals for the care provided to Medicare patients by physician residents. Within GME, there also lies what is commonly known as pass-through dollars. These dollars fund nursing and other allied health prelicensure education programs (Theis & Harper, 2004). Section 413.85 of the SSA stipulates however, that these education programs can only be supported if they "are operated by providers as specified [hospitals], enhance the quality of inpatient care at the provider; and meet the requirements of paragraph of this section for state licensure or accreditation." It is the first clause that clarifies GME pass-through dollars. The nursing programs have to be owned and operated by the hospital. Therefore, this funding has only been allocated to diploma programs and some CRNA programs operated by hospitals because of how nursing programs were administered in the 1960s (Aiken, Cheung, & Olds, 2009).

TABLE 12.3 Advanced Practice Registered Nurses (APRNs) Enrollment and Graduations (2005–2015)

Year		MASTER'S				PBDNP				PMDNP				DNP TOTAL			
		CNS	NP	CNM	CRNA	CNS	NP	CNM	CRNA	CNS	NP	CNM	CRNA	CNS	NP	CNM	CRNA
2005	Enrollment	3,992	20,965	544	2,725	–	–	–	–	–	–	–	–	–	–	–	–
	Graduation	1,035	5,920	206	840	–	–	–	–	–	–	–	–	–	–	–	–
2006	Enrollment	3,932	23,980	771	2,793	6	80	5	1	–	–	–	–	–	–	–	–
	Graduation	1,031	6,475	234	844	0	0	0	0	–	–	–	–	–	–	–	–
2007	Enrollment	3,747	26,802	797	2,908	3	152	11	0	33	391	10	19	36	543	21	19
	Graduation	1,073	6,859	229	981	0	0	0	0	1	22	0	0	1	22	0	0
2008	Enrollment	3,768	29,323	951	3,247	12	324	21	9	112	1,158	23	64	124	1,482	44	73
	Graduation	965	7,613	251	989	1	17	2	0	4	110	2	1	5	127	4	1
2009	Enrollment	3,879	33,182	759	3,308	35	813	33	30	144	1,578	23	51	179	2,391	56	81
	Graduation	930	8,354	232	1,087	5	28	4	0	14	188	3	10	19	216	7	10
2010	Enrollment	3,424	38,858	1,168	3,690	33	1,570	41	82	117	1,812	24	33	150	3,382	65	115
	Graduation	903	9,633	327	1,256	1	28	5	0	13	409	11	13	14	437	16	13
2011	Enrollment	3,139	43,475	1,272	3,614	59	2,569	61	158	137	2,021	20	63	196	4,590	81	221
	Graduation	871	10,866	345	1,289	1	95	2	0	28	535	5	20	29	630	7	20
2012	Enrollment	2,557	48,685	1,370	3,653	83	3,793	61	252	136	1,867	18	57	219	5,660	79	309
	Graduation	821	12,785	398	1,347	1	222	9	19	13	514	17	11	14	736	26	30

Year																		
2013	Enrollment	2,020	56,496	1,377	3,532	187	5,064	72	556	142	2,196	7	142	329	7260	79	698
	Graduation	761	14,416	398	1,261	9	377	16	51	24	530	5	16	33	907	21	67
2014	Enrollment	1,616	63,143	835	3,231	98	7,181	96	912	119	2,358	11	89	217	9539	107	1001
	Graduation	589	16,257	306	1,321	7	573	19	72	29	708	8	35	36	1281	27	107
2015	Enrollment	1,320	68,671	1,582	2,890	115	8,906	113	1344	83	3,036	12	196	198	11942	125	1540
	Graduation	565	19,581	483	1,272	11	934	15	148	43	942	2	25	54	1876	17	173

CNM, Certified Nurse-Midwives; CNS, Clinical Nurse Specialist; CRNA, Certified Registered Nurse Anesthetist; DNP, Doctorate of Nursing Practice; NP, Nurse Practitioner; PBDNP, post-baccalaureate DNP; PMDNP, post-master's DNP.

Source: Data from American Association of Colleges of Nursing (2004, 2006, 2008a, 2008b, 2012a, 2012b, 2016a, 2016b).

Nursing's advocacy to change the structure of this was most notable during the 1990s when the Clinton Administration was debating health care reform. Many dialogues ensued on how the American health care systems should be restructured, and nursing leaders were engaged in serious discussions concerning funding for nursing education. In the late 1990s, nursing and other health care leaders believed it was the opportune time to discuss changes to GME reimbursement. Specifically, that a portion of Medicare funding should be directed to APRN education. At that point in history diploma programs had been significantly phased out and most registered nurses obtained their nursing degree from an associate or baccalaureate program. As Aiken, Cheung, and Olds (2009) noted the "rationale for Medicare support for graduate nursing education is the same as the rationale for GME: namely, that nurses in graduate programs are providing significant clinical care to Medicare beneficiaries in hospitals and other settings" (p. w653). In 1997, the IOM released its report *On Implementing a National Graduate Medical Education Trust Fund* that made the recommendation that,

> Nursing DME (direct medical education) should be structured like physician DME and be paid to sponsoring institutions for the support of advanced practice, graduate clinical trainees. This provision should be neutral with respect to the proportion of DME that has supported nursing; diploma, undergraduate nurse education support should be phased out in 4 years or less to allow present students to complete their training. (p. 16)

Inspired by national support for APRN education, AACN, ACNP, and NONPF released the *Statement on the Redirection of Nursing Education Medicare Funds to Graduate Nurse Education* on January 29, 1998. This document, intended for the *National Bipartisan Commission on the Future of Medicare Graduate Medical Education Study Group*, urged that Medicare dollars given to entry-level nursing education be directed to graduate nursing education and specifically APRN programs (AACN, 1998). The comprehensive document outlined the role of APRNs in health care delivery, educational trends of APRN students, nursing research demonstrating the effectiveness and high quality of APRN care, as well as citing outside support for the recommendation (AACN, 1998). The report noted that the Physician Payment Review Commission in 1995 and 1997 "recommended that advanced degree nursing programs operated by 4-year colleges and universities be eligible to receive Medicare funds that otherwise would be available only to hospital-operated programs" (p. 8). The Association of Academic Health Centers also supported the allocation of Medicare dollars to APRN education as well as the coalition that represented 11 national nursing organizations (AACN, 1998).

The battle to redirect the Medicare funding from entry-level nursing to APRN education continued in the early 2000s, as AACN's department of government affairs urged Congress to make this change through a legislative fix. However, no action was taken and the health care reform discussions under the Obama Administration opened the door for a unified approach. In 2009, health care reform discussions were heating up and nursing wanted to ensure the best possible legislative results for the profession and America's patients. One entity to join the campaign to demonstrate nursing's vital role in improving the nation's health care system was a collaboration between the Robert Wood Johnson Foundation and AARP. Together, these powerful health care voices formed a new entity called the Center to Champion Nursing in America (CCNA). Their goal was to work with the nursing community to help promote the exceptional contributions of RNs to improve health care access and quality, while reducing costs. In May of 2009, AARP representatives met with nursing lobbyists to discuss the potential to secure mandatory funding for APRN education.

Initial dialogues began between AARP and AANP, AACN, AANA, ACNP, ACNM, NACNS, and NONPF. Throughout the spring and summer of 2009, they negotiated a proposal for the Medicare reimbursement for APRN education. This proposal was not to redirect the existing funding for nursing education, but a separate and distinct pot. While the nursing leaders clearly understood it would be ideal to direct the funding for APRN education to the schools of nursing, Medicare law was not structured for this type of funding allocation. Medicare reimbursed hospitals, not health professions schools. Therefore, when legislation was introduced in the Senate and House by Senator Deborah Stabenow (D-MI) and Representative Lois Capps, RN (D-CA), respectively, the bill directed the reimbursement of hospitals and affiliated schools of nursing for APRN education (S.1569, H.R. 3185, 110d Cong.). The legislation, titled *Medicare Graduate Nursing Education Act,* also clearly stated that the hospital must have an agreement with an accredited school of nursing offering APRN programs. Educational costs associated in the bill included faculty salaries, student stipends (if any), clinical instruction costs, and other direct and indirect costs (S.1569).

The coalition that worked to develop the legislation also grew to a total of 14 organizations including a number of specialty NP organizations. The next steps to secure this program included meeting with key committee staff of the Senate Finance Committee and the House Ways and Means Committee (these committees have jurisdiction over changes to Medicare) to include the *Medicare Graduate Nursing Education Act* in the final health care reform legislation. Eight months of intense negotiations with key House and Senate Committee staff, particularly Senate Finance Committee staff, proved successful. When the ACA was signed into law on March 23, 2010, by President Barack Obama, the GNE demonstration was included.

Due to necessary negotiations, the final GNE demonstration was not the original proposal that AARP and the nursing community agreed upon in the summer of 2009. Given the uncertainty of total funding, complexity of its structure, and the new model for the Centers for Medicare and Medicaid Services (CMS, which administers Medicare programs) a demonstration or test was created. Up to five hospitals would be selected and a total funding level of $200 million over a 4-year period would be allocated. The funding could only be used for the reimbursement of APRN training. The law clearly stipulated that

> Qualified training means training that provides an advanced practice registered nurse with the clinical skills necessary to provide primary care, preventive care, transitional care, chronic care management, and other services appropriate for individuals entitled to, or enrolled for, benefits under part A of Title XVIII of the Social Security Act, or enrolled under part B of such title. (P.L. 111–148, Sec. 5509)

According to the GNE solicitation, "Costs associated with the didactic training component as well as the costs for certification and/or licensure are not eligible for reimbursement under this Demonstration" (CMS, 2010, p. 3). As stipulated in the law, hospitals had to establish an agreement with at least one school of nursing and also had to include two or more nonhospital community-based care settings (P.L. 111–1148, Sec. 5509). Due to the fact that CRNA education is almost exclusively administered in acute care settings, a waiver was included in rural and medically underserved communities where 50% of the education did not occur in a community-based care site.

On March 21, 2012, CMS announced the solicitation for proposals for the GNE demonstration program with a deadline of May 21, 2012. The GNE demonstration would be run through the Centers for Medicare and Medicaid Innovation, which was created through the ACA.

In its personal communication to AACN members on March 21, 2012, the association stated, "AACN, along with our colleagues in the APRN community and AARP, have been advocating for this program since its inception and are excited to see the long-awaited solicitation for proposals released" (P. Bednash, personal communication, March 21, 2012).

On the release of the solicitation, the coalition noticed a few problems with the program that would need to be corrected, and led by AACN, quickly advocated for their change. For example, DNP programs were excluded and there was confusion concerning APRN specialties. The solicitation was changed to allow only DNP programs where the students were not already licensed as APRNs. Essentially, post-masters DNP programs were not applicable (CMS, 2010). Both the GNE coalition and CMS held webinars to help inform the hospital and nursing community about the demonstration.

After the proposals were collected (a short extension was granted), the final models were chosen and announced on July 30, 2012. They included the Hospital of the University of Pennsylvania (Philadelphia, PA), Duke University Hospital (Durham, NC), Scottsdale Healthcare Medical Center (Scottsdale, AZ), Rush University Medical Center (Chicago, IL), and Memorial Hermann-Texas Medical Center Hospital (Houston, TX). While Duke and Rush University hospitals only included their affiliated school of nursing, the proposals from Arizona and Texas included four schools of nursing and Pennsylvania included nine schools (AACN, 2012a).

By all accounts, the GNE Demonstration was a remarkable achievement for the profession as it came together under true collaboration with partners outside of nursing and a unified voice. Today, the Demonstration has completed its cycle legislated by the law with a 1-year extension. While no official report has been sent to Congress (slated for October 2017 as mandated by law), presentations given by leaders of the demonstration's work, particularly Dr. Linda Aiken, who lead the Hospital of the University of Pennsylvania, and convened the five sites, note the many benefits of the program and its impact on the community. With any demonstration, unintended consequences were inevitable, but did not outweigh the opportunity to increase the number of APRNs to serve the Medicare population. Stakeholders continue to investigate a new proposal that would create a larger scale, more sustainable program.

APRN RESIDENCIES

In 2010, the Robert Wood Johnson Foundation and the IOM released the landmark report, *The Future of Nursing: Leading Change, Advancing Health.* The report was regarded by the nursing community as monumental and quickly became the rationale and support for initiatives the profession had strived to achieve for decades. The key messages were not earth-shattering to the community. They focused on nurses practicing to the full extent of their education and training, nurses achieving higher levels of education, nurses being full partners with their colleagues in health delivery reform, and improving workforce planning and data collection (IOM, 2010). In considering the education of nurses and APRNs, the report was clear that residencies are an important part of their training.

The *Future of Nursing* report noted that in 2002, The Joint Commission "recommended the development of nurse residency programs—planned, comprehensive periods of time during which nursing graduates can acquire the knowledge and skills to deliver safe, quality care that meets defined (organization or professional society) standards of practice" (IOM, 2010, p. 5). Historically, residency programs have been focused on the acute care setting, but as the report urged, residencies must be developed and evaluated outside the acute care setting (IOM, 2010). Increasing demand for nurses who practice primary care and serve those in the rural and underserved communities required more focus on developing highly skilled practitioners. Therefore, the following recommendation was included in *The Future of Nursing* report:

> Recommendation 3: Implement nurse residency programs. State boards of nursing, accrediting bodies, the federal government, and health care organizations should take actions to support nurses' completion of a transition-to-practice program (nurse residency) after they have completed a prelicensure or advanced practice degree program or when they are transitioning into new clinical practice areas. (IOM, 2011, p. 11)

The report recommended that all levels of nurses should receive a residency program after graduation and offered a number of tactics to achieve this goal:

- State boards of nursing, in collaboration with accrediting bodies such as the Joint Commission and the Community Health Accreditation Program, should support nurses' completion of a residency program after they have completed a prelicensure or advanced practice degree program or when they are transitioning into new clinical practice areas.
- The secretary of HHS should redirect all Graduate Medical Education funding from diploma nursing programs to support the implementation of nurse residency programs in rural and critical access areas.
- Health care organizations, the HRSA and Centers for Medicare and Medicaid Services, and philanthropic organizations should fund the development and implementation of nurse residency programs across all practice settings.
- Health care organizations that offer nurse residency programs and foundations should evaluate the effectiveness of the residency programs in improving the retention of nurses, expanding competencies, and improving patient outcomes (IOM, 2011, p. 12).

The actions to achieve residency programs require a significant commitment by both public and private investors.

In November 2010, the CCNA launched the *Campaign for Action*. Their mission is "to promote implementation of recommendations in the IOM report, *The Future of Nursing: Leading Change, Advancing Health*" (CCNA, 2013, para. 2). The *Campaign for Action* established State Action Coalitions in which nursing, health care, and industry leaders have committed to implementing various portions of the report in their state. A number of state coalitions are working to implement the need for nurse residencies at all educational levels.

At the federal level, one initiative to fund APRN residencies was signed into law through the ACA. Section 5316, Demonstration Grants for Family Nurse Practitioner Training Programs, was an attempt to provide NPs with a 1-year residency after graduation from their program. These practitioners would provide primary care to those in Federally Qualified Health Centers (FQHCs) and nurse-managed health clinics (NMHCs). Grants would be awarded to eligible FQHCs and NMHCs to cover the cost of full-time paid employment and benefits of family NPs. The law authorized $600,000 for each grant and designated such sums as necessary for FYs 2011 and 2014 (P.L. 111–148, Sec. 5316).

However, like many programs and demonstrations created through the ACA, funding never came to fruition. An authorization does not equal an appropriation. When the Republicans took control of the House in 2010, new programs from the ACA were targeted, and in budget negotiations, many never saw an actual allocation. As time progressed, the debt ceiling intensified, and the Republicans took control of the Senate, making them in control of both congressional chambers, ACA programs and efforts came under continual scrutiny for effectiveness. Currently, the program has an expired authorization, making it harder to fund.

CONCLUSION

Funding for RN and APRN education has ebbed and flowed throughout history. New programs are developed given the nursing demand and phased out as they relate to the national agenda. Political factors have and will continue to play a large role in federal support for nursing education. However, nursing leaders have adapted and advocated based on the ever-changing dynamics. They have become savvier by seeking partners outside the profession and have truly invested in the importance of coalitions. For example, the work to achieve the GNE demonstration could not have been accomplished by one entity. Legislators need to know that the proposal or nursing policy is the will of the entire community, and in the best-case scenario, beyond nursing.

The health care system will continue to evolve and change. APRNs will be substantial players in ensuring access to the high-quality, cost-effective care that America's patients deserve. However, it is clear that the nation will not meet its goals of an improved system if federal investments in health professions education, including nursing, are not a priority.

DISCUSSION QUESTION

1. *Assume that all funding from the Federal government for GNE ceases. What impact will this have on nursing? On faculty? On the health care system?*

REFERENCES

Aiken, L., Cheung, R., & Olds, D. (2009). Education policy initiatives to address the nurse shortage in the United States. *Health Affairs, 28*(4), w646–w656.

American Association of Colleges of Nursing. (1998). Statement on the redirection of nursing education Medicare funds to graduate nurse education to the national bipartisan commission on the future of Medicare Graduate Medical Education Study Group. Archives of the American Association of Colleges of Nursing.

American Association of Colleges of Nursing. (2004). *2004–2005 enrollment and graduations in baccalaureate and graduate programs in nursing.* Washington, DC: Author.

American Association of Colleges of Nursing. (2006). *2006–2007 enrollment and graduations in baccalaureate and graduate programs in nursing.* Washington, DC: Author.

American Association of Colleges of Nursing. (2008a). Capitation grants: A solution for improving nursing school capacity. Archives of the American Association of Colleges of Nursing.

American Association of Colleges of Nursing. (2008b, October). *Government affairs report.* Report presented at the meeting of the American Association of Colleges of Nursing, Washington, DC.

American Association of Colleges of Nursing. (2012a). Graduate nurse education (GNE) demonstration. Retrieved from http://www.aacnnursing.org/Policy-Advocacy/GNE

American Association of Colleges of Nursing. (2012b). Sequestration: Estimating the impact on America's nursing workforce and healthcare discoveries. Archives of the American Association of Colleges of Nursing.

American Association of Colleges of Nursing. (2016a). Historical funding for Title VIII by program. Archives of the American Association of Colleges of Nursing.

American Association of Colleges of Nursing. (2016b, October). How much is too much?: A look into federal loans. Retrieved from http://www.aacnnursing.org/Portals/42/Policy/Newsletters/Inside%20Academic%20Nursing/October-2016.pdf

Buerhaus, P. I., Staiger, D. O., & Auerbach, D. I. (2009). *The future of the nursing workforce in the United States: Data, trends, and implications.* Boston, MA: Jones & Bartlett.

Center to Champion Nursing in America. (2013). About us. Retrieved from http://campaignforaction.org/about-us

Congressional Research Service. (2005). *Nursing workforce programs in Title VIII of the Public Health Service Act* (Order Code RL32805). Washington, DC: The Library of Congress.

Debisette, A. T., Martinelli, A. M., Couig, M. P., & Braun, M. (2010). U.S. Public Health Service commissioned corps nurses: Responding in times of national need. *Nursing Clinics of North America, 45*(2), 125–135.

InsideGov. (n.d.). ACA: Advanced nursing education expansion program. Retrieved from http://open-grants.insidegov.com/l/17204/ACA-Advanced-Nursing-Education-Expansion-Program-HRSA-10-281

Institute of Medicine. (1997). *On implementing a national graduate medical education trust fund.* Washington, DC: National Academies Press.

Institute of Medicine. (2010). *The future of nursing: Leading change, advancing health.* Washington, DC: National Academies Press.

Kalisch, B. J., & Kalisch, P. A. (1977). *Nurturer of nurses: A history of the U.S. public health service and its antecedents: 1798–1977.* Unpublished study prepared for the Division of Nursing.

Kalisch, B. J., & Kalisch, P. A. (1982). *Politics of Nursing.* Philadelphia, PA: J. B. Lippincott.

Medicare Graduate Nursing Education Act. (2009). S.1569, 110d Cong.

Medicare Graduate Nursing Education Act. (2009). H.R. 3185, 110d Cong.

National Health Service Corps. (2016a). Scholarships. Retrieved from http://nhsc.hrsa.gov/scholarships/index.html

National Health Service Corps. (2016b). Loan repayment. Retrieved from http://nhsc.hrsa.gov/loanrepayment/index.html

Nurse Training Act. (1964). Pub. L. No. 88–581.

Nursing Community. (2016, March). Nursing workforce development programs: Title VIII of the Public Health Service Act. Retrieved from http://www.aacn.nche.edu/government-affairs/2015-Title-VIII-Brochure.pdf

Nursing Community Consensus Document. (2008). Reauthorization priorities for Title VIII, Public Health Service Act (42 U.S.C. 296 et seq.). Archives of the American Association of Colleges of Nursing.

Patient Protection and Affordable Care Act. (2010). Pub. L No. 111–148 § 5509.

Patient Protection and Affordable Care Act. (2010). Pub. L No. 111–1148 § 5316.

Politzer, R. M., Trible, L. Q., Robinson, T. D., Heard, D., Weaver, D. L., Reig, S. M., & Gaston, M. (2000). The national health service corps for the 21st century. *Journal of Ambulatory Care Management, 23*(3), 70–85. Public Health Service Ac. Pub. L. No. 107–205.

Scott, J. M. (1967). Three years with the Nurse Training Act. *American Journal of Nursing, 67*(10), 2107–2109.

Theis, K. M., & Harper, D. (2004). Medicare funding for nursing education: Proposal for a coherent policy agenda. *Nursing Outlook, 52*(6), 297–303.

Title VIII reauthorization statutory language changes. (2009). Retrieved from https://c.ymcdn.com/sites/wocn.site-ym.com/resource/collection/031F819D-B859-4E19-9087-DB6A035C531A/Stat._Language_for_Title_VIII_Reauthorization_5-19-09.pdf

U.S. Department of Health and Human Services, Health Resources and Services Administration. (2010, June 17). Affordable Care Act, Advanced Nursing Education Expansion (ANEE), New Competition. Announcement Number HRSA-10-281, Catalog of Federal Domestic Assistance No. 93.513.

U.S. Department of Health and Human Services. (2010, September 27). HHS awards $320 million to expand primary care workforce. Retrieved from https://wayback.archive-it.org/3926/20131018160545/http://www.hhs.gov/news/press/2010pres/09/20100927e.html

U.S. Department of Health and Human Services, Centers for Medicare and Medicaid, Center for Medicare and Medicaid Innovation. (2012). Graduate nurse education demonstration solicitation. Retrieved from http://www.innovation.cms.gov/Files/x/GNE_solicitation.pdf

Yett, D. E. (1966). The nursing shortage and the Nursing Training Act of 1964. *Industrial and Labor Relations Review, 19*(2), 190–200.

Yett, D. E. (1975). *An economic analysis of the nursing shortage*. Lexington, MA: D.C. Heath.

CHAPTER 13

Implications of Health Care Reform on Independent Practice

Laura J. Thiem

Advanced Practice Registered Nurses (APRNs) experience various challenges in the practice environment. As the APRN role has evolved, inconsistencies in regulations, education, and certification hinder APRNs from practicing to the full magnitude of their education and preparation. The purpose of this chapter is to assist the reader in reviewing the historical background of APRN practice and policy changes, identifying the various definitions of APRN, and identifying the current regulations regarding APRN practice. Furthermore, the chapter discusses barriers to full and unrestricted APRN practice, as well as progress made in recent years to reduce or eliminate constraints.

A REVIEW OF THE HISTORY OF THE APRN

Historically, nurses have provided health care to underserved and needy patients. Groups of nurses including the Henry Street Settlement Visiting Nurse Service, the Frontier Nursing Service Certified Nurse-Midwives, and Indian Health Service nurses collaborated with physicians and pharmacists to expand access to patient services in areas where health care professionals were scarce (Keeling, 2015). The nurse anesthetists (NAs) were the first recognized nursing specialty, with a rich history of patient care dating to the 1870s (Bankert, 1989). Nurses provided safe anesthesia, decreasing patient morbidity, and mortality. By keeping thorough records and publishing detailed data, Alice Magaw defined and promoted the role of the NA (Bankert, 1989).

The nurse-midwives (NMs) became a recognized specialty in the late 1920s. Formal programs were developed to train RNs to perform prenatal care and deliveries. The Frontier Nursing Service provided patient care in the home with little physician interaction, while physicians and NMs provided care for the Maternity Center Association (Dawley, 2003). The NMs demonstrated safer care than their physician and lay counterparts (Dawley, 2003).

In the early 1900s, with the passage of the Nursing Registration Act, certain regulations were implemented, which delineated services that the nurses could provide (Keeling, 2015). The language stated that nurses were not to provide treatments or offer cures for illness. The definition of treatment was poorly defined, with conflicting opinions regarding common home remedies and readily available chemical compounds. Subsequently, the Food and Drug Act was implemented in 1906. This legislation began to define prescribing practices and treatment options limiting access to the home remedies and chemical compounds. The designations for access to treatments by physicians or by physician order only, controlling access by nurses, would be perpetuated for several decades (Keeling, 2015).

The NAs were also condemned for practicing medicine in the delivery of anesthesia. Physician groups attempted to define medical practice, excluding and limiting nurses from performing anesthesia. Two pivotal cases in Kentucky in 1917 and California in 1936 rendered decisions solidifying the NA role (Thatcher, 1953). Each case upheld a provision of anesthesia as a nursing role.

The Clinical Nurse Specialist (CNS) was initially an informal role that gained formal recognition in the 1950s (Peplau, 1965/2003). The role was authenticated by the need for research and development of new nursing practice strategies in evolving health care settings. The CNS would explore a health problem using observation, interpretation, and intervention with scientific methodology and advanced knowledge gleaned from education and experience (Peplau, 1965/2003). In 1976, the American Nurses Association (ANA) Congress for Nursing Practice issued a position statement identifying the CNS as a master's-degree-prepared nurse with clinical concentration (ANA Congress for Nursing Practice, 1976). By 1986 the CNS role had shifted from focused practice to include expertise in research, education, consultation, and administration (Fulton, 2002).

Expanding the Nursing Role

In an attempt to improve access to medical care for pediatric patients and families in underserved areas, Loretta Ford, RN, and Henry Silver, MD, developed an expanded role for RNs in the mid-1960s (McGivern, 1986). The new role built on the knowledge and skills of the RN to improve access to health care, provide continuity of care, and coordinate aspects of health care for pediatric patients (Ford, 1979). The programs were started as certificate continuing education programs. Graduate education in the early 1980s provided the supplemental knowledge and skills for the expanded role. The expanded role was initially named Nurse Practitioner (NP; McGivern, 1986).

After exploration of the nursing role in meeting patient needs for improved and increased access to health care, the U.S. Department of Health, Education, and Welfare provided an opinion that access to medical services could be expanded by increased usage of the RN workforce. The committee recommended the development of educational programs to prepare the current nursing workforce to provide primary care services. Regarding licensure, the committee endorsed adoption of a national licensure without state restricted barriers. A collegial, respectful, and collaborative relationship between physicians and nurses avoiding territorial concerns of the disciplines was encouraged for the benefit of the patient (Department of Health, Education and Welfare Secretary's Committee to Study Extended Roles for Nurses, 1972). While the educational programs were implemented, the other two recommendations failed.

Role Definition

The ANA, a large and respected nursing organization, defined the role of the professional RNs in 1955. The definition specifically noted that the nurses were not to diagnose or prescribe therapeutic treatments (Keeling, 2015). The description profoundly impeded nurses from providing advanced care or expanding the nursing role. Additionally, Keeling (2015) noted that the conflict between organized medical groups and nursing organizations intensified when the limiting language for nursing was presented. The restrictive language became the basis of antagonism between the fields of nursing and medicine in future years as each group claimed sole ownership of knowledge and technique unique to their professional discipline. Medicine attempted to defend its knowledge as opposed to encroachment by nursing. Ford (1979) discusses revisions in the ANA's scope-of-practice language for the NP in 1976. This language modification broadened the APRN scope of practice to include independent assessment, diagnosis, and treatment with collaboration and referral as indicated or needed (Ford, 1979).

In the 1980s the educational preparation of APRNs transitioned from the continuing education and certificate model to master's degrees or post-master's preparation (Pulcini & Wagner, 2001). The CNS role lost popularity as the NP role thrived. Dunphy, Youngkin, and Smith (2004) attribute the growth of NPs in the 1980s to third-party reimbursement, prescriptive privileges, and health care financial crisis.

In the 1990s the boards of nursing and the various certifying bodies joined to create a consistent certification for entry level performance testing. The nursing boards expressed concern that the eligibility criteria, particularly the educational requirements, for the exams were inconsistent, making the certification test a poor choice for licensure purposes. The certification inconsistencies were not legally defensible as an indicator for readiness to practice. As a result, in 2002 the unified effort created the rigorous psychometric examinations known today (National Council of State Boards of Nursing [NCSBN], n.d.-a).

Another movement occurring in the 1990s was the development of regulation of APRN practice. Identifying the need to protect and inform the public of the treating provider and reduce the risk of harm, the NCSBN encouraged each state board to develop statutes to identify and control APRNs. By 1997 each state had developed licensure, certification, or recognition for the APRN (NCSBN, n.d.-a)

In 2008 the APRN designation was further defined in the *Consensus Model for APRN Regulation: Licensure, Accreditation, Certification, and Education* (LACE) published by the NCSBN APRN Advisory Committee. This report uses the following criteria to outline the APRN role:

The definition of an APRN is a nurse:

1. Who has completed an accredited graduate-level education program preparing him/her for one of the four recognized APRN roles
2. Who has passed a national certification examination that measures APRN, role and population-focused competencies, and who maintains continued competence as evidenced by recertification in the role and population through the national certification program
3. Who has acquired advanced clinical knowledge and skills preparing him/her to provide direct care to patients, as well as a component of indirect care; however, the defining factor for all APRNs is that a significant component of the education and practice focuses on direct care of individuals
4. Whose practice builds on the competencies of RNs by demonstrating a greater depth and breadth of knowledge, a greater synthesis of data, increased complexity of skills and interventions, and a greater role autonomy
5. Who is educationally prepared to assume responsibility and accountability for health promotion and/or maintenance, as well as the assessment, diagnosis, and management of patient problems, which includes the use and prescription of pharmacologic and non-pharmacologic interventions
6. Who has clinical experience of sufficient depth and breadth to reflect the intended license
7. Who has obtained a license to practice as an APRN in one of the four APRN roles: Certified Registered Nurse Anesthetist (CRNA), Certified Nurse-Midwife (CNM), CNS, or Certified Nurse Practitioner (CNP; APRN Consensus Work Group & NCSBN APRN Advisory Committee, 2008)

This language is the foundation for current APRN practice. The report clarifies components of licensure, accreditation, credentialing, and education as applicable to APRN practice (APRN Consensus Work Group & NCSBN APRN Advisory Committee, 2008).

Legal Precedents

The Missouri legal case of *Sermchief v. Gonzales*, in 1983, set a legal precedent for the expansion of NP practice. The Board of Healing Arts filed the suit claiming two women's health NPs (WHNP) were practicing medicine without a license. The Missouri Supreme Court noted that the areas of nursing and medicine have common characteristics. Furthermore, the court stated that the Missouri Board of Healing Arts had no jurisdiction over professional nurses practicing within their licensure under the Missouri Nurse Practice Act (Blumenreich, 1998; Brent, 1997). The final verdict created the foundation for future APRN practice, encouraging the use of broad language and expanded practice indications (Keeling, 2015). This case legitimized the APRN role and acknowledged the overlap of features of nursing and medical practice.

Another case in California, *Fein v. Permanente Medical Group*, reinforced the commonality of nursing and medical practices (Brent, 1997). One aspect of note is that the APRN is to be held to the scope and standards of practice of a reasonable and prudent APRN, not professionals from medicine. The case also validated that the APRN practice is under the jurisdiction of the State Board of Nursing rather than a medical board (Brent, 1997)

APRN CORE COMPETENCIES AND PRACTICE ESSENTIALS

The Federal Guidelines for Preparation of Nurse Practitioners in 1971 was the foundation for graduate nursing education (Mezey, 1986). The guidelines identified core content for programs including philosophy and legal concepts; role within the health care system; scientific knowledge for practice; strategies for role implementation and commonalities across practice settings (Mezey, 1986). Diligent attempts to align the APRN preparation for practice have been made by the National Organization of Nurse Practitioner Faculty (NONPF). NONPF generated the core competencies for NP education in 1990 with revisions in 1995 and 2002. In the 2002 revision, the competencies were listed under seven domains. The domains included the following:

- Maintenance of patient illness/health status
- The Nurse Practitioner–patient relationship
- The teaching–coaching function
- Professional role
- Managing and negotiating health care systems
- Monitoring and ensuring the quality of health care practice
- Cultural competence (NONPF, 2002)

Each competency has additional behaviors to be exhibited by the graduates of the NP programs. Treatment may include prescription medications and therapeutic modalities (AACN, 2006, NONPF, 2002). The essential elements of APRN practice include assessing, diagnosing, and providing treatment of patients.

In 2009 NONPF presented extensive criteria for doctoral programs building on the master's level competencies (Dieter, Guberski, & Wolf, 2013). Both master's program and doctoral programs prepare the APRN for full and autonomous practice with professional accountability (NONPF, 2002). Each type of graduate degree program conveys the requisites for board certification (NONPF, 2002). The AACN makes the distinction between clinical APRN roles and research or leadership roles in nursing. The APRN roles are distinct, with different licensure, liability, and reimbursement issues than other nursing roles (AACN, 2006).

Identification of APRN Roles and Certification

Board certification serves to identify individuals who have successfully completed a course of study and have acquired the minimum skill competency for practice (Mezey, 1986). A majority of states in the United States require board certification for APRN licensure or recognition (American Association of Nurse Practitioners [AANP], n.d.). Indiana, Kansas, and Nevada license APRNs based on educational program requirements without a national certification requirement. California and New York have additional paths to licensure without national certification. APRN roles and certification are identified by the population to be served. Role and population-based foci identified in the *Consensus Model* indicate the principal education of the APRN. The population foci currently include adult/gerontology (acute or primary care), family across the life span, neonatal, pediatric (acute or primary care), psychiatric/mental health, and women's health care. APRN-designated roles include Certified Nurse Practitioner (CNP), Certified Nurse-Midwife (CNM), Certified Registered Nurse Anesthetist (CRNA) and CNS. The acute or primary care settings are currently addressed in the educational program and are not specifically outlined in the *Consensus Model*. The organizations offering APRN certifications are listed in Table 13.1 with the corresponding APRN certification foci.

APRN Regulations

Although the majority of states regulate APRN practice under the auspices of the Board of Nursing, in several states, APRN licensure falls under other regulatory boards or departments (NursingLicensure.org, n.d.). APRNs in the Virginia Commonwealth are governed jointly by the Board of Nursing and the Medical Board. Each state has statutes describing the activities approved for the APRN (AANP, n.d.). The following states use regulatory boards other than nursing:

- Connecticut, Department of Public Health
- District of Columbia, Department of Public Health
- Illinois, Department of Financial and Professional Regulation
- Indiana, Professional Licensing Agency
- Nebraska, Department of Health and Human Services
- Utah, Division of Occupational and Professional Licensing
- Washington, Nursing Care Quality Assurance Commission
- Wisconsin, Department of Safety and Professional Services (NursingLicensure.org, n.d.)

Although all states recognize a variety of APRN roles, the practice regulations vary widely regarding accepted APRN roles, the scope of practice, and physician involvement. For instance, the designation of CNSs as APRNs is not found in the statute in the states of New Hampshire and Washington, limiting the CNS to the approved activities of a RN in those states (NursingLicensure.org, n.d.). Florida has a separate process for licensing the CNS and does not include the CNS as an APRN (NursingLicensure.org, n.d.). Licensure for CRNAs is different than for other APRN roles in Nevada because of the state statute (NursingLicensure.org, n.d.). CRNAs in New York and Pennsylvania are permitted to work on their RN license without state recognition of specialty. Likewise, CNMs in New York also practice on their RN license without additional state-defined recognition. States with a distinct procedure for licensing the CNM include:

- New Jersey, Midwifery Liaison Committee
- New Mexico, Department of Public Health
- Rhode Island, Advisory Committee on Midwifery (NursingLicensure. org, n.d.)

At the time of this writing, 22 states and the District of Columbia have authorized APRNs to fully practice within the scope of their education and preparation without restriction beyond certification and licensure (AANP, n.d., NCSBN, n.d-b). The remaining states have limited APRN practice and may require interaction with professionals of other disciplines, including physicians, dentists, or podiatrists, to provide services to patients (NCSBN, n.d.-b). Each APRN should be an expert on the APRN regulations of his or her state of practice.

IDENTIFICATION OF BARRIERS TO FULL PRACTICE BY APRNS

Restrictive Regulations

In the states lacking full practice authority, restrictive regulations vary by individual state (AANP, n.d., NCSBN, n.d.-b). The statutes of many states require APRNs to have a collaborative practice or supervision arrangement with physicians. In the remaining states, practice is severely restricted, with physician oversight and involvement mandated by state statute. The statutes attempt to formalize a relationship between APRN and physician to quantify or stratify responsibilities in the provision of patient care (NCSBN, n.d.-b). The restrictions fail to recognize the education and skill of the APRN professional. Furthermore, the constraints on APRN practice do not guarantee quality, patient safety, or patient satisfaction, as purported.

After a thorough investigation of health care needs in the United States, The Institute of Medicine (IOM), now known as National Academy of Health and Medicine Division (2010), offered several recommendations to remedy the shortage of primary health care providers and improve patient access to health care. The first is permitting APRNs "to practice to the full extent of their education and training" (p. 2). The IOM (2010) noted that the discrepancies in licensure or recognition for APRNs in various states impairs APRN full usage. A variety of solutions were suggested including national incentives promoting APRN practice as evidence-based best practice (IOM, 2010). Another solution encouraged filing Federal Trade Commission complaints about cases of restraint of trade in which APRNs have been restricted in business or practice opportunities (IOM, 2010).

Inconsistent Educational Preparation

Since the inception of the APRN role, criticism has been that the various APRN programs lacked consistent content or clinical preparation. Hours spent in clinical locations and experiences varied. Initially, programs consisted of continuing education certificates (Argondizzo & Miller, 1986) progressing to formal graduate education, usually a master's degree (Keeling, 2015; Mezey, 1986). The Commission on Collegiate Nursing Education (CCNE) was created in 1998 by the AACN to address this concern (Van Ort & Butlin, 2009). The CCNE, in conjunction with various nursing education organizations, developed accreditation criteria for graduate programs to improve consistency (Van Ort & Butlin, 2009). To be nationally accredited, each graduate school or program must develop and maintain a curriculum that meets or exceeds the CCNE standards. Curriculum and outcomes are reviewed at frequent intervals by CCNE teams to assure that the standards are sustained (AACN Commission on Collegiate Nursing Education, 2008).

NONPF reviewed the clinical component of APRN education, detecting irregularity in the amounts of hours the graduate student spent in a clinical setting with a preceptor (Van Ort & Butlin, 2009). Following the *Consensus Model for APRN Regulation: LACE*, NONPF encourages nursing programs to provide clinical hours and training opportunities to deliver consistent, measurable outcomes for APRN preparation (Hain & Fleck, 2014; NONPF, 2009). The *Consensus Model* has designated the following coursework in all APRN programs:

- Advanced physiology/pathophysiology, including general principles that apply across the life span
- Advanced health assessment, which includes assessment of all human systems, advanced assessment techniques, concepts and approaches
- Advanced pharmacology, which includes pharmacodynamics, pharmacokinetics, and pharmacotherapeutics of all broad categories of agents (APRN Consensus Work Group & NCSBN APRN Advisory Committee, 2008)

Consistent preparation across accredited programs reduces the argument of dissimilar or inadequate preparation when viewed from the consumer or other disciplines.

Lack of Unity

From the inception, the APRN role met resistance from the nursing and medical professions. The APRN role was criticized by the nursing fraternity as exceeding the accepted role of the professional nurse. Although professional nurses are formally trained to perform physical assessment, diagnosis and treatment were viewed as surpassing the nursing role. At the center of the dispute, the nursing discipline experienced a philosophical upheaval. The boundaries of nursing and medicine were indistinct, and the attempts to define the boundaries led to divisiveness in nursing and animosity between nursing and organized medicine (Freund, 1986). Eventually, the focus of nursing research shifted from creating definite boundaries for nursing to how to best meet the needs of patients and improve access in the 1970s (Freund, 1986).

The ANA issued the Social Policy Statement in 1981 with limiting language (ANA, 1981). Initially, the statement defined nursing as care provided to "a response to illness" (ANA, 1981) rather than diagnosis and treatment. When nurses who provided primary care objected, stating that diagnosis and treatment were essential functions in their role, the limiting and defining language was removed in subsequent revisions (Diers & Molde, 1983).

Grindel (2006) discusses the variables in the lack of unity in the nursing profession. By sheer numbers, the nursing workforce should be able to effect change and promotion of the profession and improve health care. Grindel (2006) notes that nursing has continued to be divided based on nurses' disinterest, lack of organized effort, and lack of leadership in creating and influencing policy. Another division of nursing is the perspective that nurse educators and nursing administrators are elitist and disconnected from the nursing workforce

(Neal-Boylan, 2015). Each nursing specialty may face unique challenges as noted with the CRNAs and the reimbursement issue earlier. Nurses outside of a specialty may not join an effort to support another group of nurses.

As evidenced by the numerous organizations offering certifications for the various APRN designations, a number of professional organizations seek to engage and represent APRNs. Various organizations vie for membership at the local, state, and national level. The organizations may represent nursing as a whole or by nursing specialty. Membership fees or dues can range in the hundreds of dollars creating, a financial disincentive to join. The numerous organizations may serve the focused interest of their members, which can conflict with the goals of other nursing organizations. Moreover, the lack of coordinated lobbying for the advancement of all APRN roles may result in delayed action because of inconsistent messages presented to the legislators.

Conflicts With Organizations Beyond Nursing

Medical organizations such as the American Medical Association (AMA) promulgate the superiority of medical training as more rigorous while failing to acknowledge research that indicates patient satisfaction and outcomes are similar in physician and APRN groups (Hain & Fleck, 2014; Naylor & Kurtzman, 2010). The AMA has created scope-of-practice documents in an attempt to define and limit APRN practice (AMA, 2009; Isaacs & Jellinick, 2012). Another medical organization, The American Colleges of Physicians (Ginsburg, Taylor, & Barr, 2009), issued a position statement granting the APRN role as being complementary to that of the physician's role. As physician shortages continue, the availability of physicians to lead health care teams decreases compared to the increased needs in the health care arena. This disproportion creates an untenable position for the physician provider to remain as a leader of the health care team (Hain & Fleck, 2014). The IOM (2010) stated that "nurses should be full partners, with physicians and other health care professionals, in redesigning health care" (p. 3). This directive can only be accomplished with acknowledgment and appreciation of the scope of nursing education and preparation in the APRN scope of practice.

As a response to the IOM report, the AMA issued a statement declaring the superiority of physician education and training by length and quantity of clinical hours. The AMA continues to hold the perspective that care is best delivered by a physician-led team (Patchin, 2010). Another medical organization, American Academy of Family Physicians (AAFP), also issued a white paper touting the superiority of medical education and the necessity of a physician-led team (2012). The AAFP has published guidelines for physicians using supervisory role language in regard to APRNs (AAFP, 1990/2014, 1992/2013). These guidelines have not changed significantly since the 1990s and do not address physician shortages or studies indicating the safety and quality of care provided by APRNs.

Clarin (2007) identified physician attitude as a barrier to effective communication and collaboration between APRNs and medical professionals. She finds that physician belief of a hierarchy, with physicians positioned at the top, hinders the ability to connect and cooperate with the APRNs (Clarin, 2007). Physician attitude contributes to their lack of knowledge of the APRN scope of practice (Clarin, 2007; Hain & Fleck, 2014). Feeling that the medical knowledge is superior creates an inability to view other professionals, including APRNs, objectively.

The nursing and physician groups have a long history of incivility among them (Guidroz, Burnfield-Geimer, Clark, Schwetschenau & Jex, 2010; Rosenstein & O'Daniel, 2005). Incivility includes rudeness, discourtesy, or disrespect that may not be intended to be harmful (ANA, n.d.). Lachman (2010) expresses the need for trust and mutual respect for effective collaboration. However, attitude and incivility create acrimony between the nursing and medical professions, limiting the spirit of collaboration.

Lack of Financial Resources for Political Activity

Nursing professional organizations such as the ANA spend less than $1 million per year in lobbying activities (Center for Responsive Politics, n.d.-b) in comparison to $15 million by the AMA (Center for Responsive Politics, n.d.-a). The difference in spending may verify the influence of organized medicine in the policy-making process. The lack of cohesive lobbying may be a direct result of the fragmentation of the nursing community as noted in the "Lack of unity" section earlier. The APRN group has gained a powerful ally in AARP. AARP has assumed an advocacy role with the creation and submission of position papers and opinions on the benefit of APRNs in home health and hospice services (Brassard, 2011). AARP has also offered public opinions on lifting barriers to full practice by APRN in the Veterans Health Administration (Certner, 2016). Developing relationships with organizations seeking to improve health care creates a vehicle to advance policy.

Lack of Empaneling, Recognition, and Reimbursement of APRN Services

A long-standing hindrance to APRNs has been the lack of payment and reimbursement for services provided. Until the Omnibus Reconciliation Act of 1989 (H.R. 3299, 1989) APRNs were unable to bill for services provided to the patients. This legislation permitted narrow reimbursement of NPs and CRNAs in specific, limited situations. This act did provide employment opportunities for APRNs in Rural Health Clinics (H.R. 3299, 1989).

Some insurance companies have consistently refused to pay for services provided by APRNs and refused to credential and impanel nurses as providers (Chapman, Wides & Spetz, 2010; Naylor & Kurtzman, 2010; Yee, Boukus, Cross & Samuel, 2013). The Balanced Budget Act of 1997 provided for direct reimbursement of APRN services by Medicare and Medicaid (H.R. 2015, 1997). However, Medicare and Medicaid programs only reimburse NPs and CNSs at 85% of the physician rate for services provided (Medicare Payment Advisory Commission [MedPAC], 2002; Naylor & Kurtzman, 2010). Although the APRN services in primary care have been determined similar to the services provided by physicians, there is no parity in reimbursement (MedPAC, 2002; Naylor & Kurtzman, 2010).

Currently, CRNAs are reimbursed at 80% of the physician rate (Department of Health and Human Services, CMS, 2013). The CRNAs have met a variety of challenges in reimbursement. In the early 2000s, statutory language was introduced at the federal level requiring physician supervision of CRNAs in the hospital setting to be paid by Medicare (Malina & Izlar, 2014). This language was inconsistent with statutes in many states where CRNAs practiced without physician supervision. For the CRNAs to be reimbursed, the state government had to opt out of the program to assure anesthesia services, provided by CRNAs, were available to the constituents of their state (AANA, 2013). Malina and Izlar (2014) also noted that CRNAs were supported by CMS to be reimbursed for the provision of chronic pain management services if permitted by state statute. Chronic pain management services by CRNAs had been challenged by the American Society of Anesthesiologists (2000), who attempted to scare consumers out of CRNA service by claiming the CRNA had limited education and expertise.

CNMs gained 100% fee-for-service reimbursement with the passage of the Patient Protection and Affordable Care Act (PPACA) in 2010 (PPACA, 2010). As the previous rate had been 65% of the allowed physician Medicare charge, this legislation gave the CNM full parity in reimbursement. Additionally, the legislation created the path for CNMs to bill Medicare and other insurers directly for their services (American College of Nurse-Midwives, n.d.; PPACA, 2010).

Owing to the scope-of-practice restrictions in many states, APRNs have been forced to bill for services under a physician, effectively losing the APRN statistics regarding patient services (Chapman, Wides, & Spetz, 2010; Yee et al., 2013). Bunce and Wieske (2009) reported state by state regulations of health care coverage. Only 32 states had mandates for APRN reimbursement (Bunce & Wieske, 2009). Medicare altered the billing forms and processes to identify the rendering provider in 2007 (Department of Health and Human Services, Centers for Medicare and Medicaid Services, 2007). This alteration improved the ability to track the performance of the APRN profession by using the National Provider Identifier (NPI) of the APRN versus using the NPI of a physician (Yee et al., 2013). The IOM (2010) recommends electronic health record and billing technology to gather data, improving the identification of services provided by APRNs.

A further barrier to APRN practice is the limitations in the statute for APRNs to own and operate a business under the structure and protection of the corporate law. In many states corporations are limited by state statute from employing medical professionals as a revenue source (Michal, Pekarske, & McManus, 2006). The statutes vary significantly between states but have a significant impact on the APRN in a state requiring collaboration or supervision. In the collaborative practice states, corporate law may restrict the APRN wanting to own a practice or nurse-managed health clinic from hiring a physician to collaborate. If collaboration or supervision is a part of the APRN's nurse practice act and the corporate law prevents hiring a physician, the APRN cannot open a nurse-owned business.

IDENTIFICATION OF CURRENT ACTIVITY

Patient Protection and Affordable Care Act

With passage and implementation of the PPACA in 2010, additional opportunities are identified for APRNs to lead in models of care focused on illness prevention and health promotion (Lathrop & Hodnicki, 2014). Health promotion and preventive care activities are a cornerstone of APRN education (APRN Consensus Work Group & NCSBN APRN Advisory Committee, 2008). A shortcoming of PPACA is regulatory language increasing reimbursement for preventive screening services provided by or under the supervision of a physician (PPACA, 2010). This language is vague regarding APRNs and may result in detrimental effects for APRNs in states with full practice authority. APRNs need to take an active role to alter policy by educating and collaborating with policy makers to remove language limiting their practice and reimbursement to improve access to care for all patients.

Federal Trade Commission Policy

A policy paper was released by the Federal Trade Commission (Ramirez, Brill, Ohlhausen, & Wright, 2014) identifying the restraints to full and unencumbered practice by APRNs that may negatively impact the health care of the consumers. The paper delineates four areas of concern:

- Restrictive physician supervision requirements exacerbate well-documented provider shortages that could be mitigated by expanded APRN practice
- Excessive supervision may increase health care costs and prices
- Fixed supervision requirements may constrain innovation in health care delivery models
- Mandated collaboration agreements between APRNs and physicians are not necessary to achieve the benefits of physician–APRN coordination of care (Ramirez et al., 2016)

The policy paper recommends removal of mandated collaboration in all states (Ramirez et al., 2016).

Veterans Health Administration

The AANP conducted a grassroots campaign to remove practice restrictions for APRNs in the Veterans Health Administration (VHA) system. The VHA regulations varied by state, limiting APRNs from practicing to the full extent of their education and training (AANP, 2016; U.S. Department of Veterans Affairs, 2016). The VHA announced on December 13, 2016, that three of the APRN roles (NPs, CNSs, and CNMs) would gain full practice authority. CRNAs were not included in the amendment, which took effect January 13, 2017. Issues such as less demand and no shortage were cited by the anesthesiologist community. A full discussion of the VHA rationale for excluding CRNAs is included in the Federal Register announcement at this site (www.federalregister.gov/documents/2016/12/14/2016-29950/advanced-practice-registered-nurses). Efforts to gain full practice authority for all APRNs continue. Removal of practice restrictions in this large health care system, however, even for the three roles, sets a precedent for APRN full practice authority in other government-supported systems.

CASE IN POINT: MY PERSONAL EXPERIENCE

In 2006, I had the opportunity to open my practice as an NP when my employer sold the clinic where I had been working in a physician practice. My state has strong collaborative practice requirements meaning I would have to hire a physician to open the business. Fortunately, my state permits hiring physicians in a for-profit setting. The physician was paid $1500 per month, a significant expense to a small practice. In return, the physician appeared on site weekly, reviewed a number of charts, was available to me for questions via telephone, would serve as a hospitalist for patients requiring hospital care and provided a means to bill insurances that do not credential or impanel APRNs.

Seeing a need for psychiatric care in my rural area, I pursued education and certification in psychiatry. At that time only the psychiatric–mental health clinical nurse specialist (PMHCNS) was a reimbursable role by Medicaid in my state; the psychiatric–mental health nurse practitioner (PMHNP) credential was not. Once I had completed the coursework and certification as an adult PMHCNS, I sought a psychiatrist with whom to collaborate. There were two in the state-regulated 50 mile radius, and neither was willing to collaborate with me. As a result, I could not bill for psychiatric services as PMHCNS which may have created an additional revenue stream for the practice. Another limitation PMHCNS reimbursement in the mid-2000s was the lack of parity for psychiatric services. Often insurers did not cover psychiatric diagnoses or care. Medicare reimbursement for psychiatric services was significantly lower than medical services. I was fortunate to have the NP credential to provide limited psychiatric care in the primary care setting.

I opened and operated the clinic without loans or debt. I obtained certification for the business as a Rural Health Clinic improving the financial reimbursement for Medicare and Medicaid participants. The payor mix was unusual for a rural area, with approximately 45% private insurance, 15% Medicare, 25% Medicaid, and 15% uninsured/self-pay. The business grew although the country was in the throes of the Great Recession.

The implementation of the Affordable Care Act created a turning point for the business. Patients did not understand their insurance coverage, specifically deductibles, co-pay, and coinsurance. The patients did not pay their portions of their medical bills. As a result, the business incurred an insurmountable level of bad debt. Additional financial damage occurred when my state did not participate in Medicaid expansion. The expansion would have increased the number of covered patients and provided the business with additional revenue. The Affordable Care Act also offered incentives to physicians for health promotion activities performed under the physician's direct supervision. My business was not eligible as per the guidelines.

As a participating provider for Medicare and Medicaid, the business was incentivized to participate in the acquisition and implementation of an electronic health record and electronic billing software. The initial investment was manageable but the subsequent costs for upgrades and transition from International Classification of Diseases (ICD) version 9 to ICD-10 to participate in the second level was too expensive for my shoestring operation. Without these upgrades, the business would no longer be able to transmit bills for services rendered to insurance companies, Medicare or Medicaid.

Another aspect of my decision to close my practice involved the collaborative practice regulation and the availability of physicians to perform this service. My collaborating physician was in his 80s. I had concerns regarding the ability to find another collaborating physician should he become disabled or die. As the local physicians were employed by a hospital, none could enter into a contract or collaborative practice agreement. A business that would provide collaborative physician coverage for a fee was unaffordable. In a state with unencumbered practice hiring a physician to collaborate would not have been a concern.

(continued)

CASE IN POINT: MY PERSONAL EXPERIENCE *(continued)*

I closed my practice in 2014, after 8 years, when the business model was no longer adaptable or sustainable. Approximately half of the nurse-owned clinics in my state met a similar fate in recent years. Most of the former clinic owners claim similar factors for closure: collaborative practice restrictions, the impact of the Affordable Care Act, and the costs for participating in the electronic health record stimulus implementation. Federal and state regulations both impacted the practice and the ability to maintain viability and solvency.

TABLE 13.1 Organizations Offering Certification With the List of Certifications Offered

American Association of Nurse Practitioners Certification Program (n.d.)	Adult Nurse Practitioner (ANP) Family Nurse Practitioner Adult-Gerontology Primary Care Nurse Practitioner (AGNP)
American Nurses Credentialing Center (n.d.)	Nurse Practitioner Certifications Acute Care NP Adult Nurse NP Adult-Gerontology Acute Care NP Adult-Gerontology Primary Care NP Adult Psychiatric–Mental Health NP Family NP Gerontological NP Pediatric Primary Care NP Psychiatric–Mental Health NP School NP Adult Health CNS Adult-Gerontology CNS Adult Psychiatric–Mental Health CNS Child/Adolescent Psychiatric–Mental Health CNS Gerontological CNS Home Health CNS Pediatric CNS Public/Community Health CNS
American Midwifery Certification Board (n.d.)	Certified Nurse-Midwife
National Board of Certification & Recertification for Nurse Anesthetists (n.d.)	Certified Registered Nurse Anesthetist
National Certification Corporation (n.d.)	Neonatal Nurse Practitioner Womens Health Care Nurse Practitioner
Pediatric Nursing Certification Board (n.d.)	Primary Care Pediatric Nurse Practitioner Acute Care Pediatric Nurse Practitioner Pediatric Primary Care Mental Health Specialist

CNS, Clinical Nurse Specialist; NP, Nurse Practitioner.

CONCLUSION

Reviewing the history as related in the chapter, the reader can appreciate the steady progress being made since the origin of the APRN role in the 1960s. The history is a revealing tale of adaptation, perseverance, and progression on many fronts. Today's APRN must be aware of the regulations and impending changes that affect practice. An active role in creating change and removing restrictions provides a unified effort toward practice unfettered with artificial barriers.

DISCUSSION QUESTIONS

1. *What impact has a policy created on the development of an independent APRN role?*
2. *What barriers exist for APRNs to practice to the full extent of their educational preparation and training?*
3. *If you were going to describe the importance of your issue for policy change to potential supporters, what key issues would you stress? How would you describe this to your patients?*
4. *Consider the health policy changes discussed in this chapter or those you have described in your analysis and consider the impact that might occur if these changes are NOT enacted. In other words, what are the consequences of inaction?*

ANALYSIS, SYNTHESIS, AND CLINICAL APPLICATION

1. *Identify and describe a historical event in APRN regulation that you feel influenced the current status of APRN practice.*
2. *Based on the information in this chapter, list at least two areas of policy change you can identify where legislation could have an impact and give rationale.*

EXERCISES/CONSIDERATIONS

1. *Explore the impact on availability and delivery of patient care from an ethical standpoint.*
2. *Is it ethical to limit patient access to care due to barriers to APRN practice as described in the chapter?*

REFERENCES

Advanced Practice Registered Nurse Consensus Work Group and National Council of State Boards of Nursing Advanced Practice Registered Nurse Advisory Committee. (2008). Consensus model for APRN regulation: Licensure, accreditation, certification & education. Retrieved from https://www.ncsbn.org/Consensus_Model_for_APRN_Regulation_July_2008.pdf

American Academy of Family Physicians. (2012). *Primary care for the 21st century: Ensuring a quality physician-led team for every patient.* Kansas, MO: Author. Retrieved from http://www.aafp.org/dam/AAFP/documents/about_us/initiatives/AAFP-PCMHWhitePaper.pdf?cmpid=npp12_ad_com_na_van_1

American Academy of Family Physicians. (2013). Guidelines on the supervision of certified nurse midwives, nurse practitioners and physician assistants. Retrieved from http://www.aafp.org/about/policies/all/guidelines-nurses.html (Original work posted 1992)

American Academy of Family Physicians. (2014). Nurse midwives, certified. Retrieved from http://www.aafp.org/about/policies/all/nurse-midwives.html (Original work posted 1990)

American Association of Colleges of Nursing. (2006). The essentials of doctoral education for advanced nursing practice. Retrieved from http://www.aacnnursing.org/Portals/42/Publications/DNPEssentials.pdf

American Association of Colleges of Nursing Commission on Collegiate Nursing Education. (2008). Achieving excellence in accreditation: The first 10 years of CCNE. Retrieved from http://www .aacnnursing.org/Portals/42/CCNE/PDF/CCNE-History.pdf?ver=2017-06-26-152325-193

American Association of Nurse Anesthetists. (2013). Federal supervision rule/opt-out information. Retrieved from www.aana.com/advocacy/stategovernmentaffairs/Pages/Federal-Supervision -Rule-Opt-Out-Information.aspx

American Association of Nurse Practitioners. (n.d.). State practice environment. Retrieved from https:// www.aanp.org/legislation-regulation/state-legislation/state-practice-environment

American Association of Nurse Practitioners. (2016). AANP hails VA for advancing regulatory proposal to grant veterans full and direct access to nurse practitioners. Retrieved from https://www.aanp .org/press-room/press-releases/173-press-room/2016-press-releases/1950-aanp-hails-va-for -advancing-regulatory-proposal-to-grant-veterans-full-and-direct-access-to-nurse-practitioners

American Association of Nurse Practitioners Certification Program. (n.d.). AANPCP certification. Retrieved from http://www.aanpcert.org/certs

American College of Nurse Midwives. (n.d.). Equitable medicare reimbursement. Retrieved from http:// www.midwife.org/Equitable-Reimbursement

American Medical Association. (2009). *AMA scope of practice data series: Nurse practitioners*. Chicago, IL: Author. Retrieved from https://www.tnaonline.org/wp-content/uploads/2016/12/apn -ama-sop-1109.pdf

American Midwifery Certification Board. (n.d.). American midwifery certification. Retrieved from http://www.amcbmidwife.org

American Nurses Association. (n.d.). Incivility, bullying, and workplace violence. Retrieved from http:// www.nursingworld.org/Bullying-Workplace-Violence

American Nurses Association Congress on Nursing Practice. (1976). *Definition: Nurse practitioner, nurse clinician and clinical nurse specialist*. New York, NY: Author.

American Nurses Credentialing Center. (n.d.). AANC certification center. Retrieved from http://www .nursecredentialing.org/Certification

American Society of Anesthesiologists. (2000). ASA reports: Doctors fight for seniors' rights to keep safest anesthesia care possible. Retrieved from http://www.prnewswire.com/news-releases/ asa-reports-doctors-fight-for-seniors-rights-to-keep-safest-anesthesia-care-available-73194792 .html

Argondizzo, N. T., & Miller, M. A. (1986). Preparation of nurse practitioners in continuing educa- tion programs: The New York Hospital-Cornell Medical Center Experience. In M. Mezey & D. McGivern (Eds.), *Nurses, nurse practitioners: The evolution of primary care* (pp. 55–61). Boston, MA: Little, Brown.

Bankert, M. (1989). *Watchful care: A history of America's nurse anesthetists*. New York, NY: Continuum.

Blumenreich, G. A. (1998). The overlap between the practice of medicine and the practice of nursing. *Journal of the American Academy of Nurse Anesthetists, 66*(1), 11–15.

Brassard, A. (2011). Removing barriers to advanced practice registered nurse care: Home health and hos- pice services. *Insight on the Issues, 66*. Retrieved from http://www.aarp.org/content/dam/aarp/ research/public_policy_institute/health/removing-barriers-advanced-practice-registered-nurse -home-health-hospice-insight-july-2012-AARP-ppi-health.pdf

Brent, N. J. (1987). The nurse practitioner after Sermchief and Fein: Smooth sailing or rough waters? *Valparaiso University Law Review, 21*(2), 221–240. Retrieved from http://scholar.valpo.edu/vulr/ vol21/iss2/1

Bunce, V. C., & Wieske, J. P. (2009). *Health insurance mandates in the states 2009*. Alexandria, VA: Council for Affordable Health Insurance. Retrieved from https://www2.cbia.com/ieb/ag/CostOfCare/ RisingCosts/CAHI_HealthInsuranceMandates2009.pdf

Center for Responsive Politics. (n.d.-a). Influence & lobbying: Summary: American Medical Association. Retrieved from https://www.opensecrets.org/lobby/clientsum.php?id=D000000068&year =2016

Center for Responsive Politics. (n.d.-b). Influence & lobbying: Summary: American Nurses Association. Retrieved from https://www.opensecrets.org/lobby/clientsum.php?id=D000000173

Certner, D. (2016). Letter to the Director, Regulations Management, Department of Veterans Affairs. Retrieved from http://campaignforaction.org/wp-content/uploads/2016/07/AARP-Letter-VHA.pdf

Chapman, S. A., Wides, C. D., & Spetz, J. (2010). Payment regulations for advanced practice nurses: Implications for primary care. *Policy, Politics, & Nursing Practice, 11*(2), 89–98. doi:10.1177/1527154410382458

Clarin, O. A. (2007). Strategies to overcome barriers to effective nurse practitioner and physician collaboration. *Journal for Nurse Practitioners, 3*(8), 538–548.

Dawley, K. (2003). Origins of nurse-midwifery in the United States and its expansion in the 1940s. *Journal of Midwifery and Women's Health, 48*(2), 86–95. doi:10.1016/S1526-9523(03)00002-3

Department of Health and Human Services, Centers for Medicare and Medicaid Services. (2007, March 30). CMS Manual System: Pub 100-04 Medicare Claims Processing Transmittal 1215, Revisions to Form CMS-1500 Submission Requirements. Retrieved from https://www.cms.gov/Regulations-and-Guidance/Guidance/Transmittals/downloads/R1215CP.pdf

Diers, D., & Molde, S. (1983). Nurses in primary care: The new gatekeepers? *American Journal of Nursing, 83*(5), 742–745.

Dieter, C., Guberski, T., & Wolf, A. (Eds.). (2013). DNP NP toolkit: Process and approach to DNP competency based evaluation. Retrieved from http://c.ymcdn.com/sites/www.nonpf.org/resource/resmgr/imported/DNPNPToolkitFinal2013.pdf

Dunphy, L. M., Youngkin, E. Q., & Smith, N. K. (2004). Advanced practice nursing: Doing what had to be done: Radicals, renegades and rebels. In L. A. Joel (Ed.), *Advanced practice nursing: Essentials for role development* (p. 23). Philadelphia, PA: F. A. Davis.

Department of Health, Education, and Welfare Secretary's Committee to Study Extended Roles for Nurses. (1972). Expanding the scope of nursing practice. *Nursing Outlook, 20*, 46–52.

Ford, L. (1979). A nurse for all settings: The nurse practitioner. *Nursing Outlook, 27*, 516–521.

Freund, C. (1986). Nurse practitioners in primary care. In M. Mezey & D. McGivern (Eds.), *Nurses, nurse practitioners: The evolution of primary care* (pp. 305–333). Boston, MA: Little, Brown.

Fulton, J. S. (2002). Defining our practice. *Clinical Nurse Specialist, 16*(4), 1–3.

Ginsburg, J., Taylor, T., & Barr, M. S. (2009). Nurse practitioners in primary care: A policy monograph of the American Colleges of Physicians. Retrieved from https://www.acponline.org/advocacy/current_policy_papers/assets/np_pc.pdf

Grindel, C. (2006). The power of nursing: Can it ever be mobilized? *MedSurg Nursing, 16*(1), 5–6.

Guidroz, A. M., Burnfield-Geimer, J. L., Clark, O., Schwetschenau, H. M., & Jex, S. M. (2010). The nursing incivility scale: Development and validation of an occupation-specific measure. *Journal of Nursing Measurement, 18*(3), 176–200. doi:10.1891/1061-3749.18.3.176

H.R.2015, 105th Congress. (1997). Balanced Budget Act of 1997 (enacted). Retrieved https://www.congress.gov/bill/105th-congress/house-bill/2015

H.R.3299, 101st Congress. (1989). Omnibus Budget Reconciliation Act of 1989 (enacted). Retrieved from https://www.congress.gov/bill/101st-congress/house-bill/3299

Hain, D., & Fleck, L. M. (2014). Barriers to NP practice that impact healthcare design. *Online Journal of Issues in Nursing, 19*(2). Retrieved from http://www.nursingworld.org/MainMenuCategories/ANAMarketplace/ANAPeriodicals/OJIN/TableofContents/Vol-19-2014/No2-May-2014/Barriers-to-NP-Practice.html

Institute of Medicine of the National Academies. (2010). *The future of nursing: Leading change, advancing health.* Retrieved from http://www.nationalacademies.org/hmd/Reports/2010/The-Future-of-Nursing-Leading-Change-Advancing-Health.aspx

Issacs, S., & Jellinick, P. (2012). Accept no substitute: A report on scope of practice. *Physicians Foundation.* Retrieved from http://www.physiciansfoundation.org/uploads/default/A_Report_on_Scope_of_Practice.pdf

Keeling, A. (2015). Historical perspectives on an expanded role for nursing. *Online Journal of Issues in Nursing, 20*(2). doi:10.3912/OJIN.Vol20No02Man02

Lachman, V. D. (2010). Ethical issues in the disruptive behaviors of incivility, bullying, and horizontal/lateral violence. *MedSurg Nursing, 23*(1), 56–60. Retrieved from http://www.nursingworld.org/MainMenuCategories/EthicsStandards/Resources/Ethical-Issues-in-Disrutive-Behaviors.pdf

Lathrop, B., & Hodnicki, D. (2014). The Affordable Care Act: Primary care and the doctor of nursing practice nurse. *Online Journal of Issues in Nursing, 19*(2). doi:10.3912/OJIN.Vol198No02PPT02

Malina, D. P., & Izlar, J. J. (2014). Education and practice barriers for certified registered nurse anesthetists. *Online Journal of Issues in Nursing, 19*(2). Retrieved from http://www.nursingworld .org/MainMenuCategories/ANAMarketplace/ANAPeriodicals/OJIN/TableofContents/Vol-19 -2014/No2-May-2014/Barriers-for-Certified-Registered-Nurse-Anesthetists.html#AANA13a

McGivern, D. (1986). The evolution of primary care nursing. In M. Mezey & D. McGivern (Eds.), *Nurses, nurse practitioners: The evolution of primary care* (pp. 3–14). Boston, MA: Little, Brown.

Medicare Payment Advisory Commission. (2002, June). Report to the Congress: Medicare payment to advanced practice nurses and physician assistants. Retrieved from http://www.medpac.gov/ docs/default-source/reports/jun02_NonPhysPay.pdf?sfvrsn=0

Mezey, M. D. (1986). Issues in graduate education. In M. Mezey & D. McGivern (Eds.), *Nurses, nurse practitioners: The evolution of primary care* (pp. 101–119). Boston, MA: Little, Brown.

Michal, M. H., Pekarske, M. S. L., & McManus, M. K. (2006). Corporate practice of medicine doctrine 50 state survey summary. Retrieved from http://www.nhpco.org/sites/default/files/public/ palliativecare/corporate-practice-of-medicine-50-state-summary.pdf

National Board of Certified Registered Nurse Anesthetists. (n.d.). Certification. Retrieved from https:// www.nbcrna.com/certification/Pages/default.aspx

National Certification Corporation. (n.d.) Certification. Retrieved from https://www.nccwebsite.org/ Certification

National Council of State Boards of Nursing. (n.d.-a). History of APRN. Retrieved from https://www .ncsbn.org/737.htm

National Council of State Boards of Nursing. (n.d.-b). NCSBN's APRN campaign for consensus: State progress toward uniformity: Consensus model implementation status. Retrieved from https:// www.ncsbn.org/5397.htm

National Organization of Nurse Practitioner Faculty. (2002). *Nurse practitioner primary care competencies in specialty areas: Adult, family, gerontological, pediatric, and women's health.* Retrieved from http://c. ymcdn.com/sites/www.nonpf.org/resource/resmgr/competencies/primarycarecomps02.pdf

National Organization of Nurse Practitioner Faculty. (2009). Clarification of nurse practitioner specialty and subspecialty clinical track titles, hours, and credentialing: Report of a four-phased research project conducted by the National Organization of Nurse Practitioner Faculties. Retrieved from http://c.ymcdn.com/sites/www.nonpf.org/resource/resmgr/consensus_model/projectfinal report.pdf?hhSearchTerms=%22Position+and+paper+and+clinical+and+hours+and+nurse+and +practi%22

Naylor, M. D., & Kurtzman, E. T. (2010). The role of nurse practitioners in redefining primary care. *Health Affairs, 29*(5), 893–899. doi:10.1377/hlthaff.2010.0440

Neal-Boylan, L. (2015). Looking toward the future of nursing practice. In L. Neal-Boylan (Ed.), *The nurse's reality shift: Using history to transform the future.* Indianapolis, IN: Sigma Theta Tau International.

NursingLicensure.org. (n.d.). Nurse practitioner licensure requirements: Change is in the air. Retrieved from http://www.nursinglicensure.org/articles/nurse-practitioner-license.html

Patchin, R. J. (2010). AMA responds to IOM report on future of nursing. *Fiercenews.* Retrieved from http://www.fiercehealthcare.com/healthcare/ama-responds-to-iom-report-future-nursing

Patient Protection and Affordable Care Act. (2010). Pub. L. No. 111–148, §2702, 124 Stat. *119*, 318–319. Retrieved from www.gpo.gov/fdsys/pkg/PLAW-111publ148/pdf/PLAW-111publ148.pdf

Pediatric Nursing Certification Board. (n.d.). PNCB exams. Retrieved from https://www.pncb.org/ ptistore/control/exams/index

Peplau, H. (1965/2003). Specialization in professional nursing. *Clinical Nurse Specialist, 17*(1), 3–9.

Pulcini, J., & Wagner, M. (2001). Nurse practitioner education in the United States. Retrieved from https://international.aanp.org/Content/docs/pulciniarticle0305.pdf

Ramirez, E., Brill, J., Ohlhausen, M. K., & Wright, J. D. (2014). Policy perspectives: Competition and the regulation of advanced practice nurses. Retrieved from https://www.ftc.gov/system/ files/documents/reports/policy-perspectives-competition-regulation-advanced-practice -nurses/140307aprnpolicypaper.pdf

Rosenstein, A. H., & O'Daniel, M. (2005). Disruptive & clinical perceptions of behavior outcomes: Perceptions of nurses and physicians. *American Journal of Nursing, 105*(1), 54–64.

Thatcher, V. S. (1953). *History of anesthesia with emphasis on the nurse specialist.* Philadelphia, PA: Lippincott. Retrieved from http://www.aana.com/resources2/archives-library/Documents/0008CHP7.pdf

U.S. Department of Veterans Affairs. (2016). VA proposes to grant full practice authority to advanced practice registered nurses. Retrieved from http://www.va.gov/opa/pressrel/pressrelease.cfm?id=2793

Van Ort, S. R., & Butlin, J. (2009). *Achieving excellence in accreditation: The first 10 years of CCNE*. Washington, DC: Commission on Collegiate Nursing Education.

Yee, T., Boukus, E., Cross, D., & Samuel, D. (2013). Primary care workforce shortages: Nurse practitioner scope-of-practice laws and payment policies. NIHCR Research Brief No. 13. Retrieved from http://nihcr.org/analysis/improving-care-delivery/prevention-improving-health/pcp-workforce-nps

CHAPTER 14

The Affordable Care Act: Primary Care and the Doctor of Nursing Practice

Breanna Lathrop and Donna R. Hodnicki

The Patient Protection and Affordable Care Act (PPACA), signed into law on March 23, 2010, is the most expansive health care reform legislation in the United States since the creation of Medicare and Medicaid in 1965. The PPACA establishes a new direction for the U.S. health care system that includes an emphasis on preventive services and primary care. It provides insurance coverage to millions who are currently uninsured and attempts to address areas of the current health care system that are in need of reform so that consumer needs for safe care and improved health outcomes are met.

The Institute of Medicine (IOM, 1999) has previously reported that 44,000 deaths occurred annually as a result of medical errors. The 2001 IOM report identified deficiencies in the quality of health care received by Americans; 50 million Americans remain without health insurance (Kaiser Family Foundation, 2012), and the cost for health care is increasing. The current health care system is failing even those with insurance. With $7,538 per capita annual spending, the cost for U.S. health care is at an all-time high and is nearly double that of any other Organization for Economic Cooperation and Development (OECD) nation (Kaiser Family Foundation, 2011). The PPACA, upheld by the U.S. Supreme Court (*National Federation of Independent Businesses v. Sebelius*, 2011) will be fully implemented over the next two years.

The PPACA will initiate reform throughout the health care system and influence the provision of preventive and primary health care services. Advanced Practice Registered Nurse (APRNs) have historically been champions of preventive health care and primary care (Keeling, 2009). Implementation of the PPACA presents an unprecedented opportunity for APRNs (Nurse Practitioners, Certified Nurse-Midwives, and Clinical Nurse Specialists) to take a leadership role in offering primary care and strengthening preventive services. However, this opportunity for influence is dependent on having an appropriately educated nursing workforce which will include an increased number of nurses with doctoral education (Cleary & Wilmoth, 2011).

A relatively new member of the health care workforce, the APRN with a Doctor of Nursing Practice (DNP) degree (henceforth referred to as the DNP APRN or the DNP nurse) provides care and leadership in the areas of primary care and prevention (AACN, 2006). We will use the term DNP nurse in this article to refer to the APRNs and nurse administrators holding a DNP degree. Although the DNP nurse is prepared to work in direct patient care, academia, clinical research, or administration throughout the health care system, this discussion will focus specifically on the role of the DNP APRN in the provision of preventive services and primary care.

In this chapter, we discuss how the PPACA serves as a prevention model, describe the role of DNP nurses as primary care providers, explain how preventive health care can be enhanced through the use of a primary care model, and address challenges related to increasing preventive care in our health care system. We also consider the opportunities for DNP nurse leadership in developing community-based programs and advocating for policies to strengthen primary care delivery. We conclude by noting professional and legal barriers that need to be removed before DNP nurses are able to provide all the care they have been prepared to offer.

THE AFFORDABLE CARE ACT: A PREVENTION MODEL

A comprehensive summary of the ACA is beyond the scope of this paper, but a basic understanding of the provisions that impact primary care is essential for understanding the role of the DNP nurse as the nation implements the ACA. We have developed Table 14.1 to summarize the provisions within the ACA that have the potential to impact primary care (Patient Protection and Affordable Care Act, 2010). These provisions, designed to expand insurance, increase primary care access, and promote preventive health services, are important for improving health care outcomes. This section will discuss the ACA insurance expansion and preventive services enhanced through primary care and public health programs.

Insurance Expansion

The ACA expands and broadens the availability of health care services through health care insurance expansion for up to 32 million currently uninsured Americans (Congressional Budget Office, 2012). A state-based American Health Benefit Exchange, known as the Health Insurance Marketplace, will allow individuals to purchase private health insurance plans; individuals making 400% or less of the federal poverty level (FPL) will qualify for cost-sharing subsidies and premium tax credits to make the health plans more affordable. A state-based Small Business Health Options Program Exchange will allow for small businesses to purchase group insurance and include tax credits for those businesses providing health insurance to employees. A business with 50 or more full-time employees will be subject to fines for failing to offer insurance. By 2016, U.S. citizens and legal residents will be required to purchase insurance or pay a tax penalty equivalent to 2.5% of their taxable income. Young adults will be permitted

TABLE 14.1 Patient Protection and Affordable Care Act Provisions With the Potential to Impact Primary Care

PROVISIONS INCREASING ACCESS TO HEALTH INSURANCE	
SECTION	**PROVISION**
1311	Creates state-based American Health Benefit Exchange that allows individuals to purchase health care through state-run health plans
1402	Provides cost-sharing subsidies for individuals making between 100% and 400% of the federal poverty level (FPL)
1401	Provides premium tax credits to increase the affordability of state-based plans
1311	Establishes the Small Business Health Options Program Exchange which allows for small businesses to purchase group insurance
1421	Authorizes small business tax credits for businesses providing health insurance to employees
1501	Establishes a mandate requiring U.S. citizens and legal residents to purchase insurance or pay a tax penalty equivalent to 2.5% of their taxable income
1513	Imposes fines on employers with 50 or more full-time employees who fail to offer insurance to their employees
2101	Provides additional funding to the State Children's Health Insurance Program (SCHIP) and extends CHIP funding
2001	Encourages states to expand Medicaid to all individuals at or below 133% FPL
2714	Allows young adults to remain on their parents' insurance plan until age 26 years
Provisions increasing access to preventive health services	
2713	Requires health insurance plans to increase coverage and access to preventive services
4004	Creates a national education and outreach campaign for prevention and health promotion
4103	Provides an annual wellness visit for Medicare beneficiaries without co-pay
4104	Eliminates Medicare cost-sharing (individual co-pay) for preventive services rated "A" or "B" by the U.S. Preventive Services Task Force
4106	Provides a 1% increase in states' Federal Medical Assistance Percentage for states that eliminate Medicaid cost-sharing for "A" and "B" rated preventive services
Provisions increasing availability and access to primary care providers	
1202	Increases physician payments for primary care services provided by qualifying physicians and nonphysician providers operating under a qualifying physician's supervision
5101	Creates the Primary Care Medicine and Dentistry and the National Health Care Workforce Commission
5207, 5209, 5210	Increases funding for the National Health Service Corps and creates a Ready Reserve Corps
5301	Provides training grants for physicians in primary care specialties
5201–5203, 5308–5310	Provides funding for nursing education and loan repayment, including additional funding for APRN education
5313	Allocates funding for community health worker training

(continued)

TABLE 14.1 Patient Protection and Affordable Care Act Provisions With the Potential to Impact Primary Care   (*continued*)

PROVISIONS INCREASING ACCESS TO HEALTH INSURANCE	
5601	Allocates additional funding for community health centers
5316	Provides demonstration grants to place family nurse practitioners in Federally Qualified Health Centers and nurse-managed health centers
5208	Provides funding for nurse managed health centers
5405	Establishes the Primary Care Extension Program, which educates primary care providers and enables them to use evidence-based therapies in practice
5501	Provides a 10% payment incentive for primary care services
5509	Establishes a Graduate Nurse Demonstration Project in which Medicare dollars are used to support the education of APRNs
Provisions for preventive health and wellness programs	
4001	Establishes the National Prevention, Health Promotion and Public Health Council to coordinate federal public health efforts
4002	Establishes the Prevention and Public Health Fund to increase national investment in public health infrastructure
4101	Establishes grants for school-based health centers
4201	Allocates grant funding to support evidence-based community prevention programs
4202	Establishes grants for 5-year pilot programs providing public health interventions, screenings, and referrals for adults 55 to 64
4303	Allocates resources for employer wellness programs

Source: Patient Protection and Affordable Care Act (PPACA) Pub. L. No. 111-148, §2702, 124 Stat. 119, 318-319. (2010).

to remain on their parents' insurance plan until they are 26 years of age; lifelong spending limits and annual coverage limits will be eliminated (PPACA, 2010).

Primary Care and Preventive Services Access in Participating States

Primary care and preventive services are expanded through Medicaid and Medicare. The State Children's Health Insurance Program is reauthorized, and Medicaid is expanded to all individuals at or below 133% of FPL. ACA places new restriction on health insurance plans by requiring increased access to and coverage of preventive services. The ACA increases Medicaid payments for primary care services provided to qualifying physicians. Nonphysician providers, including Nurse Practitioners (NP), may qualify for the increased payments but only when operating under a qualifying physician's supervision. It is important to note that this payment criterion could impose a financial restriction on higher reimbursement for NPs who are already providing primary care services in states with "independent practice" legislation, meaning there is no requirement for physician collaboration to provide care. Increased funding is provided to the National Health Service Corps to support nursing and medical education that can increase placement of primary care providers in underserved areas. Funding for additional community health centers is provided (PPACA, 2010).

Public Health and Preventive Programs

The ACA establishment of the Community-Based Collaborative Care Network Program, comprised of consortiums of providers, is tasked with coordinating and integrating heath care services for low-income and uninsured populations (Kaiser Family Foundation, 2013). The National Prevention, Health Promotion, and Public Health Council has been designed to coordinate federal public health efforts, and the Prevention and Public Health Fund was created to increase a national investment in the public health infrastructure. An emphasis on evidence-based, community, prevention programs, and employer wellness programs will be provided through grant funding (Kaiser Family Foundation, 2013).

These ACA provisions offer a promising future for primary care and prevention services but will yield little tangible success without adequate funding, knowledgeable implementation of the provisions, and an increased number of primary care providers to meet the expanding numbers of persons seeking primary care and prevention services. The DNP nurse has the educational preparation to play an essential role in supporting and leading this transformation of health care to improve health care outcomes.

THE DOCTOR OF NURSING PRACTICE NURSE AS PRIMARY CARE PROVIDER

The Doctor of Nursing Practice degree is a practice doctorate, with an emphasis on the translation of research evidence to the practice context (Dreher, 2011). The focus of the degree is on demonstrating clinical practice expertise (Chism, 2010); providing both direct patient care and clinical leadership; and utilizing evidence-based practice and information technology skills to improve patient health care outcomes (AACN, 2006). DNP programs, based on the American Association of Colleges of Nursing (AACN) *Essentials of Doctoral Education for Advanced Nursing Practice* (2006), henceforth referred to as the *Essentials*, emphasize the achievement of eight essential competencies (see Table 14.2). The *Essentials* competencies include the utilization of leadership skills to improve patient outcomes, the creation of new care delivery models that will meet the increasing demand for services, and the development of policy to enhance services and remove practice barriers. In order to achieve the ACA outcomes, nurses will need to be full partners with physicians and other health care professionals to develop health care strategies that will increase primary care services to meet the consumer need for safe, quality health care (IOM, 2010).

The National Governors Association (NGA) has noted that as millions of Americans who previously lacked insurance enter the health care system over the next decade, the nation will require a concomitant increase in the number of health care providers to meet the increased health care needs arising from this influx (NGA, 2012). The U.S. Health Resources and Services Administration (HRSA) estimates that more than 35.2 million people, living within the 5,860 health professional shortage areas (HPSA) nationwide, do not currently receive adequate primary care services (HRSA, 2016). As of July 2012, an additional

TABLE 14.2 The *Essentials of Doctoral Education for Advanced Nursing Practice*

ESSENTIAL FOCUS	OUTCOME COMPETENCY
I. Scientific underpinnings for practice	Apply a strong scientific foundation to develop, implement, and evaluate health care delivery approaches.
II. Organizational and systems leadership for quality improvement and systems thinking	Use advanced communication, business, and policy skills to improve patient outcomes through the development, evaluation, and improvement of practice initiatives.
III. Clinical scholarship and analytical methods for evidence-based practice	Translate research into practice through critical literature review, evaluation, and integration and dissemination of new knowledge.
IV. Information systems/technology and patient care technology for the improvement and transformation of health care	Use information technology to manage patient information, evaluate program outcomes, and apply new knowledge to improve patient care.
V. Health care policy for advocacy in health care	Design, advocate for, critically analyze, and implement health policy to improve health care delivery and promote health equity.
VI. Interprofessional collaboration for improving patient and population health outcomes	Engage in interprofessional collaboration through effective communication, team building, and leadership skills.
VII. Clinical prevention and population health for improving the nation's health	Incorporate concepts of public health, prevention and health determinants in the integration and evaluation of evidence-based prevention strategies.
VIII. Advanced nursing practice	Demonstrate refined clinical skills as expert practitioners in the design, implementation, and evaluation of nursing interventions.

Source: American Association of Colleges of Nursing (2006).

15,168 practitioners were needed to provide primary care for the 54.5 million people living in designated, primary care HPSAs (HRSA, 2016). Underscoring the importance of primary care, the American Hospital Association (AHA) convened a roundtable of clinical and health system experts, including physician and nursing leaders, to examine the future primary-care-workforce needs as well as the role hospitals and health care systems can play in delivering primary care. The roundtable recommended a new primary care delivery model that would include the hospitals, in partnership with communities, to form primary care teams to deliver quality care (AHA, 2013).

The ACA also provides opportunities for the DNP nurse to meet primary care needs through the utilization of technology as a means to improve care delivery and measure outcomes; to identify, develop, and implement quality improvement projects; and to enhance systems thinking and evaluation (AACN, 2006). The uses of electronic health records, electronic databases, Internet searches for evidence-based-research findings, and electronic applications are technological advances that have the ability to support improved care delivery and evaluation of care outcomes. Synthesis and analysis of electronic data and subsequent identification of issues that need to be addressed can be enhanced with the use of technology.

DNP nurse leadership is needed both at the point of care delivery and at administrative levels to implement the use of technology to document care; collect and analyze essential data; and identify areas of care that need a change in their practice approach. Policy strategies are also needed to address health care disparities and implement best practices that improve health care access and the prevention of complications. DNP nurses can use their educational preparation to provide leadership in the use of technology during the nation's transition to a prevention model of health care delivery offered, within a collaborative, interdisciplinary context, to meet primary care needs.

UTILIZATION OF A PREVENTIVE HEALTH CARE MODEL IN PRIMARY CARE

Driven by rapid advancements in technology and a relentless quest for extending life, the current health care system devotes the majority of health care dollars to disease management and end-of-life care. Thorpe (2005) found that two-thirds of the increase in health care spending is a result of an increase in the treatment of disease (measured as the number of medical conditions treated multiplied by spending per case). Health care dollars are increasingly directed toward advanced treatments, yet the use of health care resources directed toward prevention has remained low. A study by the Centers for Disease Control (CDC; 2012) found that only half of U.S. adults receive recommended preventive services, such as mammography, cholesterol screenings, and colonoscopies. Individual and preventable behaviors, such as smoking and lack of exercise, account for nearly 50% of all premature deaths (Hardcastle, Record, Jacobson, & Gostin, 2011). As the United States devotes health care resources to the diagnosis and treatment of chronic diseases, opportunities for preventing both acute and chronic diseases are lost. The increased use of clinical, preventive services could save two million life-years and $3.7 billion annually (Maciosek, Coffield, Flottemesch, Edwards, & Solberg, 2010).

The ACA provides a strong emphasis on preventive medicine and primary care through insurance reform, increased reimbursement for primary care providers, funding to educate these providers, and incentives to attract providers into primary care. The DNP nurse is especially well prepared to educate providers on the use of evidence-based preventive care and to assist the U.S. health care system in its transformation toward this model.

Nursing's emphasis on preventive health care can be traced to Florence Nightingale's *Notes on Nursing*, first published in 1859. She recognized that patient care must first be focused on providing a healthy home environment, which she described as having pure air, pure water, efficient drainage, cleanliness, and light (Nightingale, 1946). Nursing has continued this focus by its attention to illness prevention, health promotion, and the teaching of self-care management (Mundinger, 2002). The primary care services provided in Nurse Managed Health Centers (NMHCs) emphasize health promotion and disease prevention (Vonderheid, Pohl, Tanner, Newland, & Gans, 2009). A survey of 60 NMHCs found that provision of health maintenance services far surpassed that of chronic illness management (Barkauskas et al., 2006). While data on NMHCs remains limited in terms of clients served and services provided (Barkauskas et al., 2006), existing data indicate that NMHCs provide greater use of preventive services along with care that is high in quality, patient satisfaction, and cost effectiveness (Coddington & Sands, 2008). Coddington, Sands, Edwards, Kirkpatrick, and Chen (2011) noted that DNP nurses at a nurse-managed pediatric clinic reported quality of care measures as meeting or exceeding national benchmarks. It is important that nurses share their strategies for encouraging and providing preventive services with other health care professionals.

Despite the ACA emphasis on prevention and primary care, there has been criticism for its considerable focus on clinical medicine and its lack of inclusion of public health priorities (Cogan, 2011; Hardcastle et al., 2011). The public health community is advocating for an increased integration of public health components along with clinical medicine. Nurses, whose education emphasizes prevention and holistic care (AACN, 1996; AACN, 2006; Tracy, 2009), are well positioned to assist in facilitating this integration. DNP nurses are prepared in the implementation of clinical prevention and population health strategies to meet the Healthy People recommendations (AACN, 2006). These nurses are prepared to lead a collaborative effort that sets a national agenda related to identifying population health outcomes, creating new models that promote prevention, and developing strategies for community outreach and education.

Although public health professionals are knowledgeable in behavioral health, health policy, and prevention, they may lack clinical training and the opportunity to work directly with patients needing preventive services. Although medical schools have started to recognize the need for a greater emphasis on primary care and prevention, the U.S. health care system remains dominated by an individual-based, curative-medicine model (Cogan, 2011). DNP nurses can bridge this gap by applying public health models of prevention to clinical medicine and educating their health care colleagues to do the same.

CHALLENGES OF IMPLEMENTING THE ACA

This section will address two challenges related to implementing the ACA. These challenges include the need for more providers and the need for more creative approaches to implement care.

Need for More Primary Care Providers

The ACA will necessitate an increase in primary care providers. A survey conducted by the Kaiser Family Foundation found that of the 24 million Americans who will likely gain health insurance through the Health Insurance Marketplace by 2019, 37% will have gone more than 2 years without a checkup, and 29% will have had no interaction with the health care system in the year prior to obtaining coverage. In addition, 13% report their health as poor or fair compared with only 6% of those currently privately insured (Trish, Damico, Claxton, Levitt, & Garfield, 2011). With the implementation of the ACA, the health care system will experience an influx of patients with complex medical needs, thus increasing the demand for clinicians who can meet these needs. DNP APRNs are increasingly available and prepared to address these needs as expert health care providers.

Additionally, most newly insured patients will access care through primary care clinics that are already experiencing a shortage of providers. Only 30% of U.S. physicians practice in primary care (Goodson, 2010); and only about 25% of current medical school graduates plan careers in primary care (Schwartz, 2012). The Agency for Healthcare Research and Quality has estimated that among NPs, 52% of all NPs were providing primary care in 2010 (Inglehart, 2012).

Need for Creative Care Management Strategies

It will be essential for health care providers to use creative strategies to incorporate prevention while also addressing the immediate needs of the millions of Americans who will be entering the health care system. Group self-care-education sessions, and the use of informatics to track the frequency of routine health screenings are strategies that can help to meet preventive care needs while using providers' time expeditiously. DNP nurses have designed, implemented, and evaluated group-care strategies to address chronic diseases, such as diabetes, metabolic syndrome, and hypertension, and have demonstrated that health outcomes can be improved using these strategies (Dickman, Pintz, Gold, & Kivlahan, 2012; Greer & Hill, 2011; Riley, 2012).

Statistics suggest that the need for primary care DNP nurses will increase with ACA implementation. Hence it is essential that these nurses be recognized for their ability to provide safe, quality, health care that improves outcomes, rather than being viewed as a physician substitute. DNP APRNs are prepared to offer a holistic approach to health care, an approach that recognizes the patient as a unique individual within an encompassing social, physical, and energy environment (Tracy, 2009).

DNP nurses have the knowledge and ability to offer a holistic and unique understanding of the challenges facing many of the newly insured, so as to provide compassionate, comprehensive, and coordinated care to meet their diverse needs. The millions of Americans who will enter the health care system with unique social and cultural backgrounds, expectations, and misconceptions, in addition to their medical needs, will present new challenges for providers. When compared with currently insured individuals, these newly insured are likely to be poorer and less educated (Trish et al., 2011). Currently more than 50% of patients seen at nurse-managed health clinics are uninsured (Van Zandt, Sloand, & Wilkins, 2008). Until recently, the majority of APRNs in the health care system frequently provided services to underserved populations (Mundinger, 2002).

LEADERSHIP IN COMMUNITY-BASED PROGRAMS

The implementation of the ACA not only provides an opportunity for DNPA PRNs to demonstrate their expertise in direct patient care, but also creates new avenues for community leadership and programmatic design. ACA nurses are prepared both to help communities understand the ACA legislation and to design new community health initiatives as described in the following.

The ACA benefits will not be fully utilized by patients without the strong presence of both providers and health educators in the community. Because the ACA is a complex law, the majority of Americans have little understanding of its components or potential impact on their lives. Unfortunately, many persons who could benefit from the provisions of the PPACA are at risk for missing this opportunity to gain coverage. A recent survey by the Kaiser Family Foundation found that 47% of the uninsured do not think the new health care reform legislation will affect them (Altman, 2011). DNP nurses are prepared to design the outreach programs needed to educate the community about the legislation and how to benefit from its provisions. For example, APRN nurses providing care to uninsured patients can help these patients understand their options for obtaining coverage, educate Medicare beneficiaries about their access to preventive health care services without cost-sharing, and encourage all patients to ask their primary care providers about obtaining these services.

The PPACA also authorizes grants for community-based, prevention programs (Community Transformation Grants), work-based wellness programs, and school-based health centers. DNP nurses have the advanced education necessary to design, implement, and evaluate such programs. They can combine their high-level clinical expertise and increased leadership competencies to create new community health initiatives. For example, the nursing-focused Transitional Care Model, created by Naylor, is already being utilized in the implementation of the PPACA (Cleary & Wilmoth, 2011). Naylor's model encompasses comprehensive hospital planning and home follow-up for older adults. Additionally, Walker's (2012) Skin Protection for Kids program, designed to educate parents and teachers about sun-damage and sun-protection strategies, has also brought health promotion activities out of the clinical setting and into the community. New ACA funding for work-based wellness programs and school-based health centers provides nursing entrepreneurs new opportunities for clinical practice.

Creation of community outreach and care prevention programs will rely heavily on interdisciplinary collaboration to improve quality of care, decrease health care costs, and enhance positive health care outcomes (Chism, 2010). The ACA actively encourages interdisciplinary collaboration within the medical home delivery model and the new Community-Based Collaborative Care Network Program. Doctorally prepared nurses are particularly equipped to lead and contribute to interdisciplinary teams practicing in medical homes (AACN, 2006; Garnica, 2009). It is essential to recognize and utilize the strengths of various health care disciplines and promote collaboration and compromise when needed. Successful interdisciplinary collaboration, along with the creation of adequate policy to support change, will ensure the best use of resources to provide direct patient care and program development to meet the need for health care services and system delivery model revision.

ADVOCACY AND POLICY DEVELOPMENT TO STRENGTHEN PRIMARY CARE DELIVERY

Although the ACA has been signed into law, health policy advocates are needed to support full implementation of its provisions. The IOM (2010) *Future of Nursing* report recommends that nurses be "full partners with physicians and other health care professionals in redesigning health care in the United States" (p.3). To accomplish this goal, nurses must serve on strategic committees and have a presence at all levels of state and national decision-making committees. The provisions and regulations established in the ACA will be enacted over this decade. During this time, modifications will be necessary as unforeseen problems are encountered.

DNP nurses are prepared to advocate for the patient, create innovative changes in the health care delivery system, and improve the context of care for health care providers during this transitional period. It is important that DNP nurses also advocate for the funding of nursing education grants and for the ability of APRNs to provide care within their full scope of practice (IOM, 2010).

DNP education emphasizes a system-wide approach and macroscopic view of health care, preparing graduates to assume leadership in changing health care systems (Talbert & Dennison, 2011). DNP nurses are currently developing policy knowledge and advocacy skills through internships and participation in professional organizations (Davis & Mangini-Vendel, 2011). Because policy makers rarely have clinical experience, they often develop policies that do not reflect or target the clinical needs of the population. Doctorally prepared nurses are needed to bridge this gap between clinical medicine and clinical nursing, and policy development.

DNP nurses involved in health care reform over the next decade need to be aware of both the strengths and the weaknesses of the ACA. Although this law engages a more macroscopic view, it is primarily a health insurance reform that leaves many important health outcomes unaddressed. Medical care prevents only 10% to 15% of premature deaths (Williams, McClellan, & Rivlin, 2010). Health and longevity are strongly influenced by other social determinants, such as education, food and housing access, and socioeconomic status (Lathrop, 2013). DNP nurses, given their holistic approach to health care and system-wide perspectives, can point out the health implications of state and national policies. They can follow the encouragement of Williams et al. (2010) to advocate for the adoption of a culture of health in which the health impact of all policy decisions is considered during policy development, to improve health care outcomes.

REMOVAL OF PROFESSIONAL AND LEGAL BARRIERS IMPEDING PRIMARY CARE DELIVERY

Now is the time for nurses to address legal restrictions and other professional barriers that limit their ability to perform within the full scope of practice for which they are prepared. The ACA offers vast opportunities for DNP nurse leadership in health care restructuring, improving direct patient care, creating innovative programmatic development, and providing political advocacy. However, barriers threaten to prevent the full realization of DNP leadership potential in health care reform. Because DNP nurses will be providing primary care to an increasing number of Americans, the IOM report (2010) explicitly noted that full scope of practice without restriction is needed. The following paragraphs both describe current barriers to DNP nurse practice, including limitations in reimbursement, collaboration, and scope of practice, and suggest ways to remove these barriers

Reimbursement Limitations

Barriers exist for the reimbursement of care provided by all APRN nurses. Nurses are actively meeting the new quality and preventive care standards established in the ACA, and they should be compensated for the services they provide in a manner equal to that of other providers offering the same services. Currently, NPs providing Medicare services to residents in long-term care facilities are reimbursed at only 85% of the Medicare physician rate for the same services (American Association of Nurse Practitioners [AANP], 2013). We encourage DNP nurses, armed with research evidence of equal abilities and equivalent patient outcomes, to advocate for equal reimbursement for all providers who give the same care.

Collaboration Barriers

DNP nurses also face barriers within their collaborative relationships. Inter-professional conflict between medicine and nursing has existed since the early 20th century (Keeling, 2009). Some physicians continue to see the expanding role of nurses as a threat and seek to limit the authority of nurses at both legislative and practice levels. As an increasing number of nurses pursue doctoral education, new conflicts are arising. In a recent editorial in the *Journal for Nurse Practitioners*, one physician argued, "The use of the prefix 'Dr.' or 'Doctor' by NPs who have completed the DNP degree could lead to confusion and misconceptions by patients" (Ralston, 2011, p. 563). We authors do not believe that this statement has any factual basis. In a recent health policy report, Iglehart (2012) suggested that the ACA may turn these turf battles between physicians and APRNs into larger public health issues if newly insured individuals have difficulty accessing care. There is a need for greater collaboration among physician and nurse leaders in addressing these issues; the impetus for this collaboration may need to come from the federal level.

Scope-of-Practice Impediments

APRNs in general lack full autonomous practice in the majority of states and the District of Columbia; only 17 states and the District of Columbia provide a full scope of practice for APRNs under the licensure authority of the state board of nursing. The remaining 33 states have a reduced or restricted scope of practice with the mandate of some degree of physician involvement (AANP, 2014). Restrictions continue without evidence to support regulations and in spite of current evidence that supports high-quality and safe care provided by NPs (Horrock, Anderson, & Salisbury, 2002; Lambing, Adams, Fox, & Divine, 2004; Munginger et al., 2000). Research has demonstrated that NPs provide comparable care by physicians in the acute care setting (Lambing et al., 2004). Mundinger et al. (2000) have noted that Nurse Practitioners and primary care physicians have comparable patient outcomes in ambulatory settings. When compared with physicians, NPs provide more information to patients, identify physical abnormalities more often, have higher communication scores, and receive higher satisfaction evaluations related to their patient consultations than do physicians (Horrock et al., 2002). Despite evidence of safe care and equivalent outcomes, state regulation of NP practice varies significantly, limiting NPs' abilities to meet the growing health care needs of the nation (Rudner, O'Grady, Hodnicki, & Hanson, 2007). With the implementation of the ACA and the resulting influx of patients needing care, the restrictions on APRN practice must be removed for patients to receive the full extent of the care they need. There is some discussion that physician groups have financial concerns in regard to broadening APRN state regulations (NGA, 2012).

However, when comparing physician salaries in states with expanded APRN practice to states without such expansion, evidence does not support this concern (Pittman & Williams, 2012).

Requiring licensure, accreditation, certification, and education in all states, as described in the *Consensus Model for APRN Regulation* (National Council of State Boards of Nursing, 2008), will provide standardization to APRN regulation through legislation. Arbitrary restrictions, which limit APRN scope of practice but are not supported by evidence, need to be removed from state nurse practice acts and health care agency policy. The NGA report has noted that although every state's board of nursing has signed onto the APRN *Consensus Model*, only five states had achieved full implementation of this model, and only 10 states had even pending legislation related to the model in their 2012 legislative sessions (NGA, 2012). APRNs will have the greatest potential for impacting care when practicing within the full scope of their education and accreditation (Rudner et al., 2007). The unrestricted contribution of APRNs will be of even greater importance as millions of newly insured Americans access health care upon implementation of the ACA. Expanding the utilization of APRNs has the potential to increase access to health care for many current and future patients, particularly in underserved areas (NGA, 2012).

Although all APRNs are prepared to advance the health care of our citizens, DNP nurses have the additional foundation needed to fully implement health care reform, the competency to meet the expanding needs for primary care and improved health care outcomes, and the skills to advocate for legislative changes. We encourage DNP nurse leaders to focus on the promotion of equal reimbursement, mutually beneficial interdisciplinary collaborative relationships, and full scope of practice in order to maximize nursing's contribution to the provision of health care.

CONCLUSION

The proliferation of DNP programs coincides with an exciting and transformative time in U.S. health care history. As of April 2013, there are currently 217 DNP programs in 40 states plus the District of Columbia, with an increase of graduates from 1,595 in 2011 to 1,858 in 2012 (AACN, 2013). The ACA provides for reform in the current health care system. Nurses are at the forefront of this health care reform, and the advanced education provided to DNP nurses will be crucial in the success of this reform. DNP nurses have the ability to provide leadership in the use of evidence-based clinical care; the restructuring of the health care system; the greater focus on prevention; and the utilization of new care delivery models, community outreach programs, and work- and school-based health centers. An increased presence in the legislative process is needed as states and the federal system prepare to adapt to new regulations for the implementation of the ACA.

In this climate of health care reform, DNP nurses have the additional preparation and the desire to serve as leaders to improve, in concert with other health care providers, the health of this nation. They are primed to eliminate barriers to APRN practice and advocate for a new age of health care with increased access to care and improved health care outcomes for all.

REFERENCES

Altman, D. (2011). Pulling it together: Uninsured but not yet informed. Retrieved from http://www.kff
.org/pullingittogether/uninsured_informed_altman.cfm

American Association of Colleges of Nursing. (1996). *The essentials of master's education for advanced practice nursing.* Washington, DC: Author.

American Association of Colleges of Nursing. (2006). *The essentials of doctoral education for advanced nursing practice.* Washington, DC: Author. Retrieved from http://www.aacnnursing.org/Portals/42/
Publications/DNPEssentials.pdf

American Association of Colleges of Nursing. (2013, April). DNP fact sheet. Retrieved from http://www
.aacnnursing.org/Portals/42/News/Factsheets/DNP-Factsheet-2017.pdf

American Association of Nurse Practitioners. (2013). Fact sheet: Medicare reimbursement. Retrieved from
www.aanp.org/legislation-regulation/federal-legislation/medicare/68-articles/325-medicare
-reimbursement

American Association of Nurse Practitioners. (2014). State practice environment. Retrieved from https://
www.aanp.org/legislation-regulation/state-legislation/state-practice-environment

American Hospital Association Primary Care Workforce Roundtable. (2013). *Workforce roles in a redesigned
primary care model.* Retrieved from http://www.aha.org/content/13/13-0110-wf-primary-care.pdf

Barkauskas, V., Schafer, P., Sebastian, J. G., Pohl, J., Benkert, R., Nagelkerk, J., . . . Tanner, C. L. (2006).
Clients served and services provided by PPAC Academic nurse-managed centers. *Journal of
Professional Nursing, 22*(6), 331–338.

Centers for Disease Control and Prevention. (2012). CDC: Half of adults get preventive health services. *Modern Healthcare, 32*(24), 4.

Chism, L. A. (2010). *The doctor of nursing practice: A guidebook for the role development and professional issues.*
Boston, MA: Jones & Bartlett.

Cleary, B., & Wilmoth, P. (2011). The affordable care act- what it means for the future of nursing. *Tar Heel
Nurse, 73*(2), 8–9, 12.

Coddington, J. A., & Sands, L. P. (2008). Cost of health care and quality outcomes of patients at nurse-
managed clinics. *Nursing Economic$, 26*(2), 75–83.

Coddington, J. A., Sands, L., Edwards, N., Kirkpatrick, J., & Chen, S. (2011). Quality of care provided
at a nurse-managed pediatric clinic. *Journal of the American Academy of Nurse Practitioners, 23*(12),
674–680. doi:10.1111/j.1745-7599.2011.00657.x

Cogan, J. A. (2011). The affordable care act's preventive service mandate: Breaking down the barriers to
nationwide access to preventive services. *Journal of Law, Medicine, & Ethics, 39*(3), 355–365.

Congressional Budget Office. (2012). Updated estimates for the insurance coverage provisions of
the Affordable Care Act. Retrieved from http://www.cbo.gov/sites/default/files/cbofiles/
attachments/03-13-Coverage%20Estimates.pdf

Davis, E., & Mangini-Vendel, M. (2011). The life of a bill: A nursing experience. *Creative Nursing,
17*(2), 74–79.

Dickman, K., Pintz, C., Gold, K., & Kivlahan, C. (2012). Behavior changes in patients with diabetes and
hypertension after experiencing shared medical appointments. *Journal of the American Academy of
Nurse Practitioners, 24*(1), 43–51. doi:10.1111/j.1745-7599.2011.00660.x

Dreher, H. M. (2011). The historical and political path of doctoral nursing education to the doctor of
nursing practice degree. In H. M. Dreher & M. E. S. Glasgow (Eds.), *Role development for doctoral
advanced nursing practice* (pp. 7–43). New York, NY: Springer Publishing.

Garnica, M. P. (2009). Coordinated primary care: "Medical home model." *Clinical Scholars Review,
2*(2), 60–64.

Goodson, J. D. (2010). Patient Protection and Affordable Care Act: Promise and peril for primary care.
Annals of Internal Medicine, 152(11), 742–744. doi:10.7326/0003-4819-152-11-201006010-00249

Greer, D. M., & Hill, D. C. (2011). Implementing an evidence-based metabolic syndrome prevention and
treatment program utilizing group visits. *Journal of the American Academy of Nurse Practitioners,
23*(2), 76–83. doi:10.1111/j.1745-7599.2010.00585.x

Hardcastle, L. E., Record, K. L, Jacobson, P. D., & Gostin, L. O. (2011). Improving the population's
health: The affordable care act and the importance of integration. *Journal of Law, Medicine, & Ethics,
39*(3), 317–327. doi:10.111/j.1748-720X.2011.00602.x

Health Resources and Service Administration. (2016). Shortage designation: Health professional shortage areas & medically underserved areas/populations. Retrieved from https://bhw.hrsa.gov/shortage-designation/hpsas

Horrock, S., Anderson, E., & Salisbury, C. (2002). Systematic review of whether nurse practitioners working in primary care can provide equivalent care to doctors. *British Medical Journal, 324*(7341), 819–823.

Iglehart, J. K. (2012). Expanding the role of advanced nurse practitioners-risks and rewards. *New England Journal of Medicine, 368*(20), 1935–1941.

Institute of Medicine. (1999). *To err is human: Building a safer health care system.* Washington, DC: Author.

Institute of Medicine. (2001). *Crossing the quality chasm: A new health system for the 21st century.* Washington, DC: Author.

Institute of Medicine. (2010). *The future of nursing: Leading change, advancing health.* Washington, DC: Author.

Kaiser Family Foundation. (2011). Snapshots: Health care spending in the Unites States and selected OECD countries. Retrieved from http://www.kff.org/insurance/snapshot/OECD042111.cfm

Kaiser Family Foundation. (2012). Five facts about the uninsured population. Retrieved at http://www.kff.org/uninsured/upload/7806-04.pdf

Kaiser Family Foundation. (2013). Summary of the Affordable Care Act. Retrieved from http://www.kff.org/healthreform/upload/8061.pdf

Keeling, A. (2009). A brief history of advanced practice nursing in the United States. In A. B. Hamric, J. A. Spross, & C. M. Hanson (Eds.), *Advanced practice nursing an integrative approach.* (pp. 3–26). St. Louis, MO: Elsevier.

Lambing, A. Y., Adams, D. L. C., Fox, D. H., & Divine, G. (2004). Nurse practitioners' and physicians' care activities and clinical outcomes with an inpatient geriatric population. *Journal of the American Academy of Nurse Practitioners, 16*(8), 343–352.

Lathrop, B. (2013). Nursing leadership in addressing the social determinants of health. Online Publication. *Policy, Politics, and Nursing Practice, 14*(1). doi:10.1177/1527154413489887

Maciosek, M. V., Coffield, A. B., Flottemesch, T. J., Edwards, N. M., & Solberg, L. I. (2010). Greater use of preventative services in U.S. health care could save lives at little or no cost. *Health Affairs, 29*(9), 1656–1660.

Mundiger, M. (2002). Twenty-first century primary care: New partnerships between nurses and doctors. *Academic Medicine, 77*(8), 9–12.

Mundinger, M. O., Kane, R. L., Lenz, E. R., Totten, A. M., Tsai, W. Y., Cleary, P. D., . . . Shelanski, M. L. (2000). Primary care outcomes in patients treated by nurse practitioners of physicians: A randomized trial. *Journal of the American Medical Association, 283*(1), 59–68.

National Council of State Boards of Nursing. (2008). Consensus model for APRN regulation: Licensure, accreditation, certification, and education. Retrieved from http://www.ncsbn.org/Consensus_Model_for_APRN_Regulation_July_2008.pdf

National Federation of Independent Business et al. v. Sebelius, Secretary of Health and Human Services. 000 U.S. 11-393 (2012). Retrieved from http://www.supremecourt.gov/opinions/11pdf/11-393c3a2.pdf

National Governors Association. (2012). The role of nurse practitioners in meeting increasing demands for primary care. Retrieved from http://www.nga.org/cms/home/nga-center-for-best-practices/center-publications/page-health-publications/col2-content/main-content-list/the-role-of-nurse-practitioners.html

Nightingale, F. (1859/1946). *Notes on nursing.* Philadelphia, PA: Edward Stern.

Patient Protection and Affordable Care Act Pub. L. No. 111-148, §2702, 124 Stat. 119, 318-319. (2010). Retrieved from www.gpo.gov/fdsys/pkg/PLAW-111publ148/pdf/PLAW-111publ148.pdf

Pittman, P., & Williams, B. (2012). Physician wages in states with expanded APRN scope of practice. *Nursing Practice and Research.* doi:10.1155/2012/671974

Ralston, F. (2011). Support for restricting the title "doctor." *Journal for Nurse Practitioners, 7*(7), 562–563.

Riley, S. B. (2012). Improving diabetes outcomes by an innovative group visit model: A pilot study. *American Academy of Nurse Practitioners Journal.* doi:10.1111/j.1745-7599.2012.00796

Rudner, N. R., O'Grady, E. T., Hodnicki, D. R., & Hanson, C. M. (2007). Ranking state NP regulation: Practice environment and consumer health care choice. *American Journal for Nurse Practitioners, 11*(4), 8–24.

Schwartz, M. D. (2012). The US primary care workforce and graduate medical education policy. *Journal of the American Medical Association, 308,* 2252–2253.

Talbert, T., & Dennison, R. D. (2011). The role of the clinical executive. In H. M. Dreher & M. E. S. Glasgow (Eds.), *Role development for doctoral advanced nursing practice* (pp. 141–157). New York, NY: Springer Publishing.

Thorpe, K. F. (2005). The rise in health care spending and what to do about it: Disease prevention/health promotion approaches are key to slowing the rise in health care spending. *Health Affairs, 24*(6), 1436–1445.

Tracy, M. F. (2009). Direct clinical practice. In A. B. Hamric, J. A. Spross, & C. M. Hanson (Eds.), *Advanced practice nursing an integrative approach* (pp.123–158). St. Louis, MO: Elsevier.

Trish, E., Damico, A., Claxton, G., Levitt, L., & Garfield, R. (2011). A profile of health insurance exchange enrollees. Retrieved from http://www.kff.org/healthreform/upload/8147.pdf

Van Sandt, S. E., Sloand, E., & Wilkins, A. (2008). Caring for vulnerable populations: Role of academic nurse-managed health centers in educating nurse practitioners. *Journal for Nurse Practitioners, 4*(2), 126–131.

Vonderheid, S. C., Pohl, J. M., Tanner, C., Newland, J. A., & Gans, D. N. (2009). CPT coding patterns at nurse-managed health centers: Data from a national survey. *Nursing Economic$, 27*(4), 211–220.

Walker, D. K. (2012). Skin protection for kids (SPF) program. *Journal of Pediatric Nursing, 27*(3), 233–243. doi:10.1016/j.pedn.2011.01.031

Williams, D. R., McClellan, M. B., & Rivlin, A. M. (2010). Beyond the affordable care act: Achieving real improvements in America's health. *Health Affairs, 29*(8), 1481–1488.

Health Policy and Special Populations: Implications

Interface of Policy and Practice in Health Care Reform: What Nurses Can Do to Improve Health Care

Kathleen R. Delaney

The Patient Protection and Affordable Care Act (PPACA) initiated the most significant upheaval in the U.S. health care system in 50 years. Now some 7 years later the reverberations of this historic legislation continue, as do the related policy issues. This chapter focuses on the PPACA provisions that significantly impacted the care of individuals with mental health issues and the mental health care system as well as the ongoing gaps in mental health care delivery. Key implications of the current health care climate for psychiatric mental health (PMH) nursing practice are highlighted along with suggestions for how PMH Advanced Practice Registered Nurses (APRNs) and RNs might thrive within service innovations and advocate for closing service gaps. Finally, how the specialty might frame the policy issues critical to both workforce development and mental health service delivery is suggested. What follows is a brief summary of the context for health care reform of 2010. This is particularly relevant because many of the cost issues continue into this decade, particularly lack of access to effective community treatment and poor overall health of individuals with serious mental illness (SMI).

DRIVERS OF HEALTH CARE REFORM

Most citizens will mark the beginning of health care reform with the signing of the PPACA. While not minimizing the innovation brought with the legislation, the APRN should understand that payment/service system reform has been a process slowly evolving for over 20 years. Looking across the last decade and costs, it is apparent that years prior to PPACA concerns existed for individuals with SMI, including access to care (Gabel et al., 2004), lack of insurance (Hadley & Holahan, 2003), and costs related to care (Druss et al., 2001); problems the industry continues to grapple with as individuals go without needed care (Osborn, Squires, Doty, Sarnak, & Schneider, 2016).

A major driver of health care reform was the cost of health care and its relatively poor outcomes, the so-called value equation (Porter, 2010), an issue which persists (Kaplan, 2016). Costs operate on two levels; one is the overall costs of health care calculated each year that examines trends in spending. Although specific sector spending varies from year to year and there has been a steady rise in health care spending (now at 17.5% of gross national product) for the last five years the rate of growth had been slowed to just about 5% (e.g., Martin, Hartman, Benson, Catlin, & National Health Expenditure Accounts Team, 2016). In addition to overall costs specific sectors of health care spending are inspected such as hospital care and pharmaceuticals which saw the most significant increases in 2014 (Martin et al., 2016).

A second level of the cost of health is the cost for the individual and specific groups, whether clustered by income, insurance status, or clinical condition (Hayes, Salzberg, et al., 2016). One group that consistently surfaces due to cost are individuals with chronic conditions; in fact 86% of all health care spending in 2010 was for people with one or more chronic medical conditions (Gerteis et al., 2014). Among these most costly conditions are ones related to mental health; the largest number of persons ages 18 years to 64 years incurring expenses was treated for mental disorders (29.6 million; Soni, 2015). Thus, the government has a history of being cost conscious and employing mechanisms to track costs and increasingly to track quality, which brings even greater pressure on mental health providers to deliver the value equation.

BRIEF HISTORICAL BACKGROUND

The PPACA instituted broad reform in how the business of health care was conducted and incentivized. With the help of public media, the PPACA has become synonymous with issues of expanding federal health insurance to the uninsured and with state development of insurance exchanges. Actually, the PPACA was a bill with 90 provisions that was phased in over more than 5 years (see www.kff.org/interactive/implementation-timeline). Taking this broader viewpoint, it becomes apparent that the PPACA was constructed to strengthen and innovate particular health care sectors such as primary care, long-term care, and mental health services; create new models of care such as the medical home; incorporate quality as an element of reimbursement; and fundamentally change the fee-for-service payment structure (Chaikind, Copeland, Redhead, & Staman, 2011). These reform elements are intertwined. For instance, strengthening primary care through payment reform is viewed as a way to address the needs of the chronically ill, reduce unnecessary hospitalization, and curtail emergency room treatment (Davis, Abrams, & Stremikis, 2011). Service models such as the patient-centered medical home were meant to encourage care coordination, which helps reduce the costs of persons with chronic illness and multiple comorbidities (Nielsen, Gibson, Buelt, Grundy, & Grumbach, 2015). Within each of these suggested practice models were provisions that changed the provider incentives from a strict fee-for-service system to one where quality becomes a factor in the payment structure (Berenson, 2010).

The PPACA also contained provisions aimed at building the workforce who would work within and engineer the service reform. For example, anticipating the need to provide services to the increasing number of citizens eligible for health care (due to the expansion of health insurance) PPACA provisions provided monies to grow the primary care workforce (Carrier, Yee, & Stark, 2011). Recognizing the role of APRNs in primary care, one of the PPACA provisions was the graduate nurse education (GNE) demonstration that tested if payment to preceptors would facilitate increased enrollment in Primary Care APRN programs (Centers for Medicare and Medicaid Services [CMS], 2013).

In line with the triple aim (Berwick, Nolan, & Whittington, 2008), the PPACA was threaded with innovative philosophies of care, such as patient-centered care (PCC), which demanded that consumer/family goals and treatment preferences be integrated into health care decision making (Epstein, Fiscella, Lesser, & Stange, 2010). The idea of PCC thrives, advanced by the Patient-Centered Outcomes Research Institute (PCORI) which funds research to advance PCC practice. Yet given the strides in implementing PPC, it is widely acknowledged that dysfunctional patient–provider communication patterns endure that silence the patient's voice and impede the development of PCC, particularly for individuals with SMI (Chang et al., 2014; Kaufman, McDonell, Cristofalo, & Ries, 2012; Tai-Seale, Foo, & Stults, 2013).

At the current time, the notion of population health has entered the lexicon of health care services (Kindig, 2016). The PPACA provisions that shifted the health care system to a focus on the health of the population, emphasizing prevention and wellness (Goodson, 2010), also created debate if the term meant population in terms of a geographic region (population health) or clinical cohort (population health management; Cashman, 2016). Even given the ongoing debate on terminology, it is clear that treatment/payment networks, such as accountable care organizations (ACO), are incentivized to keep a population of people healthy. Thus, the PPACA is a complex compilation of payment restructuring, workforce initiatives, insurance reforms, penalties, and incentives designed to fundamentally change the business of health care.

HEALTH REFORM AND MENTAL HEALTH CARE

Health care reform initiatives aimed at improving mental health care by encouraging integrated care models, parity in mental health insurance coverage, and initiatives to move Medicare and Medicaid into a capitated system (American Psychiatric Association [APA], 2012; Ebert et al., 2013). The PPACA architects also expected that the integrated primary care system would be expanded, bringing more individuals into treatment while addressing mental health and physical needs in a coordinated manner (Ebert et al., 2013). Individuals with mental illness represent a significant portion of the U.S. population and their service needs are largely unmet (Box 15.1). As individuals dealing with mental illness are more likely to be uninsured, it was thought that the PPACA provisions to expand health insurance coverage to individuals at 133% of poverty

PREVALENCE OF MENTAL ILLNESS IN THE UNITED STATES AND TREATMENT RATES	BOX 15.1

- Among adults aged 18 or older, the national rate of SMI was 4%, which equates to 9.6 million Americans (SAMHSA, 2013).
- Nationally, 42.5 million adults aged 18 or older experienced any mental illness in the past year, corresponding to a rate of 18.2% of Americans (SAMHSA, 2013).
- In 2015, an estimated 16.1 million adults aged 18 or older in the United States had at least one major depressive episode in the past year. This number represented 6.7% of all U.S. adults (NIMH, 2015).
- In the past year, 20.2 million adults (8.4%) had a substance use disorder. Of these, 7.9 million people had both a mental disorder and substance use disorder (Center for Behavioral Health Statistics and Quality, 2015).
- In 2014, an estimated 11.8 million adults aged 18 or older perceived an unmet need for mental health care in the past year, including 5.3 million adults who did not receive any mental health services in the past year (SAMHSA, 2015).

level would also expand coverage for mental health issues (Garfield, Zuvekas, Lave, & Donohue, 2011). Preliminary data confirm that this strategy has been largely successful in states that expanded Medicaid coverage (Wen, Druss, & Cummings, 2015).

The psychiatry community generally endorsed the PPACA, emphasizing the benefits of extending health coverage to 32 million more Americans, prohibitions on denying coverage based on preexisting conditions, and particularly that mental health and substance abuse disorder treatment were to be part of the basic package of benefits in the health insurance plans (APA, 2012; Mental Health America [MHA], 2011). However, concerns existed regarding coverage for mental health treatment within these new state exchanges plans; particularly that rates may be structured to discourage enrollment of individuals with high mental health needs, and that insurance packages may not contain necessary benefits for those with SMI (Barry, Weiner, Lemke, & Busch, 2012). At this point, it is difficult to ascertain if the expansion of behavioral health benefits in insurance plans has made a significant impact on outcomes of individuals with mental health issues (Jacob et al., 2015).

Now, some 7 years past the signing of the PPACA, several key provisions continue to evolve, as do mental health issues and service delivery models. These evolving issues raise concerns for all behavioral health professionals, including PMH nurses, in the areas of policy and practice. In the current health care climate four areas have significant impact on mental health service delivery and, in turn, policy, the psychiatric nursing workforce, and their future roles. Three areas of impact for mental health services directly follow from the PPACA provisions: integrated care, population health, and value-based care. An additional area of concern for PMH professionals is the gaps in mental health services, which create ongoing issues with access to services and lack of care for vulnerable/disenfranchised populations. These four areas of concern are briefly outlined, followed by their implications for the PMH workforce and policy agenda.

FOUR CRITICAL PRACTICE/POLICY AREAS
AND MENTAL HEALTH SERVICES

Integrated Care

Background

As the PPACA was being formulated, the publication of data on the medical comorbidities and decreased life expectancy of individuals with SMI hastened calls for developing systems that integrated behavioral and primary care services (Horvitz-Lennon, Kilbourne, & Pincus, 2006). Related issues emerged, including the costs of these comorbidities and the increased risk of disability and poor health outcomes, particularly for those dealing with substance abuse issues (Melek & Norris, 2008; Najt, Fusar-Poli, & Brambilla, 2011; Scott et al., 2009). On the other side of integrated care was the situation of individuals with mild to moderate mental health issues whose issues were not adequately identified or addressed in primary care (Mitchell, Vaze & Rao, 2009).

The idea of integrated care did not originate with the PPACA (see history, Collins, Hewson, Munger, & Wade, 2010), but the passage of the Affordable Care Act (ACA) accelerated the model by stipulating that essential health benefits must include mental health services and by providing state incentives to create new integrated models for specific populations (Kuramoto, 2014). Integrated care has grown over the past several years in part due to its inherent logic, that is providing behavioral health care in the system where most individuals are seen (California Primary Care Association, n.d.) and addressing consumer's preference for treatment in a less stigmatizing primary care setting (Manderscheid, 2010).

Incentives to strengthen integrated primary care were woven throughout the PPACA, such as increased payment to primary care physicians to work with families and coordinate care (U.S. Department of Health and Human Services [DHHS], 2011). The PPACA also hastened the transition to integrated care via provisions which called for expansion of insurance coverage and a reimbursement structure that favored primary care (particularly care coordination services; DHHS, 2011), by awarding grants to explore models of integrated care (CMS, 2011) and the development of the Community-Based Collaborative Care Network Program.

Current Issues

Since the passage of the PPACA, integrated care has evolved into several distinct models (e.g., co-located services, behavioral health care home) and new vehicles to integrate services, particularly telepsychiatry (Gerrity, 2016). In a recent review Gerrity notes that integrated care has been largely successful in building a systematic communication platform for primary care/psychiatric providers and that the collaborative care management model (CCM) improves outcomes for individuals with mood related disorders. Health care researchers also note continuing issues: developing outcomes, achieving patient-centered approaches, and incentivizing best practices (Goldman, Spaeth-Rublee, & Pincus, 2014; Institute for Healthcare Improvement, 2014). Integrated care rests with the treatment team so there is a recognized need for training in teamwork as well as developing competencies of team members, specific to the integrated care delivery system (Substance Abuse and Mental Health Services Administration [SAMHSA-HRSA Center for Integrated Health Solutions, 2014]). Thus the issues now rest largely with implementation, particularly isolating what factors are generating the largest positive change, for instance care coordination, which seems to be a promising intervention for helping individuals with SMI (Gerrity, 2016).

Population Health

Background

One tenet of reform was that the U.S. health care system had become increasingly geared toward treating illness and not promoting health (Fani Marvasti, & Stafford, 2012). The result was a costly system that yielded poor health outcomes for our citizens, as indicated by the greater rates of morbidity and mortality of U.S. citizens compared to other industrialized countries (Commonwealth Fund, 2008). The PPACA focused on wellness, health promotion, and prevention. It initially established a prevention fund, and recently DHHS launched its National Strategy for Quality Improvement in Health Care (DHHS, 2012), which included the key provisions they believed would make care safer, as well as more cost-effective and patient-centered. Within this document is the notion that health care organizations must focus on prevention and promoting the wellness of their members. Funding for prevention activities included state-based demonstration projects, funding for community health departments' prevention activities, and regulations stating that Medicare and Medicaid cannot impose costs on patients for services deemed beneficial by the Preventive Services Task Force (Hardcastle, Record, Jacobson, & Gostin, 2011).

In Section 2 of the Act, the National Strategy to Improve Health Care Quality, there was a call for the Secretary of Health and Human Services to devise a national strategy to improve population health. Over the ensuring years the concept of wellness and prevention became intertwined with the idea of population health in several ways. One was the need for health care providers to consider wellness in the context of patients' communities, to move health efforts out to this wider sphere of influence, and to work with community-based organizations, schools, and businesses (IOM, 2014). This approach favors the idea that population health should be understood as the distribution of health outcomes across individuals living in a geopolitical boundary (Jacobson & Teutsch, 2012; Kindig & Stoddart, 2003). An alternative view is that an organization is responsible for delivering services to a defined population guided by measurements implied in the triple aim: outcomes such as cost and the patient experience and also health, functional status, and behavioral factors such as smoking, diet, and physical activity (Lewis, 2014). It was the two lines of thinking that encouraged wellness/prevention tenets to be subsumed under the idea of population health.

For our purposes population health will be thought of as a broad concept that demands a health care organization be accountable to the populations it serves (Stoto, 2013). This accountability means that health care provider/agencies must focus not just on illness but also on prevention, promoting healthier lifestyles, and advancing well-being—an individual's appraisal that their lives are desirable and proceeding well (Diener, Oishi, & Lucas, 2015). When population health is considered in terms of the health of a geographic region the notion broadens, requiring that health care entities collaborate with schools, social services, local employers, and public health departments (Stiefel & Nolan, 2013). To boost community and individual well-being will demand providers skilled in systems of care and methods to address the upstream factors related to social determinants of health (Bacon & Newton, 2014).

Current State

The PPACA built several provisions around wellness, but a critical structural change was the creation of accountable care contracting where health care payers (e.g., insurance providers) contract with a group of health care providers, called ACO (Gourevitch, Cannell, Boufford, & Summers, 2012). The ACO is responsible for a range of services as well as care coordination, wellness and prevention. The federal insurance agencies (Medicaid and Medicare) were particular targets for accountable care contracting and moving towards managed care arrangements (Kaiser Family Foundation, 2016). In ACO arrangements quality and incentives align as the providers share in savings from reductions in procedures, and with care coordination, a decrease in preventable hospitalizations (Gourevitch et al., 2012). Since 2010 the number of ACO arrangements has increased from a few dozen to more than 600 networks and 22 million covered lives (Muhlestein, 2015).

The emphasis on population health becomes a bit more complex for patients with chronic conditions. The care of these individuals had become increasingly fragmented, ineffective, and costly (Anderson, 2010). In fact three of the five most costly health conditions in the United States are chronic, one of them being treatment for mental illness (Soni, 2015), and the approach to these individuals was often siloed, with practitioners focused on the individual chronic diseases specific to their practice (Parekh, Goodman, Gordon, & Koh, 2011). Achieving wellness and prevention with individuals dealing with SMI may also require additional effort (Gerrity, 2014). In a recent report that examined 59 recipients of SAMHSA's Primary and Behavioral Health Care Integration (PBHCI) the authors noted that sites demonstrated improved outcomes with select conditions, such as diabetes and dyslipidemia, but progress was slow with smoking cessation and obesity (Scharf et al., 2014).

Several care coordination models were strengthened by the PPACA, such as the patient-centered medical home (PCMH): a primary care based model in which a team of professionals work to coordinate care for individuals with complex health needs. As these models of care evolve, it is clear they will need modifications to comprehensively address the needs of the SMI population (Bao, Casalino, & Pincus, 2013). Other variations of the PCMH specific to mental health are the behavioral health care home (SAMHSA-HRSA Center for Integrated Health Care Solutions, 2012), the Medicaid Health Home (Medicaid.gov, n.d.), and the Certified Community Mental Health Center. All of these models aim to address not just health but also issues related to the social determinants of health such as housing. In addition, collaborative care models, often fashioned on the Wagner chronic disease model, are proving to be effective (Woltmann et al., 2012). Thus population health, wellness, and prevention are important considerations for service delivery, but health care planners will need to consider how to implement these models with individuals dealing with SMI (Bao et al., 2013).

Value-Based Care

Background

A core idea within the DHHS National Quality Strategy (2012) is the value equation, improving care of individuals and their health, all at the right cost. With this basic strategy as a backdrop, CMS began to define the outcomes they wanted to achieve from the services they purchased for their beneficiaries. These outcomes were tied to value-based purchasing (VBP) a system that rewards providers who deliver better outcomes at a lower cost (VanLare & Conway, 2012). VBP was a dramatic departure from the fee-for-service model, which pays for the amount of services that are delivered or procedures ordered. Rather the provider is rewarded for meeting defined quality standards. It should be noted that an important lever in this strategy is moving more Medicare recipients into so-called Alternative Payment Models, such as the ACO discussed earlier as well as new models for dual eligible individuals (persons eligible for both Medicare and Medicaid; DHHS, 2016).

Current Issues

Secretary Burwell recently outlined the DHHS goal that by 2016, 85% of all Medicare fee-for-service payments would be tied to quality or value and 90% by 2018 (Burwell, 2015). As VBP moves forward questions remain about the exact impact of incentives on quality of care. There are concerns that VBP may actually increase disparities if lower performing providers (who tend to care for poorer, racially diverse patients) receive lower incentives and are less able to fund quality improvement initiatives (Ryan, 2013). Establishing a value-based program for a single procedure such as a knee replacement may indeed lead to improved outcomes at a reduced cost (Lee et al., 2016). For individuals with mental illness in the recovery process, the value of services may be revealed over time, which makes measurement of a single episode of care less relevant (Porter, 2010). In addition, how the value-based system will address the "whole person" needs of individuals with SMI is unclear, particularly issues of access, helping individuals navigate complex systems and adapting a requisite social-ecologic view of the clients' issues (Ezell, Cabassa, & Siantz, 2013; Lawrence & Kisely, 2011). Finally, a critical component of understanding value is measurement, measuring, and tracking results over time. It is unclear if systems or individuals have the skill set to engineer the systematic collection of outcomes over time, particularly around mental health issues.

Gaps in Access to Care

Background

Certainly the PPACA was designed to increase care to all citizens. Its basic tenets were to improve and extend insurance coverage, to do away with exclusions, and to simplify the process so as to open the market to a great number of individuals seeking health care. The act contained a section of provisions for increasing access to mental health services, including spending for Federally Qualified Health Centers (FQHCs), modifying procedures for identification of shortage areas, and creating co-located primary care services in community mental health centers. Perhaps most important, the act included mental health services in its list of essential services a health plan must cover. In the section on state health exchanges, the PPACA contained provisions directing that plan managers must reach out to vulnerable and underserved populations. Finally, the act set down guidelines to establish Medicaid Health Homes for persons with chronic conditions, stipulating treatment should address mental health conditions and that one of the qualifying chronic conditions could be a SMI. Thus the plan, as designed, thoughtfully addressed access to services for individuals with mental health issues.

Current Issues

The initial reports on the Medicaid Health Home are emerging with select states showing cost savings, particularly a reduction in emergency department (ED) visits (Shane, Nguyen-Hoang, Bentler, Damiano, & Momany, 2016). While many of the provisions held great promise, there is the reality that the innovations have not been across all populations, particularly adults with multiple chronic conditions and a functional limitation, so-called high-needs individuals (Salzberg et al., 2016). In a recent survey, these adults were more likely to report having an unmet medical need and poor provider communication. Half of these adults who have a co-occurring mental health condition report even greater problems with access (Hayes, McCarthy, & Radley, 2016).

Access is a particular problem for persons with mental health conditions in states that did not expand Medicaid coverage, where there is less access to insurance and medical homes (Adepoju, Preston, & Gonzales, 2015). Access issues and gaps in care also arise from the shortage of behavioral health care providers (Burke et al., 2013). While the PPACA provided insurance and expanded the demand, it did little to increase the supply, particularly for psychiatrists, who are diminishing in numbers (Staff Care, 2015) and half of whom do not accept insurance as payment (Bishop, Press, Keyhani, & Pincus, 2014). This situation invites a vicious cycle: as demand and wait times grow, those that can afford it will pay out of pocket for services, as Goodman (2015) notes, providing better access to 500 patients while leaving 2000 behind.

In some respects, health care reform has left behind several disenfranchised populations, most notably, individuals incarcerated in our prison system and the homeless. The U.S. Department of Housing and Urban Development (2016) put the number of homeless in America at approximately 550,000; 15% of these individuals are considered chronically homeless— an individual who has a disability and has experienced homelessness for a year or more. While the number of homeless individuals is actually declining, those at risk are increasing. Another population of concern is the 356,000 persons in jails and state prisons who are believed to have SMI; approximately 20% of inmates in jails and 15% of inmates in state prisons (Torrey et al., 2014). A root cause in the growth of both populations is the lack of mental health services, particularly public psychiatric hospital beds, which have fallen by 17% since 2010, now standing at 11.7 available beds per 100,000 people. So while the present administration has made considerable efforts to address these issues, there remains a serious problem with lack of access to treatment and its sequelae, many individuals in need of treatment incarcerated or homeless.

PMH NURSING PRACTICE: IMPACT AND ADJUSTMENT

Integrated Care

PMH APRNs have a skill set that fits well with integrated care: They have been educated in the sciences—for example, medical, prevention, psychiatry/behavioral health, and neuroscience—and thus have the education and training to monitor co-existing physical conditions and screen for emerging physical problems (Delaney, Robinson, & Chafetz, 2013). This skill set is apparent in select community clinics, often nurse managed, which have developed best practices in effective care delivery to underserved populations with high levels of complex illness (Davis et al., 2011; Gerolamo, Kim, & Brown, 2014). While their role within traditional psychiatric models is clear, the exact function PMH APRNs have in providing assessments of medical needs and preventive care has not been well defined (Weinstein, Henwood, Cody, Jordan, & Lelar, 2011). As with other nursing specialties, PMH APRNs' competencies and scope of practice may be unclear to service organizations and payers (Delaney, 2016; Lowe, Plummer, O'Brien, & Boyd, 2012).

PMH APRNs must clearly articulate the skills they bring to new health care settings and identify the scope of their practice to providers and patients who are engaged in primary care as scope-of-practice parameters for assessment of physical issues, and integration of these issues in a plan of care, as contained in the PMH Scope and Standards of Practice (ANA, APNA, & ISPN, 2014; Delaney et al., 2013). Specific competencies are contained in the National Organization of Nurse Practitioner Faculties (NONPF), Core Competencies (NONPF, 2017), and the PMH Nurse Practitioner Competencies (NONPF, 2013). A significant workforce trend is expanding RN roles in primary care (Smolowitz et al., 2015). Given this trend, it is likely that PMH RNs will also play a greater role in integrated care. Their role within integrated care will demand new competencies including; screening for mental health/substance use conditions, telephone triage, proficiency in stepped care decisions, delivery of low intensity behavioral health interventions, wellness and engagement (Gerrity, 2014; Ladden et al., 2013; Smolowitz et al., 2015).

Population Health

The evolving behavioral health workforce must do more than standard practice. They must engineer a treatment process that connects to core metrics for health; for example, well-being, access, population health, and community engagement (IOM, 2014). This mandate has a good fit with APRN skills. Nurse Practitioners (NPs) have been recognized for their provision of preventive care, health education, health promotion, and wellness care (Hardcastle et al., 2011). PMH APRNs will also need to bring their expertise with wellness into the mental health arena (Delaney et al., 2013). PMH nurses understand that the keys to healthy behaviors are increasing an individual's sense of self-efficacy and empowering them to move toward a self-constructed vision of health (Anthony, 2006). Helping individuals make healthier choices depends on an individual's willingness to engage with a clinician and adopt particular behaviors. Thus PMH APRNs should cultivate methods to increase patients' engagement with any healthy living plan (Pelletier & Stichler, 2013). For patients with SMI, nurses must develop an understanding of their illness and lifestyle habits in the context of the social determinants of health, poverty, and the related issues of nutrition, housing, and occupational status (Onie, Farmer, & Behforouz, 2012).

Given the initial data on achieving wellness outcomes for individuals with SMI (Scharf et al., 2014), PMH nurses must advocate for the patient and the understanding that achieving wellness benchmarks for individuals with

SMI may require additional strategies, particularly given the lifestyle habits the patients may have developed to cope with their illness and its treatment. Such factors may come into play with regard to smoking, which may to some extent be "self medication" and thus cannot be adequately addressed without concurrent attention to psychiatric symptom management (Delaney et al., 2013). In each case the nurse needs to follow the individual's narrative of how smoking fits into their life, and what type of changes they might be willing to make.

For individuals with chronic conditions, population health will require active care management. Care management by PMH RNs in community-based care settings has resulted in outcomes such as improved recognition of medical conditions, reduced costs, and improved quality of life (Druss, von Esenwein, et al., 2010; Druss, von Esenwein, Compton, Zhao, & Leslie, 2011; Katon et al., 2010). Given the data on the effectiveness of nurse care managers, particularly in CCM models, one can anticipate growth in this role for PMH RNs (C. J. Miller et al., 2013). Strong support for nurses as care managers emerged from an evaluation of 12 randomized controlled trials that provided integrated care to individuals with SMI. Five sites used RN-level nurses as care managers and six sites added NPs to the care team (Gerrity, 2014). The expanded skill set required in these community-based team models will require a revising of the RN role, and establishing processes that facilitate an expanded scope of practice (Center for Excellence in Primary Care, 2015; Smolenski et al., 2015).

Value-Based Purchasing

For a health system to deliver value-based care it must track outcomes over time with a population of patients. This requires a good degree of service engagement and patient involvement in care. Persons with SMI have historically high levels of attrition from mental health services; research suggests a 50% failure to return for treatment or adherence to treatment recommendations (Gibson, Brand, Burt, Boden, & Benson, 2013). Attrition is a complex mix of perceived need for continued treatment and practical barriers that often result in premature withdrawal from mental health care (Mojtabai et al., 2011).

Nurses have the relationship-based skill set to play a critical role in building service engagement. Indeed, the interpersonal relationship is the disciplinary foundation of PMH nurses (D'Antonio, Beeber, Sills, & Naegle, 2014). Also useful in building service engagement is PMH nurses' ability to grasp a person's everyday issues and understand what a person needs in the context of their daily living (Beebe, 2010). Nurses also understand that to improve wellness and health outcomes interventions must be acceptable, feasible, and achievable within the context of the person's lived environment. Finally, one can never lose sight that an individual must be approached with a sense of a person's need to be recognized, affirmed, and valued (Spandler & Stickley, 2011).

PMH nurses must also understand how to elicit, harness, and use the consumer voice. Qualitative data document that consumers value services where what one says matters and where providers convey a sense of respect and working together to reach solutions (Knapik & Graor, 2013; Stanhope & Henwood, 2014). Consumer involvement can play a major role in solving problems that lead to attrition of individuals from mental health treatment (Gibson et al., 2013; Saxe, Heidi-Ellis, Fogler, & Navalta, 2012). Programs like the Health, Recovery, and

Peer program (HARP) show promise as consumer led teams work to increase engagement (Druss, Zhao, et al., 2010). Listening to consumers will also help refocus dialogues about best practices for designing models for diverse populations (Bridges et al., 2014). In these service engagement efforts, affiliations will be key with other professionals but more so with consumers and peer specialists, who have unique capabilities to partner with others in the recovery process (Faces and Voices of Recovery, 2013). Historically, the caring practices rendered by nurses have not been deemed reimbursable, contributing to the "economic invisibility" of this profession (Safriet, 2011). Thus PMH nurses must clearly articulate the importance of engagement, their skill set, and where it fits in effective care coordination.

Gaps in Care: Improving Access

Multiple dynamics underlie the gaps in care that result in individuals' inability to access the services they need. NPs have been recognized as an answer to the workforce needs in primary care (Naylor & Kurtzman, 2010). PMH APRNs, who are licensed to provide the full scope of mental health services, could be an equally important component of addressing the provider shortages in community-based mental health (Burke et al., 2013). PMH APRNs are a growing force: Estimates are that by 2025 there will be 17,500 practicing PMH NPs (HRSA, 2015). These APRNs could assume provider roles and leadership in CCM models as well as Health Homes. Their innate knowledge of the RN role will facilitate the functioning of effective teams where each member practices to the top of that person's scope of practice.

As PMH nurses move into new roles in service models they must be guided by the needs of consumers and their expression of what will help them lead a more meaningful life in the community. They must understand that the future is measurement-based care and outcomes will be essential to all service sectors, be it community-based mental health or integrated care. However, outcomes must be informed by a recovery perspective. Leaders lend a strong voice in shaping a service culture. Thus APRNs filling this gap provides the opportunity to build compassionate cultures of care that treat needs as legitimate (Spandler & Stickley, 2011).

EVALUATION OF APRN PRACTICE INITIATIVES

Cost, quality, and access are three of the underlying principles for evaluation of APRN practice. Cost outcomes of APRN practice are increasingly emerging in the literature (American Association of Nurse Practitioners [AANP], 2013). Cost benefits can operate at the level of savings-related factors such as decreased length of stay (Newhouse et al., 2011) or the cost benefits of an individual model (Allen, Himmelfarb, Szanton, & Frick, 2014). Similar cost outcomes of PMH APRN practice could be assessed, such as the cost savings related to care coordination and decreased use of emergency services or hospitalization.

Quality outcomes are also available in the literature, particularly for NP practice (AANP, 2013). Outcomes for integrated care are limited; mainly isolated to outcomes for specific conditions, such as somatoform and depression, and for specific models, such as Improving Mood Promoting Collaborative Treatment

(IMPACT; van der Feltz-Cornelis, Van Os, Van Marwijk, & Leentjens, 2010). What remains unknown are the effects of specific strategies and how outcomes correlate with levels of integration or care coordination processes (B. F. Miller, Kessler, Peek, & Kallenberg, 2011). By defining the scope of their practice and roles, PMH APRNs can reduce this knowledge gap and begin to measure quality metrics, such as how care coordination relates to patient satisfaction and how a particular health coaching technique relates to patient engagement in care (Pelletier & Stichler, 2013).

PMH AND POLICY: UNIFYING EFFORTS

Alignment of APRN practice with the principles of health care reform will depend on our specialty's resilience, but equally on the alliances we develop with consumers, advocacy groups, APRN professional organizations, and other behavioral health care professionals. It will require that the PMH APRNs see themselves as a single workforce with their PMH RN colleagues and other APRN groups. This perspective is essential if APRNs are to engineer systems where persons are treated holistically, and mental health, wellness, and medical needs are acknowledged with equal vigor. By bringing this focus on connectivity to the nursing community, nursing begins to address the reform ideal: to achieve a public health model of mental health care wherein individuals would receive mental health interventions at multiple points in the health care delivery system (Delaney, 2015).

Within this broad vision two policy issues demand particular attention. To create a coordinated, integrated system of care will require APRNs practicing at their full scope of practice (Newhouse et al., 2012; Stanley, Werner, & Apple, 2009). In the APRN community it is broadly acknowledged that recognizing the capacity of APRNs to improve access to and quality of care will also necessitate attention to barriers to practice arising from restrictive state regulations and payer recognition of APRNs (Poghosyan, Lucero, Rauch, & Berkowitz, 2012). PMH APRNs must join the state nursing groups that are focused on APRN issues. APRNs need to monitor government initiatives, the problems which motivate them, and how they connect to innovations and payment incentives.

The specialty must also focus on policy that removes barriers to integrated care expansion, practical considerations such as billing, coding, and broader concerns, like organizing effective interdisciplinary team, and mining national data to understand the relationship of staffing patterns, roles, and patient outcomes (Delaney et al., 2016). The ability of PMH APRNs to understand and communicate issues related to scope of practice, billing, coding, and reimbursement is paramount for their transition to integrated care.

The second critical policy area is health insurance and payment reform. There are particular concerns regarding the impact of insurance reform on access to care and benefits for persons in need of mental health services—particularly adverse selection, wherein plans "cherry pick" healthy individuals to keep the cost of services low (Barry et al., 2012). There is also concern about the actual breadth of benefits being offered in state insurance exchange plans (Garfield et al., 2011). APRNs need to embrace their advocacy role by becoming educated on each state's insurance structure and work to clarify mental health benefits within the state insurance pool.

Finally, PMH nurses must continue to build policy and advocate for access to care particularly for the vulnerable/disenfranchised population. This is particularly relevant considering the economic pressures on mental health services particularly on the state level. Between 2009 and 2012, the fiscal crisis forced cuts in states' mental health budgets of approximately $4.35 billion, and health care reform's innovations are only a partial response (National Association of State Mental Health Program Directors [NASMHPD], 2012). Because sites that provide acute care were particularly affected the entire mental health system was impacted as a reduction in hospital beds can be tied to increases in homelessness, emergency room use, and use of prisons as de facto psychiatric hospitals. PMH nurses must educate themselves and advocate for the policies that ensure access to the full range of services for individuals with mental health needs, strongly embracing an agenda of social equity (Pearson et al., 2015).

ETHICAL CONSIDERATIONS

The innovations initiated by health care reform promise to improve the health of individuals with SMI and expand access to mental health services to individuals who may not have had prior access to those services. The ensuing years have seen success, faltering efforts, and emerging problems. While there is a focus on reducing hospitalization, the need for inpatient services for those in crisis must also be recognized (NAMI, 2011). As state mental health care budgets continue to shrink, the lack of inpatient beds is recognized as a growing crisis. As PMH nurses engage in the development of integrated care, they should not lose sight of the ethical principle of professional stewardship of resources. PMH nurses should advocate for funding to maintain the mental health inpatient beds and new living room models needed by those experiencing an acute exacerbation of their illness.

Mental health records have been traditionally subject to additional privacy safeguards. Depending on the orientation, PPACA brings some degree of threat to that confidentiality. The growth of managed care will facilitate payers' access to an individual's mental health services utilization. The promise of integrated and coordinated care naturally leads to communication between clinicians and across service agencies. Integrated care networks however open up the records of those enrolled in the program (Witgert & Hess, 2012). As PMH APRNs practice within these networks, they must be mindful of confidentiality, involving patients in decisions about sharing health information and taking time to explain the ramifications of signing releases of information versus the benefits of restricting communication between providers.

For the past decade, recovery has been a grounding principle of the mental health system. According to the National Consensus Statement on Mental Health Recovery (SAMHSA, 2011), recovery is a journey of healing that enables a person with a mental health problem to live a meaningful life in his or her community. Inherent in this statement is the principle of autonomy: honoring the individual's movement along the healing trajectory. With our focus now on population outcomes and measurement-based care, the PMH nurse must be mindful of the principle of protecting that autonomy and the patient's right to map a journey toward health.

Finally, is the issue of stigma. Combating stigma is bound with the ethics of distributive justice, which requires that all citizens have access to the health care needed for living a full human life (Lamont & Favor, 2013).Stigma is an enduring ethical issue and it is the APRN's duty to be aware of how stigma operates within systems of care, both subtly and overtly (Lawrence & Kisely, 2011), and how it affects individuals with mental health issues (Corrigan, Druss, & Perlick, 2014). From a nursing perspective, the impact of stigma is ubiquitous, including unrecognized stigma nurses might hold toward both patients and their specialty (Delaney, 2012).

CONCLUSION

At this juncture, it is essential that those in the PMH specialty refine their vision, articulate it clearly, and disseminate it widely. The PMH workforce has a unique combination of education and training that makes them particularly suited for integrated care, collaborative team models, and population health. Our commitment to social justice must drive advocacy for care of disenfranchised populations. As models of care refine and payment incentives shift, nurses will undoubtedly be involved in measurement-based care and tracking the outcomes of their services. As PMH nurses expand their vision of mental health to include the community they will also become involved in building an environment that supports health, recovery, and resilience. The impact of PMH APRN practice will come from this collective vision of psychiatric nurses, working to integrate evidence-based interventions into their practice sites, and engaging with consumers and communities to build health and support their recovery journey.

DISCUSSION QUESTIONS

1. *How might changes in health care policy encourage creation of integrated care?*
2. *What is the biggest impact of your state nursing regulations on your future APRN practice?*
3. *What are the biggest hurdles to achieving effective integrated care in your state? How could policy address those hurdles?*
4. *Name one way that stigma impacts mental health care service delivery.*
5. *What are the major advocates for mental health in your state? How can you join with them to improve mental health care?*

ANALYSIS, SYNTHESIS, AND CLINICAL APPLICATION

1. *How do lifestyle and psychotropic medications combine to demand unique strategies for helping individuals achieve wellness?*
2. *What are the factors that create difficulty when isolating APRN outcomes in team-based care models?*
3. *Why would psychiatric clients be excluded from data collection on the patient experience?*
4. *Should there be a separate set of physical health benchmarks for individuals with SMI?*

EXERCISES/CONSIDERATIONS

1. *Investigate and compare among students, in the populations served by clinical practicum sites, the most common medical/psychiatric/substance use comorbidities.*
2. *What is the current policy(s) in the state legislature that will likely impact the APRN workforce?*
3. *Name one strategy used in your clinical site to promote healthy behaviors among individuals with SMI.*
4. *Investigate data in your state on access to services for individuals with mental illness.*
5. *Compare and contrast the mental health benefits in three policies in your state insurance exchange.*

REFERENCES

Adepoju, O. E., Preston, M. A., & Gonzales, G. (2015). Health care disparities in the Post–Affordable Care Act era. *American Journal of Public Health, 105*(Suppl. 5), S665–S667. doi:10.2105/AJPH.2015.302611

Allen, J. K., Himmelfarb, C. R. D., Szanton, S. L., & Frick, K. D. (2014). Cost-effectiveness of nurse practitioner/community health worker care to reduce cardiovascular health disparities. *Journal of Cardiovascular Nursing, 29*(4), 308–314.

American Association of Nurse Practitioners. (2013). Nurse practitioner cost-effectiveness. Retrieved from http://www.aanp.org/images/documents/publications/costeffectiveness.pdf

American Nurses Association, International Society for Psychiatric Nursing, & American Psychiatric Nurses Association. (2014). *Scope and standards of practice for psychiatric mental health nurses.* Silver Spring, MD: American Nurses Association.

American Psychiatric Association. (2012). *Health care reform: A primer for psychiatrists.* Washington, DC: Author.

Anderson, G. (2010). Chronic care: Making the case for ongoing care. Retrieved from https://www.rwjf.org/en/library/research/2010/01/chronic-care.html

Anthony, W. A. (2006). Personal accounts: What my MS has taught me about severe mental illnesses. *Psychiatric Services, 57*(8), 1081–1082.

Bao, Y., Casalino, L. P., & Pincus, H. A. (2013). Behavioral health and health care reform models: Patient-centered medical home, health home, and accountable care organization. *Journal of Behavioral Health Services & Research, 40*(1), 121–132.

Bacon, T. J., & Newton, W. P. (2014). Innovations in the education of health professionals. *North Carolina Medical Journal, 75*, 22–27.

Barry, C. L., Weiner, J. P., Lemke, K., & Busch, S. H. (2012). Risk adjustment in health insurance exchanges for individuals with mental illness. *American Journal of Psychiatry, 169*, 704–709.

Beebe, L. H. (2010). What community living problems do persons with schizophrenia report during periods of stability? *Perspectives in Psychiatric Care, 46*, 48–55.

Berenson, R. A. (2010). Moving payment from value to volume: What role for performance measurement—Timely analysis of immediate health policy issues. *Robert Wood Johnson, Urban Institute.* Retrieved from http://www.rwjf.org/content/dam/farm/reports/issue_briefs/2010/rwjf69037

Berwick, D. M., Nolan, T. W., & Whittington, J. (2008). The triple aim: Care, health and cost. *Health Affairs, 27*, 759–769.

Bishop, T. F., Press, M. J., Keyhani, S., & Pincus, H. A. (2014). Acceptance of insurance by psychiatrists and the implications for access to mental health care. *JAMA Psychiatry, 71*, 176–181. doi:10.1001/jamapsychiatry.2013.2862

Bridges, A. J., Andrews III, A. R., Villalobos, B. T., Pastrana, F. A., Cavell, T. A., & Gomez, D. (2014). Does integrated behavioral health care reduce mental health disparities for Latinos? Initial findings. *Journal of Latina/o Psychology, 2*(1), 37.

Burke, B. T., Miller, B. F., Proser, M., Petterson, S. M., Bazemore, A. W., Goplerud, E., & Phillips, R. L. (2013). A needs-based method for estimating the behavioral health staff needs of community health centers. *BMC Health Services Research, 13*(1), 245.

Burwell, S. M. (2015). Setting value-based payment goals—HHS efforts to improve U.S. health care. *New England Journal of Medicine, 372*(10), 897–899.

California Primary Care Association. (n.d.). Integrated behavioral health care: An effective and affordable model. Retrieved from http://www.cpca.org/cpca/assets/file/policy-and-advocacy/active-policy-issues/mhsa/integrationbrief.pdf

Carrier, E. R., Yee, T., & Stark, L. (2011). Matching supply to demand: Addressing the US primary care workforce shortage. *Policy Analysis No. 7.* Retrieved from http://nihcr.org/wp-content/uploads/2016/07/Policy_Analysis_No._7.pdf

Cashman, S. B. (2016). Accountable care organizations: Embracing a new population health? *Medical Care, 54,* 767–765

Center for Behavioral Health Statistics and Quality. (2015). Behavioral health trends in the United States: Results from the 2014 national survey on drug use and health (HHS Publication No. SMA 15-4927, NSDUH Series H-50). Retrieved from http://www.samhsa.gov/data

Center for Excellence in Primary Care. (2015). RN role reimagined: How empowering registered nurses can improve primary care. Retrieved from http://www.chcf.org/~/media/MEDIA%20LIBRARY%20Files/PDF/PDF%20R/PDF%20RNRoleReimagined.pdf

Centers for Medicare and Medicaid Services. (2011). Active projects report. Research and demonstrations in health care financing. A comprehensive guide to CMS research activities. Retrieved from http://www.cms.gov/Research-Statistics-Data-and-Systems/Statistics-Trends-andReports/ActiveProjectReports/Downloads/2011_Active_Projects_Report.pdf

Centers for Medicare and Medicaid Services. (2013). Graduate nurse education demonstration. Retrieved from http://innovation.cms.gov/ initiatives/gne

Chaikind, H., Copeland, C., Redhead, C., & Staman, J. (2011). PPACA: A brief overview of the law, implementation, and legal challenges (Congressional Research Service Report for Congress). Retrieved from http://nationalaglawcenter.org/wp-content/uploads/assets/crs/R41664.pdf

Chang, E. T., Wells, K. B., Young, A. S., Stockdale, S., Johnson, M. D., Fickel, J. J., . . . Rubenstein, L. V. (2014). The anatomy of primary care and mental health clinician communication: A quality improvement case study. *Journal of General Internal Medicine, 29*(2), 598–606.

Collins, C., Hewson, D. L., Munger, R., & Wade, T. (2010). *Evolving models of behavioral health integration in primary care.* New York, NY: Milbank Memorial Fund.

Commonwealth Fund Commission on a High Performance Health System. (2008). Why not the best? Results from the national scorecard on U.S. health system performance, 2008. Retrieved from http://www.commonwealthfund.org/Publications/Fund-Reports/2008/Jul/Why-Not-the-Best--Results-from-the-National-Scorecard-on-U-S--Health-System-Performance--2008.aspx

Corrigan, P. W., Druss, B. G., & Perlick, D. A. (2014). The impact of mental illness stigma on seeking and participating in mental health care. *Psychological Science in the Public Interest, 15*(2), 37–70.

D'Antonio, P., Beeber, L., Sills, G., & Naegle, M. (2014). The future in the past: Hildegard Peplau and interpersonal relations in nursing. *Nursing Inquiry, 21*(4), 311–317.

Davis, K., Abrams, M., & Stremikis, K. (2011). How the Affordable Care Act will strengthen the nation's primary care foundation. *Journal of General Internal Medicine, 26,* 1201–1203.

Davis, K. E., Brigell, E., Christiansen, K., Snyder, M., McDevitt, J., Forman, J., . . . Wilkniss, S. M. (2011). Integrated primary and mental health care services: An evolving partnership model. *Psychiatric Rehabilitation Journal, 34,* 317–320.

Delaney, K. R. (2012). Stigma that we fail to see. *Archives of Psychiatric Nursing, 26,* 333–335.

Delaney, K.R. (2015) Psychiatric mental health nursing at the tipping point. *Issues in Mental Health Nursing, 36,* 320–325.

Delaney, K. R. (2016). Psychiatric mental health nursing workforce agenda optimizing capabilities and capacity to address workforce demands. *Journal of the American Psychiatric Nurses Association, 22*(2), 122–131.

Delaney, K. R., Naegle, M., Flinter, M., Pulcini, J., & Hauenstein, E. J. (2016). Critical workforce issues for registered and advanced practice nurses in integrated care models. *Nursing Outlook, 64*(6), 607–609. doi:10.1016/j.outlook.2016.09.003

Delaney, K. R., Robinson, K. M., & Chafetz, L. (2013). Development of integrated mental health care: Critical workforce competencies. *Nursing Outlook, 61*(6), 384–391.

Diener, E., Oishi, S., & Lucas, R. E. (2015). National accounts of subjective well-being. *American Psychologist, 70*, 234–242.

Druss, B. G., Marcus, S. C., Olfson, M., Tanielian, T., Elinson, L., & Pincus, H. A. (2001). Comparing the national economic burden of five chronic conditions. *Health Affairs, 20*, 233–241.

Druss, B. G., von Esenwein, S. A., Compton, M. T., Rask, K. J., Zhao, L., & Parker, R. M. (2010). A randomized trial of medical care management for community mental health settings: The primary care access, referral, and evaluation (PCARE) study. *American Journal of Psychiatry, 167*, 151–159. doi:10.1176/appi.ajp.2009.09050691

Druss, B. G., von Esenwein, S. A., Compton, M. T., Zhao, L., & Leslie, D. L. (2011). Budget impact and sustainability of medical care management for persons with serious mental illnesses. *American Journal of Psychiatry, 168*, 1171–1178.

Druss, B. G., Zhao, L., von Esenwein, S. A., Bona, J. R., Fricks, L., Jenkins-Tucker, S., . . . Lorig, K. (2010). The health and recovery peer (HARP) program: A peer-led intervention to improve medical self-management for persons with serious mental illness. *Schizophrenia Research, 118*, 264–270.

Ebert, M. H., Findling, R. L., Gelenberg, A. J., Kane, J. M., Nierenberg, A. A., & Tariot, P. N. (2013). The effects of the affordable care act on the practice of psychiatry. *Journal of Clinical Psychiatry, 74*, 357–367.

Epstein, R. M., Fiscella, K., Lesser, C. S., & Stange, K. C. (2010). Why the nation needs a policy push on patient-centered health care. *Health Affairs, 29*, 1489–1495.

Ezell, J. M., Cabassa, L. J., & Siantz, E. (2013). Contours of usual care: Meeting the medical needs of diverse people with serious mental illness. *Journal of Health Care for the Poor and Underserved, 24*, 1552–1573.

Faces and Voices of Recovery. (2013). Why peer integrity and recovery orientation matters: Health reform and peer recovery support services. *Faces and Voices of Recovery, Issues Brief #3*. Retrieved from https://www.scribd.com/document/147991725/Why-Peer-Integrity-and-Recovery-Orientation-Matter

Fani Marvasti, F., & Stafford, R. S. (2012). From sick care to health care—Reengineering prevention into the US system. *New England Journal of Medicine, 367*, 889–891.

Gabel, J., Claxton, G., Gil, I., Pickreign, J., Whitmore, H., Holve, E., . . . Rowland, D. (2004). Health benefits in 2004: Four years of double-digit premium increases take their toll on coverage. *Health Affairs, 23*, 200–209.

Garfield, R. L., Zuvekas, S. H., Lave, J. R., & Donohue, J. M. (2011). The impact of national health care reform on adults with severe mental disorders. *American Journal of Psychiatry, 168*, 486–494.

Gerolamo, A. M., Kim, J. Y., & Brown, J. (2014). Integrating physical health care in behavioral health care agencies in rural Pennsylvania. Mathematica policy research. Retrieved from https://aspe.hhs.gov/sites/default/files/pdf/73206/ruralPA.pdf

Gerrity, M. (2014) Integrating primary care into behavioral health settings: What works for individuals with serious mental illness. *Milbank Memorial Fund*. Retrieved from http://www.milbank.org/uploads/documents/papers/Integrating-Primary-Care-Report.pdf

Gerrity, M. (2016). Evolving models of behavioral health integration: Evidence update 2010-2015. *Milbank Memorial Fund*. Retrieved from https://www.milbank.org/publications/evolving-models-of-behavioral-health-integration-evidence-update-2010-2015

Gerteis, J., Izrael, D., Deitz, D., LeRoy, L., Ricciardi. R., & Basu, J. (2014). *Multiple chronic conditions chartbook*. AHRQ Publications No. Q14-0038. Rockville, MD: Agency for Healthcare Research and Quality.

Gibson, S., Brand, S. L., Burt, S., Boden, Z. V., & Benson, O. (2013). Understanding treatment nonadherence in schizophrenia and bipolar disorder: A survey of what service users do and why. *BMC Psychiatry, 13*, 153. doi:10.1186/1471-244X-13-153

Goldman, M. L., Spaeth-Rublee, B., & Pincus, H. A. (2015). Quality indicators for physical and behavioral health care integration. *Journal of the American Medical Association, 314*, 769–770. doi:10.1001/jama.2015.6447

Goodman, J. (2015). Six problems with the ACA that aren't going away. *Health Affairs Blog*. Retrieved from http://healthaffairs.org/blog/2015/06/25/six-problems-with-the-aca-that-arent-going-away

Goodson, J. D. (2010). Patient protection and affordable care act: Promise and peril for primary care. *Annals of Internal Medicine, 152,* 742–744.

Gourevitch, M. N., Cannell, T., Boufford, J. I., & Summers, C. (2012). The challenge of attribution: Responsibility for population health in the context of accountable care. *American Journal of Preventive Medicine, 42*(6, Suppl. 2), S180–S183. doi:10.1016/j.amepre.2012.03.012

Hadley, J., & Holahan, J. (2003). How much medical care do the uninsured use, and who pays for it? *Health Affairs, W3,* w66–w81.

Hardcastle, L. E., Record, K. L., Jacobson, P. D., & Gostin, L. O. (2011). Improving the population's health: The Affordable Care Act and the importance of integration. *Journal of Law, Medicine & Ethics, 39,* 317–327.

Hayes, S. L., McCarthy, D., & Radley, D. C. (2016). The impact of a behavioral health condition on high-need adults. *To the Point.* Retrieved from http://www.commonwealthfund.org/publications/blog/2016/nov/behavioral-health-high-need-adults

Hayes, S. L., Salzberg, C. A., McCarthy, D., Radley, D., Abrams, M. K., Shah, T., & Anderson, G. F. (2016). High-need, high-cost patients: Who are they and how do they use health care—A population-based comparison of demographics, health care use, and expenditures. *The Commonwealth Fund.* Retrieved from http://www.commonwealthfund.org/publications/issue-briefs/2016/aug/high-need-high-cost-patients-meps1

Health Resources and Services Administration. (2015). Projecting the supply of non-primary care specialty and subspecialty clinicians: 2010–2025. Retrieved from https://bhw.hrsa.gov/sites/default/files/bhw/nchwa/projections/clinicalspecialties.pdf

Horvitz-Lennon, M., Kilbourne, A. M., & Pincus, H. A. (2006). From silos to bridges: Meeting the general health care needs of adults with severe mental illnesses. *Health Affairs, 25,* 659–669.

Institute for Healthcare Improvement. (2014). *Integrating behavioral health and primary care: 90-day R&D project final summary report.* Cambridge, MA: Author. Retrieved from http://www.ihi.org

Institute of Medicine. (2014). *Population health implications of the Affordable Care Act.* Retrieved from https://www.nap.edu/catalog/18546/population-health-implications-of-the-affordable-care-act-workshop-summary

Jacob, V., Qu, S., Chattopadhyay, S., Sipe, T. A., Knopf, J. A., Goetzel, R. Z.; Community Preventive Services Task Force. (2015). Economic effects of legislations and policies to expand mental health and substance abuse benefits in health insurance plans: A community guide systematic review. *Journal of Mental Health Policy and Economics, 18*(1), 39–48.

Jacobson, D. M., & Teutsch, S. (2012). An environmental scan of integrated approaches for defining and measuring total population health by the clinical care system, the government public health system, and stakeholder organizations. Retrieved from http://www.improvingpopulationhealth.org/PopHealthPhaseIICommissionedPaper.pdf

Kaiser Family Foundation. (2016). Total Medicaid MCO enrollment. Retrieved from http://kff.org/other/state-indicator/total-medicaid-mco-enrollment/?currentTimeframe=0

Kaplan, J. G. (2016). Cost is the big item in the value equation of health care and here's why. *Managing Managed Care.* Retrieved from https://www.managingmanagedcare.com/story/cost-big-item-value-equation-health-care-and-heres-why

Katon, W. J., Lin, E. H. B., Von Korff, M., Ciechanowski, P., Ludman, E., Young, B., . . . McCulloch, D. (2010). Collaborative care for patients with depression and chronic illnesses. *New England Journal of Medicine, 363,* 2611–2620. doi:10.1056/NEJMoa1003955

Kaufman, E. A., McDonell, M. G., Cristofalo, M. A., & Ries, R. K. (2012). Exploring barriers to primary care for patients with severe mental illness: Frontline patient and provider accounts. *Issues in Mental Health Nursing, 33*(3), 172–180.

Kindig, D. (2016). What are we talking about when we talk about population health? *Health Affairs Blog.* Retrieved from http://healthaffairs.org/blog/2015/04/06/what-are-we-talking-about-when-we-talk-about-population-health

Kindig, D., & Stoddart, G. (2003). What is population health? *American Journal of Public Health, 93*(3), 380–383.

Knapik, G. P., & Graor, C. H. (2013). Engaging persons with severe persistent mental illness into primary care. *Journal for Nurse Practitioners, 9*(5), 283–287.

Kuramoto, F. (2014). The Affordable Care Act and integrated care. *Journal of Social Work in Disability & Rehabilitation, 13,* 44–86.

Ladden, M. D., Bodenheimer, T., Fishman, N. W., Flinter, M., Hsu, C., Parchman, M., & Wagner, E. H. (2013). The emerging primary care workforce: Preliminary observations from the primary care team: Learning from effective ambulatory practices project. *Academic Medicine, 88,* 1830–1834.

Lamont, J., & Favor, C. (2013, Spring). Distributive justice. In E. N. Zalta (Ed.), *The Stanford encyclopedia of philosophy.* Retrieved from https://plato.stanford.edu/entries/justice-distributive

Lawrence, D., & Kisely, S. (2011). Inequalities in healthcare provision for people with severe mental illness. *Journal of Psychopharmacology, 24,* 61–68.

Lee, V. S., Kawamoto, K., Hess, R., Park, C., Young, J., Hunter, C., . . . Graves, K. K. (2016). Implementation of a value-driven outcomes program to identify high variability in clinical costs and outcomes and association with reduced cost and improved quality. *Journal of the American Medical Association, 316*(10), 1061–1072.

Lewis, N. (2014). Populations, population health, and the evolution of population management: Making sense of the terminology in US health care today. Retrieved from http://www.ihi.org/communities/blogs/_layouts/15/ihi/community/blog/itemview.aspx?List=81ca4a47-4ccd-4e9e-89d9-14d88ec59e8d&ID=50

Lowe, G., Plummer, V., O'Brien, A. P., & Boyd, L. (2012). Time to clarify—The value of advanced practice nursing roles in health care. *Journal of Advanced Nursing, 68,* 677–685.

Manderscheid, R. W. (2010). Evolution and integration of primary care services with specialty services. In B. Levin, K. Hennessy, & J. Petrila (Eds.), *Mental Health Services: A Public Health Perspective* (3rd ed., pp. 389–400). New York, NY: Oxford University Press.

Martin, A. B., Hartman, M., Benson, J., Catlin, A., & National Health Expenditure Accounts Team. (2016). National health spending in 2014: Faster growth driven by coverage expansion and prescription drug spending. *Health Affairs, 35*(1), 150–160.

Medicaid.gov. (n.d.). Guide to medicaid health home design and implementation. Retrieved from https://www.medicaid.gov/state-resource-center/medicaid-state-technical-assistance/health-homes-technical-assistance/guide-to-health-homes-design-and-implementation.html

Melek, S., & Norris, D. (2008). *Chronic conditionsand comorbid psychological disorders.* Seattle, WA: Milliman.

Mental Health America. (2011). Position statement 71: Health care reform. Retrieved from http://www.mentalhealthamerica.net/positions/health-care-reform

Miller, B. F., Kessler, R., Peek, C. J., & Kallenberg, G. A. (2011). *A national agenda for research collaborative care: Papers from the collaborative care research network. Research development conference.* AHRQ Publication No. 11-0067. Rockville, MD: Agency for Healthcare Research and Quality.

Miller, C. J., Grogan-Kaylor, A., Perron, B. E., Kilbourne, A. M., Woltmann, E., & Bauer, M. S. (2013). Collaborative chronic care models for mental health conditions: Cumulative meta-analysis and meta-regression to guide future research and implementation. *Medical Care, 51*(10), 922–930.

Mitchell, A. J., Vaze, A., & Rao, S. (2009). Clinical diagnosis of depression in primary care: A meta-analysis. *The Lancet, 374*(9690), 609–619.

Mojtabai, M., Olfson, N. A., Sampson, R., Jin, B., Druss, P. S., Wang, K. B., . . . Kessler, R. C. (2011). Barriers to mental health treatment: Results from the national comorbidity survey replication. *Psychological Medicine, 41,* 1751–1761.

Muhlestein, D. (2015). Accountable care growth in 2014: A look ahead. *Health Affairs Blog.* Retrieved from http://healthaffairs.org/blog/2014/01/29/accountable-care-growth-in-2014-a-look-ahead

Najt, P., Fusar-Poli, P., & Brambilla, P. (2011). Co-occurring mental and substance abuse disorders: A review of the potential predictors and clinical outcomes. *Psychiatry Research, 186,* 159–164.

National Alliance on Mental Illness. (2011). State mental health cuts: A national crisis. Retrieved from https://www.nami.org/getattachment/About-NAMI/Publications/Reports/NAMIState BudgetCrisis2011.pdf

National Association of State Mental Health Program Directors. (2012). Proceedings on the state budget crisis and the behavioral health treatment gap: The impact on public substance abuse and mental health treatment systems. Retrieved from https://www.nasmhpd.org/sites/default/files/SummaryCongressional%20Briefing_2012(6).pdf

National Institute of Mental Health. (2015). Major depression among adults. Retrieved from https://www.nimh.nih.gov/health/statistics/prevalence/major-depression-among-adults.shtml

National Organization of Nurse Practitioner Faculties. (2013). Population focused nurse practitioner competencies: Psychiatric-mental health nurse practitioner competencies. Retrieved from http://www.nonpf.org/associations/10789/files/PopulationFocusNPComps2013.pdf

National Organization of Nurse Practitioner Faculties. (2017). Nurse practitioner core competencies. Retrieved from http://c.ymcdn.com/sites/www.nonpf.org/resource/resmgr/competencies/2017_NPCoreComps_with_Curric.pdf

Naylor, M. D., & Kurtzman, E. T. (2010). The role of nurse practitioners in reinventing primary care. *Health Affairs, 29*(5), 893–899.

Newhouse, R. P., Stanik-Hutt, J., White, K. M., Johantgen, M., Bass, E. B., Zangaro, G., . . . Weiner, J. P. (2011). Advanced practice nurse outcomes 1990–2008: A systematic review. *Nursing Economics, 29*(5), CNE series, 1–21.

Newhouse, R. P., Weiner, J. P., Stanik-Hutt, J., White, K. M., Johantgen, M., Steinwachs, D., . . . Bass, E. B. (2012). Policy implications for optimizing advanced practice registered nurse use nationally. *Policy, Politics, & Nursing Practice, 13*, 81–89.

Nielsen, M., Gibson, L., Buelt, L., Grundy, P., & Grumbach, K. (2015). The patient-centered medical home's impact on cost and quality: Annual review of evidence, 2013–2014. Retrieved from https://www.pcpcc.org/resource/patient-centered-medical-homes-impact-cost-and-quality-annual-review-evidence-2013-2014

Onie, R., Farmer, P., & Behforouz, H. (2012). Realigning health with care. *Stanford Social Innovation Review, 10*, 28–35. Retrieved from http://www.ssireview.org/articles/entry/realigning_health_with_care

Osborn, R., Squires, D., Doty, M. M., Sarnak, D. O., & Schneider, E. C. (2016). In new survey of eleven countries, US adults still struggle with access to and affordability of health care. *Health Affairs, 10*, 1377.

Parekh, A. K., Goodman, R. A., Gordon, C., & Koh, H. K. (2011). Managing multiple chronic conditions: A strategic framework for improving health outcomes and quality of life. *Public Health Reports, 126*, 468–471.

Pearson, G. S., Hines-Martin, V. P., Evans, L. K., York, J. A., Kane, C. F., & Yearwood, E. L. (2015). Addressing gaps in mental health needs of diverse, at-risk, underserved, and disenfranchised populations: A call for nursing action. *Archives of Psychiatric Nursing, 29*(1), 14–18.

Pelletier, L. R., & Stichler, J. F. (2013). Action brief: Patient engagement and activation: A health reform imperative and improvement opportunity for nursing. *Nursing Outlook, 61*, 51–54.

Poghosyan, L., Lucero, R., Rauch, L., & Berkowitz, B. (2012). Nurse practitioner workforce: A substantial supply of primary care providers. *Nursing Economic$, 30*, 268–274, 294.

Porter, M. E. (2010). What is value in health care? *New England Journal of Medicine, 363*(26), 2477–2481.

Ryan, A. M. (2013). Will value-based purchasing increase disparities in care? *New England Journal of Medicine, 369*(26), 2472–2474.

Safriet, B. (2011). Federal options for maximizing the value of advanced practice nurses in providing quality, cost-effective health care. In Committee on the Robert Wood Johnson Foundation Initiative on the Future of Nursing, at the Institute of Medicine (Ed.), *The future of nursing: Leading change, advancing health* (pp. 443–476). Washington, DC: National Academies Press. Retrieved from https://www.nap.edu/read/12956/chapter/20

SAMHSA-HRSA Center for Integrated Health Care Solutions. (2012). Behavioral health homes for people with mental health & substance use conditions: The core clinical features. Retrieved from http://www.integration.samhsa.gov/clinical-practice/CIHS_Health_Homes_Core_Clinical_Features.pdf

SAMHSA-HRSA Center for Integrated Health Solutions. (2014). Core competencies for integrated behavioral health and primary care. Retrieved from http://www.integration.samhsa.gov/workforce/Integration_Competencies_Final.pdf

Salzberg, C. A., Hayes, S. L., McCarthy, D., Radley, D. C., Abrams, M. K., Shah, T., & Anderson, G. F. (2016). Health system performance for the high-need patient: A look at access to care and patient care experiences. *Issue Brief (Commonwealth Fund), 27*, 1.

Saxe, G. N., Heidi-Ellis, B., Fogler, J., & Navalta, C. P. (2012). Innovations in practice: Preliminary evidence for effective family engagement in treatment for child traumatic stress–trauma systems therapy approach to preventing dropout. *Child and Adolescent Mental Health, 17*(1), 58–61.

Scharf, D. M., Eberhart, N. K., Schmidt, N., Horvitz-Lennon, M., Beckman, R., Han, B., . . . Burnam, M. A. (2014). Improving the physical health of adults with serious mental illness. Retrieved from http://www.rand.org/pubs/research_briefs/RB9789.html

Scott, K. M., Von Korff, M., Alonso, J., Angermeyer, M. C., Bromet, E., Fayyad, J., . . . Williams, D. (2009). Mental–physical co-morbidity and its relationship with disability: Results from the world mental health surveys. *Psychological Medicine, 39*, 33–43.

Shane, D. M., Nguyen-Hoang, P., Bentler, S. E., Damiano, P. C., & Momany, E. T. (2016). Medicaid health home reducing costs and reliance on emergency department: Evidence from Iowa. *Medical Care, 54*, 752–758.

Smolowitz, J., Speakman, E., Wojnar, D., Whelan, E. M., Ulrich, S., Hayes, C., & Wood, L. (2015). Role of the registered nurse in primary health care: Meeting health care needs in the 21st century. *Nursing Outlook, 63*, 130–136. doi:10.1016/j.outlook.2014.08.004

Soni, A. (2015). Top five most costly conditions among adults age 18 and older, 2012: Estimates for the U.S. civilian noninstitutionalized adult population. *Statistical Brief #471*. Rockville, MD: Agency for Healthcare Research and Quality. Retrieved from http://www.meps.ahrq.gov/mepsweb/data_files/publications/st471/stat471.shtml

Spandler, H., & Stickley, T. (2011). No hope without compassion: The importance of compassion in recovery-focused mental health services. *Journal of Mental Health, 20*(6), 555–566.

Staff Care. (2015). Behavioral health: "The silent shortage". Retrieved from http://www.staffcare.com/uploadedFiles/StaffCare/Content/Resources/Blogs/white-paper-behavioral-health-silent-shortage.pdf

Stanhope, V., & Henwood, B. F. (2014). Activating people to address their health care needs: Learning from people with lived experience of chronic illnesses. *Community Mental Health Journal, 50*(6), 656–663.

Stanley, J. M., Werner, K. E., & Apple, K. (2009). Positioning advanced practice registered nurses for health care reform: Consensus on APRN regulation. *Journal of Professional Nursing, 25*(6), 340–348.

Substance Abuse and Mental Health Services Administration. (2011). National consensus statement on mental health recovery. Retrieved from https://store.samhsa.gov/shin/content//SMA05-4129/SMA05-4129.pdf

Substance Abuse and Mental Health Services Administration. (2013). *Behavioral health barometer: United States, 2013*. HHS Publication No. SMA-13-4796. Rockville, MD: Author.

Substance Abuse and Mental Health Services Administration. (2015). Receipt of services for behavioral health problems: Results from the 2014 national survey on drug use and health. Retrieved from https://www.samhsa.gov/data/sites/default/files/NSDUH-DR-FRR3-2014/NSDUH-DR-FRR3-2014/NSDUH-DR-FRR3-2014.htm

Stiefel, M., & Nolan, K. (2013). Measuring the triple aim: A call for action. *Population Health Management, 16*, 219–220. doi:10.1089/pop.2013.0025

Stoto, M. A. (2013). Population health in the Affordable Care Act era. Retrieved from http://www.academyhealth.org/files/publications/files/AH2013pophealth.pdf

Tai-Seale, M., Foo, P. K., & Stults, C. D. (2013). Patients with mental health needs are engaged in asking questions, but physicians' responses vary. *Health Affairs, 32*, 259–267.

Torrey, E. F., Zdanowicz, M. T., Kennard, A. D., Lamb, H. R., Eslinger, D. F., Biasotti, M. C., & Fuller, D. A. (2014). The treatment of persons with mental illness in prisons and jails: A state survey. *Treatment Advocacy Center*. Retrieved from http://www.treatmentadvocacycenter.org/storage/documents/treatment-behind-bars/treatment-behind-bars.pdf

U.S. Department of Health and Human Services. (2011). HHS launches new initiative to strengthen primary care. Retrieved from http://www.maineafp.org/docs/PCMH/HHS-launches-new-Affordable-Care-Act-Initiative-to-Strengthen-Primary-Care.pdf

U.S. Department of Health and Human Services. (2012). 2012 annual progress report to congress: National strategy for quality improvement in health care. Retrieved from https://www.ahrq.gov/workingforquality/reports/2012-annual-report.html

U.S. Department of Health and Human Services. (2016). HHS fact sheet: Delivery system reform: Progress and the future. Retrieved from https://wayback.archive-it.org/3926/20170127192819/https://www.hhs.gov/about/news/2016/10/25/hhs-fact-sheet-delivery-system-reform-progress-and-future.html

U.S. Department of Housing and Urban Development. (2016). The 2016 annual homeless assessment report (AHAR) to congress. Retrieved from https://www.hudexchange.info/resources/documents/2016-AHAR-Part-1.pdf

VanLare, J. M., & Conway, P. H. (2012). Value-based purchasing—National programs to move from volume to value. *New England Journal of Medicine, 367*(4), 292–295.

van der Feltz-Cornelis, C. M., Van Os, T. W., Van Marwijk, H. W., & Leentjens, A. F. (2010). Effect of psychiatric consultation models in primary care: A systematic review and meta-analysis of randomized clinical trials. *Journal of Psychosomatic Research, 68*(6), 521–533.

Weinstein, L. C., Henwood, B. F., Cody, J. W., Jordan, M., & Lelar, R. (2011). Transforming assertive community treatment into an integrated care system: The role of nursing and primary care partnerships. *Journal of the American Psychiatric Nurses Association, 17,* 64–71.

Wen, H., Druss, B. G., & Cummings, J. R. (2015). Effect of medicaid expansions on health insurance coverage and access to care among low-income adults with behavioral health conditions. *Health Services Research, 50*(6), 1787–1809.

Witgert, K., & Hess, C. (2012). Including safety-net providers in integrated delivery systems: Issues and options for policymakers. *Commonwealth Fund, Issues Brief.* Retrieved from http://www.common wealthfund.org/publications/issue-briefs/2012/aug/including-safety-net-providers

Woltmann, E., Grogan-Kaylor, A., Perron, B., Georges, H., Kilbourne, A. M., & Bauer, M. S. (2012). Comparative effectiveness of collaborative chronic care models for mental health conditions across primary, specialty, and behavioral health care settings: Systematic review and meta-analysis. *American Journal of Psychiatry, 169,* 790–804.

CHAPTER 16

The Aging Population

Evelyn Duffy

Older adults represent a segment of the population that has the greatest dependence on government policies, whether they are national, state, or local. Advanced Practice Registered Nurses (APRNs) who care for this population need to understand the impact policy has on the health care and the daily lives of their older patients. These policies also impact the practice of APRNs and may erect barriers that prevent the provision of the quality of care they have the skills and training to give. In this chapter demographics of this population, a review of key legislation, and discussion of strategies to take advantage of opportunities to participate in the policy process will be presented.

Adults older than the age of 65 comprised 15% of the population of the United States in 2014, and they account for a disproportionate percentage of health care expenditure—34% in 2010, which was 2.6 times the national average and one-third of all U.S. medical spending (De Nardi, French, Jones, & McCauley, 2015; Mather, Jacobson, & Pollord, 2015; Meltack & Noel-Miller, 2012). The majority of these health care dollars, 65%, comes from government programs, Medicare, or Medicaid. Control of these dollars is in the hands of the politicians at the national and state levels. APRNs caring for older adults owe it to their patients to be active participants in the political process that not only directly affects their patients' care, but also can erect barriers to APRN's ability to practice to the full extent of their expertise and preparation. Understanding the government programs on which their patients depend is a key to participation in the process.

The median age of the population, not only in the United States but worldwide, is increasing. This trend has been referred to as the Silver Tsunami, Aging Wave, Graying of America. This is the result of a decline in the birthrate, an increase in average life expectancy, and the Baby Boom generation reaching the age of retirement. The average age of older adults is also increasing, the over-85 age group is the fastest growing segment of the U.S. population. These growing numbers will increase demands for medical care and social services and increase the need for caregiving and expenditure of health care dollars. This reality is putting a strain on national and state budgets, and legislators are concerned about finding ways to continue to provide these services.

MEDICARE AND MEDICAID

In 1965, two of the most significant changes to the Social Security Act of 1935 occurred when on July 30th President Lyndon Johnson signed into law amendments Title XVIII and Title XIX establishing Medicare and Medicaid (Klees, Wolfe, & Curtis, 2009). Almost 96% of adults older than the age of 65 have Medicare coverage. However, Medicare is not just for older adults; those with permanent disability also qualify for Medicare benefits and represent approximately 17% of the total Medicare population. Medicare covers the health care costs of some of the United States' sickest individuals. Medicaid is a program for low-income individuals that is jointly administered by the federal and state governments using a system of cost sharing. Twenty-one percent of Medicare recipients are also receiving Medicaid.

The Medicare program initially included two parts: Part A, which is coverage for hospitalization and provided to everyone, and Part B, Medical coverage, which was offered as an option and requires an additional premium. The Balanced Budget Act of 1997 added an option for a managed care plan, Part C, known as Medicare + Choice, now labeled the Medicare Advantage Plans. The Medicare Prescription Drug, Improvement, and Modernization Act of 2003 added coverage for outpatient medications. Further modifications were made as a result of the passage of the Patient Protection and Affordable Care Act of 2010 (ACA). The ACA includes Nurse Practitioners (NPs) and Clinical Nurse Specialists (CNSs) as primary care practitioners and contains extensive provider-neutral language that may serve to support the removal of restrictions on scope of practice. The future of the ACA is in question, and APRNs need to stay engaged and be carefully observing the changes and replacements to assure that the advantages gained will not be lost. Changes to the ACA could open up opportunities to remove existing barriers to full practice.

SOCIAL SECURITY

APRNs have sometimes been accused of advocating only for issues that affect their practice, but the very nature of the biopsychosocial model of nursing means they understand that managing chronic illness and the conditions associated with aging requires a complex set of skills and continuous management, which is an integral part of APRN education. Having health care covered by Medicare and Medicaid is a key to the health of older adults, but there are other social determinants of health that require adequate resources. The original Social Security Act brought about some of the greatest improvements in the life of adults older than the age of 65. The Social Security Act resulted in part from the social changes occurring at the beginning of the 20th century. Industrialization resulted in a transition from a society predominated by family farms and extended families that provided a safety net to older adults, to an urban society with nuclear families leaving older adults to manage on their own. After the Great Depression in 1934 it was estimated that over half of older adults were unable to support themselves.

The Social Security Act of 1935 was House Resolution 7760 and contained benefits for older adults as well as provisions for unemployment compensation, aid to dependent children, maternal and child welfare, crippled children, the blind, and vocational rehabilitation. The implementation of this act saw a rapid improvement in the welfare of older adults (O'Brien, Wu, & Baer, 2010). By 1968 the number of older adults living in poverty had decreased to 25% and further decreased to 14% in 1978 and in 2013 the official poverty rate of adults older than 65 was 10%. Poverty is not equal among all demographic groups. Women, especially those older than the age of 80, are almost twice as likely as men to live in poverty. Regarding race and ethnicity, Hispanics have the highest poverty rate, 20%, followed by Blacks, 18%, and Whites, 7%. Poverty impacts health and perception of health. Those living in poverty are more likely to describe their health as fair/poor than excellent/very good/good (Cubanski, Casillas, & Damico, 2015).

THE OLDER AMERICANS ACT

The Older Americans Act (OAA) is another important piece of legislation that impacts adults over the age of 60. It was passed in 1965, the same year as the Medicare Amendments to Social Security. It provides essential programs for many older adults living in the community. A goal of the law is to support the dignity of older adults by facilitating their engagement in the community. The programs of the OAA can help older adults avoid hospitalization and nursing home placement.

The original law established the Federal Agency on Aging, which is now part of the Administration for Community Living, a branch of the Department of Health and Human Services. In April 2016, the OAA Reauthorization Act was signed into law. Previous reauthorization expired in 2011 and it took 5 years of negotiation to develop the current version of the law. The OAA supplies money to the states to administer programs that provide services such as home delivered meals, community nutrition services, in-home services, transportation, legal services, elder abuse prevention, and caregiver support. These programs are administered through 56 state agencies on aging, 629 area agencies on aging, nearly 20,000 service providers, 244 tribal organizations, and 2 Native Hawaiian organizations representing 400 tribes. While the OAA was reauthorized, it was funded under a continuing resolution until April 2017. When Congress is unable to pass a federal budget, continuing resolutions are a means of keeping the government running. They often offer a modest increase in spending across the board. The continuing resolution will temporarily stall some attacks on the OAA programs. For example, the Senate version of the 2017 budget would have eliminated funding for State Health Insurance Assistance Program or SHIP, a program to help older adults on Medicare determine which of the plan options is most cost effective while still meeting their health care needs. SHIP helped older adults on Medicare save millions of dollars. Each time the federal budget is being developed APRNs have an opportunity to speak on behalf of their patients and provide examples of the benefits their patients receive from the programs funded by the OAA, as well as the risks to these patients if these supports are eliminated.

BARRIERS TO APRN PRACTICE CARING FOR OLDER ADULTS

As a result of the ACA there has been an increase of insured across the life span that has put a strain on the primary care system. APRNs offer a solution to this increased demand, they have proven ability to provide services in homes, community health centers, nurse-managed clinics, and other traditional and non-traditional settings and can address the unmet need for primary care, disease management, and care coordination (www.rwjf.org/newsroom, 2011). Access, however, can only increase if there is modernization of the regulations and administrative mandates that limit their scope of practice and thus impact their availability or how they function in various settings of care. While individual advocacy is the key to change and removal of barriers, monitoring the barrage of laws introduced in legislatures and the rules that guide the implementation of the laws requires the assistance of policy professionals. Involvement in professional organizations is essential so that APRNs who care for older adults can receive timely alerts to the need for activation in response to laws or rules. One advocacy group, the APRN Workgroup, includes policy advocates from 14 organizations that represent APRNs. The group created a document with a listing of barriers to practice that is updated and reviewed at each monthly meeting. It can be utilized as talking points when meeting with legislators, and connection with your professional organization is one way to get more details about that document. Many of these barriers result from the fact that the Medicare and Medicaid amendments of 1965 occurred before the advent of CNSs or NPs. While Certified Nurse Anesthetists have been credentialed since 1956, the first NP program was introduced in 1965 and CNSs were first recognized by the American Nurses Association in 1976. Language in the Medicare and Medicaid amendments often specified "physician" and this terminology has resulted in barriers to the full practice authority of APRNs.

The barrier's document specifies multiple examples of the need to eliminate costly and unnecessary supervision requirements. Examples that particularly affect the care of older adults include the requirement for physician certification of APRNs ordering home health and hospice and oversight of the care of patients receiving these services. Another example is the requirement that physicians conduct the admission physical for patients in skilled nursing facilities. A fix to this problem was introduced by a previous Physician Fee Schedule and allowed an APRN to bill for a medically necessary visit prior to the admission physical. APRNs that provide care to patients in skilled nursing facilities often have to see patients for some medical crisis before the physician does the admitting exam and while previously they could not charge for these visits the rule change now allows it. Another barrier is the requirement that a physician perform every other regulatory visit in long-term care (not skilled care). This requirement, along with the regulation that precludes APRNs from being designated as the primary care provider in long-term care facilities prevents an APRN from practicing independently even in states that would allow that. These role impediments restrict access to patients and may well inhibit a wellness, quality of life approach for a very vulnerable group of older adults that would benefit from that type of care model. An important document for all APRNs to be aware of is the Federal Trade Commission's Policy Perspectives: Competition and the Regulation of Advanced Practice Nurses, accessible at www.ftc.gov/system/files/documents/reports/policy-perspectives-competition-regulation-advanced-practice-nurses/140307APRNpolicypaper.pdf.

Amendments to resolve the barrier to APRNs providing certification and oversight of home health care have been introduced in both the Senate and the House since at least June 2007. While always acquiring good bipartisan support, they have never made it to the floor of either chamber for a vote. For APRNs who care for older adults understanding how laws are applied and interpreted can mean the difference of being able to practice to the greatest benefit to their patients. One obstacle to these laws being brought to a vote by Congress is the lack of a cost estimate by the Congressional Budget Office (CBO). When a bill has been introduced into committee, members of the committee have to put a dollar figure on the bill. They rely on what is referred to as a CBO score. Recently Congress had to demonstrate that any new bill would be budget neutral. If it cost money they would have to show where the money would come from. On the other hand, if it saved money it could be highly desirable to offset some other expenditure. Without data to demonstrate the ways that APRNs currently manage to facilitate home health care for their patients, Congress assumes that opening up the option for more providers to certify for home health care would increase costs. APRNs need to document the cost savings that would be realized if they were not required to find physicians to attest to their face-to-face visits and to sign the forms for certification and recertification. They also need to share their stories of patients that have suffered as a result of the delay of services because of the delay in acquiring the physician signature. Independent assessment of the cost of passing the home health bills indicates millions of dollars of savings, but to date there has not been an official CBO score.

Many APRNs are the initial provider of care for patients in skilled nursing facilities. While they are not eligible to bill for the admitting exam, they often are the ones getting the history and performing a physical in order to assure that the proper care is provided in the period before the physician arrives to document the "Official Admission Exam," which may be primarily based on the work of the APRN. The reimbursement for this admission visit by the physician is paid at a higher level than that for the reimbursement of the APRN, who in reality does the exam and can only bill at a follow-up visit rate. APRNs need to continue to work to be recognized and reimbursed for the work that they do.

APRNs need to help legislators understand the reality of these and other situations where their work is not acknowledged because of the administrative requirements of outdated laws. APRNs are capable of providing safe, effective care to those with acute and chronic conditions. They are better at communicating with patients about self-managing their conditions, offering advice, providing screenings, counseling, and ensuring follow-up care (Naylor & Kurtzman, 2010). Duplication of the work that occurs in the skilled nursing facility and delays in care that may result because of the home health restrictions are not cost effective or patient centered.

Other key issues affecting the care of older adults include the never events that affect reimbursement for care resulting from those events, the 30-day readmission rule, the repeal of the sustainable growth rate, the initiation of the Medicare Access and CHIP Reauthorization Act (MACRA) which changes reimbursement from pay-for-service to pay-for-outcomes, the requirement for electronic medical records, the privatization of Medicare as more of the implementation of the program is provided by private insurance with capitated programs through the Medicare Advantage Part C programs, and the dual eligible demonstration where older adults on Medicare and Medicaid are assigned to managed care programs with private insurance companies. Managed care plans vary widely. Capitated programs receive a set amount of money whether they need it to provide care or not. Because these companies are in the business of making money they need to balance what they offer with what they will not include. For example, it may be more cost effective to offer hearing aids than to cover an expensive new-generation pharmaceutical therapy.

Dual eligible patients may decide to keep traditional Medicare while choosing a provider for their Medicaid benefit. However, in many of the states that are participating in the demonstration projects, dual eligible older adults have been assigned to a plan that subsumed their traditional Medicare and have not been well-informed about their ability to "opt out" and either keep their traditional Medicare or choose a different plan that may meet their personal needs. For example, the managed care plan may offer benefits that exceed traditional Medicare, but not cover items that traditional Medicare would cover such as electric wheelchairs. Few APRNs have an available social worker to help their patients sort through this confusing change in their health insurance; the burden falls on the APRNs to be aware of what is possible to best meet the needs of their patients.

PHYSICIAN FEE SCHEDULE

When the barriers to practice are in statute, they require an amendment so the law can be changed or modified. There are also rules that guide the practice of APRNs, and some of these are the result of the yearly Physician Fee Schedule. The Physician Fee Schedule was introduced in 1992 and provides information about what will be reimbursed by Medicare and at what rate. The Physician Fee Schedule is posted in the Federal Register for public comment. The 2017 fee schedule included 393 pages; the expertise of APRN advocacy groups that closely watch these yearly guidelines is invaluable. Professional organizations may mobilize their membership to submit comments on the Federal Register if there are specific concerns. The details of the fee schedule can result in barriers to practice simply because of a carelessly inserted term, but they can also result in the removal of barriers to practice. A recent example was a rule that required portable x-rays ordered by a physician, podiatrist, or dentist to have the service covered by Medicare. The intention of the rule was to prevent portable x-ray companies from performing services that may have been ordered by the nurse on duty rather than the provider. Because this was a rule and not in law, a subsequent year Physician Fee Schedule was able to clarify that eligible providers within their scope of practice could order portable x-rays and the company would be eligible to be paid for that service. Whether at the national or state level when advocating for changes in the law, keeping them more generalized and leaving the specifics to the rules written later can be a real advantage when the environment in health care changes.

MEDICARE PAYMENT ADVISORY COMMISSION

MedPAC is a nonpartisan committee that provides Congress with analysis and policy advice on Medicare. Details regarding their comments and the dates of their public meetings as well as their membership are available on their website, medpac.gov. The committee includes 17 members that serve 3-year staggered terms, appointed by the Comptroller General. The current commission includes one registered nurse, but not an APRN. Professional organizations can recommend candidates for these positions and suggestions may be sought from their membership. Commissioners have reached out to APRN advocacy groups and leadership seeking help to understand the APRN perspective on issues regarding the barriers to the care they provide to older adults that result from Medicare policy. When APRNs share their stories about these barriers it helps to paint a more comprehensive picture of their patients' experience. The presence of an APRN on the MedPAC committee could make a difference in the advice this committee offers Congress and key leaders involved in policy, so APRNs should be alert to opportunities to be nominated to serve. Nominations have been submitted, but to date an APRN who was submitted has not been selected to serve.

NEW PAYMENT MODELS, NEW OPPORTUNITIES

There is a major change in reimbursement strategy that was brought about by the "permanent doc fix" to the Medicare sustainable growth rate (SGR). Now in addition to fee-for-service reimbursement, increases will be based on outcomes. The growing number of older adults eligible for Medicare combined with increasing costs of care created an urgent need to find a way to contain costs (De Nardi, French, Jones, & McCauley, 2015). The SGR was an attempt to decrease Medicare costs that resulted from the Balanced Budget Act of 1997. The SGR linked Medicare expenditure per patient to the growth in the gross domestic product (GDP). If the total expenditures for the year exceeded the projected expenditures there was a conversion factor that would result in decrease in the payments to providers for the next year. The recommended change in payment as a result of this conversion factor was almost always unacceptable so it would be adjusted by Congress with what was referred to as the "doc fix." Almost from the beginning Congress worked to find ways to repeal the legislation, and finally in 2015 a permanent fix was implemented with the passage of the Medicare Access and Children's Health Insurance Plan (CHIP) Reauthorization Act of 2015 (MACRA). This legislation created the Quality Payment Program (QPP) for care under Medicare Part B with two new payment strategies: Merit-Based Incentive Payment System (MIPS) and Advanced Alternative Payment Models (APMs). Practices that participate in APMs are assuming more risk but at a greater reward. These new payment models have their roots in the Physician Quality Reporting System (PQRS), the Electronic Health Record Incentive Program (Meaningful use), and the bundled payment programs such as the accountable care organizations (ACOs) and Bundled Payment for Care Initiative (BPCI) that began in 2007. Participation in these early programs was voluntary, but it will be difficult to avoid participation in the new QPPs. APRNs are eligible for the MIPS program, but to be included they must be in an APM or bill Medicare for $30,000 a year and care for more than 100 Medicare patients a year. MIPS creates four new categories of measurement: quality, resource use, advancing care information, and improvement activities. The program's initial reporting period may begin any time between January 1, 2017 and October 2, 2017 and those results will be reflected in payments in 2019. For providers who are eligible for MIPS but do not submit any data in 2017 their payment will be reduced by 4% in 2019; those who sign up early are eligible for greater reward. The Centers for Medicare and Medicaid Services (CMS) offer resources to understand this new system with detailed information on their website, qpp.cms.gov. Vigilance on the part of APRNs will be necessary to assure that incentives are distributed appropriately and that they are involved in decision making as changes and expansion of the program are inevitable in the years ahead. MACRA is a separate piece of legislation that resulted from historic bipartisan support; it is not an amendment to the ACA and although changes may occur it is unlikely to be a victim of the proposed repeal of the ACA.

Another new opportunity for increased revenue was made available to primary care providers including APRNs who care for complex patients with multiple chronic conditions. Since 2015 Medicare has paid for chronic care management (CCM) separately under the Physician Fee Schedule using CPT codes 99490 or 99487 and 99489, when that care meets specific guidelines. These codes assume that the provider spends at least 15 minutes a month caring for the patient, but it allows the provider to bill for the work of others that they oversee. For example, the CCM code 99490 would be used when at least 20 minutes of clinical staff time in a month is required to implement a comprehensive plan of care. The complex CCM codes include 99487, which requires greater medical complexity and at least 60 minutes of clinical staff time a month, and 99489, which can be used for each additional 30 minutes of staff time required to implement the plan. These codes can help APRNs capture the time it takes to communicate with clinical staff and provide oversight and coordination of the care of this special patient population. There are extensive guidelines and considerations which are addressed in detail on the CMS website www.cms.gov/ Outreach-and-Education/Medicare-Learning-Network-MLN/MLNProducts/ Downloads/ChronicCareManagement.pdf. The decision to reimburse for these codes was addressed in the 2015 Physician Fee Schedule. Decisions like this require continued monitoring for any proposed changes that may be included in the Fee Schedule and require new constraints that create barriers for APRN practice. When APRNs avoid using available opportunities to demonstrate their skill in providing primary care, they abdicate the ability to document the contribution they make to quality patient-centered care.

CMS demonstration projects may offer APRNs opportunities to participate and contribute to the data that can result in the future of reimbursement. Previous projects resulted in the bundled payments, medical homes, and ACOs. APRNs should be monitoring for additional opportunities to participate in these projects and advocate for inclusion if necessary. Projects include new methods of service delivery, reimbursement for new types of service, and new payment strategies. The data collected as a result of these innovation projects are available to researchers, and existing data offer opportunities for APRN research and analysis. More information about the CMS Innovation Center as well as a full list of current projects and those in individual states is available on their website: innovation.cms.gov/index.html.

THE FUTURE FOR THE AGING POPULATION

For lack of a crystal ball the ability to predict the future of health care and social support programs for our aging population is not feasible. We are ushering in a new administration with agendas that are certain to shake up the current environment. How this administration will respond to the needs of the adults who depend on government programs is not at all clear. Proposals range from privatizing Medicare to keeping it as is. The age of eligibility for full social security has already increased and will continue to increase in the future. There is an income ceiling for Social Security taxes, which is $127,200 in 2017, at which point taxes are no longer deducted for payment into the system. If the ceiling were eliminated there would be an increase in the amount collected each year as higher earners would still have the tax withheld from all of their income. This ceiling does not apply to the Medicare tax. The ceiling for Social Security deductions exists in part because there is a maximum monthly retirement benefit which depends on previous contributions and age at retirement. For 2017 that amount is $2,687 a month. Medicare benefits are not modified due to income. When privatization of Medicare is discussed it is important to evaluate the privatization that is already in place in the Medicare Advantage Plans and the dual-eligible demonstration projects. In 2016, 31% of Medicare recipients were enrolled in Medicare Advantage Plans. Those recipients forgo their traditional Medicare for additional benefits that may be offered by the capitated systems. However, these systems may also omit benefits that are offered by traditional Medicare. A voucher program has been proposed as a way to contain Medicare costs. Seniors would receive a voucher for a specific amount that they could use to pay for traditional Medicare or purchase private insurance. The amount of the voucher would make cost of care predictable, but skeptics are concerned that the voucher amount would not continue to be able to purchase the same quality of care currently offered by Medicare programs. Over time, recipients may have to supplement these vouchers in order to receive the same services or be satisfied with less coverage.

A strategy that has been proposed to contain the costs of Medicaid is the use of block grants. Block grants would be used in the place of the current revenue sharing. Block grants allow states to shift funds to other programs if the demand for a certain program decreases. So if more jobs are created and fewer people are on Medicaid, money that would have been used to pay for that program could be applied to another program. The intent would be to apply to a program that would benefit a similar population, but historically in block grant programs such as the Temporary Assistance for Needy Families (TANF) initiated in 1996, states often used the money to fill other budget holes or to cover existing programs provided by the states. The population the TANF block grants were intended to help did not always realize the benefit.

APRNs should be part of the conversation as future proposals to change the system of coverage for care of older adults evolve. Staying engaged in professional organizations and responding to calls to contact legislators and comment on the Federal Register can make a difference in the future of their care. It cannot be left to the health policy staff. APRNs need to share their clinical experience with policy experts who often lack that clinical knowledge. Considering the unintended consequences of changes and the lessons from the historical use of similar strategies are important in shaping any response. APRNs can share the stories of the effects

---

THE STORIES

Mr. H, an 89-year-old, lives alone in senior subsidized housing. He receives his primary care from a NP. His family assists with his personal care, he receives meals on wheels, and he gets weekly visits from a home health nurse. He has multiple chronic conditions including chronic heart failure, atrial fibrillation, hypertension, and chronic kidney disease. He is on multiple medications, and the home health nurse checks his vital signs, international normalized ratio (INR), reviews his medications, and records his weight. It was time for his recertification for home health care and a physician signature was needed on the form. While the NP was the primary care provider, reviewed and made appropriate changes on the form without a physician signature, the recertification was not complete. The home health agency had recently instated a policy that if the form was not received by the start of the new certification period, they would not continue to provide care. The physician that routinely signed the forms was away on an extended medical leave. Without the signed form, the home health agency cancelled the service. This story would have a very sad ending had the nurse that provided the gentleman care for several years not made an unpaid visit when she saw it had been 2 weeks since he was on her regular schedule, because she knew how vulnerable he was. She found him ill, with a supratherapeutic INR, a 10-pound weight gain, and a pulse oximetry reading of 88%. A call to the primary care NP resulted in his transfer to the emergency department and subsequent admission to the hospital. He was treated for an acute exacerbation of his failure and had a complete recovery. Had the NP been able to sign the form recertifying for home health, the patient could have received the visit on the usual schedule and the decompensation may have been avoided. This story is probably repeated regularly across the country because of delays in care as APRNs seek physician signatures for the certification and recertification forms for their patients.

---

policies have had on their patients' health and well-being. These stories can personalize a discussion that is otherwise based on ideology and theory.

CMS Innovation projects need involvement of APRNs to help illustrate the contribution that they make to the health and well-being of their patients. The Care Transitions Program launched in 2012 was funded by the ACA for 5 years. Programs such as these respond to the needs of individuals such as Mr. N, who is an 82-year-old living in an apartment with his wife. He has a history of peripheral vascular disease with a left below-knee amputation, chronic obstructive pulmonary disease, and diabetes. Despite having a lower-leg prosthesis, he is nonambulatory and unable to shop, do housekeeping, drive, or use public transportation. He is taking eight medications and has been admitted to several hospitals and long-term care facilities over the past 2 years on multiple occasions for respiratory infections. He has no provider of record and uses the emergency room for acute issues. During his last visit to the emergency room he was seen by an acute care NP who initiated treatment for an upper respiratory infection and referred him to a house call program available through the hospital system. He was seen at his home within 24 hours of discharge and ongoing care was launched. Since then his primary care has been provided on a regular basis by an NP with an expertise in geriatric care, and after 6 months of continuing care he has had no exacerbations and no hospital admissions nor has he had to utilize the emergency room. This patient required much more than medical care. His wife needed caregiver support, they needed increased community services, and the NP helped them to get the Medicare and Medicaid benefits they were entitled to but had not been accessing.

These case examples help bring home the realities of the barriers that APRNs face in providing care to older adults. Not only do the barriers threaten excellent health care, but they also drive up costs. The Triple Aim which has been promoted by the Institute for Healthcare Improvement includes three dimensions: population health, patient experience, and cost of care. Barriers to the practice of APRNs prevent the realization of these goals. Legislators need to hear the stories of patient experience that was compromised because of the barriers to practice. APRNs need to keep it about the patient and speak up about the work they do on a daily basis that provides patient-centered care and saves the system money because it is holistic and appropriate. This applies to all APRNs, but those who care for older adults have an added responsibility because of the dependence their patients have on the government to make the right decisions regarding the laws and rules that touch every aspect of their lives.

Essential V of the Doctor of Nursing Practice essentials addresses health care policy for advocacy in health care (American Association of Colleges of Nursing, 2006). The following questions are intended to assess the accomplishment of this objective.

DISCUSSION QUESTIONS

1. *Describe three ways that current Medicare law limits the practice of APRNs. Provide rationale for why those barriers should be removed. Who would you contact to raise your concerns?*
   a. *Concepts to include*
      - *Certification and recertification of home health care*
      - *Ability to perform and bill for the admitting physical exam in skilled nursing facilities*
      - *Ability to be the PCP and perform the face-to-face for home health, but needing a physician to sign off on all orders and on the face-to-face. How would this be especially burdensome in a full practice authority state?*
      - *The need for a physician to be the PCP of a patient in long-term care and do every other regulatory visit*
   b. *Identify the committees in the House and the Senate that are responsible for Medicare law. Who sits on those committees? If your representative is a member, contact that person with your concerns or contact the chair.*
2. *Explore the history of block grants when used to control costs. Would you or would you not support the use of block grants to fund Medicaid in the future? Provide your rationale. Give some examples of the state decisions with regard to implementation of the ACA to identify strengths or weaknesses of the system. Discuss the use of a surplus of money from a block grant to meet the basic services. How have states dealt with these surpluses?*

ANALYSIS, SYNTHESIS, AND CLINICAL APPLICATION

1. *Review the titles under the Older Americans Act. If you had to distribute a finite amount of money to fund the act where would you put the priorities? What considerations and rationale do you use to set these priorities?*

2. *The Supreme Court struck down the mandatory Medicaid expansion component of ACA and as a result, most states that held a Republican majority in power (Red States) chose not to expand it on principle. Medicaid being a shared federal/state program is not the same everywhere, as traditional Medicare is. Select two states, one with Republican and one with Democratic majorities and compare/contrast the use of Medicaid funds. Which states provide more comprehensive care for the elderly through Medicaid?*

EXERCISES/CONSIDERATIONS

1. *Download the latest version of the Physician Fee Schedule. Go to the Federal Register and review some of the comments. What could you add? (This is usually released for the next year in the spring, if the class is prior to release, look at the current schedule and comments on it even though the period is over.)*
2. *Using the website www.ssa.gov/history/briefhistory3.html, describe the environment in 1935 when the Social Security Act was passed. What were the precursors to the act? Compare and contrast the political environment in 1935 with that of 1965 when the Medicare and Medicaid amendments were added. What were huge social concerns in those two periods? Can you find similarities and differences in those time periods?*
3. *Create an elevator speech to defend your right to certify and recertify for home health care. Include concepts of the Triple Aim and the FTC document. Keep it patient centered.*

REFERENCES

American Association of Colleges of Nursing. (2006). *The essentials of doctoral education for advanced nursing practice.* Washington, DC: Author.

Cubanski, J., Casillas, G., & Damico, A. (2015). Poverty among seniors: An updated analysis of national and state level poverty rates under the official and supplemental poverty measures. *The Kaiser Family Foundation.* Retrieved from http://kff.org/medicare/issue-brief/poverty-among-seniors-an-updated-analysis-of-national-and-state-level-poverty-rates-under-the-official-and-supplemental-poverty-measures

De Nardi, M., French, E., Jones, J. B., & McCauley, J. (2015). Medical spending of the U.S. elderly. National Bureau of Economic Research. Working Paper 21270. Retrieved from http://www.nber.org/papers/w21270

Klees, B. S., Wolfe, C. J., & Curtis, C. A. (2009). Brief summaries of Medicare & Medicaid: Title XVIII and Title XIX of the Social Security Act. Retrieved from https://www.cms.gov/Research-Statistics-Data-and-Systems/Statistics-Trends-and-Reports/MedicareProgramRatesStats/downloads/MedicareMedicaidSummaries2009.pdf

Mather, M., Jacobsen, L., & Pollard, K. M. (2015). Aging in the United States. *Population Bulletin, 70*(2). Retrieved from http://www.prb.org

Meltack, M., & Noel-Miller, C. (2012). Who relies on Medicare? Profile of the Medicare population. Fact Sheet 259. Retrieved from http://www.AARP.org/ppi

Naylor, M. D., & Kurtzman, E. T. (2010). The role of nurse practitioners in reinventing primary care. *Health Affairs, 29*(5), 893–899.

O'Brien, E., Wu, K. B., & Baer, D. (2010). Older Americans in poverty: A snapshot. Retrieved from http://www.AARP.org/ppi

Health Policy Implications for Advanced Practice Registered Nurses Related to End-of-Life Care

Judy Lentz

The process of dying and the ultimate death experience over the past 100 years have changed dramatically (Table 17.1). In the early 20th century, generally deaths followed short-term illnesses such as pneumonia, end-stage cancers, and strokes. In the 21st century, those diseases are either cured or controlled for prolonged periods of time.

In 1900, the average life span was 48.23 years as compared with 78.8 in 2016, more than a century later, and more than 70% who die each year are 65 years old or older (Centers for Disease Control and Prevention [CDC], 2016; Coyle, 2015; Infoplease, 2016; Wei, Anderson, Curtin, & Arias, 2012; West, Cole, Goodkind, & He, 2014). Only 4% of Americans in the early 1900s were older than 65 years of age (Hoefler, 2010). Today, more than 12.8% of Americans are 65 years and older, and this percentage is projected to increase to 19.3% by 2030, more than quadrupling in the past 100 years (CDC, 2014; Jackson et al., 2012). Again, in the early 20th century, the dying trajectory was short term following an acute illness. However, in mid-century, a short 50 years later, circumstances changed. With the advent of antineoplastics, antimicrobial agents, and technological advances, acute illnesses were treatable and life-threatening illnesses could be ameliorated. Many life-threatening acute illnesses became chronic in nature and Americans began to believe most diseases could be cured or at least controlled for long periods. The extended life span in the 21st century has confirmed this belief.

As a result of these advances, illnesses progressed more slowly, treatment options caused more suffering, pain was frequently unrelieved, and the dying process became protracted. Physicians who had taken the Hippocratic Oath sought to prolong life, and family members became death-denying by urging the medical staff to try "one more" approach. Dying with dignity became an unfulfilled wish. In its place, there was isolation, pain, and suffering.

TABLE 17.1 Changes in Death Processes in the Past 100 Years

CRITERIA	1900	2016
Average life expectancy	48.23 years	78.8 years
Place of death	Majority at home	Majority at long-term care facility or home
Family acceptance	Openly discussed	Death-denying society
Expenses paid by	Family	Medicare
Disease trajectory prior to death	Acute—short term	Chronic—long term

Today, more than 2.5 million people die in the United States annually (CDC, 2016). Most of these deaths are caused by heart disease, cancer, cerebrovascular diseases, pulmonary diseases, and renal syndromes. Providing quality end-of-life care is a huge challenge, given the many variations of disease processes, ages, settings, and health care professionals, for those who face these challenges daily.

Assuring palliative care services begin at the time of diagnosis and include hospice care over the final 6 months for every one of the 2.5 million people is the goal of the palliative care health care professionals.

DRIVING FORCES

Changes in the way Americans view end-of-life care have been influenced over the past six decades by a death-denying society, family value changes, financial cost escalations, geography, and political influences. Let us begin with why Americans are a death-denying society. Technology has driven this sociological change. Americans have witnessed an explosion of technology and advanced treatment modalities. With the development of automatic implantable cardiac defibrillators (AICDs), the perfection of transplantation of organs and bone marrow, the advancements in surgical procedures through robotics, as well as the advancement of genomics, Americans believe any disease can be cured and life can be prolonged hopefully indefinitely. Just look at the statistics describing the number of people living well beyond 100 years of age. The centenarian population has grown by 65.8% from 1980 to 2010 especially for females (U.S. News, 2013). As we continue to perfect and advance medical management of diseases, we strengthen this myth of infinite living.

Family value changes are evidenced by egocentricity, belief of the rights of individuals, an educated society, and family advocacy. Again, technological advances through social media, the Internet, global communication, and natural inquisitiveness drive the individual to expect a certain level of medical treatment regardless of cost.

The financial impact of this level of care is driving our country into extreme debt. In 2016, health care in the United States is 17.5% of the gross national product (Centers for Medicare and Medicaid Services [CMS], 2016a; Coyne, Smith, & Lyckholm, 2015). This level of cost is unsustainable. Even within this high percentage and unsustainable cost, end-of-life care in the United States is inferior to other developed countries due to the use of high-technology interventions. For example, more than 40% of those individuals dying of cancer are admitted to intensive care at some point in the final 6 months of their life (Penn Medicine, 2016). The Hospice Medicare Benefits (HMBs) spending in 2013 was approximately 15.1 billion. The average length of stay for these patients was 72.6 days, for an estimated 1.6 million to 1.7 million patients who received hospice care in 2014, which represents only half of Medicare recipients (National Hospice and Palliative Care Organization [NHPCO], 2015). The cost is expected to be double for the same number of people over the next 5 years (Buck, 2011). Extrapolating from this, if all dying Americans received end-of-life care, the costs would quadruple. Ironically, studies have demonstrated that cost savings of nearly $1,700 per admission for live discharges and $5,000 per admission for patients who died can be realized through hospital-based palliative care teams who through advance care planning (ACP) allow the patient to shift the chosen course of care (Morrison et al., 2008). For an average 400-bed hospital, these savings translate to nearly $1.3 million net savings per year.

Where one lives can also influence end-of-life care (Buck, 2011; Giovanni, 2012; Sherman & Cheon, 2012). For example, statistics of those dying in hospitals in rural areas of the western and northwestern states were lower as compared with southern and eastern states, where large urban medical centers were easily accessible (Giovanni, 2012; Sherman & Cheon, 2012).

The political environment has also negatively influenced end-of-life care in the United States. Understandably, as legislators and their aides are representatives of the death-denying society in which they live, they are naturally influenced by their constituencies. When the 2010 Patient Protection and Affordable Care Act (ACA) recommended reimbursement for ACP, adversaries interpreted this recommendation as rationing care and the language was removed from the final document (Coyne et al., 2015; Giovanni, 2012; Zeytinoglu, 2011). The positive impact on quality of end-of-life care is directly dependent on having the conversations with the patient, the family, and the legislators who create laws that determine the right to have life-saving or ending treatment. Removing the incentives to do so negatively impacts the outcomes of care—physically, psychosocially, and economically. Paying for conversations is just one of many changes needed, and fortunately with the outcry from the palliative care community, legislative changes allowed for end-of-life conversations reimbursement beginning in January, 2016 (Lowes, 2016). Ironically, according to a survey of more than 700 physicians in 2016, only 14% have actually billed Medicare for having the conversation. Seventy-five percent of respondents believe having end-of-life conversations is their responsibility, but less than one-third of them acknowledged receiving any formal training (Kaiser Health News, 2016; Ostrov, 2016). This is a perfect example of the value of the Advanced Practice Registered Nurse (APRN) being able to have the conversations when physicians are unable to do so.

NEED FOR POLICY CHANGES IN END-OF-LIFE CARE

Although there has been extensive political debate about end-of-life care, the number of policy changes has been negligible. According to the *Approaching Death: Improving Care at the End-of-Life* report written by a panel from the Institutes of Medicine in 2007, "people have come both to fear a technologically over-treated and protracted death and to dread the prospect of abandonment and untreated physical and emotional distress" (Zeytinoglu, 2011). A recent report by the Kaiser Health News indicated overtreatment occurs in the elderly in five areas: Two areas are breast and prostate screenings and three additional areas occur in end-of-life care: hospice referrals, feeding tubes, and intensive care stays that occur in contrast to patient preferences (Kaiser Health News, 2016).

Several studies have suggested that patients and families believe end-of-life care is inadequate (Center to Advance Palliative Care [CAPC], 2015; Giovanni, 2012; Hoefler, 2010; Jackson et al., 2012; Sherman & Cheon, 2012). Access alone is a major problem. Millions of Americans are denied palliative care services because none are available where they live even though we have experienced tremendous growth in the number of programs over the past decade. According to the 2008 CAPC Report Card published in 2015, 90% of large hospitals with 300 or more beds have a palliative care team (CAPC, 2015). Palliative care is most prevalent in New England and lowest in the east, south, and central states (CAPC, 2015). The overall grade for palliative care across the nation improved from a C in 2008 to a B in 2011 and has remained at this level (CAPC, 2015). No states received failing grades in the most recent report card and 17 states received an A grade (CAPC, 2015).

Just as in the 1980s when legislators saw the opportunity to improve quality and to reduce the cost of care at end of life by establishing the Medicare Hospice Benefit, we once again saw the opportunity to advance palliative care nationally through policy change. What those changes should be is a national debate that continues currently.

Studies continue to show that treatments fail to align with patient wishes (Giovanni, 2012; Jackson et al., 2012; Morrison et al., 2008). Having conversations with patients and family members when serious illnesses have been detected provides the insight to what the patient/family preferences are, allows the burden of decision making for the family to be decreased, and assures the treatments to match the patient's wishes. Although these conversations are difficult for the generalist, experienced palliative care professionals are experts and can make all the difference in achieving quality of dying and death in end-of-life care (Boucher et al., 2010; Kaiser Health News, 2016; Ostrov, 2016).

HISTORY

In the early 1960s, as Dr. Elisabeth Kübler-Ross was beginning her teaching career at the University of Colorado Medical School, she was distressed to find nothing in the medical school curricula regarding how to care for the dying. In an effort to introduce medical students to the needs and concerns of the dying patient, she invited a young 16-year-old girl with leukemia to come to her lecture. Dr. Kübler-Ross encouraged the students to ask the young girl anything they would like. Their questions were directed only to her medical condition. The young girl became angry and began talking about what mattered most to her— like what it would be like to never get married or have children or even attend her senior prom. This encounter led Kübler-Ross to extensively study and publish research regarding the responses of those who were experiencing the dying process (Biography.com, 2012).

At the same time, Dame Cicely Saunders, who started the hospice movement in England, was invited to Yale University to lecture about her new philosophy of care for the dying. Dean of the School of Nursing at Yale University at that time was Dr. Florence Wald. Dr. Wald was so impressed after hearing Dame Saunders's lecture, she resigned her position at Yale and returned to her beloved public health nursing where she focused on the care of young dying breast cancer patients. In her effort to improve their quality of life, she, along with other health care professionals, initiated the Connecticut Hospice in 1972 (Buck, 2011). This occurrence determined the inauguration of the hospice philosophy in the United States.

Soon after, legislators began to look for ways to reimburse this new model of care. In 1986, the Medicare Hospice Benefit was made a permanent entitlement under Medicare (Buck, 2011). Those hospices receiving reimbursement for medical care have to be certified through the CMS and are required to strictly adhere to the Conditions of Participation (CoPs) to prevent sanctions (Department of Veterans Affairs, 2016). The CoPs are frequently revised through the Federal Registry and continue to serve as the regulatory standards of hospice care. Nonadherence leads to financial penalties and certification removal.

This was the same period of time that the Hospice Nurses Association was incorporated. Thirty-eight hospice nurses established the specialty nursing organization to "lead the way" in hospice nursing through education. The organization quickly grew and soon thereafter spawned the National Board for Certification of Hospice Nurses in 1992. In 1998, both of these organizations added the word "palliative" to their name, becoming the Hospice and Palliative Nurses Association (HPNA) and the National Board for Certification of Hospice and Palliative Nursing (NBCHPN®) recognizing the significance of palliative care that was simply providing the hospice philosophy earlier in the disease trajectory. (In 2013, NBCHPN changed their name to the Hospice and Palliative Certification Center [HPCC].)

As legislators worked to improve end-of-life care in America, a new policy was written called the Patient Self-Determination Act of 1990 (Congress 101st, 1990). The intent of the act was to give Americans a voice in end-of-life decisions through the completion of advance directives (Giovanni, 2012). The law required every Medicare-participating organization to ask patients upon admission if they had an advance directive and if not, would they like assistance in completing one. The advance directive was then supposed to become a part of the permanent medical record. As well intentioned as it was, the law failed miserably. Despite more than 25 years of promoting advance directives, more than 25% of individuals of all ages have given no thought to their end-of-life preferences (Institute of Medicine, 2011, 2015; Morham & Pollack, 2013).

In 1995, a study underwritten by Robert Wood Johnson Foundation became the first of three sentinel studies to serve as springboards to the introduction of palliative care in America. The study was called *The SUPPORT Study: A Controlled Trial to Improve Care for Seriously Ill Hospitalized Patients—The Study to Understand Prognoses and Preferences for Outcomes and Risks of Treatment* (Connors et al., 1995; Coyle, 2015; Pace & Lunsford, 2011). The objectives of this study were to seek ways to improve the end-of-life decision making and improve the quality of life of the dying. Several outcomes highlighted the abysmal circumstances that existed for the dying. Communications were lacking regarding patient preferences and choices, do-not-resuscitate orders were being written within 2 days of death, patients wanted to die at home yet were dying in intensive care units (ICUs), and patients/family members were reporting excessive levels of pain being experienced by their dying loved ones.

Soon thereafter, the Institute of Medicine published the second sentinel study called *Approaching Death: Improving Care at the End-of-Life*. One outcome of this study confirmed the findings of the SUPPORT Study—pain was under-treated in the dying. Other outcomes focused on the need to gather more data, remedy the impediments to quality care, and research the many gaps in scientific knowledge (Coyle, 2015; Pace & Lunsford, 2011).

The third sentinel study was the Last Acts report called *Means to a Better End: A Report on Dying in America Today* again underwritten by the Robert Wood Johnson Foundation. This study graded each state in the nation on eight criteria that described the availability and quality of end-of-life care in America (Pace & Lunsford, 2011). The results of this study were very discouraging. Our nation was failing to meet the needs of those facing serious illnesses.

These three sentinel studies launched a national campaign for moving hospice care upstream. In 2001, Dr. Diane Meier convened a group of national leaders in palliative care and challenged them to create a set of palliative care guidelines. With representation from the four leading organizations— American Academy of Hospice and Palliative Medicine (AAHPM), CAPC, HPNA, and the NHPCO—the National Consensus Project (NCP) work began. The first edition of the *Clinical Practice Guidelines for Quality Palliative Care* was published in 2004 and revised in 2009. A third edition was published in 2013 (Dahlin, 2015; National Consensus Project for Quality Palliative Care, 2013). These guidelines are intended to be initiated at the time of diagnosis and continue throughout the disease trajectory providing curative, restorative, or comfort care that waxes and wanes as indicated by patient-driven goals and preferences. This is meant to continue through the final 6 months, and the death and bereavement period thereafter, therefore, inclusive of hospice care if the patient desires representing the end of the palliative care continuum (Figure 17.1). The guidelines espouse eight domains of care—structure and process, physical aspects, psychosocial and psychiatric aspects, social aspects, spiritual/religious/existential aspects, cultural aspects, care of the imminently dying, and ethical/legal aspects of care (Dahlin, 2015; National Consensus Project for Quality Palliative Care, 2013). For more details, visit www.national-consensusproject.org. These core elements serve as the conceptual framework of quality palliative care in America.

In 2006, the National Quality Forum (NQF), the nonprofit agency charged with building consensus on performance improvement through measurement, reporting, education, and outreach programs, developed a more formal definition by naming 38 preferred practices in a document known as *A National Framework and Preferred Practices for Palliative and Hospice Care Quality* that can be found at www.qualityforum.org (National Consensus Project for Quality Palliative Care, 2013; NQF, 2006).

The preferred practices were synergistic to the NCP Clinical Practice Guidelines and can be easily cross-walked with the eight domains. This document becomes the first step toward the development of quality indicators as required by CMS.

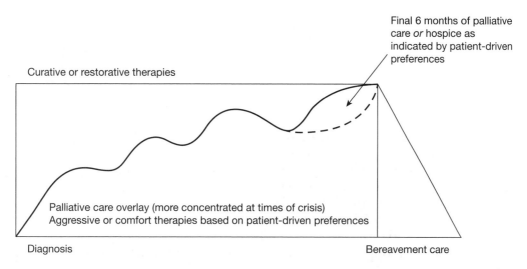

FIGURE 17.1 The continuum of palliative care.

Source: Adapted from National Consensus Project for Quality Palliative Care (2009).

PALLIATIVE CARE IN THE 21ST CENTURY

Over the past decade, palliative care has achieved significant momentum spurred by the negative outcomes of the SUPPORT Study (Coyne et al., 2015; Forero et al., 2012). The development of the clinical practice guidelines by the NCP and the preferred practices published by the NQF generated a great deal of attention among health care professionals. A broad dissemination of the guidelines with requests for endorsement yielded positive responses. The work of the CAPC to establish palliative care delivery models in hospitals across the nation created the incentives to establish these highly successful programs (CAPC, 2015). The momentum gave great hope to the leaders in the field. But were the programs reflective of the tenets of the hospice philosophy as described in the clinical practice guidelines?

The tenets of palliative care are many: holistic care inclusive of mind, body, and spirit aspects; 24/7 coverage; interprofessional team specifically including the physician, nurse, social worker, chaplain, and any other health care professionals indicated; ACP as a continuous and dynamic process; patient/family as the unit of care; and assurances that treatments match the patient-stated wishes. To ensure that program development matched the guidelines, The Joint Commission established a palliative care certification initiated in August 2011. The written standards for this certification match the 2013 clinical practice guidelines. Thus far, several hospital programs have achieved palliative care certification recognition as an add-on option. The rights of the dying supersede all others' issues, and palliative care professionals are the team to assure these rights are acknowledged and honored. "The Hospice Patient's Bill of Rights" that covers the topics of dignity, respect, decision making, privacy, financial obligations, quality of care, and responsibilities of patient and caregiver is widely used by practitioners in the field of hospice/palliative care (Hospice Association of America, 2016).

Several successful programs have come out of demonstration projects, research studies, and exemplar practice settings. These programs have served as pioneers, role models, and benchmarks for new developing programs. Take, for instance, the Safe Conduct Study performed from 2000 to 2002. Awarded a demonstration project from Robert Wood Johnson Foundation, the Ireland Cancer Center in Cleveland, Ohio, and the Hospice of the Western Reserve teamed together to offer a unique palliative care service for newly diagnosed stage 4 lung cancer patients. Patients were randomized into the study group or the control group. This study group received care by a palliative care nurse practitioner, social worker, and chaplain every visit they made to the facility from the time of diagnoses throughout the disease trajectory, death, and bereavement thereafter. The control group received standard care. The outcomes of this study were most surprising. Not only did patients and families rate the quality of their care as highly satisfactory but also they rated their quality of life highly satisfactory, while the control group rated the quality of their care much lower (Pitorak & Armour, 2003).

A similar study was conducted in 2009 by Dr. Jennifer Temel at the Massachusetts General Hospital Palliative Care service. Although the outcomes of the Temel study replicated those of the Safe Conduct Study, one additional benefit was noted in the Temel study. For unexplainable reasons, the patients in the study group lived 2.7 months longer than the control group (Kelley & Meier, 2010). Although unexplainable, it is believed that the reasons may be because the patient's symptoms were better controlled, the patient's depression was treated, and there was a reduction in patient hospitalizations (Kelley & Meier, 2010). This was a landmark study because it refuted the general public suspicions that those receiving palliative care may have life shortened by withdrawal or withholding of care by the medical team.

Other studies conducted by leading researchers demonstrate the value of palliative care in terms of cost savings, growth, and improved quality of life (Dumanovsky et al, 2016; Giovanni, 2012; Kelley & Morrison, 2015; May et al., 2016; Ranganathan et al., 2013).

CONCEPTUAL AND THEORETICAL FRAMEWORK

Historically, palliative care has been based on the hospice philosophy. The core elements for hospice are replicated in palliative care. The management of serious illness is very different from the management of acute care. The theoretical framework recommends introduction of palliative care at the time of diagnosis, increasing the concentration of the palliative care team based on the disease progression and the patient wishes, ultimately assuming 100% of the care management through the dying phase, death, and bereavement thereafter (National Consensus Project for Quality Palliative Care, 2013).

Two distinct elements make palliative care unique—the interprofessional team and ACP. Care is delivered by an interprofessional team composed of the physician, nurse, social worker, and chaplain at a minimum of health care professionals as required by the Medicare Hospice Benefit CoPs and replicated by palliative care as written in the clinical practice guidelines (Otis-Green & Fineberg, 2015). The nurse becomes pivotal to this team, serving as the care coordinator, assures the care plan reflects the patient and family wishes and goals, assures the team is informed and honors the patient's stated care goals, coordinates the plan-of-care meetings, and continually evaluates the effectiveness of treatments prescribed to relieve the physical, psychosocial, and spiritual distresses experienced by the patient.

The success of the interprofessional team is assured by hiring the right people, demonstrating mutual respect and humility, building a quality team, and assuring healthy group dynamics occur during debriefing sessions. The conceptual framework for the interprofessional team is based on interprofessional collaboration that is defined by Bronstein as "an interpersonal communication process leading to the attainment of specific goals not achievable by any single team member alone" (Baldwin, Wittenberg-Lyles, Oliver, & Demiris, 2011, p. 173). Team training, conflict resolution, and team building are critical processes to define for a successful team. Seeking ways to support one another, balancing workloads, and providing self-care options are some examples of team building (Dahlin & Wittenberg, 2015; Larsen & Jense, 2015).

ACP is a process of conversations based on the needs and preferences of the patient and family. In palliative care, this mantra is frequently heard: "it's all about the conversation." Make no mistake, it sounds simple but is far from it. Acquiring skill in these kinds of conversations is what makes palliative care professionals unique.

The American Academy of Nursing published a policy brief (Tilden et al., 2012) titled *Advance Care Planning as an Urgent Public Health Concern*. Collaborating with HPNA leaders, the task force made several recommendations: (a) to pay for the conversations, (b) to utilize the electronic medical record to record the patient's preference, (c) to update the advance directives and expand the requirements of the Patient Self-Determination Act of 1990, and finally (d) to provide health professionals with education and training for caring of the dying (Tilden et al., 2012). After 6 years and many letters to support this position, legislation made this possible beginning in 2016.

Even though death is inevitable, discussing the possibility is difficult for all of us. And yet, when diagnosed with a serious illness, patients and families will emphatically say, decision making is simplified by ACP discussions. These discussions occur frequently based on the individual and the situation, beginning with the first conversation to establish the patient/family goals of care. In palliative care, the patient is the driver of the treatment directions. There are several steps to each conversation, beginning with knowing what the patient/family understands about the situation. Next, the palliative care professional must establish how much the patient wants to know and who will make decisions if he or she is unable. The conversations from then on should be frequent, transparent, based on what the patient/family wants and cover the benefits and burdens of each treatment being considered. Shared decision making from patients/families that have been fully informed is the hallmark of quality palliative care. It is a dying patient's right (Giovanni, 2012; Hospice Association of America, 2016; HPNA, 2014a; Schaffer et al., 2012; Zeytinoglu, 2011).

Studies have shown little evidence that treatments match patient wishes. Why? Access, fear, educational curricula failing to address end-of-life care, and workforce issues are some of the reasons (Giovanni, 2012). Providing the right care to the right patient at the right time defines quality according to Giovanni.

HEALTH POLICY

Because of the inception of hospice in America, health policy has served as an impetus for change in the care of the dying. Health policy is often guided by the research. Although the availability of quantitative and qualitative research has the potential to drive decisions in health policy, in a field as new as palliative care, there is as yet a paucity of research (Lunney, 2011). But this trend is changing as evidence-based research is growing rapidly. However, the research continues to have a minimum impact indicated by a low level of attention (Forero et al., 2012).

Several noted nursing researchers have contributed heartily to the field of hospice/palliative care in the past 40 years—Jeanne Quint Beneliel, Florence Wald, Ida Martinson, Marylin Dodd, Elizabeth Clipp, Virginia Tilden, Pam Hinds, Betty Ferrell, Joy Buck, Mary Ersek, and June Lunney are several notable historic end-of-life nursing research leaders. A 2010 review of the published research literature revealed that 14% had been contributed by nursing in that year (Lunney, 2011). With increased emphasis on the need for more research, additional research leaders including Mi-Kyung Song, Harleah Buck, Marie Bakitis, Judith Baggs, Lisa Lindley, Deborah McGuire, and others have emerged.

In 2010, a group of leading researchers met to establish a cooperative research body to overcome many of the barriers to palliative care research—namely lack of funds, small provider sites, data heterogeneity, and so on. The outcome of this gathering was the establishment of the Palliative Care Research Cooperative (PCRC; Abernethy et al., 2010; Ferrell, Grant, & Sun, 2015).

The majority of funds received for early research came from private funders—Robert Wood Johnson Foundation and George Soros contributed millions of research dollars (Martinez, 2011). Although funding from governmental sources was limited in the early years, the National Institutes of Health has substantially increased its support to the study of hospice and palliative research over the recent years. Funded projects increased from less than 50 in 1990 to more than 350 in 2010 (Lunney, 2011). The National Institute of Nursing Research (NINR) is the agency that provides the focus of all palliative care research currently—medical and nursing. In 2011, NINR funded two initiatives, one called the *End-of-Life and Palliative Care Needs Assessment* and the other a *Summit on the Science of Compassion: Future Directions in End-of-Life and Palliative Care* (Lunney, 2011). These initiatives helped lead the way to significant increases in palliative research in the past 5 years. Newer initiatives such as *Palliative Care: Conversations Matter* and *Because of Nursing Research: End of Life Care in the ICU* have provided frameworks for improved pediatric palliative care as well as adult palliative care in the ICUs (Lunney, 2011; National Institute of Nursing Research, 2016; National Institutes of Health, 2016).

The HPNA Scope and Standards of Practice document has always defined research as an expected area of participation for hospice and palliative nurses. Hospice nurses in the earlier years hesitated to allow their patients to participate in research because of the severity of their illness. It was later discovered that patients wanted the opportunity to participate in an effort to advance the field for their loved ones. Defining areas of research need has long been attributed to the clinician as well as assisting with data collection (Lunney, 2011). Every hospice and palliative nurse can contribute to research in meaningful ways.

Until 2009, the HPNA had no research agenda even though the organization's leaders valued the need (HPNA, 2015a). Through the efforts of a core group of palliative nursing researchers, the first HPNA research agenda was published in 2011. The focus was to encourage research on dyspnea, fatigue, constipation, and heart failure (Lunney, 2011). In 2012, the HPNA Board of Directors published the second research agenda focusing on Domains 1 (structure and processes), 2 (physical aspects of care), and 3 (psychological and psychiatric aspects of care) of the Clinical Practice Guidelines in Quality Palliative Care. Again, in 2015, the third research agenda continues this same focus (HPNA, 2015a).

Nurses led the policy changes with hospice care. As noted earlier, it was Dr. Florence Wald who spearheaded the hospice movement in America. Through stories told by nurses, many policies have been generated in an effort to improve the care of the dying (Buck, 2011). The HMB reimbursement was probably the most significant change so far. Although offering financial security for hospices in America at the time the HMBs were initiated, these benefits have been attributed as the cause for many reimbursement issues that exist today (Buck, 2011; CMS, 2015).

In 2004, the HPNA Board of Directors, recognizing the critical need for nursing advocacy, established a Public Policy Committee. One of the very first efforts of this committee was to recommend "Public Policy Guiding Principles." Originally written in 2006 and revised in 2010 (Box 17.1), they continue today as written at that time (HPNA, 2014a).

HPNA PUBLIC POLICY GUIDING PRINCIPLES, 2014A   **BOX 17.1**

HPNA acts independently and with collaborating organizations to address hospice and palliative care issues at the national, state, local, and regional levels. HPNA bases its public policy positions and actions on the following guiding principles.

1. HPNA asserts that it is the responsibility and obligation of clinicians to address hospice/palliative care public policy and regulatory issues that impact the health-related quality of life of patients and caregivers living with serious illness.
2. HPNA takes a leadership and advocacy role to ensure equitable access to comprehensive palliative care as defined by the NCP Clinical Practice Guidelines for Quality Palliative Care, across the life span and illness continuums. HPNA serves on the Steering Committee of the National Coalition for Hospice and Palliative Care. HPNA also works collaboratively with other national coalitions.
3. HPNA works independently and collaboratively to promote ethical and competent provision of hospice and palliative care based upon the expressed goals of the patient and family caregivers.
4. HPNA takes a leadership and advocacy role in regulatory issues and public education regarding the legitimate use and appropriate access to medications.
5. HPNA advocates for nursing workforce funding and professional education issues as they impact hospice and palliative care.
6. HPNA advocates for equitable funding for hospice and palliative care research.
7. HPNA supports improved access to comprehensive health care for appropriate management of physical and emotional symptoms that allows patients to achieve the highest quality of life through the relief of suffering in all of its manifestations.

HPNA, Hospice and Palliative Nurses Association; NCP, National Consensus Project.

The public policy issues that continue to hinder the field of hospice/palliative care are many. Access is the most significant one. Access is impacted in three ways—insurance coverage, availability of services, and public awareness. Although the PPACA has decreased the numbers of uninsured and underinsured, 28 million individuals do not have health care insurance and another 3 million are underinsured and therefore fall into the "coverage gap" (Betancourt, 2016). Availability of care has improved based on the CAPC Report Card, but gaps are noted in this area as well (CAPC, 2015). Awareness is the final issue. Because many health care professionals do not understand what palliative care is, how can we expect the lay public to comprehend its complexity? We are a death-denying society that precludes having the conversations, so improving these access issues is slow.

Other public policy issues focus on pain management, workforce issues, educational needs, physician and APRN fellowships, ACP, comparative effectiveness research, health information technology, payment reform, health delivery reform, and chronic care coordination (CAPC, 2015). The list is long and much work is needed.

ROLE OF THE PALLIATIVE CARE APRN

The role of the advanced practice palliative care nurse is growing rapidly as indicated by the increased demand. Historically, the American Academy of Nurse Practitioners argued that APRNs demonstrated their ability to be cost-effective and provide high-quality care (Reifsnyder & Yeo, 2011). In palliative care, APRNs spearhead the palliative care delivery service through development, implementation, and evaluation of services and are considered highly valued members of the interprofessional team (Sherman & Cheon, 2012; Wiencek, 2015). Dr. Ira Byock, a highly acclaimed palliative care physician, has often stated, "If you want a good palliative care service, you need to find a good palliative care nurse" (personal communication, August 12, 2011).

The significance to the value of palliative care increased in January 2009 when the CMS finally recognized the new specialty. With this approval came a new code for physicians and nonphysician practitioners to bill for their services (Pace & Lunsford, 2011). Advanced practice palliative care nurses are poised for success with the recognition of the palliative care specialty in the medical community, regulatory recognition by CMS for palliative care billing purposes, and legal recognition by CMS in terms of the approval of the palliative care nursing certification body (HPCC formally NBCHPN) that finally occurred under the direction of the author of this chapter while serving as the executive director of the certification organization.

In addition to their clinical practice role, APRNs serve as administrators, educators, health policy makers, and researchers (Box 17.2; Sherman & Cheon, 2012). As administrators, they assure the implementation and evaluation of the programs and assure that they remain viable and eventually eligible for The Joint Commission certification. As educators, they are called on to assist staff with the dying process and to educate the patient and family to be fully informed and able to understand the disease process and the subsequent prognosis and treatment options in terms of benefits and burdens. They also educate the lay public

PALLIATIVE CARE ADVANCED PRACTICE ROLES	BOX 17.2

Clinical consultant

- Leads the team as coordinator, leads family conferences, updates plan of care, monitors and revises treatments to achieve stated patient goals

Administrator

- Designs, implements, and evaluates program delivery
- Advocates business model to administration

Educator

- Educates staff, patients, family members, other health care professionals, and lay public

Health care policy maker

- Advocates for policy changes internally and externally on the local, state, and national levels

Researcher

- Recommends clinical issues to study
- Advocates for research participation and assists in data collection
- Designs research studies, seeks funding, and implements research

Source: Sherman and Cheon (2012).

about the value of palliative care and educate other health care professionals to improve communication and quality of life for all patients (Jackson et al., 2012).

As health policy advocates, the adage "all politics are local" becomes a mantra of nursing advocacy (Meier & Beresford, 2009). Reaching out locally, influencing state lawmakers as well as federal senators and representatives can be very effective. The more committed nurses are to public policy, the louder our voice of advocacy will be heard. It is through stories told by nurses that regulatory and legislative changes occur. For example, in 2009, the Food and Drug Administration (FDA) mandated that morphine can be pulled from the manufacturing process to comply with current approval requirements of new drugs.

Morphine, a long-established drug, therefore had no previous approval requirements. The FDA had no idea of the unintended consequences of their mandate. Pain management for the terminally ill became a nightmare. Opioid shortages occurred as a ripple effect. Opioid rotations became more difficult. Practitioners scrambled to achieve pain control. In an effort to effectively communicate the subsequent havoc, letters with attached surveys were sent to nurses and physicians. The survey data achieved were significant, but it was the impact of the dramatic stories told by the nurses in the field that reversed the new FDA mandate and morphine became immediately available once again. According to Dr. Douglas Throckmorton of the FDA, it was the stories from the nurses that convinced the FDA of the need to make a sudden process change. Finally, in terms of research, the role of the APRN is not only to define areas of needed research but also to participate in research through data collection, prevention of "gatekeeper" mentality of coworkers, and education of the patient/family in terms of participation to increase the base of evidence for practice.

In July 2012, HPNA held a congressional briefing with legislative aides discussing the importance of being able to make informed choices in palliative care. A panel of patients and family members participated, expressing their concerns. An issue brief titled *Assuring Choice for Seriously and Progressively Ill Patients* was distributed that recommended the following: "Include in future legislative language a requirement that advanced practice nurses and physicians offer seriously, progressively ill patients information and counseling concerning palliative and end-of-life options for care and treatment" (HPNA, 2014b).

The education of advanced practice palliative care nurses began with Ursuline College in 1997. Soon after, New York University established an advanced degree program. Although additional programs followed, many have since converted to postgraduate certificate programs or have become tracks in the adult-geriatric programs that currently exist (HPNA, 2012). APRNs work in all arenas of palliative care, and therefore it is difficult to identify the total number because of expansiveness of care settings. As a result of the Advanced Practice Registered Nursing Consensus Work Group with what is referred to as the Licensure, Accreditation, Certification, and Education (LACE) project, subspecialty emphasis lies outside the mandated educational components. The four groups represented by the LACE acronym began working collaboratively in 2006 to design an advanced practice model that satisfies all four advanced practice nursing roles (Dahlin, 2013; HPCC, 2014; Pace & Lunsford, 2011). In this model, palliative care is defined as a specialty. Beginning in 2015, APRN education focused on one of the four roles and one of six primary population foci. Certification for licensure purposes is focused on the two components of role and population (e.g., adult-gerontology nurse practitioner), and then the individual is permitted to become certified in a specialty (e.g., palliative care). As a result, the educational curricula have been modified accordingly, and any emphasis on specialties becomes self-education, postgraduate, or at the discretion of the faculty (HPCC, 2014).

Certification for the APRN is critical to practice. The HPCC (formally NBCHPN) offers an advanced practice certification with the credential ACHPN, the acronym for advanced certified hospice and palliative nurse (HPCC, 2016; Wiencek, 2015). As of 2016, 1,392 advanced practice palliative care nurses hold this credential (HPCC, 2016; Lentz & Sherman, 2010). The ACHPN exam is accredited by the Accreditation Board of Specialty Nursing Certification (ABSNC; HPCC, 2015). Accreditation is an important distinction not only acknowledging the adherence to 18 stringent standards (ABSNC, 2015; Martinez, 2011) but also being required by the state to achieve recognition for advanced practice licensure as well as being approved for billing by CMS.

Although certification is the focus of its mission, in 2010, HPCC (formally NBCHPN) undertook a major initiative seeking a singular broadly endorsed definition for continuing competence for nurses at all levels of practice, recognizing the need to apply this definition to certification. In the field of nursing education, competence usually represents the knowledge, skills, and ability to practice in one's specialty. Competency refers to the skillful art of actual practice. Both competence and competency are especially important to the APRN as well as the safety of the public. As noted in the Institute of Medicine report (2011) titled *The Future of Nursing: Leading Change, Advancing Health,* lifelong learning is one of the recommendations. The American Nurses Association (ANA), the National Council of State Boards of Nursing (NCSBN), the American Board of Nursing Specialties (ABNS), and the Citizen Advocacy Coalition (CAC) have long sought ways to prove continuing competence through portfolios, self-assessments, examinations, simulated judgment exams, and personal improvement plans (Martinez, 2011).

As HPCC sought to implement a plan to establish continuing competence, they recognized the variations of definitions in the literature and decided to undertake this initiative. With a team of experts from both inside and outside of hospice and palliative care, the work began. Nearly a year later, the agreed-upon definition titled "Statement on Continuing Competence for Nursing: A Call to Action" was presented to the Accreditation Board for Specialty Nursing Certification (ABSNC) and ABNS for endorsement. ABNS further committed themselves to seek an even broader endorsement through their member organizations (HPCC, 2011). The American Association of Colleges of Nursing (AACN) has also voted to endorse this definition that will drive the implementation throughout the graduate programs for APRNs nationally.

With this milestone, complete HPCC launched a yearlong study of how the newly endorsed definition (Box 17.3) could be implemented in palliative care. The study included a variety of methodologies, a feedback loop for the certificant, and a certification renewal process that clearly defines the individual's unique continuing education and competence.

Simultaneously, a new initiative is under way with AACN in terms of continuing education. Spawned from the Institute of Medicine report conducted in 2009 indicating the need to revamp the entire educational process for health care professionals, AACN has joined five other major organizations to provide recommendations to establish a new approach—interprofessional education (Interprofessional Education Collaborative Expert Panel, 2011). Ironically, palliative care has long participated in interprofessional education being a hallmark for the field and thus for advanced practice nursing. For example, for the past 14years, physicians, nurses, social workers, chaplains, pharmacists, and others copresent and attend the annual cosponsored educational conference. This mirrors the education occurring daily clinically in the field.

OUTCOME MEASURES

Starting in 2014, under the current PPACA, hospices are required to publicly report quality data to the federal government (National Quality Forum, 2012b). The NQF developed the Triple Aim that defined directions for this new

---

DEFINITION OF CONTINUING COMPETENCE	BOX 17.3

"Continuing competence is the ongoing commitment of a registered nurse to integrate and apply the knowledge, skills, and judgment with the attitudes, values, and beliefs required to practice safely, effectively, and ethically in a designated role and setting."

Source: HPCC (2011).

requirement and extended the public reporting to the hospice community similar to the requirements for other practice settings. The Triple Aim represents: (a) healthier people, (b) better care, and (c) more affordable care. In 2011, NQF convened a group of 60 organizations called the Measure Applications Partnership (MAP) to function as an advisory role to the Department of Health and Human Services. MAP offered 28 measures, nearly half of which are ready for immediate use (NQF MAP Partnership, 2012a). Two of the nonclinical measures are person- and family-centered care and care coordination—easily prioritized to hospice care. Of the other measures, seven of the recommended measures apply to both hospice and palliative care, three apply only to hospice, and three apply only to palliative care (Table 17.2).

A group of experts convened by the CAPC agreed with many of these measures and suggested specific ways to assess the needs of patients at admission with a potentially life-limiting or life-threatening condition. They recommend beginning with a checklist that contains primary criteria (Weissman & Meier, 2011). The primary criteria are the minimum indicators that hospitals should use in screening patients on admission, and they include palliative care's most effective question called the "surprise question"—"would you be surprised if the patient died within 12 months or before adulthood" (Weissman & Meier, 2011, p. 19). Other criteria include frequent admissions, admissions due to uncontrolled

TABLE 17.2 Measure Application Partnership (MAP) Measures

MEASURE	HOSPICE CARE	PALLIATIVE CARE	BOTH
Experience of care			×
Comprehensive assessment (holistic)			×
Physical aspects–pain, dyspnea, constipation, etc.			×
Care planning			×
Implement patient/family goals			×
Prevent avoidable admissions to ED and hospital			×
Manage anxiety, depression, delirium, other psychological			×
Timeliness/responsiveness of care	×		
Access to health care team on 24-hour basis	×		
Avoiding unwanted treatments	×		
Sharing medical records and advance directives		×	
Patient education and support		×	
Access to palliative care		×	

ED, emergency department.

Adapted from National Quality Forum (2012a).

symptoms, complex care requirements, and a significant decline in function, weight, or feeding.

The Patient-Centered Outcomes Research Institute (PCORI) was also established during this same period of time as part of the ACA of 2010. The purpose of this effort is to change how clinical questions are worded, how the questions are pursued and what happens to the data gathered (Frank, Basch, & Selby, 2014).

IMPLICATIONS FOR APRN PRACTICE

Future implications for palliative APRNs can be enumerated most clearly by following the 2010 Institute of Medicine Report's eight recommendations as paraphrased and combined subsequently (Institute of Medicine, 2011).

Recommendation 1,8—Remove Practice Barriers

In 2016, the Veterans Administration (VA) proposed to grant full practice authority to APRNs employed by the VA in an effort to improve access to care in light of the current staffing shortages (Department of Veterans Affairs, 2016). These shortage concerns extend to the public in the next decade. Aging nurses, as well as shortages of others in associated fields, have caused a projected 2.3 million jobs to be added to the health care and social assistance employment sector in the next decade (U.S. Department of Labor, 2015).

Recommendation 2, 7—Leadership

In 2014, a joint strategy council was established to adopt a shared position regarding palliative nursing leadership. Their joint position is that palliative nursing leadership is transformative, should be recognized at all levels and in all aspects of palliative nursing, and is advanced by involvement, collaboration, and engagement in education, practice, and research (HPNA, 2015b, 2015c).

Recommendation 3, 4, 5, 6—Addresses Education

Nursing education in palliative care has grown in many ways. In 2000, The End of Life Nursing Education Consortium (ELNEC) was initiated. A "train the trainer" model curriculum for end-of-life care was developed. In the first 14 years, 20,000 nurses became approved educators and have gone on to educate 480,000 individuals nationally and internationally using this curriculum (Malloy, 2015). Simultaneously, HPNA has published numerous palliative care courses, resources, continuing education e-courses, and so on to aid their membership in self-education as well as teach others. Additionally, HPNA has partnered with the AAHPM to cosponsor annual interdisciplinary educational conferences. Physician education and therefore education also appropriate for APRNs has been enhanced by the Palliative Care and Hospice Education and Training Act passed by Congress in 2015 (Kamal, LeBlanc, & Meier, 2016). CAPC also provides a new interactive palliative care curriculum called Vital Talk (Morrison, Bowman, Meier, & Back, 2016).

Other areas impacting APRNs in palliative care are in quality measurement, addressing quality of care associated with access, cost, and providing a "good death." HPNA has partnered with AAHPM to provide a consensus framework of 10 measures called "Measuring What Matters." Included in the measures are issues such as pain, dyspnea, spiritual and emotional concerns, and treatment and care preferences (HPNA, 2016).

Nurses can also be instrumental in educating the public about palliative care. Although 90% of the public indicate they know nothing about palliative care, most of them responded they wanted this kind of care when they were read a definition (Kelley & Morrison, 2015). In terms of cost, one study found a significant cost reduction when palliative care consults were secured within 2 days of admission (May et al., 2016). APRNs are a critical member of the team to assure consults are secured and effected. Five triggers for consultations have been identified in oncology patients in one study with outcomes demonstrating increased patient satisfaction, decreased costs, and decreased 30-day readmissions. The triggers were Stage IV solid tumor malignancies, Stage III pancreas or liver cancers, poorly controlled physical or emotional symptoms, more than two admissions in previous 6 months, and the presence of distress in the family (Meier, 2015).

A recent delivery model was released by CMS called the Medicare Care Choices Model that allows the patient to receive curative treatment as well as hospice care simultaneously. This innovative model has opened quality palliative care for pediatrics as well as adults alike (Sopcheck, 2016). Rep. Earl Blumenaurer and Rep. Phil Roe recently introduced a bipartisan proposal called Personalize Your Care Act in the House of Representatives. APRNs can impact the approval of this legislative proposal by offering their written support. Several points are included in this bill to increase access as well as increase public awareness (NHPCO, 2016). Additionally, CMS has issued a proposed rule change to measure the number of hospice visits in the last week of life. APRNs are invaluable when they take the time to comment on these proposals during the public comment period (CMS, 2016b).

The impact on APRNs who currently or futuristically practice in palliative care is pivotal to leading the way to change the quality of life of every individual facing serious illnesses.

ETHICS

Due to the complexity of the patient's condition as well as the vulnerability of these patients, ethical dilemmas can be expected. How we handle these situations is an area needing a great deal of attention in hospice and palliative care directly led by palliative APRNs.

Ethical dilemmas such as double effect, competency versus capacity, benevolent deception with informed consents, futility, withholding/withdrawing, goals of care, compassion fatigue, and substituted judgment are just a few of the myriad of ethical concerns facing hospice and palliative nurses daily as they assist the terminally ill patients and their families through critical decisions (Prince-Paul & Daly, 2015). Moral distress occurs in nurses who have neither the power of autonomy nor the power of futility (Hayes, 2004; Prince-Paul & Daly, 2015).

Dr. Ira Byock stated it best: "Clinicians can serve the dying person by being present. We may not have the answers for the existential questions of life and death any more than the dying person does. We may not be able to assuage all feelings of regret or fears of the unknown. But it is not our solutions that matter. The role of the clinical team is to stand by the patient, steadfastly providing meticulous physical care and psychological support, while people strive to discover their own answers" (Hayes, 2004, p. 43).

The advanced practice palliative care nurse is the coordinator of the inter-professional team and therefore uniquely positioned to assure the meticulous care to which Byock refers and thereby allowing the patient and family to discover their own answers. As an APRN in palliative care, offering nonjudgmental support, genuine compassion, education about the benefits and burdens of options, and most important, having the expertise to relieve physical, emotional, and spiritual suffering provides the experience and knowledge to advocate for health policy changes that improve the quality of life for these most vulnerable patients.

CONCLUSION

With a $3.2 trillion health care industry that fails to meet the needs of those experiencing end of life, the need for health care reform and availability of palliative care is obvious. Unacceptable outcomes continue to exist—unrelieved suffering, failure to acknowledge and honor wishes, benevolent deception, and death without dignity (Pear, 2016). The need for change is now.

What should that change look like? The call to action white paper called *Call to Action: Health Care Reform 2009* offered one model emphasizing three legs of reform. The design advocates weeding out waste and overpayment; focusing on quality, value, and less costly care; and finally ensuring meaningful coverage and care to all Americans (Meier & Beresford, 2009).

Others recommend changing the educational preparation of all health care professionals creating a new culture. A cultural change is needed in the lay public as well. It is the belief of many in the field of palliative care that the baby boomers will be instrumental in creating this cultural change. As a sandwich generation, they struggle to meet the needs of aging parents as they raise their young children. The 55-year-old daughter who is working full time is frustrated with the complexity of the health care system and the compassion needed to meet the demands of her dying parents. In fear of losing her job, she searches Google for answers. Once she is guided to palliative care and recognizes the value palliative care has offered her loved ones as well as herself, she becomes an ambassador for having palliative care available for all. It is just a matter of time until the tipping point is reached and the consumer becomes the driver of change.

Again, the sage advice of Byock guides us in our thinking with this statement of his:

> Our field knows a great deal that would be of value in the health care reform process. We know where the excesses are, and the deficiencies that should be addressed—if only we were asked. The public clearly wants what we have to offer. But if there's no voice speaking for the public on these matters, who is going to advance these goals? Unless and until our field is able to translate what we know is possible to improve care into

terms that can be used by a consumer-driven movement, we will not realize what is possible in health care reform. We must make key expectations about care for frail elders and the seriously ill part of the citizen and consumer rights agenda, that patients' wishes are known and honored, that continuity of care is assured, that pain is managed, and that families are supported in their caregiving and in their grief. (Meier & Beresford, 2009, p. 595)

APRNs possess the skills, knowledge, and ability to teach the public so the public can give "sound" to the silent consumer voice. In the meantime, palliative care APRNs will continue to start the conversations and continue to talk as needed, learn about patient/family wishes, preferences, and goals, and advocate to assure these wishes are honored and treatments matched. They will continue to keep the patient/family fully informed, be fully transparent, and coordinate the interprofessional team to achieve the patient-stated goals. Palliative care APRNs are experts and as such serve as the beacon to lead social change through policy change so that palliative care and therefore "good deaths" are accessible to all.

DISCUSSION QUESTIONS

1. *Discuss the regulatory impact on managing pain in palliative care.*
2. *What are examples of barriers to practice for the palliative care APRN?*

ANALYSIS, SYNTHESIS, AND CLINICAL APPLICATION

1. *If you were going to describe the importance of your issue for policy change to potential supporters, what key issues would you stress. How would you describe this to your patients?*
2. *How can a palliative care APRN get involved in policy on a local level?*
3. *Consider the health policy changes discussed in this chapter or those you have described in your analysis and consider the impact that might occur if these changes are NOT enacted. In other words, what are the consequences of inaction?*
4. *What do you do to facilitate research in your work setting?*
5. *Discuss your concerns for the need for caregiver support in palliative care.*
6. *How can changes in legislation improve quality of end-of-life care?*
7. *Talk to an ACHPN to get ideas on how you can get involved in advocacy.*

EXERCISES/CONSIDERATIONS

1. *Based on the information in this chapter, list at least two areas of policy change you can identify where legislation could have an impact.*
2. *Name three major workforce issues in palliative care.*

REFERENCES

Abernethy, A. P., Aziz, N. M., Basch, E., Bull, J., Cleeland, C. S., Currow, D. C., . . . Kutner, J. S. (2010). A strategy to advance the evidence base in palliative medicine: Formation of a palliative care research cooperative group. *Journal of Palliative Medicine, 13*(12), 1407–1413.
American Board for Specialty Nursing Certification. (2015). ABSNC accreditation. Retrieved from http://www.nursingcertification.org/absnc/accreditation

Baldwin, P. K., Wittenberg-Lyles, E., Oliver, D. P., & Demiris, G. (2011, May/June). An evaluation of inter-disciplinary team training in hospice care. *Journal of Hospice and Palliative Nursing, 13*(3), 172–182.

Betancourt, M. (2016). The devastating process of dying in America without insurance. *The Nation.* Retrieved from https://www.thenation.com/article/the-devastating-process-of-dying-in-america-without-insurance

Biography.com. (2012). *Elisabeth Kübler-Ross—Biography: Facts, birthday, life story.* Retrieved from http://www.biography.com/people/elisabeth-kubler-ross-262762

Boucher, J., Bova, C., Sullivan-Bolyai, S., Theroux, R., Klar, R., Terrien, J., & Kaufman, D. (2010, January/February). Next-of-kin's perspectives of end-of-life care. *Journal of Hospice and Palliative Nursing, 12*(1), 41–50.

Buck, J. (2011). Policy and the re-formation of hospice: Lessons from the past for the future of palliative care. *Journal of Hospice and Palliative Nursing, 13*(6), S35–S43.

Center to Advance Palliative Care. (2015). *America's care of serious illness.* Retrieved from https://reportcard.capc.org/wp-content/uploads/2015/08/CAPC-Report-Card-2015.pdf

Centers for Disease Control and Prevention. (2016). *FastStats death.* Retrieved from http://www.cdc.gov/nchs/fastats/deaths.htm

Centers for Medicare and Medicaid Services. (2015). *Medicare benefit policy manual: Chapter 9—Coverage of hospice services under hospital insurance.* Retrieved from https://www.cms.gov/Regulations-and-Guidance/Guidance/Manuals/Downloads/bp102c09.pdf

Centers for Medicare and Medicaid Services. (2016a). National health expenditure data. Retrieved from https://www.cms.gov/research-statistics-data-and-systems/statistics-trends-and-reports/nationalhealthexpenddata

Centers for Medicare and Medicaid Services. (2016b). Retrieved from https://www.cms.gov/Newsroom/MediaReleaseDatabase/Fact-sheets/2016-Fact-sheets-items/2016/04/3.html

Congress 101st. (1990). H.R.4449—Patient Self Determination Act of 1990. Retrieved from https://www.congress.gov/bill/101st-congress/house-bill/4449

Connors, A. F., Dawson, N. V., Desbiens, N. A., Fulkerson, J., Goldman, L., Knaus, W. A., . . . Ransohoff, D. (1995). A controlled trial to improve care for seriously ill hospitalized patients. The study to understand prognosis and preferences for outcomes and risks of treatments (SUPPORT). *Journal of the American Medical Association, 274*(20), 1591–1598. Retrieved from http://jama.jamanetwork.com/article.aspx?articleid=391724

Coyle, N. (2015). Introduction to palliative nursing care. In B. R. Ferrell, N. Coyle, & J. A. Paice (Eds.), *Oxford textbook of palliative nursing* (4th ed., pp. 3–10). New York, NY: Oxford University Press.

Coyne, P. J., Smith, T. J., & Lyckholm, L. J. (2015). Clinical interventions, economic impact, and palliative care. In B. R. Ferrell, N. Coyle, & J. A. Paice (Eds.), *Oxford textbook of palliative nursing* (4th ed., pp. 1048–1055). New York, NY: Oxford University Press.

Dahlin, C. (2013). A national perspective of advanced practice registered nursing. In *APRN VERVE,* HPNA monthly newsletter. Retrieved from https://issuu.com/verve-magazine/docs/vervemayebook2013

Dahlin, C. M. (2015). National consensus project for quality palliative care: Promoting excellence in palliative nursing. In B. R. Ferrell, N. Coyle, & J. A. Paice (Eds.), *Oxford textbook of palliative nursing* (4th ed., pp. 11–19). New York, NY: Oxford University Press.

Dahlin, C., & Wittenberg, E. (2015). Communication in palliative care: An essential competency for nurses. In B. R. Ferrell, N. Coyle, & J. A. Paice (Eds.), *Oxford textbook of palliative nursing* (4th ed., pp. 81–109). New York, NY: Oxford University Press.

Department of Veterans Affairs. (2016). 81 FR 33155. Retrieved from https://www.federalregister.gov/articles/2016/05/25/2016-12338/advanced-practice-registered-nurses

Dumanovsky, T., Augustin, R., Rogers, M., Lettang, K., Meier, D. E., & Morrison, R. S. (2016). The growth of palliative care in U.S. hospitals: A status report. *Journal of Palliative Medicine, 19*(1), 8–15.

Federal Register. (2012). Medicare and Medicaid programs; reform of hospital and critical access hospital conditions of participation. Retrieved from https://www.federalregister.gov/documents/2012/05/16/2012-11548/medicare-and-medicaid-programs-reform-of-hospital-and-critical-access-hospital-conditions-of

Ferrell, B. R., Grant, M., & Sun, V. (2015). Nursing research. In B. R. Ferrell, N. Coyle, & J. A. Paice (Eds.), *Oxford textbook of palliative nursing* (4th ed., pp. 1028–1038). New York, NY: Oxford University Press.

Forero, R., McDonnell, G., Gallego, B., McCarthy, S., Mohsin, M., Shanley, C., . . . Hillman, K. (2012). A literature review on care at the end-of-life in the emergency department. *Emergency Medicine International, 2012*, 486516. doi:10.1155/2012/486516

Frank, L., Basch, E., & Selby, J. V.; Patient-Centered Outcomes Research Institute. (2014). The PCORI perspective on patient-centered outcomes research. *Journal of the American Medical Association, 312*(15), 1513–1514.

Giovanni, L. A. (2012). End-of-life care in the United States: Current reality and future promise—A policy review. *Nursing Economic$, 30*(3), 127–134; quiz 135.

Hayes, C. (2004, January–March). Ethics in end-of-life care. *Journal of Hospice and Palliative Nursing, 6*(1), 36–43.

Hoefler, J. M. (2010). United States lags on palliative care at the end of life. *Journal of Pain and Symptom Management, 40*(6), e1–e3.

Hospice and Palliative Certification Center. (2014). *Consensus model for APRN regulation: Licensure, accreditation, certification & education*. Retrieved from http://hpcc.advancingexpertcare.org/wp-content/uploads/2014/09/consensus-model-for-APRN-regulation.pdf

Hospice and Palliative Certification Center. (2016). *Certification map*. Retrieved from http://www.gohpcc.org/certificants_map.aspx?cert=APRN

Hospice and Palliative Certification Center. (2015). *CHPN candidate handbook*. Retrieved from http://hpcc.advancingexpertcare.org/wp-content/uploads/2014/11/CHPN-Handbook-March-2015.pdf

Hospice and Palliative Certification Center. (2011). Statement on continuing competence for nursing: A call to action. Retrieved from http://hpcc.advancingexpertcare.org/wp-content/uploads/2015/02/Statement-on-Continuing-Competence-for-Nursing.pdf

Hospice and Palliative Nurses Association. (2012). *Palliative care graduate programs*. Retrieved from http://hpna.advancingexpertcare.org/education/graduate-program-listing

Hospice and Palliative Nurses Association. (2014a). *HPNA public policy guiding principles*. Retrieved from http://hpna.advancingexpertcare.org/advocacy/guiding-principles

Hospice and Palliative Nurses Association. (2014b). *Congressional issues brief: Assuring choice for seriously and progressively ill patients*. Retrieved from http://hpna.advancingexpertcare.org/wp-content/uploads/2014/10/HPNA-Issue-Brief.AC_.pdf

Hospice and Palliative Nurses Association. (2015a). *HPNA research agenda*. Retrieved from http://www.hpna.advancingexpertcare.org/research/research-agenda

Hospice and Palliative Nurses Association. (2015b). *Role of hospice and palliative nurses in research* [Position Statement]. Retrieved from http://hpna.advancingexpertcare.org/wp-content/uploads/2015/08/Role-of-Hospice-and-Palliative-Nurses-in-Research.pdf

Hospice and Palliative Nurses Association. (2015c). *Palliative nursing leadership* [Position Statement]. Retrieved from http://hpna.advancingexpertcare.org/wp-content/uploads/2015/02/Position-Statement-on-Palliative-Nursing-Leadership.pdf

Hospice and Palliative Nurses Association. (2016). Measuring what matters. Retrieved from http://www.advancingexpertcare.org/research/measuring-what-matters

Hospice Association of America. (2016). *Hospice patient's bill of rights*. Retrieved from http://www3.nahc.org/haa/attachments/BillofRights.pdf

Infoplease. (2016). *Life expectancy by age, 1850–2004*. Retrieved from http://www.infoplease.com/ipa/A0005140.html

Institute of Medicine. (2011). *The future of nursing: Leading change, advancing health*. Retrieved from https://www.nap.edu/read/12956/chapter/1

Institute of Medicine. (2015). *Dying in America: Improving quality and honoring individual preferences near the end of life*. Retrieved from https://www.nap.edu/read/18748/chapter/1

Interprofessional Education Collaborative Expert Panel. (2011). *Core competencies for interprofessional collaborative practice: Report of an expert panel*. Retrieved from http://www.aacnnursing.org/Portals/42/Population%20Health/IPECReport.pdf?ver=2017-08-03-134812-943

Jackson, J., Derderian, L., White, P., Ayotte, J., Fiorini, J., Hall, R. O., & Shay, J. T. (2012). Family perspectives on end-of-life care. *Journal of Hospice & Palliative Nursing, 14*(4), 303–311.

Kaiser Health News. (2016). *Report details senior health care that misses the mark*. Retrieved from http://khn.org/news/report-details-senior-health-care-that-misses-the-mark

Kamal, A. H., LeBlanc, T. W., & Meier, D. E. (2016). Better palliative care for all improving lived experience with cancer. *Journal of the American Medical Association, 316*, 29–30. doi:10.1001/jama.2016.6491

Kelley, A. S., & Meier, D. E. (2010). Palliative care—A shifting paradigm. *New England Journal of Medicine, 363*(8), 781–782.

Kelley, A. S., & Morrison, R. S. (2015). Palliative care for the seriously ill. *New England Journal of Medicine, 373*(8), 747–755.

Larsen, P., & Jense, S. (2015). Interdisciplinary collaborative practice in hospice and palliative settings. In H. Martinez & P. Berry (Eds.), *Core curriculum for hospice and palliative registered nurse* (4th ed., pp. 17–32). Dubuque, IA: Kendall Hunt.

Lentz, J., & Sherman, D. W. (2010). Development of the specialty of hospice and palliative care nursing. In M. Matzo & D. W. Sherman (Eds.), *Palliative care nursing: Quality care to the end of life* (3rd ed., pp. 107–117). New York, NY: Springer Publishing.

Lowes, R. (2016). Medicare approves payment for end-of-life counseling. Retrieved from http://www.medscape.com/viewarticle/853541

Lunney, J. (2011, November/December). Hospice and palliative nursing research: 25 years of progress. *Journal of Hospice and Palliative Nursing, 13*(6S), S3–S7.

Malloy, P. (2015). Nursing education. In B. R. Ferrell, N. Coyle, & J. A. Paice (Eds.), *Oxford textbook of palliative nursing* (4th ed., pp. 1010–1027). New York, NY: Oxford University Press.

Martinez, J. (2011, November/December). Hospice and palliative nursing certification: The journey to defining a new nursing specialty. *Journal of Hospice and Palliative Nursing, 13*(6S), S29–S34.

May, P., Garrido, M. M., Cassel, J. B., Kelley, A. S., Meier, D. E., Normand, L. S., . . . Morrison, R. S. (2016). Palliative care teams' cost-saving effect is larger for cancer patients with higher numbers of comorbidities. *Health Affairs, 35*(1), 44–53. doi:10.1377/hlthaff.2015.0752

Meier, D. E. (2015). Palliative medicine and patient satisfaction. *Healthcare Executive, 30*(1), 54–57.

Meier, D. E., & Beresford, L. (2009). Palliative care seeks its home in national health care reform. *Journal of Palliative Medicine, 12*(7), 593–597.

Morham, D. D., & Pollack, K. M. (2013). End-of-life care issues: A personal, economic, public policy, and public health crisis. *American Journal of Public Health, 103*(6), e8–e10. Retrieved from http://www.ncbi.nlm.nih.gov/pmc/articles/PMC3698717

Morrison, R. S., Bowman, B., Meier, D. E., & Back, A. L. (2016). Educational offerings and technology. *Journal of Palliative Medicine, 19*(5), 481. doi:10.1089/jpm.2016.0042

Morrison, R. S., Penrod, J. D., Cassel, J. B., Caust-Ellenbogen, M., Litke, A., Spragens, L., & Meier, D. E.; Palliative Care Leadership Centers' Outcomes Group. (2008). Cost savings associated with US hospital palliative care consultation programs. *Archives of Internal Medicine, 168*(16), 1783–1790.

National Consensus Project for Quality Palliative Care (2009). Clinical practice guidelines for quality palliative care (2nd ed.). Pittsburgh, PA: Author.

National Consensus Project for Quality Palliative Care. (2013). *Clinical practice guidelines for quality palliative care* (3rd ed.). Pittsburgh, PA: Author.

National Hospice and Palliative Care Organization. (2015). *The medicare hospice benefit.* Retrieved from http://www.nhpco.org/sites/default/files/public/communications/Outreach/The_Medicare_Hospice_Benefit.pdf

National Hospice and Palliative Care Organization. (2016). Personalize Your Care Act by Rep. Earl Blumenhauer and Rep. Phil Roe, U.S. House of Representatives Hospice Action Network. Retrieved from https://www.nhpco.org/press-room/press-releases/nhpco-applauds-personalize-your-care-act-2016

National Institute of Nursing Research. (2016). NIH resources to help families navigate pediatric palliative care. Retrieved from https://www.nih.gov/news-events/news-releases/nih-resources-help-families-navigate-pediatric-palliative-care

National Institutes of Health. (2016). Because of nursing research: End of life care in the ICU. Retrieved from https://www.ninr.rnih.gov/newsandinformation/because-of-nursing-research-curtis-eol

National Quality Forum. (2006). *A national framework and preferred practices for palliative and hospice care quality.* Retrieved from http://www.qualityforum.org/publications/2006/12/A_National_Framework_and_Preferred_Practices_for_Palliative_and_Hospice_Care_Quality.aspx

National Quality Forum. (2012a, June). *Measure application partnership: Performance measurement coordination strategy for hospice and palliative care* [Final Report] (pp. 2–25). Washington, DC: Author.

National Quality Forum. (2012b). *Mission and vision.* Retrieved from http://www.qualityforum.org/About_NQF/Mission_and_Vision.aspx

Ostrov, B. F. (2016). End-of-life care discussions are challenging for doctors, study finds. *Kaiser Health News*. Retrieved from http://www.cnn.com/2016/04/19/health/end-of-life-care-discussions

Otis-Green, S., & Fineberg, I. C. (2015). Enhancing team effectiveness. In B. R. Ferrell, N. Coyle, & J. A. Paice (Eds.), *Oxford textbook of palliative nursing* (4th ed., pp. 1039–1047). New York, NY: Oxford University Press.

Pace, J. C., & Lunsford, B. (2011, November/December). The evolution of palliative care nursing education. *Journal of Hospice and Palliative Nursing, 13*(6S), S8–S19.

Palliative Care and Hospice Education and Training Act. (2015). HR 3119, S.2748, 114th Congress, 1st Session, 2015.

Pear, R. (2016). National health spending to surpass $10,000 a person in 2016. Retrieved from http://www.nytimes.com/2016/07/14/US/national-health-spending-to-surpass-10000-per-person-in-2016.html?mcubz=3

Penn Medicine. (2016). *Cost of end-of-life care in the U.S. is comparable to Europe and Canada, finds New Penn Study*. Retrieved from http://www.uphs.upenn.edu/news/News_Releases/2016/01/emanuel

Pitorak, E., & Armour, M. B. (2003). Project safe conduct integrates palliative goals into comprehensive cancer care. *Journal of Palliative Medicine, 6*(4), 645–655.

Prince-Paul, M., & Daly, B. J. (2015). Ethical considerations in palliative care. In B. R. Ferrell, N. Coyle, & J. A. Paice (Eds.), *Oxford textbook of palliative nursing* (4th ed., pp. 987–1000). New York, NY: Oxford University Press.

Ranganathan, A., Dougherty, M., Waite, D., & Casarett, D. (2013). Can palliative home care reduce 30-day readmissions? Results of a propensity score matched cohort study. *Journal of Palliative Medicine, 16*(10), 1290–1293.

Reifsnyder, J., & Yeo, T. P. (2011). Continuity of care. In D. B. Nash, J. Reifsnyder, R. J. Fabius, & V. P. Pracilio (Eds.), *Population health: Creating a culture of wellness* (pp. 63–88). Sudbury, MA: Jones & Bartlett.

Schaffer, M. A., Keenan, K., Zwirchitz, F., & Tierschel, L. (2012, January/February). End-of-life discussion in assisted living facilities. *Journal of Hospice and Palliative Nursing, 14*(1), 13–24.

Sherman, D. W., & Cheon, J. (2012). Palliative care: A paradigm of care responsive to the demands for health care reform in America. *Nursing Economic$, 30*(3), 153–162, 166.

Sopcheck, J. (2016). Social, economic and political issues affecting end-of-life care. *Policy, Politics & Nursing Practice, 17*(1), 32–42. doi:10.1177/1527154416642664

Tilden, V., Corless, I., Dahlin, C., Ferrell, B., Gibson, R., & Lentz, J. (2012). Advance care planning as an urgent public health concern. Nursing Outlook, 60, 418–419. Retrieved from http://www.nursing-outlook.org/article/S0029-6554(12)00250-3/pdf

U.S. Department of Labor Bureau of Labor Statistics. (2015). Employment projections—2014–2024. USDL-15-2327. Retrieved from http://www.bls.gov/emp/tables.htm

U.S. News. (2013). *What people who live to 100 have in common*. Retrieved from https://money.usnews.com/money/retirement/articles/2013/01/07/what-people-who-live-to-100-have-in-common

Wei, R., Anderson, R. N., Curtin, L., & Arias, E. (2012). U.S. decennial life tables for 1999–2001: State life tables. *National Vital Statistics Report, 60*(9). Retrieved from https://www.cdc.gov/nchs/data/nvsr/nvsr60/nvsr60_09.pdf

Weissman, D. E., & Meier, D. E. (2011). Identifying patients in need of a palliative care assessment in the hospital setting: A consensus report from the Center to Advance Palliative Care. *Journal of Palliative Medicine, 14*(1), 17–23.

West, L. A., Cole, S., Goodkind, D., & He, W. (2014). *65+ in the United States: 2010*. Retrieved from https://www.census.gov/content/dam/Census/library/publications/2014/demo/p23-212.pdf

Wiencek, C. (2015). The advanced practice registered nurse. In B. R. Ferrell, N. Coyle, & J. A. Paice (Eds.), *Oxford textbook of palliative nursing* (4th ed., pp. 961–968). New York, NY: Oxford University Press.

Zeytinoglu, M. (2011). Talking it out: Helping our patients live better while dying. *Annals of Internal Medicine, 154*(12), 830–832. Retrieved from http://www.lynnlauner.com/yahoo_site_admin/assets/docs/The_Dying_Persons_Bill_of_Rights.114130706.pdf

CHAPTER 18

Health Policy Implications of Genetics and Genomics on Advanced Practice Nursing

Elizabeth L. Pestka and Karen L. Zanni

Genetics, focusing on individual genes, and genomics, which involves the broader study of genes and their interactions with other genes and environmental influences, have gained much greater relevance to health and to the risk for both rare and common diseases and treatment responsiveness (Calzone et al., 2013; Camak, 2016; Feero, Guttmacher, & Collins, 2010). Identification of genomic differences that influence disorders provides information that is enhancing understanding about the biology of disease, resulting in more precise interventions influencing health care decisions (Burke, Love, Jones, & Fife, 2016; Calzone et al., 2010; Feero et al., 2010).

Nursing brings an important and essential perspective to the utilization of genetics and genomics through focus on health promotion, caring, and the understanding of individuals, including their relationships with families, the community, and society (Calzone et al., 2013). The integration of genetics and genomics into pharmacotherapeutics and treatment guidelines for many diseases and disorders has been the catalyst for advancing integration into nursing practice (Camak, 2016). Nurses play an essential role in creating an infrastructure that supports delivery of services that maximize utilization of genomic information (Calzone et al., 2013). Nurses also can influence policies related to the utilization of genomic information associated with ethical, legal, and social issues (Calzone et al., 2013; Lea, 2008). With a comprehensive understanding of the relevance as well as appreciation of the limitations of genomic information, nurses can be influential in the application of genomics to clinical care (Calzone et al., 2013; Thompson & Brooks, 2011).

This chapter provides historic information explaining how genetics and genomics information has become increasingly relevant and important to health care and nursing. Competencies, standards, and outcome measures related to the use of genetics/genomics information and interventions by Advanced Practice

Registered Nurses (APRNs) are identified. In addition, areas within genetics and genomics involving ethical and health policy issues that are important to APRNs are presented. For each area discussed an overview of current and/or emerging ethical and health policy issues is the focus. Approaches are described so that APRNs can integrate timely knowledge into practice to most fully meet the needs of their clients, families, and society.

HISTORICAL BACKGROUND

In the distant past, philosophers and scientists conjured up theories of how transmission of traits to offspring occurred. Gregor Mendel, a monk in central Europe who is posthumously recognized as the father of modern genetics, studied pea plants and described the laws of inheritance in a scientific publication in 1866 (De Castro, 2016). While Mendel's research was with plants, the basic principles of heredity that he discovered also apply to humans because the mechanisms of genetic transmission are essentially the same for all complex life forms (De Castro, 2016). For a long time, a rather small number of health care professionals specialized in genetics and focused on the relatively rare disorders caused by single gene mutations.

The impact of genetics was significantly broadened in 1999 when international funding support was made available for mapping of the entire human genome as part of the Human Genome Project (HGP; Collins, 1999). This international effort, completed in 2003, created a map of the approximately 80,000 genes to 100,000 genes that contain basic DNA information that directs the structure and function of the human body (Jenkins, 2000). The mapping and sequencing of the human genome enhanced opportunities for rapidly evolving research technologies leading to pathology in health related to both rare and common disorders (Lea, Skirton, Read, & Williams, 2011). It is important to note that as the first director of the National Centre for Human Genome Research overseeing use of the HGP data, James Watson pledged that 3% to 5% of the project's budget was devoted to addressing ethical, legal, and social issues that arose from study of the human genome (Lorentz, Wieben, Tefferi, Whiteman, & Dewald, 2002).

Since the mapping of the human genome was completed in 2003, research efforts are rapidly improving understanding of the functions and interactions of all genes in the genome as well as interactions with each other and environmental influences (American Nurses Association [ANA] & International Society of Nurses in Genetics [ISONG], 2016). This has resulted in a shift from the focus on single genes, genetics, to a much broader use of inheritance information, genomics, affecting all areas of health care and nursing practice (ANA & ISONG, 2016; Calzone et al., 2010; Camak, 2016; Lea et al., 2011). Genetic and genomic research findings and technologies are now routinely used in health care, and nurses are challenged to incorporate this important information into their clinical practice.

Genetics nursing practice in the United States has historical roots in public health nursing, prenatal and neonatal screening, and pediatrics mostly through maternal and child health programs. In the 1960s, nurses in North America and Europe began to discuss their observations and the implications of genetics/genomics for professional nursing practice while providing care for individuals, families, and communities (ANA & ISONG, 2016). In the United States, the passage of the Genetic Diseases Act in 1976 supported funding of state and federal programs to provide prenatal and pediatric genetics/genomics services, and the nursing profession was an important aspect of this initiative. In response, a nursing consensus conference was held in 1980 to identify the level of genetics education received by undergraduate and graduate nurses, to describe knowledge needed by all nurses, and to make recommendations for programs to address the gaps between knowledge and practice (Forsman, 1994).

From 1980 to 1984 a growing number of nurses were involved in local, state, and federal genetics services programs. Focus on activities included development of educational resources on genetics, facilitation of community support groups for individuals and their families with a genetic condition, and support of public policy on behalf of those whose lives were affected by genetic disorders. A few nurses were certified as genetic counselors by the American Board of Medical Genetics. In 1984, the Genetics Nurses Network was formed which brought together nurses who identified their practice as genetics nursing. The focus on this group was to provide educational programs that highlighted the unique practice challenges encountered in genetics nursing (ANA & ISONG, 2007; ISONG & ANA, 1998).

A nursing organization with a broader scope, ISONG was established in 1988 to promote the scientific, professional, and personal development of genetics nurses worldwide in the management of genetics information, and it continues as an important professional nursing resource. ISONG's original vision was, "Caring for people's genetic health," and has been enhanced to a current vision of, "Caring for people's genetic and genomic health." Throughout the 1990s nurses continued to define the requisite knowledge and scope of genetics nursing practice. In 1997, the ANA conferred specialty practice status on genetics nursing in the United States. In 1998, the initial publication of the scope and standards of genetics nursing practice and in 2007 an updated edition broadened the specialty to genetics/genomics nursing (ANA & ISONG, 2007; ISONG & ANA, 1998).

In 1999, ISONG created a credentialing committee to oversee a process for providing recognition of competence in genetics/genomics nursing. Working from the ISONG scope and standards of genetics/genomics nursing practice, the committee established a list of core competencies and assessment measures and a professional portfolio method for credentialing genetics/genomics nurses at the baccalaureate and master's level (Cook, Kase, Middleton, & Monsen, 2003). In 2002, the Genetics Nursing Credentialing Commission was created to oversee the credentialing of nurses in genetics/genomics (Monsen, 2005). The credentialing process for genetics/genomics nursing further evolved in 2014 when oversight was transitioned to the American Nurses Credentialing Center with a professional portfolio method used to demonstrate specialty knowledge and competence (American Nurses Credentialing Center, n.d.).

Nursing education has also focused on inclusion of genetics and genomics in both undergraduate and graduate curriculums. The American Association of Colleges of Nursing revised the *Essentials of Baccalaureate Education for Professional Nursing Practice* in 2008, which now integrates genetic/genomic concepts as foundational for baccalaureate nursing curriculum (American Association of Colleges of Nursing, 2008). Similarly, graduate nursing education also is requiring inclusion of genetic/genomic information in all accredited programs (American Association of Colleges of Nursing, 2011).

FRAMEWORK FOR GENETICS AND GENOMICS NURSING

The overall framework for genetics and genomics nursing requires an understanding of the basic principles of inheritance and developing a philosophy of care that has this information at its core (Lea & Smith, 2003). This means always including in a nursing assessment how genetics/genomics factors are influencing an individual's health. Each person's health is influenced over time through complex psychological processes that include biological and genetic aspects, cognitive development, and experiential events within relationships (Jenkins & Lea, 2005).

The International Council of Nurse's *Code of Ethics for Nurses* (2012) provides a framework for ethical inclusion of genetics/genomics information in nursing practice worldwide. In addition, in the United States, *The Code of Ethics for Nurses with Interpretive Statements* (ANA, 2015) provides guidance for ethical individualized care. When assessing, planning, and providing services for persons with genetic/genomic conditions sensitivity to cultural, lifestyle, racial, and ethnic diversity is imperative.

APRNs are in an excellent position to be coordinators of genetics/genomics health care. They oftentimes have intimate knowledge of a client's, family's, and community's perspectives on health and disease. Nurses possess an understanding of biologic underpinnings of health conditions and skills in communication and building relationships. Across the entire life span, nursing focuses on health promotion and disease prevention. To gain the most benefit from genetic/genomic discoveries, APRNs must be competent to obtain comprehensive family histories and recognize risk factors, identify individuals and family members at risk for developing genomic influenced conditions and for genomic influenced drug reactions, help people make informed decisions about genetics/genomics tests and therapies, and refer at-risk persons to appropriate health care professionals for specialized care.

APPLICATION TO ALL APRNs

Advances in genetics and genomics over the past 20 years have necessitated initiatives on the part of all health care disciplines including nursing. Nursing has responded by developing core competencies for all nurses (Consensus Panel on Genetic/Genomic Nursing Competencies, 2009) and then more specific competencies for APRNs (Greco, Tinley, & Siebert, 2012). Baseline genetic and genomic competencies for all nurses who are functioning at a graduate level in nursing were developed in 2012 by a diverse panel of nursing leaders and genetics experts representing professional nursing organizations, academic institutions, regulatory bodies, and government agencies (Greco et al., 2012). The process for establishing competencies followed a structured, methodical approach with validation by consensus of 31 nursing leaders. These graduate nursing competencies build upon a set of core competencies for all nurses, *Essentials of Genetics and Genomic Nursing: Competencies, Curricula Guidelines, and Outcome Indicators* (Consensus Panel on Genetic/Genomic Nursing Competencies, 2009) and assume that graduate nurses have already achieved the basic genetic/genomic competencies.

Greco et al. (2012) conducted a comprehensive review of the literature between 1997 and 2009 for key published articles and documents related to genetic/genomic competencies as part of the development process. They also reviewed 11 exam guidelines from six graduate-nursing certification bodies for genetic/genomic content:

- American Nurses Credentialing Commission: (Family Nurse Practitioner [NP], Adult NP, Pediatric NP, Gerontological NP, and Clinical Nurse Specialist [CNS] "Core" exam) www.nursecredentialing.org
- National Certification Corporation: Women's Health Care NP and Neonatal NP www.nccwebsite.org
- American Academy of Nurse Practitioners: Family NP www.aanp.org/Certification
- Pediatric Nursing Certification Board: Primary Care Pediatric NP www.pncb.org/ptistore/control/index
- American Midwifery Certification Board: Midwifery www.amcbmidwife.org
- National Board of Certification & Recertification for Nurse Anesthetists www.nbcrna.com/Exams/Pages/Exams.aspx

Table 18.1 lists the essential competencies in genetics and genomics identified for all nurses with graduate degrees and additional items specific to nurses functioning in APRN roles.

APPLICATION TO GENETICS/GENOMICS SPECIALTY NURSING PRACTICE

The ANA and the ISONG collaborated to identify six standards of practice to describe a competent level of genetics/genomics nursing care for nurses specializing in this area as demonstrated by the critical thinking model known as the nursing process (ANA & ISONG, 2016). This process encompasses all significant actions taken by registered nurses. The standards for practice are:

Standard 1. Assessment: The genetics/genomics nurse collects comprehensive data pertinent to the client's health and/or the situation.
Standard 2. Diagnosis: The genetics/genomics nurse analyzes the assessment data to determine the diagnoses or the issues.
Standard 3. Outcomes identification: The genetics/genomics nurse identifies expected outcomes for a plan individualized to the client or the situation.
Standard 4. Planning: The genetics/genomics nurse develops a plan that prescribes strategies and alternatives to attain expected outcomes.
Standard 5. Implementation: The genetics/genomics nurse implements the identified plan.
   5A: Coordination of care
   5B: Health teaching and health promotion
   5C: Consultation
   5D: Prescriptive authority and treatment
Standard 6. Evaluation: The genetics/genomics nurse evaluates progress toward attainment of outcomes.

TABLE 18.1 Essential Competencies in Genetics and Genomics for Nurses With Graduate Degrees

	ALL NURSES WITH GRADUATE DEGREES	IN ADDITION FOR NURSES WITH GRADUATE DEGREES FUNCTIONING IN ADVANCED PRACTICE REGISTERED NURSE (APRN) ROLES
Professional Practice: Risk Assessment and Interpretation	Identify clients with inherited predispositions to diseases as appropriate to the nurse's practice setting.	Analyze a pedigree to identify potential inherited predispositions to disease. Estimate risks for Mendelian and multifactorial disorders in affected families as appropriate. Use family history and pedigree information to plan and conduct a targeted physical assessment. Interpret the findings from the physical assessment, family history, laboratory findings, diagnostic tests, and/or radiology results that may indicate a genetics/genomics referral. Refer at-risk family members for assessment of inherited predisposition to disease.
Professional Practice: Genetic Education, Counseling, Testing, and Results Interpretation	Incorporate clients' attitudes, values, and beliefs rooted in varying ethnic, cultural, social, and religious backgrounds when communicating genetic/genomic information. Provide genetic/genomic information that is appropriate to client's level of health literacy and numeracy. Educate clients about possible risks, benefits, and limitations of genetic testing and/or therapy. Provide anticipatory guidance to assist clients in the decision-making process related to genetics/genomics. Obtain informed consent for genetic/genomic testing and/or therapy. Assess the influence of genetic/genomic risk and disease on family communication and functioning. Assess the clinical and psychosocial outcome, including benefits, limitations, and risk of genetic/genomic information and/or therapies, for clients. Support client coping and client use of genetic/genomic information in promoting health, reducing risk, managing symptoms, and/or preventing illness.	Provide genetic/genomic education and counselling appropriate to practice setting. Select appropriate genetic/genomic tests and/or studies. Communicate results of genetic/genomic screening and/or testing at a level that clients can understand.
Professional Practice: Clinical Management	Apply knowledge about the interaction of genetic/genomic and environmental factors to the care of clients. Make appropriate referrals to genetic professional or other health care resources. Evaluate effectiveness of prevention, risk reductions, health promotion, and disease management interventions related to genetics/genomics.	Manage care of clients, incorporating genetic/genomic information and technology (e.g., risk-based genetic screening and testing, prescription of pharmacogenomics-based drugs, gene-targeted therapy, and use of genetic/genomic information in symptom management). Collaborate with genetic specialists, health professionals, and those in relevant disciplines to develop a comprehensive plan to evaluate and manage clients with genetic/genomic disease or risk.

Professional Practice: Ethical, Legal, and Social Implications (ELSI)	Facilitate ethical decision-making related to genetics/genomics congruent with the client's values and beliefs. Inform health care and research policy related to ELSI issues in genetics/ genomics. Implement effective strategies to resolve ELSI issues in genetics/ genomics. Apply ethical principles when making decisions regarding management of genetic/genomic information identified through clinical or research technologies.		
Professional Responsibilities: Professional Role	Integrate best genetic/genomic evidence into practice that incorporates client values and clinical judgment. Mentor other nurses in the application of genetics/genomics to nursing care within their practice setting. Identify genetic/genomic learning needs of other health professionals and disciplines. Conduct educational interventions to address the genetic/genomic learning needs of health professionals and clients. Participate in the development of professional practice guidelines related to genetics/genomics.		
Professional Responsibilities: Leadership	Contribute a nursing perspective to genetic/genomic clinical and policy discussions. Facilitate an organizational climate that is responsive to genetic/genomic discoveries. Use care delivery strategies which incorporate genetic/genomics. Influence health policy at the local, state, national, and international levels related to genetics/genomics.		
Professional Responsibilities: Research	Participate in the application and translation of genetic/genomic research in nursing practice and/or education. Identify genetic/genomic health care methods and outcomes that can be influenced by nursing. Collaborate with researchers in relevant disciplines in the conduct, dissemination, and/or translation of genomics inquiry and research.		

Source: Greco, Tinley, and Seibert (2012).

EVALUATION OF ADVANCED PRACTICE NURSING OUTCOMES

Establishing genetic and genomic competencies is the first step toward ensuring that nurses with graduate degrees are prepared to deliver genetic/genomic care. The next major initiative is to develop performance, or outcome, indicators related to each identified competency. The plan, which is not yet completed, is to use a process similar to the one used for the basic competencies which identified measurable outcomes for each competency item (Consensus Panel on Genetic/Genomic Nursing Competencies, 2009).

A study of one defined group of 211 advanced practice genetics nurses in the United States who were members of the ISONG provides a snapshot of integration of genetics/genomics into practice (Lea et al., 2006). The most common specialty areas were oncology, neonatal, and pediatric. However, all specialty areas of professional nursing were identified. Most survey respondents provided key services including information on genetics/genomics, psychosocial counseling or support, pedigree construction and family history analysis, and genetic counseling. Proportion of professional time by activity revealed that education or teaching represented 39% of time, followed by patient care (20%), research (19%), administration (16%), and community health (7%). Nurses reported that they are considered colleagues of other genetic/genomic specialists and participate in numerous venues to advance genetics care (Lea et al., 2006).

ETHICAL CONSIDERATIONS

Molecular genetic techniques developed during the HGP are transforming research, clinical practice, and health care delivery. Progress in the identification of genes involved in monogenic disorders and multifactorial inheritance, pharmacotherapy metabolism and dose-response, as well as the detection of single nucleotide polymorphisms (SNPs), make evident the promise of genetic testing (Collins & McKusick, 2001; National Human Genome Research Institute, 2012; Subramanian, Adams, Venter, & Broder, 2001). Although these new advances raise expectations for disease prevention and treatment, they also present equally challenging ethical and health policy issues to clients and health care providers (Figure 18.1).

The National Human Genome Research Institute's (NHGRI) Ethical, Legal, and Social Implications (ELSI) Research Program was established in 1990 as a part of the HGP to promote basic and applied research on the ethical, legal, and social implications of genetic and genomic research for individuals, families, and communities. This early focus on ELSI recognized the importance of health policies to ensure ethical management of genetic and genomic technologies and information (Lorentz et al., 2002). *Nature* magazine published the NHGRI's strategic plan for the future of human genomics research called *Charting a Course for Genomic Medicine: From Base Pairs to Bedside*. This strategic plan was developed to stimulate researchers to advance genomic understanding through research in several areas (Green, Guyer, & NHGRI Affiliations, 2011). Based on these areas, the NHGRI has developed four broad research priorities (Table 18.2).

APRNs often take part in genetic and genomic-based practice activities such as taking a family history, managing gene-based therapies, and attaining

Genetic privacy and confidentiality	• Should individuals be able to control access to the results of their tests? • Who owns genetic information?
Genetic discrimination	• Should there be more comprehensive provisions of the Genetic Information Nondiscrimination Act (GINA) that prohibit discrimination based on phenotype? • Should employers be able to require or request an individual undergo genetic testing or disclose the results of a genetic test as a condition of employment?
Equitable access to genomic technologies	• How might genomic technologies be made available to those with fewer resources, especially resource-poor nations, the uninsured, rural and inner-city communities?
Genetic information and the impact on individuals and society	• How does a person's genetic information affect that individual and society's perception of that individual? • How does genetic and genomic information affect members of minority communities?

FIGURE 18.1 Ethical challenges for health care providers.

Source: Adapted from National Human Genome Research Institute (2015).

TABLE 18.2 National Human Genome Research Institute Research Priorities

• **Genomic research**: Issues that arise in the design and conduct of genomic research, particularly as it involves the production, analysis, and sharing of individual genomic information that is frequently coupled with detailed health information.
• **Genomic health care**: Rapid advances in genomic technologies and the availability of increasing amounts of genomic information influence how health care is provided and how it affects the health of individuals, families, and communities.
• **Broader societal issues**: Beliefs, practices, and policies regarding genomic information and technologies, as well as the implications of genomics for how we conceptualize and understand health, disease, and individual responsibility.
• **Legal, regulatory, and public policy issues**: Existing genomic research, health and public policies and regulations; new policies and regulatory approaches.

Source: Adapted from Green, Guyer, and National Human Genome Research Institute (2011).

informed consent for genetic testing. APRNs also have an important role in educating, supporting, counseling, and advocating for clients and families who are making genetic and genomic-based health care decisions (Greco et al., 2012). The promise of genetically informed, personalized clinical care is now a possibility and APRNs need to translate genetic and genomic information in an understandable way to their clients and families. One of the greatest challenges is translating unfamiliar language from the genetics and genomics field into language that providers can understand, and take action on, and then convey to clients. This new direction in health care calls for APRNs to integrate the evolving capabilities of personalized genetic and genomic information into their scope of practice.

If genetics and genomics approaches are to become part of standard health care, providers, including APRNs, will need to know more about molecular genetics and these new technologies. APRNs will increasingly find themselves needing to interpret the results of genetic tests, understand how that information is relevant to treatment or prevention approaches, and convey this knowledge to clients and families (Vorderstrasse, Hammer, & Dungan, 2014). Advanced practice nursing competencies have been established but specific measurement of competent integration into practice still needs to be completed and promoted.

INFORMED DECISION MAKING AND INFORMED CONSENT

As personal genetic information becomes increasingly accessible and available, the protection of such data challenges APRNs to understand the ethical concerns associated with processes such as informed decision making and informed consent. Genetic technologies, including molecular genetic testing, can now be used for client screening and diagnosis, to guide therapy, as well as for health and reproductive decision making. Benefits of genetic testing may include early detection for some treatable disorders to enable prevention, before the onset of symptoms for those individuals who are at risk for a genetic condition are manifested. Genetic testing may also be used to enable parents to make reproductive decisions. Consumers of genetic technologies may also appreciate the psychological and social benefit of knowing their genetic risks. APRNs need to understand possible adverse effects of genetic testing, which can include psychosocial distress, altered family functioning, misinterpretation of the meaning of results, discrimination, and additional health care resource use (NHGRI, 2015). APRNs have a central role in providing accurate information and support to clients in the process of genetic testing. With knowledge related to genetics and genomics, APRNs can advocate, educate, counsel, and support clients during the informed decision-making process. Health policies must ensure and support ongoing informed decision making and informed consent for all clients.

APRNs have a responsibility to alert clients prior to consenting to genetic testing of their right to make an informed decision (ANA, 2015). Informed decision making and informed consent involve making sure the individual understands the benefits and risks of the procedure, and that the individual gives consent without coercion (ANA, 2015). The increasing availability of genetic information and technology means that clients and their family members will be learning more about their distinct genetic status and making decisions based on this information. The consequence for APRNs is that they will increasingly be involved in counseling clients about these issues during the process of obtaining consent. APRNs are often a part of a collaborative process of genetic testing and need to advocate for the informed decision-making authority of the client to make their own choice whether to accept or reject testing. Pivotal to completing this process is a dialogue between the client and the provider in a joint endeavor to facilitate informed decision making through open discussion and an honest exchange of relevant information at the level of language comprehensible to the client. The dialogue needs to include encouraging clients to seek information and identify concerns before undergoing genetic testing. The nursing process can be universally utilized to assist clients contemplating any type of genetic testing to ascertain whether essential information is understood and is part of the decision-making process. Routine activities that have genetic/genomic implications include collecting and assessing a family history and requesting medical/patient health information, and clients need to understand how this information will be used for their care.

ENSURING PRIVACY AND CONFIDENTIALITY OF GENETIC AND GENOMIC INFORMATION

The clinical use of genetic and genomic information is becoming an increasingly common aspect of today's health care delivery. According to the Genetic Information Nondiscrimination Act (GINA), "genetic information" means information about a person's genetic tests, genetic tests of a person's family members, any manifestation of a disease or disorder in a family member, participation of a person or family member in research that includes genetic testing, counseling, or education (NHGRI, 2016). Genetic information can be identified at any point throughout an individual's life course from pre-conception until after death. Genetic technologies are generating new sources of health information for clients, their families, and communities that elicit important ethical, legal, and social issues. While this information has the potential to provide health benefits, it may also increase risk of harm. APRNs need to be comfortable with the nature and sources of genetic information so that they can ensure privacy and confidentiality for their clients. Of major concern is the potential for misuse of genetic information resulting in any kind of discrimination or stigmatization. Continued vigilance on the part of APRNs is required as genetic technologies and discoveries are increasingly translated into clinical application and practice, assuring privacy and confidentiality of genetic information. Comprehensive health policies supporting privacy and confidentiality of genetic and genomic information are essential.

The current ANA *Code of Ethics for Nurses* (ANA, 2015) is clear in intent and meaning as it relates to the nurse's role in promoting and advocating for patients' rights related to privacy and confidentiality. Privacy, as defined by the ANA *Code of Ethics for Nurses* (2015) involves the right of the individual to control his or her own body, actions, and personal information. Confidentiality refers to the nurse's duty to protect, and not to disclose, personal information provided in confidence to another. Genetic information acquired from family history and genetic testing, nevertheless, may reveal knowledge not only about the health risks of the individual client being seen, but also of other family members who may not be aware of the health condition. APRNs must recognize that each individual in a family is autonomous with respect to genetic matters that may be compromised by decisions of other family members.

When an individual is identified as being at risk for a genetic condition, the entire family may be affected by this information. Communication within families about genetic risk is important because it is essential to independent decision making. Whether a person discloses genetic information, even to family members, depends on many factors. In order to help individuals and families make decisions about disclosing genetic information regarding risk, and avoid undue distress in the process, APRNs must understand the issues that affect families when genetic risk is discussed. An ethical issue can occur for nurses and other health care providers when a client does not choose to share genetic information with other family members when it may be valuable to that person's health. This produces a dilemma for the health care provider, who on the one hand must respect the client's confidentiality, while on the other hand recognizes a responsibility to inform other family members of their potential health risk. It is currently accepted that a provider needs to inform the client of the benefit of sharing risk information with family members. In the clinical setting, policies must be developed and followed to protect patient information, and APRNs can help ensure that the policies meet current needs and circumstances. Maintaining client privacy and confidentiality when managing genetic information and providing genomic care is essential in meeting the needs of clients and families.

AVOIDING GENETIC DISCRIMINATION

Many individuals fear that undergoing genetic testing or participating in genetic or genomic research will lead to discrimination based on test results. Such fears may lead to refusing genomics-based clinical tests or dissuade people from volunteering to participate in research studies necessary for the development of new tests, therapies, and cures. To address this, in 2008 the GINA was passed into law, prohibiting discrimination in the workplace and by health insurance issuers. In addition, there are other legal protections against genetic discrimination by employers, issuers of health insurance, and others. In this act, genetic information refers to information about a person's genetic tests, the genetic tests of a person's family members, and the incidence of diseases in a person's family. GINA also includes information about any person's or family's request for, or receipt of, genetic services or their participation in clinical research that involves genetic services (NHGRI, 2016).

APRNs must have an understanding of how genetic testing will impact their clients' lives, financially, emotionally, and otherwise. APRNs must understand exactly what GINA does and does not cover in order to responsibly advise their clients in regard to genetic testing. Prior to GINA's inception, professional careers and insurance coverage were potentially at risk. Even with GINA, not all clients are fully protected. Simply stated, GINA prohibits employers and health insurers from using genetic information to discriminate. At this time, however, GINA has important limitations of which clinicians also need to be aware. GINA does *not* cover an individual's manifested disease or condition—a condition which an individual is experiencing, is being treated for, or has been diagnosed with (NHGRI, 2016).

GINA is a step in the right direction toward protecting individuals; however, its limitations pose specific opportunities for genetic discrimination. In order to truly protect clients from discrimination, GINA must be more comprehensive to address the limitations identified in Table 18.3. Health policies must take into consideration limitations posed by GINA.

EQUITABLE ACCESS TO GENETIC AND GENOMIC TECHNOLOGIES

Genomics has become an essential element of biomedical research and clinical care. Early examples of the potential of genomic medicine have already emerged. By using genomic technologies and findings, clinical care can be precisely tailored to an individual's unique, genetically influenced predisposition to disease

TABLE 18.3 Limitations of the Genetic Information Nondiscrimination Act

• Does not cover life, disability, or long-term care insurance.
• Does not apply to members of the military, veterans obtaining care through the Veterans Administration, or the Indian Health Service.
• Applies only to employers covered under the Americans with Disabilities Act (ADA) and Title VII of the Civil Rights Act of 1964; therefore, it does not cover employers with fewer than 15 employees.
• Does not cover an individual's manifested disease or conditions–a condition from which an individual is experiencing symptoms, is being treated for, or that has been diagnosed.
• Does not interfere with an employee's ability to qualify for family or medical leave under state or federal Family Medical Leave laws, nor to participate in an employer-sponsored wellness program or other genetic services offered by an employer.
• Does not restrict genetic services, the practice of medicine, or the authority of health care professionals, whether or not they are affiliated with a health plan or insurer or an employer. Clinicians and health care providers can recommend that an individual or an individual's family member undergo a genetic test for the purposes of that individual's medical benefit.
• Does not pre-empt state law; therefore, if a state's genetic discrimination law provides more extensive protections than GINA, GINA does not change it.

Source: Adapted from National Human Genome Research Institute (2016).

and disability. Announced in 2015, the Precision Medicine Initiative in the United States gives voice to the complex task with a call to create a million-citizen cohort, assembled largely from existing cohorts, to contribute and share extensive health data including genetic and genomic information (Collins & Varmus, 2015). Researchers will need to find ways to standardize collection of data from more than one million volunteers from hospitals and clinics around the United States. They will also need to find ways to safely and securely store a large amount of private data. Then they will need to identify clinical applications for using this data to precisely provide care for a wide array of conditions and circumstances.

Cost is a concern with expanding use of genetic and genomic information. Technologies such as sequencing large amounts of DNA are still expensive, although the cost of sequencing is decreasing. Moreover, some drugs that are developed to target an individual's genetic characteristics are very expensive. Reimbursement from health care payers, such as private insurance companies, is not universally available to all individuals and therefore access to services poses an ethical issue. Receiving new precision tests and treatments needs to be equally available to all persons regardless of their wealth or social status. Health policies are needed to address this concern.

GENETIC AND GENOMIC INFORMATION AFFECTING INDIVIDUALS AND SOCIETY

There are many concerns about how a person's genetic information might affect that individual and society's perception of that individual. There are also many questions and concerns about how genetic and genomic information might affect members of minority communities (NHGRI, 2015). Establishing an ELSI focus from the inception of the HGP has helped to keep these questions in the forefront. Adhering to strict confidentiality of genetic and genomic information, demanding that all individuals need to give informed consent to testing and research, maintaining and strengthening policies to prohibit genetic discrimination, and focusing on aiming for equitable access to genomic technology for all persons is the best way to ensure positive use of this information.

To support initiatives to provide genetics and genomics services to clients, many APRNs need additional education. The technology of this field is evolving so rapidly that keeping up with new developments creates another challenge. Moreover, the brevity of current clinical encounters and time spent with clients coupled with the cost and time associated with interpreting and incorporating precision medicine data could constrain utilization. If these challenges are to be addressed, appropriate resources and training for all health care providers, including APRNs, are needed.

SUMMARY

We are in an era of identification of genetic and genomic differences that influence disorders, providing information that is enhancing understanding about the biology of disease, resulting in more precise interventions influencing health care decisions. APRNs bring an important and essential perspective to the utilization of this information through focus on health promotion, caring, and the understanding of individuals, including their relationships with families, the community, and society. APRNs have an opportunity and responsibility to influence health policies related to the utilization of genomic information associated with ethical, legal, and social issues. Areas of most concern are maintaining privacy and confidentiality of genetic/genomic information, avoiding discrimination based on genetic risks, advocating for equitable access to genomic technologies and treatments, and understanding and protecting the effects of genetic and genomic information on individuals and society.

DISCUSSION QUESTIONS

1. *Based on the information in this chapter on the advances in genetics and genomics, list at least two areas of policy change you can identify where legislation could have an impact.*
2. *If you were asked to describe the importance of health care policy changes related to genetics and genomics, what key issues would you stress?*
3. *According to the Human Genome Project Information, Privacy in Genomics, what are the primary ethical challenges for health care providers and how do they affect advanced practice nursing?*
4. *What are the consequences of no changes to health care policies regarding the use of genetic and genomic technologies and information?*
5. *Discuss the importance of the GINA.*
6. *How can health care policies promote more equal access to genetic testing and precision medicine?*

ANALYSIS, SYNTHESIS, AND CLINICAL APPLICATION

1. *Determine how to obtain informed consent for genetics/genomics testing and/or therapy.*
2. *Using your own client case example, evaluate effectiveness of prevention, risk reductions, health promotion, and disease management interventions related to genetics/genomics.*
3. *Using your own client case example, apply ethical principles when making decisions regarding use of genetics/genomics information identified through clinical evaluation and interventions.*
4. *Participate in the development of professional practice guidelines related to genetics/genomics.*

EXERCISES/CONSIDERATIONS

1. *Nurses have an essential role in supporting utilization of genomics information, interventions, and policy development.*
2. *Advanced practice nurses have developed competencies, standards, and outcome measures to guide implementation of relevant interventions into clinical practice.*
3. *Research priorities for advanced practice nurses related to genomics include designing and conducting clinically relevant studies, evaluating how genomics information affects the health of individuals, families, and communities, looking a broader societal implications associated with genomics information, and providing input on legal, regulatory, and public policy issues.*

REFERENCES

American Association of Colleges of Nursing. (2008). *The essentials of baccalaureate education for professional nursing practice.* Washington, DC: Author.

American Association of Colleges of Nursing. (2011). *Essentials of master's education in nursing.* Washington, DC: Author.

American Nurses Association. (2015). *Code of ethics for nurses with interpretive statements.* Silver Spring, MD: Nursebooks.org

American Nurses Association & International Society of Nurses in Genetics. (2007). *Genetics/genomics nursing: Scope and standards of practice.* Silver Spring, MD: Nursebooks.org

American Nurses Association & International Society of Nurses in Genetics. (2016). *Genetics/genomics nursing: Scope and standards of practice* (2nd ed.). Silver Spring, MD: Nursebooks.org

American Nurses Credentialing Center. (n.d.). Advanced genetics nursing. Retrieved from http://www.nursecredentialing.org/Certification/NurseSpecialties/AdvancedGenetics

Burke, E., Love, R., Jones, P., & Fife, T. (2016). Pharmacogenetic testing: Application in mental health prescribing. *Journal of the American Psychiatric Nurses Association, 22*(3), 185–191.

Calzone, K. A., Cashion, A., Feetham, S., Jenkins, J., Prows, C. A., Williams, J. K., & Wung, S. (2010). Nurses transforming health care using genetics and genomics. *Nursing Outlook, 58*(1), 26–35.

Camak, D. J. (2016). Increasing importance of genetics in nursing. *Nurse Education Today, 44,* 86–91.

Collins, F. (1999). Shattuck lecture: Medical and societal consequences of the human genome project. *New England Journal of Medicine, 341,* 28–36.

Collins, F. S., & McKusick, V. A. (2001). Implications of the human genome project for medical science. *Journal of the American Medical Association, 285*(5), 540–544.

Collins, F. S., & Varmus, H. (2015). A new initiative on precision medicine. *New England Journal of Medicine, 372,* 793–795.

Consensus Panel on Genetic/Genomic Nursing Competencies. (2009). *Essentials of genetic and genomic nursing: competencies, curricular guidelines, and outcome indicators* (2nd ed.). Silver Spring, MD: American

Nurses Association. Retrieved from http://www.nursingworld.org/MainMenuCategories/ EthicsStandards/Resources/Genetics_1/EssentialNursingCompetenciesandCurriularGuidelines forGeneticsandGenomics.pdf

Cook, S. S., Kase, R., Middleton, L., & Monsen, R. B. (2003). Portfolio evaluation for professional competence: Credentialing in genetics for nurses. *Journal of Professional Nursing, 19*(2), 85–90.

De Castro, M. (2016). Johan Gregor Mendel: Paragon of experimental science. *Molecular Genetics & Genomic Medicine, 4*, 3–8. doi:10.1002/mgg3.199

Feero, W. G., Guttmacher, A. E., & Collins, F. S. (2010). Genomic medicine—An updated primer. *New England Journal of Medicine, 362*(21), 2001–2011.

Forsman, I. (1994). Evolution of the nursing role in genetics. *Journal of Obstetric, Gynecologic, and Neonatal Nursing, 23*(6), 481–486.

Greco, K. E., Tinley, S., & Seibert, D. (2012). *Essential genetic and genomic competencies for nurses with graduate degrees.* Silver Spring, MD: American Nurses Association and International Society of Nurses in Genetics.

Green, E. D., Guyer, M. S., & National Human Genome Research Institute. (2011). Charting a course for genomic medicine from base pairs to bedside. *Nature, 470*, 204–213.

International Council of Nurses. (2012). *The ICN code of ethics for nurses.* Geneva, Switzerland: Author.

International Society of Nurses in Genetics & American Nurses Association. (1998). *Statement on the scope of standards of genetics clinical nursing practice.* Washington, DC: American Nurses Publishing.

Jenkins, J. F. (2000). An historical perspective on genetic care. *Online Journal of Issues in Nursing, 5*(3), Manuscript 1. Retrieved from www.nursingworld.org/MainMenuCategories/ANAMarketplace/ ANAPeriodicals/OJIN/TableofContents/Volume52000/No3Sept00/HistoricalPerspective.aspx

Jenkins, J. F., & Lea, D. H. (2005). *Nursing care in the genomic era: A case-based approach.* Sudbury, MA: Jones & Bartlett.

Lea, D. H. (2008). Genetic and genomic healthcare: Ethical issues of importance to nurses. *Online Journal of Issues in Nursing, 13*(1), Manuscript 4. doi:10.3912/OJIN.Vol13No01Man04

Lea, D. H., Skirton, H., Read, C. Y., & Williams, J. K. (2011). Implications for educating the next generation of nurses on genetics and genomics in the 21st century. *Journal of Nursing Scholarship, 43*(1), 3–12.

Lea, D. H., & Smith, R. (2003). *The genetics resource guide: A handy reference for public health nurses.* Scarborough: Maine Department of Human Services Genetics Program.

Lea, D. H., Williams, J. K., Cooksey, J. A., Flanagan, P. A., Forte, G., & Blitzer, M. G. (2006). U.S Genetics nurses in advanced practice. *Journal of Nursing Scholarship, 38*(3), 213–218.

Lorentz, C. P., Wieben, E. D., Tefferi, A., Whiteman, D. A., & Dewald, G. W. (2002). Primer on medical genomics part 1: History of genetics and sequencing of the human genome. *Mayo Clinic Proceedings, 77*, 773–782.

Monsen, R. B. (Ed.). (2005). *Genetics nursing portfolios: A new model for credentialing.* Silver Spring, MD: Nursebooks.org

National Human Genome Research Institute. (2012). Personalized medicine: How the human genome era will usher in a health care revolution. Retrieved from https://www.genome.gov/13514107

National Human Genome Research Institute. (2015). Project information: Privacy in genomics. Retrieved from https://www.genome.gov/27561246/privacy-in-genomics

National Human Genome Research Institute. (2016). Issues in genetics. Genetic discrimination. Retrieved from https://www.genome.gov/10002077

Subramanian, G., Adams, M. D., Venter, J. C., & Broder, S. (2001). Implications of the human genome for understanding human biology and medicine. *Journal of the American Medical Association, 286*(18), 2296–2307.

Thompson, H. J., & Brooks, M. V. (2011). Genetics and genomics in nursing: Evaluating essentials implementation. *Nurse Education Today, 31*, 623–627.

Vorderstrasse, A., Hammer, M. J., & Dungan, J. R. (2014). Nursing implications of personalized and precision medicine. *Seminars in Oncology Nursing, 30*(2), 130–136.

CHAPTER 19

Oncology

Kelly J. Brassil, Garry Brydges, Cynthia Abarado, and Joyce E. Dains

"To infinity and beyond." This quote from a popular Pixar animated feature accurately captures the current and future direction for oncology Advanced Practice Registered Nurses (APRNs) in the context of the National Cancer Moonshot (National Cancer Institute [NCI], 2016a). This policy-driven initiative announced by former President Barack Obama during his State of the Union address on January 28, 2016, aims to "accelerate progress towards prevention, treatment, and a cure—to double the rate of progress in the fight against cancer—and put ourselves on a path to achieve in just 5 years research and treatment gains that otherwise might take a decade or more" (The White House Office of the Press Secretary, 2016c). The National Cancer Moonshot initiative, while research driven, impacts all aspects of cancer care delivery, focusing on expanding clinical trials, enhanced data sharing, cancer immunology and prevention, implementation sciences, pediatric cancer, precision prevention and early detection, tumor progression and evolution (NCI, 2017). This includes the integration of proteomics, immunotherapy, and precision medicine (Conrads & Petricoin, 2016), for each of which the oncology APRN has an integral role in the education and clinical management of cancer patients. From identifying patients for clinical trials to the management of side effects from new and emerging treatments, the role of oncology APRNs will be influenced now and in the future as a result of this significant policy-driven initiative (Kennedy Sheldon, 2016). Because of their engagement in oncology care across the cancer continuum and in a diversity of settings, oncology APRNs are well positioned to support the implementation and execution of the goals of the National Cancer Moonshot.

This chapter presents an overview of the role of oncology APRNs and how their education, training, and practice are influenced by health policy, most notably that associated with the National Cancer Moonshot. Specific emphasis is given to the influence of health policy on oncology APRNs' prescriptive authority and their unique role in cancer prevention and survivorship. Ultimately, the National Cancer Moonshot seeks to take all oncology providers, including

APRNs, to infinity and beyond, as we engage in the next major evolution of cancer treatment, care, and prevention.

ONCOLOGY AS A SPECIALTY NURSING PRACTICE

Oncology APRNs are a unique cohort of health care providers, specialized through education, certification, the population with whom they work, or a combination of these factors. The oncology APRN has a distinct place in a health care specialty that provides for 14.5 million individuals living with cancer in the United States (American Cancer Society, 2016). Cancer impact and incidence (Box 19.1) continue to grow, with an estimated 1.6 million new cases expected to be diagnosed each year (American Cancer Society, 2016), yet the availability of specialized advanced practice providers is challenged by policy-related changes in how these professionals are educated, certified, and licensed from state to state. Further, evolving prescribing practices, with great variability between states, can contribute to challenges in care coordination and provision.

The APRN *Consensus Model* and Its Impact on Licensure, Accreditation, Credentialing, and Education

As outlined in Chapter 6, the APRN *Consensus Model* guides the licensure, accreditation, certification, and education of APRNs (APRN Consensus Work Group & the National Council of State Boards of Nursing APRN Advisory Committee, 2008). Because oncology is defined as a specialty area, preparation as an oncology specialist is optional and must build on the APRN role and population focus. Competency for oncology specialization will be assessed and regulated by professional organizations instead of the state board of nursing (APRN Consensus Work Group & the National Council of State Boards of Nursing APRN Advisory Committee, 2008). As a result, oncology specialization in the form of education, certification, and licensure is significantly affected by changes associated with this regulatory model.

Education

As a result of the APRN *Consensus Model*, educational institutions have moved away from specialized degree programs, although optional concentrations or postmaster's certification are still offered (Duke University School of Nursing,

---

CANCER BURDEN IN THE UNITED STATES	BOX 19.1

- Each year more than 1.6 million individuals are diagnosed with cancer
- Annual cancer-related deaths are estimated at 595,690 for 2016
- Cancer accounts for $88.7 billion in medical costs annually
- Nearly 15.5 million individuals are living with a cancer history
- The lifetime risk of developing cancer is approximately 42% for men and 37% for women in the United States.

Source: American Cancer Society (2016).

2016; Yale University School of Nursing, 2016). Such changes require individuals to pursue additional credits in order to obtain specialized oncology education and may prove to be both time- and cost-prohibitive, thereby limiting the number of oncology APRNs specialized by virtue of educational preparation.

The transition away from specialty-focused educational preparation of the APRN raises the question of whether fellowship training can provide a viable avenue for specialized oncology APRNs, similar to the training of medical fellows. Oncology APRN fellowships such as those offered at The Ohio State University Comprehensive Cancer Center–James (The Ohio State University, 2016), The University of Texas MD Anderson Cancer Center (The University of Texas MD Anderson Cancer Center, 2016), and Memorial-Sloan Kettering Cancer Center (Memorial Sloan Kettering Cancer Center, 2016) provide avenues for APRNs interested in specializing after receiving their degree to develop clinical expertise and to prepare for oncology certification through focused clinical rotations within this patient population.

Certification and Competencies

Specialty certification is not regulated by or recognized for practice by licensing boards; instead, it is granted through specialty organizations, such as the Oncology Nurse Certification Corporation (ONCC). Currently, three oncology advanced-practice certifications are supported by the ONCC—Advanced Oncology Certified Nurse Practitioner (AOCNP®), Advanced Oncology Certified Clinical Nurse Specialist (AOCNS®), and Advanced Oncology Certified Nurse (AOCN®). However, the AOCN®, and as of 2017, the AOCNS certifications, will be available only for maintenance and renewal (Oncology Nursing Certification Corporation, 2016a). Although pediatric oncology certification is available for registered nurses, no advanced practice pediatric oncology certification exists at this time. In addition, Certified Registered Nurse Anesthetists (CRNAs), who function in a specialized capacity distinct from other APRNs, may obtain oncology certification as AOCNPs. However, no distinct certification specific to anesthetists practicing in oncology exists at this time. One of the challenges of obtaining specialty certification within an increasingly generalist educational focus is that specialty education obtained concurrently with the generalist curriculum may not provide the number of clinical hours necessary for certification. Currently, oncology certification for both Nurse Practitioners (NPs) and CNSs requires 500 hours to 1,000 hours of adult oncology nursing practice within the 5 years preceding the test registration date (Oncology Nursing Certification Corporation, 2016b).

The Oncology Nursing Society (ONS), a professional organization of more than 39,000 nursing and health care professionals, establishes the competencies for oncology nurse practitioners and Clinical Nurse Specialists (Table 19.1; The Oncology Nursing Society, 2016). The focus on health promotion, disease prevention, and managing illness, as well as the emphasis on negotiating health care systems, is well aligned with the aims and goals of the National Cancer Moonshot, the implications of which are presented as follows.

TABLE 19.1 Oncology Nursing Society Advanced Practice Registered Nurse Competencies

NURSE PRACTITIONER (ONCOLOGY NURSING SOCIETY, 2007)	OUTCOMES	CLINICAL NURSE SPECIALIST (ONCOLOGY NURSING SOCIETY, 2008)	OUTCOMES
Health promotion, health protection, disease prevention and treatment	Increased access to care; decreased health care costs	The patient/client sphere of influence Assessment and diagnosis of health status Development of plan of care and interventions Evaluation of outcomes	Improved delivery of care through individualized care planning that leads to increased patient satisfaction and improved health outcomes
Nurse Practitioner–patient relationship	Improved patient satisfaction achieved through fostering collaborative relationships with patients and their caregivers as partners in care	The nursing practice sphere of influence Assessment, diagnosis, outcomes identification, and planning related to oncology nursing practice Intervention and evaluation of evidence-based oncology nursing practice Professional role development in oncology nursing	Generation of evidence for and implementation of evidence-based practice; development of self and colleagues toward competence and excellence in oncology nursing
Teaching–coaching function	Patient compliance; improved patient satisfaction	The organization/system sphere of influence Assessment, diagnosis, outcomes identification and planning related to organization practice settings Intervention and evaluation of oncology care delivery systems	Improvement in work environmental outcomes that impact the ability of the oncology APRN and interdisciplinary colleagues to deliver high-quality oncology care
Professional role	Generation of evidence for and implementation of evidence-based practice		
Negotiating health care delivery systems	Delivery of clinical services within an integrated system of health care that improves health outcomes for patients		
Monitoring and ensuring the quality of health care practice	Decreased length of stay, admission rates, emergency care visits and health care costs		
Caring for diverse populations	Provision of culturally competent care that incorporates evidence-based practice to best meet population needs and reduce health disparities		

APRN, Advanced Practice Registered Nurse.

THE NATIONAL CANCER MOONSHOT: NEW FRONTIERS FOR ONCOLOGY ADVANCED PRACTICE

Legislation and Implications

The National Cancer Moonshot is an initiative launched by the Obama administration in January 2016 to provide concerted, collaborative efforts to accelerate cancer research. Former President Barack Obama established a Cancer Moonshot Task Force, with membership from governmental agencies and chaired by former Vice President Joe Biden, which was charged with making recommendations in an advisory capacity related to the investment of resources in support of research and clinical advances in cancer care (The White House Office of the Press Secretary, 2016c). This major initiative includes nearly $1 billion funding to be appropriated through fiscal year 2017 in support of cancer-related research activities (The White House Office of the Press Secretary, 2016b). A Blue Ribbon Panel was assembled, consisting of 28 content experts, and five ex-officio members from scientific concentrations including biology, immunology, genomics, diagnostics, bioinformatics, nursing, cancer treatment, and prevention, as well as industry representatives from pharmaceutical and biotechnology companies, and representatives from cancer advocacy groups (NCI, 2016b). The Blue Ribbon Panel made recommendations for working groups related to seven priority topics (Table 19.2). These working groups then made 10 recommendations to guide the focus of collaborative, innovative research across industries, and practice settings (Table 19.3; NCI, 2017).

The next step for the Cancer Moonshot involves activity in the public and private sector. Collaborative, innovative cancer research is at the forefront of these

TABLE 19.2 Cancer Moonshot Working Group Content Areas

WORKING GROUP	FOCUS
Expanding Clinical Trials	Increase clinical trial participation
Enhanced Data Sharing	Increase data sharing to improve access, analysis, and clinical trial outcomes
Cancer Immunology and Prevention	Advance immunotherapy development, improve access, and expand use to cancer prevention
Implementation Sciences	Increase population studies to measure the impact of cancer that influences practices, policies, and programs that directly affect public health
Pediatric Cancer	Conduct more studies to understand molecular biology in childhood cancer and develop less toxic cancer treatments
Precision Prevention and Early Detection	Develop more genomic and molecular assay using blood diagnostics to control cancer throughout the cancer continuum
Tumor Progression and Evolution	Understand the mutations that occur in cancer cells and non-cancer cell microenvironment within the concept of tumor initiation and progression to develop more strategies in cancer control

Source: National Cancer Institute (2015).

TABLE 19.3 Blue Ribbon Panel Recommendation Topics

TOPIC	CONTENT
Establish a network for direct patient involvement	Engage patients to contribute their comprehensive tumor profile data to expand knowledge about what therapies work, in whom, and in which types of cancer.
Create a translational science network devoted exclusively to immunotherapy	Establish a cancer immunotherapy network to discover why immunotherapy is effective in some patients but not in others.
Develop ways to overcome cancer's resistance to therapy	Identify therapeutic targets to overcome drug resistance through studies that determine the mechanisms that lead cancer cells to become resistant to previously effective treatments.
Build a national cancer data ecosystem	Create a national ecosystem for sharing and analyzing cancer data so that researchers, clinicians, and patients will be able to contribute data, which will facilitate efficient data analysis.
Intensify research on the major drivers of childhood cancers	Improve our understanding of fusion oncoproteins in pediatric cancer and use new preclinical models to develop inhibitors that target them.
Minimize cancer treatment's debilitating side effects	Accelerate the development of guidelines for routine monitoring and management of patient-reported symptoms to minimize debilitating side effects of cancer and its treatment.
Expand use of proven cancer prevention and early detection strategies	Reduce cancer risk and cancer health disparities through approaches in development, testing, and broad adoption of proven prevention strategies.
Mine past patient data to predict future patient outcomes	Predict response to standard treatments through retrospective analysis of patient specimens.
Develop a 3-D cancer atlas	Create dynamic 3-D maps of human tumor evolution to document the genetic lesions and cellular interactions of each tumor as it evolves from a precancerous lesion to advanced cancer.
Develop new cancer technologies	Develop new enabling cancer technologies to characterize tumors and test therapies.

Source: National Cancer Institute (2017).

goals fueled by funding such as the Vice President's Exceptional Opportunities in Cancer Research Fund, which promotes high-risk, high-return research to propel cancer treatment forward (The White House Office of the Press Secretary, 2016b). Numerous public and private sector initiatives already exist, including cancer prevention activities through the promotion of the human papillomavirus (HPV) vaccination; collaborative research on the quality and efficacy of oncology nurse navigation, and the expansion of programs like the Extension for Community Healthcare Outcomes (ECHO) to foster partnerships between health care providers at National Cancer Institute (NCI)–designated comprehensive cancer centers and community-based settings (The White House Office of the Press Secretary, 2016a). In this context, robust opportunities exist for oncology APRNs to contribute to National Cancer Moonshot–related, policy-driven initiatives.

Directions for Advanced Practice Providers

The National Cancer Moonshot platform provides diverse opportunities for health care providers and researchers to support the program's aims. However, oncology APRNs are uniquely positioned to engage in cancer screening and prevention activities, as well as survivorship support.

Cancer Screening and Prevention

The Patient Protection and Affordable Care Act (PPACA) provides coverage for annual wellness visits, including the creation of a personalized prevention plan; an individualized health risk assessment, including medical and family history; evaluation of current providers and medications; physical and cognitive assessment; and review of a screening schedule (U.S. Department of Health and Human Services, 2010). The ACA provides mandatory coverage of evidence-based prevention services, including those that contribute to the prevention of cancer such as smoking cessation, obesity screening and counseling, and diet counseling. The cancer screening provisions of the ACA support early detection of breast, cervical, and colorectal cancers, as well as detection of lung cancers in individuals at high risk. In the context of cancer care, this approach focuses on identifying and remediating behavioral, environmental, and genetic risk factors—areas in which oncology APRNs can use their expertise and skills to influence patient behavior. While these support services are important for cancer control, the uptake of prevention services and screening interventions depends largely on provider input to patients (Yabroff, 2008), an area in which APRNs can also use their expertise, skills, and communication strategies.

Tobacco cessation is an example of a cancer prevention initiative strongly supported by policy. The U.S. Preventive Services Task Force (USPSTF) recommends with an "A" rating that clinicians ask all adults about tobacco use, advise them to stop using tobacco, and provide behavioral interventions and U.S. Food and Drug Administration (FDA)–approved pharmacotherapy for cessation to adults who use tobacco (USPSTF, 2015). The U.S. Public Health Service recommends tobacco cessation medications and counseling without cost sharing or prior authorization (Agency for Health Care Research and Quality, 2008). The U.S. Departments of Health and Human Services, Labor, and Treasury have issued guidance on tobacco cessation under the ACA to clarify that insurance plans should offer access to all U.S. Public Health Service–recommended tobacco cessation medications and counseling without cost sharing or prior authorization (American Lung Association, 2016). The National Cancer Moonshot initiative highlights tobacco cessation as an important strategy for reducing largely preventable cancer deaths. The Commission on Cancer (CoC) includes a standard that addresses smoking/chewing tobacco cessation and smoking prevention in adolescents (CoC, 2015). The American Lung Association has assembled an ACA Tobacco Cessation Guidance Toolkit to help ensure tobacco cessation opportunities (American Lung Association, 2016). Armed with both this policy and practical support, APRNs are empowered to facilitate tobacco cessation strategies for their patients and their communities.

Human papilloma virus (HPV) vaccination is another area strongly driven by policy, with recommendations by the Advisory Committee on Immunization Practices (ACIP) and the Centers for Disease Control and Prevention (CDC) for vaccination of preadolescent and adolescent girls and boys and young adults who have not been previously vaccinated (Markowitz et al., 2014; Petrosky et al., 2015). The American College of Obstetricians and Gynecologists (ACOG; 2015) recommends routine vaccination for both boys and girls aged 11 and 12. ACOG (2015) also recommends education of patients and parents about the safety and benefits of the HPV vaccination. Most private insurance plans cover HPV vaccination. The ACA requires all new private insurance plans to cover recommended preventive services including HPV vaccination with no co-pay, deductible, or co-insurance. The CoC includes a standard that addresses the use of strategies to modify attitudes and behaviors to reduce the chance of developing cancer including vaccination for HPV (CoC, 2015). Under the ACA, the bivalent and quadrivalent HPV vaccines are covered for adolescents and young adults of either sex, and over time. Medicaid covers HPV vaccination in accordance with the ACIP recommendations, and immunizations are a mandatory service under Medicaid for eligible individuals under age 21. In addition, the federal Vaccines for Children Program provides immunization services for children 18 and under who are Medicaid eligible, uninsured, underinsured, receiving immunizations through a Federally Qualified Health Center or Rural Health Clinic, or are Native American or Alaska Native (U.S. Department of Health and Human Services, 2010). The Blue Ribbon Panel report from the National Cancer Moonshot includes HPV vaccination as a target (NCI, 2016c).

However, despite overwhelming evidence that the vaccine is both safe and an effective primary prevention for cervical cancer, vaccination data from the 2015 National Immunization Survey-Teen (NIS-Teen) demonstrates that vaccination rates remain relatively low at 60% for girls and 50% for boys (Reagan-Steiner et al., 2016). Completion of the recommended three doses is even lower, with only 40% among girls and 22% among boys in the United States (NCI, 2016c). Missed opportunities result from assumptions about the timing of vaccination relative to sexual activity and the relationship of the vaccine to sexual promiscuity (Bailey et al., 2016). APRNs have the responsibility to be knowledgeable about the HPV vaccine. They have the opportunity to educate parents about the diseases that can be prevented by preadolescent and adolescent vaccines and to talk about the vaccine in terms of cancer prevention rather than HPV as a sexually transmitted infection. As with other cancer prevention measures, strong vaccine recommendations from primary care providers and pediatricians are the key to HPV vaccine uptake (Bailey et al., 2016). The CDC provides ready-to-use tools and resources for clinicians to successfully communicate with parents about HPV vaccination (Centers for Disease Control and Prevention, 2015). The American Academy of Pediatrics (AAP) provides a toolkit to assist clinicians in educating other health professionals, discussing HPV vaccination with parents, and making practice changes to increase vaccination rates (American Academy of Pediatrics, 2016).

Cancer Risk Assessment

A significant component of cancer prevention is risk assessment. The NCI defines a risk factor as a behavioral, environmental, biological, or hereditary factor that increases an individual's predisposition toward developing a disease (NCI, 2015). Comprehensive cancer risk assessment includes clinical assessment, genetic/genomic testing when appropriate, and risk management (NCI, 2015). An APRN competency, as defined by the ONS, includes performance of a relevant cancer risk assessment for general populations, at-risk populations, newly diagnosed patients with cancer, cancer survivors, and patients with a past, current, or potential diagnosis of cancer (Oncology Nursing Society, 2007). APRNs are also charged with educating patients, caregivers, and the community about cancer risk, screening, and early detection (Oncology Nursing Society, 2007, 2008).

Oncology APRN practice may include comprehensive cancer genetic risk assessment, education, facilitation and interpretation of genetic testing, pretest and posttest counseling and follow-up, and provision of personally tailored cancer risk recommendations and management, along with psychosocial counseling and supportive services. The American Nurses Association (ANA) has specified practice and education essentials in its Essentials of Genetic and Genomic Nursing: Competencies, Curricula Guidelines, and Outcome Indicators (American Academy of Colleges of Nursing, 2009). ONS (Oncology Nursing Society, 2012) has endorsed these essentials for oncology care and further specifies in their position statement that oncology APRNs also provide patient and community education and nursing practice that is consistent with the ANA Essentials and with the International Society of Nurses in Genetics *Essential Genetic and Genomic Competencies for Nurses With Graduate Degrees* (Greco, Tinley, & Seibert, 2012). The CoC has a standard that requires cancer risk assessment, genetic counseling, and genetic testing services to be provided to patients either on-site or by referral to a qualified genetics professional. Qualified professionals include a Genetics Clinical Nurse (GCN), an Advanced Practice Nurse in Genetics (APNG), or an Advanced Genetics, Nursing–Board Certified (AGN-BC) individual credentialed through the American Nurses Credential Center (ANCC), and an Advanced Practice Oncology Nurse who is prepared at the graduate level (master's or doctorate) with specialized education in cancer genetics and hereditary cancer predisposition syndromes (CoC, 2015). These guidelines constitute a powerful policy imperative for APRNs involved in oncology care to demonstrate educational preparation in the principles of human genetics and genomics, to integrate evidence-based genetic and genomic information into their practice, and to be cognizant of the ethical, legal, social, emotional, and advocacy issues in the application of personalized health care in oncology.

Survivorship

The Institute of Medicine (IOM) landmark report, *From Cancer Patient to Cancer Survivor: Lost in Transition* (Hewitt, Greenfield, & Stovall, 2005) established survivorship care as a priority and paved the way for practice changes that have occurred in survivorship. The report established cancer survivorship as a distinct phase of cancer care and identified components of care that include a follow-up care plan (Survivorship Care Plan [SCP]), evidence-based clinical practice guidelines, assessment tools, and screening instruments to help identify and manage late effects of cancer and its treatment.

In 2014, the CoC, which accredits cancer programs in the United States and Puerto Rico and provides data for the National Cancer Database, established a standard reporting requirement for SCPs. The SCP standard (Standard 3.3) was updated in 2016 and requires cancer treatment facilities to provide a treatment summary and follow-up plan to patients who have completed treatment that had a curative intent (CoC, 2015). The CoC references the American Society of Clinical Oncology (ASCO) definitions of the minimum data elements to be included in a treatment summary and SCP. The CoC also identifies health care provider(s) from the oncology care team who will be responsible for approving and discussing the SCP. Identified appropriate providers include RNs and APRNs (CoC, 2015).

A second IOM report, *Delivering High-Quality Cancer Care: Charting a New Course for a System in Crisis* (Levit et al., 2013) endorses a team-based approach to cancer care and recommends legislation and regulatory mechanisms that eliminate reimbursement and scope-of-practice barriers to enable all members of the cancer care team practice at the highest level of their licensure. The report highlights cancer survivorship as an area in which alternate models of care have been successful. These alternate models include APRNs as the providers of choice for survivorship patients. ASCO also presents recommendations (Box 19.2) and models for survivorship care (ASCO, 2016a), including models in which the APRN is a primary provider of care.

These recommendations, requirements, and models support the development of cancer survivorship clinics, set the standards for survivorship care, and strengthen the role of the APRN in survivorship. The ONS nurse practitioner practice competencies (Oncology Nursing Society, 2007) include cancer risk assessment for cancer survivors and assessment of actual and potential late effects of cancer, as well as the establishment of collaborative, interdisciplinary relationships to provide optimal care to patients with cancer. These competencies align with the core elements of survivorship care as outlined by the IOM report: prevention and detection of new primary cancers, surveillance for recurrence, assessment and interventions for the management of long-term and late effects, and coordination of care between cancer specialists and primary care providers (Hewitt et al., 2005).

Evidence-based practice algorithms can serve as guidelines for managing survivorship care. These algorithms help guide clinical practice; define patient eligibility for survivorship care; and delineate disease-specific surveillance

---

AMERICAN SOCIETY OF CLINICAL ONCOLOGY RECOMMENDATIONS FOR IMPROVING SURVIVOR CARE	BOX 19.2

- Promote patient-centered coordinated care through the use of shared-care models, which allow for collaboration among practitioners of different disciplines or with different skills and knowledge
- Increase adoption of quality improvement programs, such as ASCO's Quality Oncology Practice Initiative (QOPI®), which help physicians monitor and improve care for all survivors
- Expand research on long-term and late effects to expand the evidence base required to define optimal survivor care
- Strengthen education of health care providers on survivorship care to keep pace with growing evidence on the long-term follow-up care needs of patients with different types of cancers
- Educate and empower cancer survivors and their families to advocate for their unique needs and to ensure optimal long-term health

strategies, preventive services, late effects of treatment, and psychosocial issues that the patient could face. ASCO provides guidelines on surveillance and screening, as well as management of long-term effects for select cancers (ASCO, 2016b). The National Cancer Comprehensive Network presents guidelines that address general survivorship principles, late effects, psychosocial and physical problems, and preventive health (National Comprehensive Cancer Network, 2016).

Coverage of and reimbursement for survivorship services are not standardized, and there are no specific billing survivorship codes. Coverage and reimbursement are subject to Medicare, Medicaid, and third-party payer benefit plans. Most payers reimburse for follow-up visits, but not all survivorship providers can bill in all states. Services provided by APRNs are reimbursable although regulations may vary by state.

Summary

The National Cancer Moonshot is a governmental initiative that holds potential for tremendous contributions by oncology APRNs, particularly in the areas of cancer prevention, screening, and survivorship. In addition, the ability to refer patients to clinical trials emerging from Cancer Moonshot Research, as well as support detailed documentation of patient assessments as part of a larger database, will contribute to the advancement of these research-driven initiatives. Regardless of role or practice setting, oncology APRNs are uniquely poised to participate in the next great advancement of oncology science and clinical practice.

PRESCRIPTIVE AUTHORITY

Overview

Historically, limitations to prescriptive authority are one of the major barriers to APRN practice (Kaplan & Brown, 2007; Phillips, 2016). APRNs confront a fragmented regulatory system with high variability between states, especially related to prescriptive authority. Prescriptive authority is a component of oncology APRN practice that involves both clinical and licensure considerations. Managing the cancer patient offers additional challenges due to the disease progression, increased pain management requirements, and treatment complexities. Limiting APRN prescriptive authority contributes to untimely and undertreated pain management needs of the cancer patient (Hudspeth, 2016).

Barriers to Practice

APRN scope of practice, state nursing practice acts, limited prescriptive authority through state laws and regulations, and limited financial reimbursement are legislative barriers limiting APRN prescriptive authority (Plank, 2011). In many states, APRNs are not permitted to prescribe schedule II controlled substances, which are a mainstay of practice for oncology APRNs who manage acute and chronic pain and hospice care. Prescribing authority in states that permit APRNs to prescribe schedule II controlled substances can still be complicated by federal, local, and institutional requirements. Drug Enforcement Agency (DEA) registration is mandatory for prescribing APRNs, with some states requiring further state-regulated registrations prior to applying for a DEA number (Plank, 2011).

The practice barriers, including prescriptive authority restrictions on prescribing schedule II controlled substances, are multidimensional and impede scope-of-practice, particularly related to end-of-life care (DuBois & Reed, 2014).

Health care facility policy and procedures for APRN privileges must comply with federal laws, state laws, state board of nursing regulations, and APRN organizational scopes of practice. Ultimately, health care facility policy and procedures govern what an APRN is able to prescribe in that facility and can limit APRNs' full prescriptive authority through restrictive institutional policies. Some health care entities maintain policies stricter than those established by state law. A landmark policy change to remove APRN supervision in Veterans Administration facilities is currently under way, which will set the precedent for APRNs across the nation (U.S. Department of Veterans Affairs, 2016).

Physician opposition to full prescriptive authority, which may reflect lack of knowledge, reluctance to collaborate, and lack of professional respect for the APRN roles in health care, also serves as a barrier (Brown, 2012; Plank, 2011). Physician rationale for limiting full prescriptive authority is the increased prescribing practice for modalities such as schedule II agents and concerns about the opioid abuse endemic. Schirle and McCabe (2016) found the opposite to be true. Restricting APRN full prescriptive authority resulted in significantly increased prescriptions for opioids and benzodiazepines when compared to full prescriptive authority.

APRNs may contribute to barriers of their own with respect to prescriptive authority by resisting independent practice, increased accountability, and responsibility for health care delivery (Kaplan & Brown, 2007). Despite physician opposition, studies continue to document the high-quality, safety, and cost-effectiveness profiles of APRNs (Stanik-Hutt et al., 2013).

Given the extent to which cancer patients may experience pain throughout treatment and into survivorship and palliative care, policy restrictions that limit an APRN's caring for an oncology patient pose significant challenges to effective care. Other limitations include restrictions on prescribing for investigational drugs, chemotherapeutic agents, radiation therapy, and radiopharmaceuticals, and for patients receiving in-home hospice care (Kelvin et al., 1999; Lynch, Cope, & Murphy-Ende, 2001). One example of the critical nature of prescriptive authority to oncology APRNs is in the area of radiation therapy. APRNs are critical in radiation therapy delivery and symptom management during radiation treatment (Kelvin et al., 1999). For example, anxiolytics and pain management are mainstays in the management of patients undergoing radiation therapy (Carper & Haas, 2006). Although radiation oncologists perform the core prescription of radiation therapy, APRNs are integral in the education and management of this patient population.

Medical Marijuana

Medical marijuana is an increasingly prominent topic in the management of cancer patients. The prescribing of medical marijuana in the context of cancer care is a source of significant debate. Although cannabinoids have shown anti-emetic, appetite-stimulating properties and efficacy in alleviating moderate neuropathic pain in cancer patients, concern remains about associated upper respiratory tract cancers resulting from their use (Hall, Christie, & Currow, 2005). California was the first state to legalize marijuana for medical use in 1985 (O'Rourke, 2016). In

2013, Washington and Colorado became the first states to legalize recreational marijuana. Medical marijuana is considered a schedule I controlled substance, or an illegal drug. It is important to recognize that marijuana is not legal under federal law for any reason, due in part to a lack of rigorous trial and scientific scrutiny, as required by the FDA (Brown, 2012; Kaplan, 2015).

Synthetic marijuana analogs, dronabinol and nabilone, have been rigorously researched and available since 1985. Dronabinal, a schedule III medication, is prescribed for chemotherapy-induced nausea and vomiting. Similarly, nabilone, a schedule II medication, is prescribed for refractory chemotherapy-induced nausea and vomiting (Kaplan, 2015). Therefore, state laws that provide immunity from prosecution for practitioners who appropriately recommend the use of medical marijuana to oncology patients do not extend the same immunity to practitioners under federal law. Currently, 23 states, the District of Columbia, and Guam maintain medical marijuana laws (Brown, 2012; Kaplan, 2015). Maine, Minnesota, New Hampshire, New Mexico, Vermont, and Washington are the only six states that allow APRNs to be involved in the process of prescribing medical marijuana (Brown, 2012; Kaplan, 2015). Other states, such as Massachusetts and New York, are moving toward APRNs prescribing medical marijuana (Brown, 2012). Medical marijuana is an expanding adjunctive therapy for cancer and pain management (Brown, 2012). Such pharmacological adjuncts are limited to physicians in all states except Washington and New Mexico. Although an increasing number of states allow APRNs to prescribe medical marijuana, APRNs must familiarize themselves with the nurse practice act within their state. Resources, like the National Council of State Legislatures and National Council of State Boards of Nursing, are available to review legislation by state (www.ncsl.org/research/health/state-medical -marijuana-laws.aspx#1 and www.ncsbn.org/47.htm; Kaplan, 2015).

SUMMARY

Despite numerous barriers, APRNs have made significant legislative progress in all areas of practice between 2014 and 2016 (Phillips, 2016). In 2015, Delaware, Maryland, and Nebraska moved to full practice authority with forms of a post-licensure period of supervision, collaboration, or mentorship (Phillips, 2016). Also, more than eight states enhanced APRN prescriptive authority rules related to controlled substances (Phillips, 2016). APRNs can have a significant role in expanding prescriptive authority through active engagement with professional organizations and lobbying for policy change at the local, state, and national level. Nurses (more than 3.4 million) are the largest single group of health professionals possessing one of the greatest potentials to influence policy and legislation, if they participate (ANA, 2016).

CONCLUSION

The context of oncology care is constantly changing, and we are now in a time of unprecedented clinical and research advances in support of cancer treatment and cure. With an ever-growing number of individuals living with cancer, the need for APRNs who are trained in oncology and can serve as advocates for progressive health policy related to academic preparation, licensure, clinical practice, research and prescriptive authority, is paramount to both the future success

1. CANCER CARE CASE STUDY

Trisha is a 25-year-old daughter of a woman diagnosed with *BRCA+* breast cancer. She presents to Kathleen, an APRN who is her primary care provider, for her well visit with questions about genetic testing and risk assessment. Trisha asks if she should be tested for the *BRCA* mutation and if there is anything that can be done to reduce her risk for cancer.

1. According to the ACA, what costs are associated with Trisha's well visit?
   a. The visit should be covered without co-pay by Trisha's insurance
2. Given Trisha's age, what assessments and recommendations might be appropriate for Trisha to make?
   a. Assessing Trisha for healthy eating, exercise, and lifestyle choices (smoking and alcohol use), as well as completion of the HPV vaccination series would be consistent with preventive care recommendations outlined in the ACA.

In conducting the standard wellness assessment, Kathleen discusses healthy diet, exercise, and smoking prevention with Trisha, who reports that while she smoked "maybe five cigarettes with friends when I was a teenager" she has no current smoking history, consumes one to two alcoholic beverages per week socially with friends, and exercises 45 minutes to 1 hour daily at least 5 days per week. When discussing prevention, Kathleen discovers that while sexually active, Trisha has never received the HPV vaccine.

1. Based on her age, is Trisha still a candidate for the HPV vaccine?
   a. Yes, individuals not vaccinated in the recommended age range may receive catch-up vaccination through age 26.

Trisha agrees to receive the first of the three-shot HPV vaccination series at this appointment. She now asks about genetic testing related to her mother's breast cancer diagnosis.

1. What recommendations should Kathleen make related to genetic testing for Trisha?
   a. The NCI supports genetic testing and risk assessment for individuals with high-risk profiles, such as the presence of cancer with genetic features in first-degree relatives. As such, Kathleen would be an appropriate candidate for genetic testing.
2. What is Kathleen's role in the genetic testing process?
   a. Depending on her training and background, Kathleen may support the facilitation and interpretation of genetic testing, pre- and posttest counseling and follow-up, and provision of personally tailored cancer risk recommendations and management, along with psychosocial counseling and supportive services, consistent with recommendations from the ONS and the American Nurses Association.
3. What recommendation might Kathleen make to Trisha related to the use of her genetic testing data consistent with the National Cancer Moonshot?
   a. Kathleen might suggest Trisha consent for her test results to be integrated into a national database of patient data that can be used to analyze trends in the risk for, occurrence, and outcomes of cancer. Data mining through the use of a national cancer data ecosystem may contribute to profound findings related to trends in cancer risk and occurrence that can inform the prevention and treatment of cancer in future individuals.

Kathleen refers Trisha to a licensed genetic counselor for further follow-up and writes a prescription for her to receive her subsequent HPV vaccinations at 1 month and 6 months after the first injection, consistent with Centers for Disease Control guidelines.

of the profession and the well-being of oncology patients. The National Cancer Moonshot is a policy-driven platform through which such progress may be made. Ensuring APRN familiarity and engagement with the Moonshot initiative will provide the foundation for their practice now and in the future.

DISCUSSION QUESTIONS

1. *Based on the information in this chapter, list at least two areas of policy change you can identify where legislation could have an impact.*
2. *If you were going to describe the importance of your issue for policy change to potential supporters, what key issues would you stress? How would you describe this to your patients?*

ANALYSIS AND SYNTHESIS EXERCISES

1. *What are particular areas of the Moonshot platform that affect my practice?*
2. *What are the medical marijuana prescribing laws in my state?*
3. *What are the restrictions on my practice related to medical marijuana?*
4. *What can I do from a policy perspective to further cancer prevention initiatives such as HPV vaccination?*

CLINICAL APPLICATION

1. *What policy changes are needed to advance APRN prescriptive authority for cancer patients?*
2. *How can I incorporate survivorship care into my practice? What resources are needed? What policy elements are essential to consider?*
3. *How can I strategically utilize the Moonshot platform to enhance my clinical practice?*

ETHICAL CONSIDERATIONS

1. *Consider the health policy changes discussed in this chapter and consider the impact that might occur if these changes are NOT enacted. In other words, what are the consequences of inaction?*

REFERENCES

Agency for Healthcare Research and Quality. (2008). *Treating tobacco use and dependence—2008 Update.* Rockville, MD: Author. Retrieved from http://www.ahrq.gov/sites/default/files/wysiwyg/professionals/clinicians-providers/guidelines-recommendations/tobacco/clinicians/update/treating_tobacco_use08.pdf

American Academy of Pediatrics. (2016). HPV champion toolkit. Retrieved from https://www.aap.org/en-us/advocacy-and-policy/aap-health-initiatives/immunizations/HPV-Champion-Toolkit/Pages/HPV-Champion-Toolkit.aspx

American Cancer Society. (2016). *Cancer facts and figures 2016.* Retrieved from http://www.cancer.org/acs/groups/content/@research/documents/document/acspc-047079.pdf

American College of Obstetricians and Gynecologists. (2015). *Human papillomavirus vaccination.* Committee Opinion No. 641. Washington, DC: Author.

American Lung Association. (2016). Affordable Care Act tobacco cessation guidance toolkit. Retrieved from http://www.lung.org/our-initiatives/tobacco/cessation-and-prevention/affordable-care-act-tobacco.html

American Nurses Association. (2016). Advocacy—Becoming more effective. Retrieved from http://www.nursingworld.org/MainMenuCategories/Policy-Advocacy/Advocacy ResourcesTools

American Nurses Association Consensus Panel. (2008). *Essentials of genetic and genomic nursing: Competencies, curricula guidelines and outcome indicators* (2nd ed.). Silver Spring, MD: Author. Retrieved from https://www.genome.gov/pages/careers/healthprofessionaleducation/genetic-scompetency.pdf

American Society of Clinical Oncology. (2016a). Models of long-term follow-up care. Retrieved from https://www.asco.org/practice-guidelines/cancer-care-initiatives/prevention-survivorship/survivorship/survivorship-3

American Society of Clinical Oncology. (2016b). Survivorship compendium. Retrieved from https://www.asco.org/practice-guidelines/cancer-care-initiatives/prevention-survivorship/survivorship/survivorship-compendium

APRN Consensus Work Group & the National Council of State Boards of Nursing APRN Advisory Committee. (2008). *Consensus model for APRN regulation: Licensure, accreditation, certification & education.* Chicago, IL: National Council of State Boards of Nursing. Retrieved from https://www.ncsbn.org/Consensus_Model_for_APRN_Regulation_July_2008.pdf

Bailey, H. H., Chuang, L. T., duPont, N. C., Eng, C., Foxhall, L. E., Merrill, J. K., . . . Blanke, C. D. (2016). American Society of Clinical Oncology Statement: Human papillomavirus vaccination for cancer prevention. *Journal of Clinical Oncology, 34*(15), 1803–1812.

Brown, M. A. (2012). *The advanced practice registered nurse as a prescriber.* Chichester, England: Wiley Blackwell.

Carper, E., & Haas, M. (2006). Advanced practice nursing in radiation oncology. *Seminars in Oncology Nursing, 22*(4), 203–211.

Centers for Disease Control and Prevention. (2015). Human papillomavirus (HPV). Retrieved from http://www.cdc.gov/hpv

Commission on Cancer. (2015). *Cancer program standards: Ensuring patient-centered care* (2016 ed.). Chicago, IL: American College of Surgeons.

Conrads, T. P., & Petricoin, E. F. (2016). The Obama Administration's Cancer Moonshot: A call for proteomics. *Clinical Cancer Research, 22*(18), 4556–4558.

DuBois, J. C., & Reed, P. G. (2014). The nurse practitioner and policy in end-of-life care. *Nursing Science Quarterly, 27*(1), 70–76.

Duke University School of Nursing. (2016). Oncology specialty. Retrieved from https://nursing.duke.edu/academics/programs/msn/oncology-specialty

Greco, K. E., Tinley, S., & Seibert, D. (2012). *Essential genetic and genomic competencies for nurses with graduate degrees.* Silver Spring, MD: American Nurses Association and International Society of Nurses in Genetics.

Hall, W., Christie, M., & Currow, D. (2005). Cannabinoids and cancer: Causation, remediation, and palliation. *The Lancet Oncology, 6*(1), 35–42.

Hewitt, M., Greenfield, S., & Stovall, E. (2005). *From cancer patient to cancer survivor: Lost in transition.* Washington, DC: National Academies Press.

Hudspeth, R. S. (2016). Safe opioid prescribing for adults by nurse practitioners: Part 2. Implementing and managing treatment. *Journal for Nurse Practitioners, 12*(4), 213–220.

Kaplan, L. (2015). Medical marijuana: Legal and regulatory considerations. *The Nurse Practitioner, 40*(10), 46–54; quiz 54.

Kaplan, L., & Brown, M. A. (2007). The transition of nurse practitioners to changes in prescriptive authority. *Journal of Nursing Scholarship, 39*(2), 184–190.

Kelvin, J. F., Moore-Higgs, G. J., Maher, K. E., Dubey, A. K., Austin-Seymour, M. M., Daly, N. R., . . . Kuehn, E. F. (1999). Non-physician practitioners in radiation oncology: Advanced practice nurses and physician assistants. *International Journal of Radiation Oncology, Biology, Physics, 45*(2), 255–263.

Kennedy Sheldon, L. (2016). Oncology nurses and the Cancer Moonshot 2020. *Clinical Journal of Oncology Nursing, 20*(4), 355–356.

Levit, L. A., Balogh, E., Ganz, P. A., & Nass, S. (2013). *Delivering high-quality cancer care: Charting a new course for a system in crisis.* Washington, DC: National Academies Press.

Lynch, M. P., Cope, D. G., & Murphy-Ende, K. (2001). Advanced practice issues: Results of the ONS Advanced Practice Nursing survey. *Oncology Nursing Forum, 28*(10), 1521–1530.

Markowitz, L. E., Dunne, E. F., Saraiya, M., Chesson, H. W., Curtis, C. R., Gee, J., . . . Unger, E. R.; Centers for Disease Control and Prevention. (2014). Human papillomavirus vaccination: Recommendations of the Advisory Committee on Immunization Practices (ACIP). *Morbidity and Mortality Weekly Report. Recommendations and Reports, 63*(RR-05), 1–30.

Memorial Sloan Kettering Cancer Center. (2016). Pain and palliative care nursing fellowship. Retrieved from https://www.mskcc.org/hcp-education-training/fellowships/pain-and-palliative-care -nursing-fellowship

National Cancer Institute. (2015). *Cancer trends progress report.* Bethesda, MD: U.S. Department of Health and Human Services.

National Cancer Institute. (2016a). Cancer Moonshot. Retrieved from https://www.cancer.gov/research/ key-initiatives/moonshot-cancer-initiative

National Cancer Institute. (2016b). Cancer Moonshot Blue Ribbon Panel members. Retrieved from https://www.cancer.gov/research/key-initiatives/moonshot-cancer-initiative/blue-ribbon -panel/members

National Cancer Institute. (2016c). Cancer Moonshot Blue Ribbon Panel report 2016. Retrieved from https:// www.cancer.gov/research/key-initiatives/moonshot-cancer-initiative/blue-ribbon-panel/blue -ribbon-panel-report-2016.pdf

National Cancer Institute. (2017). Cancer Moonshot Blue Ribbon Panel. Retrieved from https://www .cancer.gov/research/key-initiatives/moonshot-cancer-initiative/blue-ribbon-panel

National Comprehensive Cancer Network. (2016). NCCN guidelines. Retrieved from https://www .nccn.org/professionals/physician_gls/f_guidelines.asp

Ohio State University. (2016). Acute care oncology fellowship program. Retrieved from https:// cancer.osu.edu/cancer-specialties/nursing/acute-care-oncology-fellowship-program

Oncology Nursing Certification Corporation. (2016a). Advanced oncology certified clinical nurse spe- cialist examination to sunset in 2017 [Press release]. Retrieved from http://www.oncc.org/about -oncc/news/advanced-oncology-certified-clinical-nurse-specialist-examination-sunset-2017

Oncology Nursing Certification Corporation. (2016b). *Advanced oncology certified nurse practitioner & advanced oncology certified clinical nurse specialist test candidate handbook.* Retrieved from http:// www.oncc.org/files/AOCNPAOCNSHandbook_2016.pdf

Oncology Nursing Society. (2007). *Oncology nurse practitioner competencies.* Pittsburgh, PA: Author. Retrieved from https://www.ons.org/sites/default/files/npcompentencies.pdf

Oncology Nursing Society. (2008). *Oncology clinical nurse specialist competencies.* Pittsburgh, PA: Author. Retrieved from https://www.ons.org/sites/default/files/cnscomps.pdf

Oncology Nursing Society. (2013). Oncology nursing: The application of cancer genetics and genomics throughout the oncology care continuum. *Oncology Nursing Forum, 40*(1), 10–11. doi:10.1188/13 .ONF.10-11

The Oncology Nursing Society. (2016). About ONS. Retrieved from https:// www.ons.org/about

O'Rourke, K. (2016). Medical marijuana: Tips for ensuring safer use. Retrieved from http://www.pain medicinenews.com/Web-Only/Article/07-16/Medical-Marijuana-Tips-for-Ensuring-Safer-Use/ 37153/ses=ogst

Petrosky, E., Bocchini, J. A., Hariri, S., Chesson, H., Curtis, C. R., Saraiya, M., . . . Markowitz, L. E. (2015). Use of 9-valent human papillomavirus (HPV) vaccine: Updated HPV vaccination recommenda- tions of the advisory committee on immunization practices. *Morbidity and Mortality Weekly Report, 64*(11), 300–304.

Phillips, S. J. (2016). 28th annual APRN legislative update: Advancements continue for APRN practice. *The Nurse Practitioner, 41*(1), 21–48.

Plank, L. S. (2011). Governmental oversight of prescribing medications: History of the U.S. Food and Drug Administration and prescriptive authority. *Journal of Midwifery & Women's Health, 56*(3), 198–204.

Reagan-Steiner, S., Yankey, D., Jeyarajah, J., Elam-Evans, L. D., Curtis, C. R., MacNeil, J., . . . Singleton, J. A. (2016). National, regional, state, and selected local area vaccination coverage among ado- lescents aged 13-17 years—United States, 2015. *Morbidity and Mortality Weekly Report, 65*(33), 850–858.

Schirle, L., & McCabe, B. E. (2016). State variation in opioid and benzodiazepine prescriptions between independent and nonindependent advanced practice registered nurse prescribing states. *Nursing Outlook, 64*(1), 86–93.

Stanik-Hutt, J., Newhouse, R. P., White, K. M., Johantgen, M., Bass, E. B., Zangaro, G., . . . Heindel, L. (2013). The quality and effectiveness of care provided by nurse practitioners. *Journal for Nurse Practitioners, 9*(8), 492–500, e413.

The University of Texas MD Anderson Cancer Center. (2016). APRN post-graduate oncology fellowship.

U.S. Department of Health and Human Services. (2010). Preventive services covered under the Affordable Care Act. Retrieved from http://www.hhs.gov/healthcare/facts-and-features/fact-sheets/preventive-services-covered-under-aca

U.S. Department of Veterans Affairs. (2016). VA proposes to grant full practice authority to advanced practice registered nurses [Press release]. Retrieved from http://www.va.gov/opa/pressrel/pressrelease.cfm?id=2793

U.S. Preventative Services Task Force. (2015). Tobacco smoking cessation in adults, including pregnant women: Behavioral and pharmacotherapy interventions. Retrieved from https://www.uspreventiveservicestaskforce.org/Page/Document/UpdateSummaryFinal/tobacco-use-in-adults-and-pregnant-women-counseling-and-interventions1

White House Office of the Press Secretary. (2016a). Fact sheet: At Cancer Moonshot Summit, Vice President Biden Announces New Actions to Accelerate Progress Toward Ending Cancer As We Know It [Press release]. Retrieved from https://www.whitehouse.gov/the-press-office/2016/06/28/fact-sheet-cancer-moonshot-summit-vice-president-biden-announces-new

White House Office of the Press Secretary. (2016b). Fact sheet: Investing in the National Cancer Moonshot [Press release]. Retrieved from https://www.whitehouse.gov/the-press-office/2016/02/01/fact-sheet-investing-national-cancer-moonshot

White House Office of the Press Secretary. (2016c). Memorandum—White House Cancer Moonshot Task Force [Press release]. Retrieved from https://www.whitehouse.gov/the-press-office/2016/01/28/memorandum-white-house-cancer-moonshot-task-force

Yabroff, K. R. (2008). Interventions to improve cancer screening: Commentary from a health services research perspective. *American Journal of Preventive Medicine, 35*(1, Suppl.), S6–S9.

Yale University School of Nursing. (2016). Adult oncology concentration. Retrieved from http://nursing.yale.edu/node/207

Health Policy and Its Impact on APRN-Driven Quality and Research

Moving Toward Accountable Care: A Policy Framework to Transform Health Care Delivery and Reimbursement

Susan Kendig

Concerns regarding quality of care, inefficiencies, and rising health care continue to drive calls for "delivery system reform." Innovative reimbursement models designed to encourage providers to improve quality and value through care coordination are recognized as one mechanism with the potential to transform health care delivery. The Patient Protection and Affordable Care Act, Public Law 111–148 ("PPACA" or "the Act"), enacted in 2010, provided a legislative attempt to curb health care costs and improve health care quality by linking payment to quality outcomes through the development of alternate care delivery models and payment structures (PPACA, 2010a). In addition to introducing the "Medicare Shared Savings Program" (MSSP), which provided one framework for the accountable care organization (ACO) model, the Act also authorized the Secretary of the U.S. Department of Health and Human Services (the Secretary) to initiate programs and demonstration projects designed to control costs and improve the quality of care provided to Medicare, Medicaid, and Children's Health Insurance Program (CHIP) beneficiaries. During the intervening years, learnings from implementation of the MSSP, and demonstration projects focused on medical home and bundled payment models are beginning to inform strategies and identify challenges associated with calculating savings (Baseman, 2016).

The MSSP framework is codified within the PPACA, whereas the Medical Home and Bundled Payment strategies exist as demonstration projects within the statute. In January 2015, the Centers for Medicare and Medicaid Services (CMS) set a goal of shifting 30% of Medicare fee-for-service payments to a value-driven model by the end of 2016. CMS estimates that this goal was achieved in early March 2016 (USDHHS, 2016). Given changes in the political landscape, questions arise as to how ACOs will be affected (Slonim & Maraccini, 2016). As of March 2016, approximately 840 ACOs were operational across the United States, of which 477 had been established under CMS (Tu, 2016). Although the current ACO nomenclature and some elements of health care delivery reform may change, the need for improved quality and efficiency in health care is likely to continue, with attention to alternate care delivery and reimbursement models as mechanisms to achieve such goals (Slonim & Maraccini, 2016). Recognizing the changing policy landscape, this chapter provides an overview of PPACA's ACO provisions as of 2016, with examples of programs and demonstration projects that may inform further development of alternate care delivery and payment mechanisms.

POLICY-DRIVEN ALTERNATE HEALTH CARE REIMBURSEMENT MODELS: THE EVOLUTION OF ACOS

Over the past two decades Congress has passed legislation designed to move the CMS from a passive purchaser of volume-based health care to an active purchaser of value-based, high-quality health care. Earlier Medicare programs and demonstration projects authorized by Congress have targeted health care quality and efficiency improvements through payment reform. For example, the Medicare Prescription Drug and Modernization Act of 2003 (MMA), extended by the Deficit Reduction Act of 2005 (DRA), linked Medicare payments to hospital quality reporting. Under these statutes, hospitals reporting on specific quality measures received their full Medicare annual payment update; whereas those who failed to participate in the quality reporting initiative saw a 2% reduction in their annual payment update (Deficit Reduction Act of 2005, 2006a; MMA, 2003). Similarly, the Tax Relief and Health Care Act of 2006 (2006) and the Medicare Improvements for Patients and Providers Act of 2008 (2008) linked the Medicare value-based purchasing initiatives to physicians, providing bonuses to physicians reporting on specific quality measures. In 2009, the American Recovery and Reinvestment Act (ARRA, 2009) provided for financial incentives to providers that "meaningfully use" electronic health records as a quality improvement tool. These are but a few of the policy driven attempts to improve health care quality and efficiency that were under way well before PPACA's passage.

When PPACA became law in 2010, it authorized the secretary to further explore provider reimbursement models aimed at driving down health care costs while maintaining or improving patient outcomes through quality and efficiency improvements. Under PPACA, new programs and demonstration projects were established, and current demonstration projects with implications for payment reform were extended. The Medicare Access and CHIP Reauthorization Act of 2015 (MACRA), Public Law 114–110, further advances mechanisms to incorporate quality measurement into payments, and incentivize provider participation in alternate payment models (APMs). MACRA provides a framework for health care providers to participate in the value-based CMS Quality Payment Program through Advanced Alternative Payment Models (Advanced APMs) or a Merit-based Incentive Payment System (MIPS; USDHHS, 2016).

RELEVANT DEMONSTRATION PROJECTS AUTHORIZED BY PPACA

Over the past decade, delivery system reform under Medicare has focused on value-based APMs that fell into three categories: bundled payments, ACOs, and medical homes. The Centers for Medicare and Medicaid Innovation (CMMI) was created within the Act to support testing these innovative payment and delivery models, intended to improve quality and decrease costs. The models were designed to address a defined population for which there are deficits in care leading to poor clinical outcomes or avoidable expenditures. CMMI's overall goal is to test innovative, comprehensive payment models that drive down health care costs through improved quality and efficiency (PPACA, 2010c).

Through PPACA, $10 billion was appropriated to CMMI to support innovation activities from 2011 to 2019. Since its inception, CMMI has been responsible for awarding funding to test innovations throughout the country. CMMI's portfolio includes Innovation Models in seven categories: accountable care, Bundled Payments for Care Improvement, primary care transformation, initiatives focused on the Medicaid and CHIP population, initiatives focused on Medicare-Medicaid enrollees, initiatives to accelerate development and testing of new payment and service delivery models, and initiatives to speed adoption of best practices (CMMI, 2011).

Common throughout the PPACA initiatives is a theme of payment reform moving from a fee for service to payment for quality and value (CMMI, 2010). Given the significant amount of funding appropriated to and immediately available from CMMI, these opportunities sparked new collaborative efforts to achieve cost and quality goals. Although preliminary results are mixed, learnings from the demonstration projects enumerated in the statute, and the CMMI initiatives, are helping to inform successful ACO and other APMs in both the public and private sectors.

Overview of Current Alternate Payment Models

Bundled Payments

Bundled payments establish an overall budget for services provided in a discreet episode of care for a specified clinical condition over a defined period. Instead of paying for each service individually, as occurs in a fee-for-service model, bundled payments incentivize providers to coordinate care to improve efficiency for the defined episode of care (Baseman, 2016).

The National Pilot Program on Payment Bundling is designed to develop and evaluate bundled payments for integrated care that includes acute, inpatient, and post-acute care for an episode of care beginning 3 days before hospital admission and continuing for 30 days postdischarge. The program goal is to improve coordination, quality, and efficiency of services around a hospitalization related to selected conditions (PPACA, 2010e).

CMS has tested four different bundled payment models under the Bundled Payments for Care Improvement (BPCI) initiative. Model 1 bundles only inpatient hospital charges. In contrast, Model 2 bundles inpatient hospital services with physician services, post-acute services, Medicare Part A and B services accessed post-hospital discharge, and hospital readmissions. Model 3 bundles only the post-acute care, postdischarge Medicare Part A and B services, and readmissions. Model 4 bundles all inpatient and physician services and subsequent readmissions, but excludes post-acute care (Baseman, 2016). Variation in models tested allows for more complete learning with regard to elements of success. Although quality outcomes did not differ among the four models, Model 2 showed a decline in Medicare payments for orthopedic surgery involving hip and knee replacements during year one (Lewin Group, February 2015).

Primary Care Health Home

Health homes generally refer to team-based models of care with an emphasis on primary care and care coordination. Typically, Primary Care Health Home (PCHH) payment models include fee-for-service reimbursements as well as additional payments, such as monthly care management fees or capitated per-member-per-month payments, to support patient care and coordination activities (Baseman, 2016).

The Health Home for Medicaid and Medicare Beneficiaries with Chronic Disease initiative was created under section 2703 of the PPACA. Under this provision, states, through a state plan amendment, could choose to provide medical care to Medicaid beneficiaries with chronic disease through a "health home," under different reimbursement models designed to promote quality and efficiency of care. Individuals eligible to participate in the health home include those who have two chronic conditions; those who have one chronic condition and are at risk for developing a second chronic condition; or persons with one serious and persistent mental health condition. Health home services are comprehensive, timely services provided by a designated provider working within a health care team. Services are designed to include comprehensive care management, care coordination, health promotion, comprehensive transitional care, patient and family support, and referral to relevant community and social support services. Health information technology is used to link services, track data, and guide quality improvement (PPACA, 2010b).

In addition to the Health Home for Medicaid and Medicare Beneficiaries with Chronic Disease initiative, CMMI has tested a variety of health home models. Under the Multi-Payer Advanced Primary Care (MPAPC) Practice model, and Comprehensive Primary Care (CPC) initiative, CMMI tested whether receipt of care management fees for most patients across multiple payers would result in improved quality and efficiency as compared to models where fees are not aligned. Similarly, the Federally Qualified Health Center Advanced Primary Care Practice (FQHC-APCP) provided monthly care management fees to FQHCs engaged in PCHH activities, while supporting participating FQHCs in attaining National Committee for Quality Assurance (NCQA) recognition as a level-3 medical home. While these three CMMI initiatives have had mixed results in terms of quality and efficiency (Baseman, 2016), the Independence at Home (IAH) model has shown promising results.

The IAH Demonstration Project tested a payment incentive and service delivery model that utilizes physician and Nurse Practitioner directed teams to deliver home-based primary care services to high-need Medicare beneficiaries. Participating IAH practices teams did not receive monthly management fees, but shared in savings accomplished by reducing preventable hospitalizations and readmissions and other improvements in efficiencies of care and patient outcomes (PPACA, 2010f). During the first 2 years, the IAH program saved over $25 million and $10 million, respectively (CMS, June 2015; CMS, August 2016).

THE ACCOUNTABLE CARE MODEL ORGANIZATION

ACOs are "provider groups that accept responsibility for the cost and quality of care delivered to a specific population of patients cared for by the groups' clinicians," and provide data to assess performance on cost and quality criteria (Shortell, 2010). The organizational model has three features:

- Local accountability for effective management of the full continuum of care
- Shared savings based on historical trends as adjusted for different populations
- Performance measurement including clinical outcomes, quality, and patient experience (Drake & Guterman, 2010)

Rather than focusing on providing singular care and billing for volume of services provided to an individual patient, the ACO model seeks to influence the health and wellness of a defined population, throughout the continuum of care. By accepting risk for a defined population, ACOs can receive a share of the savings accrued when efficiency of care is increased through quality and service delivery improvements. This is referred to as "upside" risk. Likewise, if such quality and cost benchmarks are not met, at a minimum the ACO receives no shared savings, or may lose revenues through "downside" risk.

The ACO model may seem strikingly similar to the early health maintenance organization (HMO) or managed care organization (MCO) models that sought to drive down escalating health care costs by using financial incentives for managing populations in a less costly manner (Table 20.1). However, accountable care models differ from the HMOs and MCOs of the past by assigning care management to a group of health care providers instead of payers, focusing on measurable outcomes, and leveraging technology advancements for risk adjustment, advanced analytics, and health data management (Muhlestein, 2013). Rather than focusing on cost containment, the ACO is premised on health management that generates improved patient outcomes, which in turn will result in decreased cost.

The Medicare Shared Savings model is built on earlier initiatives, including CMS's Physician Group Practice (PGP) demonstration. The PGP demonstration included 10 provider groups ranging from free-standing PGPs to integrated delivery systems. The groups continued to receive their usual fee-for-service payments, and received bonuses for improving care through improved service delivery and care coordination, driven by quality and efficiency improvements. By year three, all 10 sites had achieved success on most quality measures, with two

TABLE 20.1 Comparison of Core Requirements of Traditional Versus Accountable Care

	TRADITIONAL CARE	ACCOUNTABLE CARE
Reimbursement Model	Fee-for-service payment for individual visits, services, or procedures	Bears financial risk for a defined population
Patient Care	Focus on individual patient at point of access to care	Coordinated, patient-focused system of clinical care for a defined population across the health care service continuum
Quality	Focus on individual patient and/or site-specific outcomes; cost and quality not linked	Provides measured outcomes related to both population health outcomes and cost efficiencies

groups meeting benchmarks on all 32 quality measures, and five groups achieving savings sufficient to trigger the shared savings bonus (CMS, 2009; McClellan, McKethan, Lewis, Roski, & Fisher, 2010). At the end of the fifth year, seven of the 10 groups had met benchmarks on all 32 quality measures, and four met cost-efficiency benchmarks (CMS, July 2011).

THE MEDICARE SHARED SAVINGS PROGRAM

In their 2009 Report to Congress, the Medicare Payment Advisory Commission (MedPAC) identified the ACO model as one tool for achieving payment and delivery system reform (MedPAC, 2009). Further, MedPAC recommended that ACOs be compensated through a model that combines fee-for-service with financial incentives to reduce cost, improve quality, and achieve information transparency (MedPAC, 2009).

Consistent with the MedPAC recommendation, PPACA specifies a voluntary ACO program to better align financial incentives with quality and cost goals. The MSSP is unique within PPACA. Unlike the National Pilot Program on Payment Bundling and other pilots and demonstration projects authorized under PPACA, the MSSP creates, in statute, a new clinical model and accompanying payment strategy premised on meeting quality and cost efficiency metrics.

The Act directed CMS to create the national voluntary program for ACOs by January, 2012, and to set forth eligibility requirements for ACO participation in the federal program (PPACA, 2010d). The ACO framework provided in PPACA § 3022 outlines the eligibility criteria to participate as an ACO, required elements for ACO activities, reporting requirements, and a payment methodology. The following paragraphs provide a summary of key ACO requirements as presented in § 3022.

ACO Providers

The following groups of service providers that have established a mechanism for shared governance are eligible to participate as an ACO:

- ACO professionals in group practice arrangements
- Networks of individual practices of ACO professionals
- Partnerships or joint venture arrangements between hospitals and ACO professionals
- Hospitals employing ACO professionals
- Other groups as deemed appropriate by the secretary

PPACA defines ACO professionals according to XVIII of the Social Security Act (PPACA, 2010d). Under this definition, an ACO professional is defined as a physician, including a doctor of medicine or osteopathy, doctor of dental surgery or medicine, a podiatrist, optometrist, or chiropractor licensed by the state (42 U.S.C. § 1861(r)(l), 2010). Practitioners, defined as a physician assistant, Nurse Practitioner, Clinical Nurse Specialist, Certified Registered Nurse Anesthetist, clinical social worker, clinical psychologist, or registered dietitian or nutrition professional are also eligible to participate as ACO professionals (42 U.S.C. §1842(b)(18)(C)(i), 2010).

General Requirements

To qualify for recognition as a Medicare ACO, the MSSP identify the following general requirements. The Medicare ACO must:

- Be willing to be accountable for quality, cost, and overall care of their assigned Medicare fee-for-service beneficiaries
- Agree to participate for 3 years
- Have a formal legal structure to allow for receipt and distribution of shared savings payments
- Include a sufficient number of ACO professionals to care for assigned Medicare beneficiaries
- Have a minimum of 5,000 assigned Medicare beneficiaries
- Have sufficient ACO professionals as determined necessary by the Secretary to support the assignment of Medicare fee-for-service beneficiaries, and implementation of the quality and administrative requirements
- Have in place a leadership and management structure that includes clinical and administrative systems
- Have defined processes to promote evidence-based medicine and patient engagement, reporting on quality and cost measures, and care coordination and
- Meet patient-centeredness criteria as defined by the secretary (U.S. Code of Federal Regulations, 2010b).

Quality and Reporting Requirements

Participating ACOs are required to report data to CMS for evaluation of the quality of care furnished by the ACO. Medicare ACOs are required to report on 33 quality measures, as well as a survey of patient experience of care. The quality measures are divided into four domains: Patient/caregiver experience, care coordination/patient safety, preventive health, and at risk populations. The "At Risk Population" domain specifically targets metrics relevant to diabetes, hypertension, ischemic vascular disease, and coronary artery disease (U.S. Department of Health and Human Services [USDHHS], 2011). To be eligible for the shared savings, ACOs must meet minimum attainment levels in each domain. Failure to report quality data accurately, completely, and in a timely manner may result in the ACO's termination from the MSSP, and loss of financial incentives (42 C.F.R. § 425.502(d), 2011).

Payments and Treatment of Savings

At the start of each agreement period, the secretary will set the ACO's established benchmark using the ACO's most recent available 3 years of per-beneficiary expenditures for Medicare Parts A and B services. Participating ACOs will be eligible to receive payment for shared savings if the ACO meets the established quality performance standards and its estimated average Medicare expenditure for each Medicare fee-for-service beneficiary for Medicare Part A and B services is at least the established percent below the established benchmark. If the ACO meets the accepted performance standards, a percent of the difference between the established benchmark and the average per capita annual Medicare expenditures may be paid to the ACO as shared savings. In 2016, revisions in the MSSP rules created benchmarking methodologies less dependent on the ACO's historical spending, and more reflective of spending in the ACO's region (42 C.F.R. § 425.603, 2016).

Attribution of ACO Beneficiaries

MSSP ACOs are required to have a minimum of 5,000 beneficiaries, who are assigned, or "attributed to" a specific ACO based on a formula described in the ACO regulations (PPACA, 2010e). Despite the inclusion of Advanced Practice Registered Nurses (APRNs) within the definition of ACO professionals, the statute and its implementing regulations effectively limit APRN practices from joining or establishing ACOs within the MSSP by basing assignment of beneficiaries solely on primary care services provided by a physician (PPACA, 2010d). Although APRNs can participate in ACOs as ACO professionals, patients who choose an APRN as their primary care provider cannot be counted as beneficiaries for Medicare Shared Savings purposes. Because the statute explicitly defines "primary care services provided by a physician" as the sole predicate for beneficiary assignment to an ACO, the APRN's patients are precluded from being assigned to an ACO and any resulting benefits from ACO participation. CMS could not change this statutory language within the rule-making process. However, recognizing that APRNs and other nonphysician health care providers can be significant assets to ACO success in achieving quality and cost-efficiency improvements, CMS sought a solution to this issue in the ACO rules through a stepwise approach to beneficiary assignment (USDHHS, 2011). Under the final rule, beneficiaries are first assigned to an ACO if the allowable charges for primary services accessed by the patient were provided by a primary care physician within the ACO, and such charges were greater than the allowable charges for primary care services accessed through other ACOs or non-ACO providers. In step 2, among the remainder of beneficiaries who have received at least one primary care physician service within the ACO, and have not accessed other primary care services by any other primary care physician either within or outside of the ACO, the beneficiary will be assigned to the ACO if the allowable charges for primary care services by all ACO professionals who are providers (such as APRNs) within the ACO are greater than charges for such services by ACO professionals working in another ACO, or by physicians, Nurse Practitioners, and other nonphysician providers working in a non-ACO setting (42 C.F.R. § 425.402, 2011). Although an imperfect solution, this regulatory "fix" provides a mechanism for recognition of care by physician specialists, APRNs, and other nonphysician providers in driving assignment of beneficiaries to a specific ACO. In addition to placing an unnecessary barrier to patient participation in ACOs, the stepwise approach to assignment of beneficiaries may have implications for the ACO's overall success in meeting some of the general ACO requirements.

NON–MEDICARE SHARED SAVINGS PROGRAMS

Although the "accountable care" concept existed well before PPACA's passage in March 2010, the Act generated renewed interest in the ACO model. Two such accountable care–based models that preceded PPACA are the Group Health Cooperative of Puget Sound's and Geisinger Health Systems's approach to integration.

The Group Health Cooperative of Puget Sound (Group Health) was founded in 1947. True to the founders' belief that "health was everybody's business and everybody's right," Group Health is one of only a few consumer-governed health plans in the United States. Most Group Health members receive care through the cooperative's integrated network of primary care, specialty care, and hospital providers. Consumer-based governance and reimbursement strategies that reward better care through quality and cost-efficiency improvements drive the innovation (Larson, 2009).

Geisinger is an integrated health system serving a large swath of central and northeastern Pennsylvania. This predominantly rural area is covered by Geisinger's employed primary care and specialty physicians, acute and specialty care hospitals, ambulatory surgery campuses, the Geisinger Health Plan (GHP), and other clinical and community-based outreach programs. The Geisinger model is an organized system of care with many examples of clinical integration. Geisinger leverages the patients for whom Geisinger is both financially responsible, through their health plan (GHP) and clinically, through their care providers to foster innovation (Paulus, 2008). Geisinger's ProvenCare model for managing acute episodes of care is looked to as a successful model of what application of evidence driven standardized care paths, aligned with significant financial incentives, can achieve.

The requirements for ACO participation as set forth in the Act create a broad framework for ACO implementation. Thus, several ACO models have been suggested, ranging from integrated delivery systems to "virtual ACOs" that encompass a wide range of small practices and providers in disparate locations. Despite variation in suggested organizational structures, the core concept of joint accountability for quality and cost improvement remains constant.

Emerging ACOs are also focused on factors other than medical illness with potential to impact health outcomes and the quality and efficiency of care delivery. For example, patients with behavioral health disorders generally have worse health outcomes and higher health care utilization metrics as compared to individuals without behavioral health conditions. Linking behavioral health referral mechanisms and embedding behavioral health providers in primary care practices in one large academic medical center resulted in a 13% decrease in emergency department utilization among patients with behavioral health needs (Clarke, 2016). Social determinants of health also have a significant impact on health outcomes. Social factors such as education, racial segregation, lack of social support, and poverty have been linked to increased at-risk health behaviors and the likelihood of living in an environment that poses barriers to health (Heiman & Artiga, 2015). Recognizing the impact of social determinants on health outcomes, population health management that addresses both medical and non-medical services is gaining attention. As such, some ACOs have begun to consider ways to identify patients with nonmedical needs and to begin to address those needs through individualized pathways, or well-defined, targeted approaches, such as linkage to housing resources or transportation options (Fraze, 2016).

IMPLICATIONS FOR APRNs IN AN ERA OF ACCOUNTABLE CARE

Although Medicare's version of ACOs has been formalized in statute and regulation, a variety of non-Medicare ACO models have emerged. In addition to the CMS-recognized ACOs, private accountable care models sponsored by providers, such as hospital systems or independent provider associations, or insurance companies are present in the health care market. Many of this first wave of ACOs are centered in areas with larger populations. Although hospital system led ACOs remain the majority model, physician group led models continue to grow (Muhlestein, 2013). While the framework for the Medicare ACOs is more proscriptive by the statutory and regulatory requirements, private models have more leeway to experiment with different approaches to population management and reimbursement.

APRNs Within the ACO Framework

APRNs should be aware of key concepts and their potential impact on APRN practice and ACO success. Specifically, the requirements related to number of patients receiving care within the ACO, the ability to achieve quality and cost benchmarks, and patient-centeredness criteria may be influenced by the treatment of APRNs within the ACO framework, as well as their utilization within the ACO itself.

Patient Activation and Engagement

The Institute of Medicine (IOM) lists patient-centeredness as one of six aims for health care system improvement (IOM & Committee on Quality of Health Care in America, 2001). In 2008, the National Priorities Partnership (NPP) identified patient and family engagement as one of six priorities with the most potential to reduce harm, eliminate disparities, decrease disease burden, and remove inefficiencies in health care delivery (NPP, 2008). Given the significance placed on patient-centeredness by these and other similar national recommendations, it is not surprising that ACOs are required to define processes to promote patient engagement and demonstrate that they meet patient-centeredness criteria (PPACA, 2010d).

Patient-centeredness means "providing care that is respectful of and responsive to individual patient preferences, needs, and values, and ensuring that patient values guide all clinical decisions" (IOM & Committee on Quality of Health Care in America, 2001). The aim focuses on the patient's experience of illness and health care and the effectiveness of health care delivery systems in meeting the patient's individual needs. Patient-centeredness, as defined by the IOM, encompasses the qualities of compassion, empathy, and responsiveness to the patient's *expressed* needs and preferences related to the health care experience (IOM & Committee on Quality of Health Care in America, 2001). Within the context of the ACO statute and it's implementing regulations, patient-centeredness criteria means that patient-centered care must be promoted by the ACO's governing body and integrated into practice by leadership and management working with the ACO's health care teams (USDHHS, 2011).

Since inception of the term by the IOM, health care providers have struggled to identify, incorporate, and evaluate patient-centeredness in practice. Patient surveys of satisfaction with the health care experience are frequently used to evaluate patient-centered care (Davies, 2008). Criteria regarding ease of access to care, provider–patient communication, provider knowledge of the patient's history, responsiveness of office staff, care coordination, and general satisfaction with the health care provider and staff are examples of surrogates for patient-centered care (Davies, 2008; Rodriguez, Scoggins, von Glahn, Zaslavsky, & Safran, 2009). Consistent with these criteria, the ACO regulations cite eight elements as surrogates for proof of patient centeredness:

- A beneficiary experience of care survey with an accompanying quality improvement plan
- Patient involvement in ACO governance
- A culturally competent process, and description of such process, for evaluating the health needs of the assigned population
- Systems to identify high risk individuals and processes to develop individualized care plans that integrate community resources, for the targeted population
- Care coordination processes which include electronic technologies consistent with meaningful use criteria
- Health literacy processes to support communication of clinical knowledge to beneficiaries that allow for beneficiary engagement and shared decision-making
- Written standards and processes for beneficiaries to access their medical records
- Internal processes to measure physician clinical or service performance across practices that are used to drive a quality improvement plan (42 C.F.R. § 425.112(2), 2011)

A recent IOM report suggests team-based models of care as a response to an increasingly complex health care delivery system and the shift toward clinically integrated, value-based payment models, such as those associated with ACOs (IOM, 2013). This attention to team-based models of care has prompted professional organizations to weigh in on how such models might be developed. In 2015, an interdisciplinary task force convened by the American College of Obstetricians and Gynecologists (ACOG) released *Collaboration in Practice: A Framework for Team-Based Care*. The document, endorsed and supported by over 20 professional organizations, including six APRN organizations, sets forth an equitable approach to team-based care that encourages "all health care providers to function to the full extent of their education, certification, and experience" (ACOG Task Force on Collaborative Practice, 2016). Former CMS Director Berwick suggests that proper incorporation of patient-centeredness into new health care designs will "involve some radical, unfamiliar, and disruptive shifts in control and power, out of the hand of those who give care and into the hands of those who receive it" (Berwick, 2009). While the new reimbursement models resulting from the shift to value-based care support a team-based approach to care, the type of radical change Berwick describes as necessary to achieving patient-centeredness may be difficult to achieve if existing research on primary care structure and culture holds true. Evidence suggests that when practices attempt change, they often maintain existing structures without fundamentally evaluating and redefining team members' roles (Chesluck & Holmboe, 2010). Successful transition to a care model that utilizes each member to that member's full scope of practice and ability will require substantial communication, collaboration, and flexibility among health care providers and staff, explicit communication with patients regarding team members' roles and responsibilities, and an organizational culture that fosters collaboration.

Although "patient-centeredness" is only one of eight ACO requirements listed in the Act, it has the potential to significantly impact benchmarking criteria. Evidence suggests that emphasis on clinical quality and patient experience criteria, as opposed to productivity and efficiency, is associated with greater improvement in care coordination and office staff interaction (Rodriguez, von Glahn, Elliott, Rogers, & Safran, 2009). Patient and family centeredness is a core guiding principle in an equitable model of team-based care. Reliable, high quality decision aids, and decision-support tools can help to support patient engagement and activation (ACOG Task Force on Collaborative Practice, 2016). Care planned by highly functioning teams, in partnership with patients, can positively impact outcomes (Mitchell, 2012). Attention to patient experience measures will be important in meeting ACO quality performance benchmarks.

Meeting Quality and Cost Efficiency Measures

Generally, ACOs must meet quality benchmarks in addition to efficiency metrics, in order to qualify for shared savings. Poor care coordination and discretionary medical interventions contribute to inefficient utilization of health care resources and higher health care costs. Regional variations in health care spending are associated with variability in primary care provider discretionary decision making. Patients receive approximately half of the recommended processes for leading acute and chronic conditions (McGlynn et al., 2003). Care coordination and communication failures are linked to increased hospitalizations and readmission rates, contributing to large Medicare expenditures (Jencks, Williams, & Coleman, 2009; Piekes, Chen, Schore, & Brown, 2009). APRNs consistently demonstrate positive rankings on overall levels of patient satisfaction, consultation time, and preventive screenings (Lenz, Mundinger, Kane, Hopkins, & Lin, 2004). It is likely that effective integration of APRNs into accountable care models will have a positive effect on cost and quality metrics.

Efficient, cost-effective care delivery requires access to patient information, decision support, and timely access to benchmarking data. The ACO serves as the information and data center for its population. Information technologies (IT) and analytical resources are necessary to achieve the level of clinical integration necessary to improve quality, reduce costs, and track performance against explicit quantitative benchmarking targets. Accurate and complete ACO-specific quality and cost information will be essential to maximizing the financial incentives. Appropriate IT systems and tools, such as disease registries that enable population-based decision making and predictive modeling to identify high-risk patients in need of care coordination, will be critical in facilitating the level of communication, data collection, monitoring, evaluation, and reporting activities necessary to fully support and capture the ACOs quality and cost improvements (Fields, 2010).

CONCLUSION

In response to the multisector interest in APMs and the CMS goal of moving to a value driven health care delivery system, CMS launched the CMS Alliance to Modernize Healthcare (CAMH), a federally funded research and development center. The Health Care Payment Learning & Action Network (HPLAN) was created as part of the CAMH initiative to drive alignment in payment approaches across the public and private sector. HPLAN guiding principles, informed by wide stakeholder involvement, recognize that provider incentives alone are not enough to move the needle to patient-centered care. Rather, patients must be integral partners in transforming health care. Further, APMs that do not include quality in the payment equation are not recognized within the HPLAN APM framework. Value-based incentives should be sufficient to motivate practice change and should reach the providers who deliver care. Finally, care delivery models, such as ACOs and medical homes, are examples of care delivery systems, rather than the end-point of an alternate payment model (Alternative Payment Model and Progress Tracking [APM FPT] Workgroup, 2016).

As new care models are developed in both the public and private markets, barriers to full utilization of APRNs must be identified and addressed. First, while most Medicare and non-Medicare ACOs currently reside in more densely populated areas and are hospital led, as success is demonstrated in improved outcomes and cost efficiencies, it is likely that variations of the model will spread into more rural areas and to more vulnerable populations accessing care among safety net providers. Given current provider shortages, and decreased access to care, APRNs provide a logical solution to expanding care in these areas.

Health care transformation to a quality and value driven system, informed by best practices gleaned from evolving clinical integration demonstrations, has the potential to improve both individual and population health. Organizational structure, information technology capabilities, and strong quality improvement strategies are priorities in preparing for transition to an accountable care model. Practice patterns and patient factors are important considerations to inform the process. Evaluation of these factors and implementation of changes to support intra- and interpractice team collaboration and coordination are necessary to assure success in meeting quality and efficiency benchmarks, and ultimately transforming health care service delivery to a patient centric, value driven model.

DISCUSSION QUESTIONS

1. *Consider the ACO framework, using the MSSP as set forth in PPACA, as an example.*
   a. *Describe the points where APRNs seem to be most included in the framework.*
   b. *Discuss areas where APRNs could make the greatest impact within the framework.*
   c. *Discuss areas where APRNs are least included within the framework.*
   d. *With reference to areas that are less supportive of APRN inclusion, discuss how APRNs may affect policy change that is more favorable to APRN practice.*
2. *The ACO and ACO-like models are premised on the proposition that providers will access a share of "savings" that are directly attributable to meeting and exceeding quality and cost benchmarks. Such models are often referred to as "provider incentives."*
   a. *If a practice is participating in a "shared savings model" how should APRNs be included?*

    b. *How could you broach the subject of APRN access to shared savings if you were employed by an ACO?*

ANALYSIS, SYNTHESIS, AND CLINICAL APPLICATION

1. *The APRN skill set could be critical to the success of an ACO, or clinical integration model. Consider the following:*
   a. *What types of unique skills does the APRN bring to the table that would significantly contribute to ACO's successful achievement of quality and cost efficiency benchmarks?*
   b. *How can APRNs best articulate the necessity for their skill sets within the ACO team?*
   c. *Consider one clinical example where an APRN led intervention could contribute to the practice achieving their quality and efficiency metrics.*

EXERCISES/CONSIDERATIONS

1. *The emphasis on improved population health outcomes through improved quality and efficiency seeks to improve health care delivery. Do you think there are potential negative implications associated with this approach? If so, discuss how such concerns might be mitigated to meet the intent of the law?*

REFERENCES

ACOG Task Force on Collaborative Practice. (2016). Executive summary: Collaboration in Practice: Implementing team-based care. *Obstetrics & Gynecology, 127*(3), 612–617.

Alternative Payment Model Framework and Progress Tracking Workgroup. (2016). Alternative payment model (APM) framework final white paper. *The MITRE Corporation.* Retrieved from https://hcp-lan.org/workproducts/apm-whitepaper-total.pdf

American Recovery and Reinvestment Act. (2009). (Pub. L. 111–115).

Baseman, S. B. (2016). *Payment and delivery system reform in Medicare: A primer on medical homes, accountable care organizations, and bundled payments.* Menlo Park, CA: Kaiser Family Foundation.

Berwick, D. M. (2009). What 'patient-centered' should mean: Confessions of an extremist. *Health Affairs, 28*(4), w555–w565.

Centers for Medicare and Medicaid Innovation. (2010, June 1). The CMS innovation center. Retrieved from http://innovation.cms.gov

Centers for Medicare and Medicaid Innovation. (2011). Pioneer ACO model. Retrieved from http://innovation.cms.gov/initiatives/Pioneer-ACO-Model

Centers for Medicare and Medicaid Services. (2009). *Fact sheet: Medicare physician group demonstration: Physician groups continue to improve quality and generate savings under Medicare physician pay for performance demonstration.* Baltimore, MD: Author.

Centers for Medicare and Medicaid Services. (2011, July). *Fact sheet: Medicare physician group demonstration: Physician groups continue to improve quality and generate savings under Medicare physician pay for performance demonstration.* Retrieved from http://www.cms.gov/Medicare/Demonstration-Projects/DemoProjectsEvalRpts/downloads/PGP_Fact_Sheet.pdf

Centers for Medicare and Medicaid Services. (2015, June 18). Affordable Care Act payment model saves more than $25 million in first performance year. Retrieved from https://www.cms.gov/Newsroom/MediaReleaseDatabase/Press-releases/2015-Press-releases-items/2015-06-18.html

Centers for Medicare and Medicaid Services. (2016, August 9). Independence at home demonstration performance year 2 results. Retrieved from https://www.cms.gov/Newsroom/MediaReleaseDatabase/Fact-sheets/2016-Fact-sheets-items/2016-08-09.html

Chesluck, B. J. & Holmboe, E. S. (2010). How teams work—or don't—in primary care: A field study on internal medicine practices. *Health Affairs, 29*(5), 874–879.

Clarke, R. J. (2016). Beivering on accountable Care: Lessons from a behavioral health program to improve access and outcomes. *Health Affairs, 35*(8), 1487–1493.

Davies, E. S.-L. (2008). Evaluating the use of a modified CAHPS survey to support improvements in patient-centered care: Lessons from a quality improvement collaborative. *Health Expectations, 11*, 160–176.

Deficit Reduction Act of 2005. (2006a). Pub. L. 109–171 § 5001(a).

Drake, H., & Guterman, S. (2010). *Developing innovative payment approaches: Finding the path to high performance*. Washington, DC: Commonwealth Fund.

Fields, D. L. (2010). Analysis & commentary: Driving quality gains and cost savings through adoption of medical homes. *Health Affairs, 29*(5), 819–826.

42 C.F.R. § 425.112(2) (2011).

42 C.F.R. § 425.402 (2011).

42 C.F.R. § 425.502(d) (2011).

42 C.F.R. § 425.603 (2016).

42 U.S.C. § 1842(b)(18)(C)(i) (2010).

42 U.S.C. § 1861(r)(l) (2010).

Fraze, T. L. (2016). Housing, transportation, and food: How ACOs seek to improve population health by addressing nonmedical needs of patients. *Health Affairs, 35*(11), 2109–2115.

Heiman, H. J., & Artiga, S. (2015). *Beyond health care: The role of social determinants in promoting health and health equity*. Menlo Park, CA: The Kiaser Family Foundation.

Institute of Medicine, Committee on Quality of Health Care in America. (2001). *Crossing the quality chasm: A new health system for the 21st century*. Washington, DC: National Academies Press.

Institute of Medicine. (2013). *Best care at lower cost: The path to continuously learning health care in America*. Washington, DC: National Academies Press.

Jencks, S. W., Williams, M. V., & Coleman, E. A. (2009). Rehospitalizations among patients in the Medicare fee-for-service program. *New England Journal of Medicine, 360*, 1418–1428.

Larson, E. (2009). Group health cooperative—one coverage and delivery model for accountable care. *New England Journal of Medicine, 36*(17), 1620–1622.

Lenz, E. M., Mundinger, M. O., Kane, R. L., Hopkins, S. C., & Lin, S. X. (2004). Primary care outcomes in patients treated by nurse practitioners or physicians: Two-year follow-up. *Medical Care & Research Review, 61*(3), 332–351.

Lewin Group. (2015, February). CMS bundled payments for care improvement initiative models 2-4: Year 1 Evaluation & Monitoring Annual report. Retrieved from https://innovation.cms.gov/files/reports/bpci-evalrpt1.pdf

McClellan, M. M., McKethan , A. N., Lewis , J. L., Roski , J., & Fisher , E. S. (2010). A national strategy to put accountable care into practice. *Health Affairs, 29*(5), 982–990.

McGlynn, E. A., Asch, S. M., Adams, J., Keesey, J., Hicks, J., DeCristofaro , A., & Kerr, E. A. (2003). The quality of health care delivered to adults in the United States. *New England Journal of Medicine, 348*, 2635–2645.

Medicare Improvements for Patients and Providers Act of 2008, Pub. L. 110–275, § 131(b) (2008).

Medicare Prescription Drug and Modernization Act. (2003). (Pub. L. 108–173) § 501(b).

MedPAC. (2009, June). Report to Congress: Improving incentives in the Medicare Program. Retrieved from http://www.medpac.gov/documents/jun09_entirereport.pdf

Mitchell, P. W. (2012). *Core principles and values of effective team-based health care. Discussion paper: The best practices innovation collaborative of the IOM roundtable on value & science-driven health care*. Washington, DC: Institute of Medicine.

Muhlestein, D. C. (2013). *The accountable care paradigm: More than just managed care 2.0*. Salt Lake City, UT: Leavitt Partners. Retrieved from https://leavittpartners.com/2013/03/the-accountable-care-paradigm-more-than-just-managed-care-2-0

National Priorities Partnership. (2008). *National priorities and goals: Aligning our efforts to transform America's healthcare*. Washington, DC: National Quality Forum.

Paulus, R. D., Davis, K., & Steele , G. D. (2008). Continuous innovation in health care: Implication of the Geisinger experience. *Health Affairs, 27*(5), 1235–1245.

Patient Protection and Affordable Care Act, Pub. L. 111–148 (2010a).

Patient Protection and Affordable Care Act, Pub. L. 111–148 § 2703 (2010b).

Patient Protection and Affordable Care Act, Pub. L. 111–148 § 3021 (2010c).

Patient Protection and Affordable Care Act, Pub. L. 111–148 § 3022 (2010d).

Patient Protection and Affordable Care Act, Pub. L. 111–148 § 3023 (2010e).

Patient Protection and Affordable Care Act, Pub. L. 111–148 § 3024 (2010f).

Piekes, D. C., Chen , A., Schore , J., & Brown, R. (2009). Effects of care coordination on hospitalization, quality of care, and health expenditures among Medicare beneficiaries. *Journal of the American Medical Association, 301*(6), 603–618.

Rodriguez, H. P., Scoggins, J. F., von Glahn, T., Zaslavsky, A. M., & Safran, D. G. (2009). Attributing sources of variation in patients' experiences of ambulatory care. *Medical Care, 47*(8), 835–841.

Rodriguez, H. P., von Glahn, T., Elliott, M. N., Rogers, W. H., & Safran, D. G. (2009). The effect of performance-based incentives on improving patient care experiences: A statewide evaluation. *Journal of General Internal Medicine, 24*(12), 1281–1288.

Shortell, S. C. (2010). How the Centers for Medicare and Medicaid innovation should test accountable care organizations. *Health Affairs, 29*(3), 1293–1298.

Slonim, A., & Maraccini, A. M. (2016, December). The post-election future of ACOs. *The American Journal of Accountable Care,* 52–53. Retrieved from http://www.ajmc.com/journals/ajac/2016/2016-vol4 -n4/the-post-election-future-of-acos

Tax Relief and Health Care Act of 2006, Pub. L. 109-432, Div. B, § 101(b) (2006).

Tu, T. (2016, March 1). CMS ACOs and the future of the movement. Retrieved from http://leavitt partners.com/2016/03/cms-acos-and-the-future-of-the-movement-2/

U.S. Department of Health and Human Services. (2011, November 2). Medicare program: Medicare shared savings program: Accountable care organizations. Retrieved from http://www.gpo.gov/ fdsys/pkg/FR-2011-11-02/pdf/2011-27461.pdf

U.S. Department of Health and Human Services. (2016, March 3). HHS reaches goal of tying 30 percent of Medicare payments to quality ahead of schedule. Retrieved from https://www.hhs.gov/ about/news/2016/03/03/hhs-reaches-goal-tying-30-percent-medicare-payments-quality-ahead -schedule.html

U.S. Department of Health and Human Services. (2016, October 14). Medicare program: Merit-based incentive payment system (MIPS) and alternative payment model (APM) incentive under the physician fee schedule and criteria for physician-focused payment models. Retrieved from https://qpp.cms .gov/docs/QPP_Executive_Summary_of_Final_Rule.pdf

CHAPTER 21

A Systemic Approach to Containing Health Care Spending

Ezekiel Emanuel, Neera Tanden, Stuart Altman, Scott Armstrong,
Donald Berwick, François de Brantes, Maura Calsyn, Michael Chernew,
John Colmers, David Cutler, Tom Daschle, Paul Egerman, Bob Kocher,
Arnold Milstein, Emily Oshima Lee, John D. Podesta,
Uwe Reinhardt, Meredith Rosenthal, Joshua Sharfstein,
Stephen Shortell, Andrew Stern, Peter R. Orszag, and Topher Spiro

National health spending is projected to continue to grow faster than the economy, increasing from 18% to about 25% of the gross domestic product (GDP) by 2037 (Congressional Budget Office, 2012). Federal health spending is projected to increase from 25% to approximately 40% of total federal spending by 2037 (Congressional Budget Office, 2012). These trends could squeeze out critical investments in education and infrastructure, contribute to unsustainable debt levels, and constrain wage increases for the middle class (Emanuel, 2012; Emanuel & Fuchs, 2008).

Although the influx of baby boomers increases the number of Medicare beneficiaries, growth in per capita health costs increasingly drives growth in federal health spending over the long term (Congressional Budget Office, 2012). This means that health costs throughout the system drive federal health spending. Reforms that shift federal spending to individuals, employers, and states fail to address the problem. The only sustainable solution is to control overall growth in health costs.

Although the Affordable Care Act (ACA) significantly reduced Medicare spending over the decade after its passage (Sisko et al., 2019), health costs remain a major challenge. To effectively contain costs, solutions must target the drivers of both the level of costs and the growth in costs—and both medical prices and the quantity of services play important roles. Solutions need to reduce costs not only for public payers but also for private payers. Finally, solutions need to root out administrative costs that do not improve health status and outcomes.

The Center for American Progress convened leading health policy experts with diverse perspectives to develop bold and innovative solutions that meet these criteria. Although these solutions are not intended to be exhaustive, they have the greatest probability of both being implemented and successfully controlling health costs. The following solutions could be implemented separately or, more effectively, integrated as a package.

PROMOTE PAYMENT RATES WITHIN GLOBAL TARGETS

Under our current fragmented payment system, providers can shift costs from public payers to private payers and from large insurers to small insurers (Reinhardt, 2011). As each provider negotiates payment rates with multiple insurers, administrative costs are excessive. Moreover, continued consolidation of market power among providers increases prices over time (Berenson, Ginsburg, Christianson, & Yee, 2012). For all these reasons, the current system is not sustainable.

Under a model of self-regulation, public and private payers would negotiate payment rates with providers, and these rates would be binding on all payers and providers in a state. Providers could still offer rates lower than the negotiated rates.

The privately negotiated rates would have to adhere to a global spending target for both public and private payers in the state. After a transition, this target should limit growth in health spending per capita to the average growth in wages, which would combat wage stagnation and resonate with the public. We recommend that an independent council composed of providers, payers, businesses, consumers, and economists set and enforce the spending target.

We suggest that the federal government award grants to states to promote this self-regulation model. States could phase in this model, one sector (e.g., hospitals) at a time. To receive grants, states would need to report measures of quality, access, and cost publicly, and would receive bonus payments for high performance. For providers, the negotiated rates would be adjusted for performance on quality measures, which should be identical for public and private payers.

Funding for research, training, and uncompensated care—currently embedded in Medicare and Medicaid payments—should be separated out and increased with growth in the global spending target. These payments must be transparent and determined through negotiations or competitive bidding.

ACCELERATE USE OF ALTERNATIVES TO FEE-FOR-SERVICE PAYMENT

Fee-for-service payment encourages wasteful use of high-cost tests and procedures. Instead of paying a fee for each service, payers could pay a fixed amount to physicians and hospitals for a bundle of services (bundled payments) or all the care that a patient needs (global payments).

Payers need to accelerate the use of such alternative payment methods. As soon as possible, both public and private payers should adopt the bundles for 37 cardiac and orthopedic procedures used in the Medicare Acute Care Episode Program (Cutler & Ghosh, 2012; Mechanic, 2011). The bundles also need to include rehabilitation and post-acute care for 90 days after discharge. Within

5 years, Medicare should make bundled payments for at least two chronic conditions, such as cancer or coronary artery disease. Within 10 years, Medicare and Medicaid should base at least 75% of payments in every region on alternatives to fee-for-service payment.

Together, these policies would remove uncertainty about transitions from fee-for-service payment, allowing sufficient time for investment in infrastructure and technology by payers and providers.

USE COMPETITIVE BIDDING FOR ALL COMMODITIES

Evidence suggests that prices for many products, such as medical equipment and devices, are excessive (Government Accountability Office, 2012). Instead of the government setting prices, market forces should be used to allow manufacturers and suppliers to compete to offer the lowest price. In 2011, such competitive bidding reduced Medicare spending on medical equipment such as wheelchairs by more than 42% (Centers for Medicare and Medicaid Services, 2012). The ACA requires Medicare to expand competitive bidding for equipment, prosthetics, orthotics, and supplies to all regions by 2016 (Patient Protection and ACA, 2010). We suggest that Medicare immediately expand the current program nationwide.

As soon as possible, Medicare should extend competitive bidding to medical devices, laboratory tests, radiologic diagnostic services, and all other commodities (Office of Management and Budget, 2008). Medicare's competitively bid prices would then be extended to all federal health programs (Office of Management and Budget, 2011).

To oversee the process, we recommend that Medicare establish a panel of business and academic experts. Finally, we recommend that exchanges— marketplaces for insurance starting in 2014—conduct competitive bidding for these items on behalf of private payers and state employee plans.

REQUIRE EXCHANGES TO OFFER TIERED PRODUCTS

The market dominance of select providers often drives substantial price variation (Commonwealth of Massachusetts, 2011a, 2011b). To address this problem, insurers can offer tiered plans. These insurance products designate a high-value tier of providers with high quality and low costs and reduce cost sharing for patients who obtain services from these providers. For instance, in Massachusetts, one-tiered product lowers copayments by as much as $1,000 if patients choose from 53 high-value providers (Commonwealth of Massachusetts, 2011a, 2011b). We suggest that exchanges and state employee plans offer at least one-tiered product at the bronze and silver levels of coverage. This requirement can be implemented by 2016 or sooner if feasible. To encourage participation in the tiered product, it must achieve a minimum premium discount. For instance, in Massachusetts, insurers must offer at least one tiered product with a premium that is at least 12% lower than the premium for a similar nontiered product (Commonwealth of Massachusetts, 2010).

Transparency and consumer education are essential (Sinaiko & Rosenthal, 2010). Quality and cost measures must be standardized and publicly disclosed, and standards must be set for how these measures are used to create tiers. Whenever possible, quality measures should use data from all payers. Finally, in contracts between insurers and providers, clauses that inhibit tiered products must be prohibited.

REQUIRE ALL EXCHANGES TO BE ACTIVE PURCHASERS

If exchanges passively offer any insurance product that meets minimal standards, an important opportunity is lost. As soon as reliable quality reporting systems exist and exchanges achieve the adequate scale, it is critical that federal and state exchanges engage in active purchasing—leveraging their bargaining power to secure the best premium rates and promote reforms in payment and delivery systems.

The ACA provides bonus payments to Medicare Advantage plans with four- or five-star ratings on the basis of their performance on measures of clinical quality and patients' experience (Health Care and Education Reconciliation Act, 2010). We recommend that exchanges adopt this or a similar pay-for-performance model for participating plans and award a gold star to plans that provide high quality at a low premium.

SIMPLIFY ADMINISTRATIVE SYSTEMS FOR ALL PAYERS AND PROVIDERS

The United States spends nearly $360 billion a year on administrative costs (Institute of Medicine [IOM], 2010), accounting for 14% of excessive health spending (Farrell et al., 2008). Section 1104 of the ACA requires uniform standards and operating rules for electronic transactions between health plans and providers (Patient Protection and ACA, 2010). Although plans must comply with these standards and rules, the law does not require providers to exchange information electronically.

First, we suggest that payers and providers electronically exchange eligibility, claims, and other administrative information as soon as possible. Second, public and private payers and providers should use a single, standardized physician credentialing system. Currently, physicians must submit their credentials to multiple payers and hospitals. Third, payers should provide monthly explanation-of-benefits statements electronically but allow patients to opt for paper statements. Fourth, electronic health records should integrate clinical and administrative functions—such as billing, prior authorization, and payments—over the coming 5 years. For instance, ordering a clinical service for a patient could automatically bill the payer in one step.

Most important, we recommend that a task force consisting of payers, providers, and vendors set binding compliance targets, monitor use rates, and have broad authority to implement additional measures to achieve systemwide savings of $30 billion a year (U.S. Healthcare, 2010).

REQUIRE FULL TRANSPARENCY OF PRICES

Prices for the same services vary substantially within the same geographic area (Commonwealth of Massachusetts, 2011a, 2011b). However, consumers almost never receive price information before treatment. Price transparency would allow consumers to plan ahead and choose lower cost providers, which may lead high-cost providers to lower prices. Although price transparency could facilitate collusion, this risk could be addressed through aggressive enforcement of anti-trust laws.

Moreover, both private and public models can achieve meaningful price transparency without leading to collusion (Government Accountability Office, 2011). Aetna provides the price it negotiated with a specific provider to members through an internet website. Similarly, New Hampshire has a public website that provides the median price paid by an insurer to a specific provider on the basis of claims data.

It is important that all private insurers and states provide price informa-tion that reflects negotiated discounts with specific providers. The information should include one price that bundles together all costs associated with a service, individualized estimates of out-of-pocket costs at the point of care, and informa-tion on the quality of care and volume of patients so that consumers can make informed decisions by value.

In contracts between insurers and providers, many providers prohibit insur-ers from releasing price information to their members (Government Accountability Office, 2011). These so-called gag clauses and other anticompetitive clauses must be prohibited. Finally, we recommend that state insurance commissioners and exchanges collect, audit, and publicly report data on prices and claims.

MAKE BETTER USE OF NONPHYSICIAN PROVIDERS

Restrictive state scope-of-practice laws prevent nonphysician providers from practicing to the full extent of their training. For instance, 34 states do not allow Advanced Practice Registered Nurses (APRNs) to practice without physician supervision (Pittman & Williams, 2012). Making greater use of these providers would expand the workforce supply, which would increase competition and thereby lower prices.

We recommend that the federal government provide bonus payments to states that meet scope-of-practice standards delineated by the IOM. Medicare and Medicaid payments to nonphysician providers should allow them to prac-tice to the full extent permitted by state law.

EXPAND THE MEDICARE BAN ON PHYSICIAN SELF-REFERRALS

Many studies show that when physicians self-refer patients to facilities in which they have a financial interest, especially for imaging and pathology services, they drive up costs and may adversely affect the quality of care (Medicare Payment Advisory Commission, 2009; Mitchell, 2012). Under the so-called Stark law, phy-sicians are prohibited from referring Medicare and Medicaid patients to facilities in which they have a financial interest. However, an exception allows physicians to provide "in-house ancillary services," such as diagnostic imaging, in their offices (42 C.F.R. § 411.355, 2011).

We believe that the Stark law should be expanded to prohibit physician self-referrals for services that are paid for by private insurers. In addition, the loop-holes for in-office imaging, pathology laboratories, and radiation therapy should be closed. Physicians who use alternatives to fee-for-service payment should be exempted because these methods reduce incentives to increase volume.

LEVERAGE THE FEDERAL EMPLOYEES PROGRAM TO DRIVE REFORM

The Federal Employees Health Benefits Program (FEHBP) provides private health insurance to 8 million federal employees and their families. Although the FEHBP has encouraged various reforms to improve the quality of care (U.S. Office of Personnel Management, 2012), it could be much more innovative.

We recommend that the FEHBP align with Medicare by requiring plans to transition to alternative payment methods, reduce payments to hospitals with high rates of readmissions and hospital-acquired conditions, and adjust payments to hospitals and physicians by their performance on quality measures. In addition, the FEHBP should require carriers to offer tiered products and conduct competitive bidding on behalf of plans for all commodities. Finally, the FEHBP should require plans to provide price information to enrollees and prohibit gag clauses in plan contracts with providers.

REDUCE THE COSTS OF DEFENSIVE MEDICINE

More than 75% of physicians—and virtually all physicians in high-risk specialties—face a malpractice claim over the course of their career (Jena, Seabury, Lakdawalla, & Chandra, 2011). Regardless of whether a claim results in liability, the risk of being sued may cause physicians to practice a type of defensive medicine that increases costs without improving the quality of care.

Strategies to control costs associated with medical malpractice and defensive medicine must be responsible and targeted. These strategies must not impose arbitrary caps on damages for patients who are injured as a result of malpractice. According to the Congressional Budget Office, arbitrary caps on damages would reduce national health spending by only 0.5% (Congressional Budget Office, 2009a, 2009b). Although such caps would have a barely measurable effect on costs; they might adversely affect health outcomes (Congressional Budget Office, 2009a, 2009b; Lakdawalla & Seabury, 2009).

A more promising strategy would provide a so-called safe harbor, in which physicians would be presumed to have no liability if they used qualified health-information-technology systems and adhered to evidence-based clinical practice guidelines that did not reflect defensive medicine. Physicians could use clinical decision-support systems that incorporate these guidelines.

Under such a system, the physician could use the safe harbor as an affirmative defense at an early stage in the litigation and could introduce guidelines into evidence to avoid a courtroom battle of the experts. The patient could still present evidence that the guidelines were not applicable to the particular situation, and the judge would still determine their applicability.

It is critical to develop guidelines with credibility. A promising step is an initiative called Choosing Wisely, in which leading physician groups released guidelines on 45 common tests and procedures that might be overused or unnecessary (Cassel & Guest, 2012). Given the important role of guidelines, physicians who participate in developing them must be free from financial conflicts of interest.

CONCLUSION

These are the types of large-scale solutions that are necessary to contain health costs. Although many in the health industry perceive that it is not in their interest to contain national health spending, it is a fact that what cannot continue will not continue.

Americans, therefore, face a choice. Payers could simply shift costs to individuals. As those costs become more and more unaffordable, people would severely restrict their consumption of health care and might forgo necessary care. Alternatively, governments could impose deep cuts in provider payments unrelated to value or the quality of care. Without an innovative alternative strategy, these options become the default. They are not in the long-term interests of patients, employers, states, insurers, or providers.

We present alternative strategies to contain national health spending that allow Americans to access necessary care. Our approach addresses the system as a whole, not just Medicare and Medicaid. It is the path to rising wages, a sustainable federal budget, and the health system that all Americans deserve.

REFERENCES

Berenson, R. A., Ginsburg, P. B., Christianson, J. B., & Yee, T. (2012). The growing power of some providers to win steep payment increases from insurers suggests policy remedies may be needed. *Health Affairs, 31,* 973–981.

Cassel, C. K., & Guest, J. A. (2012). Choosing wisely: Helping physicians and patients make smart decisions about their care. *Journal of the American Medical Association, 307,* 1801–1802.

Centers for Medicare and Medicaid Services. (2012). Competitive bidding update—one year implementation update. Retrieved from http://www.cms.gov/Medicare/Medicare-Fee-for-Service-Payment/DMEPOSCompetitiveBid/Downloads/Competitive-Bidding-Update-One-Year-Implementation.pdf

Commonwealth of Massachusetts. (2010). S.2585, an act to promote cost containment, transparency, and efficiency in the provision of quality health insurance for individuals and small businesses: Approved. Retrieved from http://www.malegislature.gov/Laws/SessionLaws/Acts/2010/Chapter288

Commonwealth of Massachusetts. (2011a). Office of Attorney General Martha Coakley. Examination of health care cost trends and cost drivers: Report for annual public hearing. Retrieved from http://www.mass.gov/ago/docs/healthcare/2011-hcctd.pdf

Commonwealth of Massachusetts. (2011b). Recommendations of the special commission on provider price reform. Retrieved from http://www.mass.gov/eohhs/docs/dhcfp/g/p-r/special-commppr-report.pdf

Congressional Budget Office. (2009a). Letter to the Honorable John D. Rockefeller: Additional information on the effects of tort reform. Retrieved from http://www.cbo.gov/publication/41812

Congressional Budget Office. (2009b). Letter to the Honorable Orrin G. Hatch: CBO's analysis of the effects of proposals to limit costs related to medical malpractice ("tort reform"). Retrieved from http://www.cbo.gov/publication/41334

Congressional Budget Office. (2012). The 2012 long-term budget outlook. Retrieved from http://cbo.gov/publication/43288

Cutler, D. M., & Ghosh, K. (2012). The potential for cost savings through bundled episode payments. *New England Journal of Medicine, 366,* 1075–1077.

Emanuel, E. J. (2012). What we give up for health care. *New York Times.* Retrieved from http://opinionator.blogs.nytimes.com/2012/01/21/what-we-give-up-for-health-care

Emanuel, E. J., & Fuchs, V. R. (2008). The perfect storm of overutilization. *Journal of the American Medical Association, 299,* 2789–2791.

Farrell, D., Jensen, E., Kocher, B., Bradford, J. W., Knott, D. G., Levine, E. H., & Zemmel, R. N. (2008). Accounting for the cost of US health care: A new look at why Americans spend more. *McKinsey Global Institute.* Retrieved from http://www.mckinsey.com/insights/mgi/research/americas/accounting_for_the_cost_of_us_health_care

42 C.F.R. § 411.355 (2011).

Government Accountability Office. (2011). Health care price transparency: Meaningful price information is difficult for consumers to obtain prior to receiving care. Retrieved from http://www.gao.gov/products/GAO-11-791

Government Accountability Office. (2012). Lack of price transparency may hamper hospitals' ability to be prudent purchasers of implantable medical devices. Retrieved from http://www.gao.gov/products/GAO-12-126

Health Care and Education Reconciliation Act of 2010. Public Law 111–152. 111th Congress. Section 1102(c) (2010).

Institute of Medicine. (2010). *The healthcare imperative: Lowering costs and improving outcomes: Workshop series summary.* Washington, DC: National Academies Press.

Jena, A. B., Seabury, S., Lakdawalla, D., & Chandra, A. (2011). Malpractice risk according to physician specialty. *New England Journal of Medicine, 365,* 629–636.

Lakdawalla, D. N., & Seabury, S. A. (2009). *The welfare effects of medical malpractice liability.* Cambridge, MA: National Bureau of Economic Research (working paper wl5383). Retrieved from http://www.nber.org/papers/wl5383

Mechanic, R. E. (2011). Opportunities and challenges for episode-based payment. *New England Journal of Medicine, 365,* 777–779.

Medicare Payment Advisory Commission. (2009). Report to the Congress: Improving incentives in the Medicare program. Retrieved from http://www.medpac.gov/documents/jun09_entirereport.pdf

Mitchell, J. M. (2012). Urologists' self-referral for pathology of biopsy specimens linked to increased use and lower prostate cancer detection. *Health Affairs, 31,* 741–749.

Office of Management and Budget. (2008). Major savings and reforms in the President's 2009 budget. Retrieved from http://www.whitehouse.gov/sites/default/files/omb/assets/omb/budget/fy2009/savings_reform.html

Office of Management and Budget. (2011). Living within our means and investing in the future: The president's plan for economic growth and deficit reduction. Retrieved from http://www.whitehouse.gov/sites/default/files/omb/budget/fy2012/assets/ jointcommitteereport.pdf

Patient Protection and Affordable Care Act Public Law 111–148, 111th Congress, Section 6410 (2010).

Pittman, P., & Williams, B. (2012). Physician wages in states with expanded APRN scope of practice. *Nursing Research and Practice, 2012,* 67197–67194.

Reinhardt, U. E. (2011). The many different prices paid to providers and the flawed theory of cost shifting: Is it time for a more rational all-payer system? *Health Affairs, 30,* 2125–2133.

Sinaiko, A. D., & Rosenthal, M. B. (2010). Consumer experience with a tiered physician network: Early evidence. *American Journal of Managed Care, 16,* 123–130.

Sisko, A. M., Truffer, C. J., Keehan, S. P., Poisal, J. A., Clemens, M. K., & Madison, A. J. (2019). National health spending projections: The estimated impact of reform through 2019. *Health Affairs, 29,* 1933–1941.

U.S. Healthcare. (2010). Efficiency index: National progress report on healthcare efficiency. Retrieved from http://www.ushealthcareindex.org/ resources/USHEINationalProgressReport.pdf

U.S. Office of Personnel Management. (2012). FEHBP program carrier letter: Letter no. 2012-09. Retrieved from http://www.opm .gov/carrier/carrier_letters/2012/2012-09.pdf

CHAPTER 22

Connecting Research Priorities, the Research Agenda, and Health Policy

Jennifer M. Manning and Tracy Pasek

WHAT IS A RESEARCH AGENDA?

A research agenda is a list of short- and/or long-term goals that aims to guide research priorities, funding decisions, and policy formation. A research agenda may typically include a list of unique and timely topics intended to steer further investigation. "Timely" implies current trends in nursing, populations, health care, and policy. A research agenda can be developed for a person, community, group, organization, school, or profession. Typically, research agendas are developed by a group of people with similar interests who may or may not actually conduct the research (Reedy, 2009).

The overarching purpose of a research agenda is to guide those who have research interests and plans to pursue them (e.g., a university may develop a research agenda to guide faculty and students regarding certain topics of inquiry that align with a strategic plan or funding opportunities). Research agendas should be updated on a regular basis as they naturally change over time as knowledge develops, trends change, and new research questions emerge. When perusing a research agenda, the reader should have no doubt about what the recommended research priorities are, and researchers should be able to easily discern if their own interests and the agenda priorities align. Research agendas can be valuable in informing the scope of a problem and can be used to substantiate policy proposals.

UTILIZATION OF RESEARCH AGENDAS

A research agenda may be developed for or by an individual. The purpose of a personal research agenda is primarily to guide a researcher with staying on schedule with work and achieving academic milestones or project goals that are timely and relevant. An organized researcher could develop a research agenda independently to guide his or her personal research agenda. Likewise, faculty could craft a research agenda that is similar for all students—a roadmap of sorts—with the express purpose of fulfilling graduation criteria.

Elements of a personal research agenda may include writing drafts of proposals and submission of a project to an ethics board for review and approval. Allotting time to collect data, dedicating time to write, seeking grant funding, and planning for the dissemination of findings are also potential items that could be listed on a personal research agenda.

There are numerous resources available to researchers when developing an individual agenda. Some may consider the process akin to project management. A personal research agenda is vital to systematic and successful scientific inquiry. However, a personal research agenda has less to do with broader research priorities, policy, and advocacy than that associated with a larger organization. An example of potential catalysts for the development of a research agenda are listed in Table 22.1.

EXAMPLES OF RESEARCH AGENDAS

One could look to important research agendas that have been established in the past as examples of how to model new research agendas. For example, the Fellows of the American Association of Nurse Practitioners (FAANP) regularly update their research agenda, most recently in 2015, and share it with Nurse Practitioners nationally (American Association of Nurse Practitioners, 2015). The FAANP research agenda identifies priority topics, thereby serving many Nurse Practitioners in a variety of ways. Potential ways the research agenda can serve Nurse Practitioners is to provide a starting point for Doctorate of Nursing Practice (DNP) projects or to serve as a source of ideas for a quality improvement

TABLE 22.1 Catalysts for the Development of a Research Agenda

• Alignment of research goals with a strategic plan
• Clinical practice application (e.g., patient-centered outcomes, comparative effectiveness)
• Health care system (e.g., care delivery, nurse-sensitive indicators)
• Health promotion (e.g., quality of life, work environment)
• Procurement of research funding
• Emergence of new epidemiologic trends (e.g., viral epidemic, chronic illness)
• Validation of underserved populations
• Validation of vulnerable populations
• Impact of technology and innovation
• Regulatory mandates
• Health care policy (e.g., scope of practice)
• Education (e.g., nursing students, communities)
• Potential and actual threats to human rights (e.g., stigma-associated disease)

project in the clinical setting. A full report is available on the organization's website, and the research agenda is divided into four major areas of interest for Nurse Practitioners: (a) workforce characteristics, (b) education, (c) policy regulation, and (d) practice models.

Another important research agenda was developed by the National Association of Clinical Nurse Specialists (NACNS). The overarching purpose of the NACNS-developed research agenda was to advance the expertise of Clinical Nurse Specialists (CNSs) as well as support increased contributions of CNSs to health care, specifically nursing research.

Clearly, it is vital to not only have varied expertise on a task force that develops a research agenda but vision as well. For example, during a presidential election year, nurses must be able to anticipate, to the best of their ability, how the direction of policy may move. An organization that enjoys members with varied expertise will likely have a broader agenda that spans populations or the lifespan. It is no surprise that the two research priorities of the NACNS are clearly representative of CNSs' practice.

APPLICATION TO APRN PRACTICE—NACNS RESEARCH AGENDA DEVELOPMENT

Development of a research agenda for an organization requires a systematic process or methodology. A group of key stakeholders should be gathered to provide expert input. The working group must be established at the onset. Additionally, the group should be fully apprised of the working plan, time involved, and goals. Epidemiology may be the foundation of a research agenda, as will the context and operational definitions (Melvin et al., 2013). For example, a disease-focused research agenda will likely be grounded in prevalence rates, risk factors, and disparities (Melvin et al., 2013). Contextual factors may include patient demographics (e.g., race and ethnicity), socioeconomic status, or health care insurance status (Melvin et al., 2013). Stakeholders may also need to reach a consensus on operational definitions early in the research agenda development process. Examples of important operational definitions could include "obesity," "urban," "vulnerable population," or "underserved." Information from stakeholders can be informally gathered or gathered via survey.

In 2004, NACNS developed its first national research agenda. The research agenda has undergone revision several times since its initial version. In 2016, the NACNS board of directors assembled a task force to create research priorities that would promote the role functions of the CNS and further the organization's mission.

In late 2015, the work of the NACNS research priorities task force commenced. A chair of the task force was appointed. The task force chair was given the charge of developing a research agenda for NACNS. Volunteers to join the chair were solicited from NACNS members and 10 NACNS members volunteered to join the task force. Task force members represented a variety of research experience, practice settings, and geographical locations.

The task force convened via a virtual meeting and reviewed a summary of the forum results from the 2016 annual meeting. After the task force was convened, a review of the literature was conducted to evaluate what research was currently being conducted and to guide the development of the new research agenda. The literature review included an evaluation of multiple research organization websites, major nursing organization websites, nurse-sensitive quality indicators, patient-centered outcome measures, nurse-centered intervention measures, and The Joint Commission patient safety goals.

Following the review of literature, the task force identified several potential areas for inclusion in the research agenda. At the annual NACNS meeting in early 2016, an open-ended forum was convened to gather input from members regarding key research priorities identified by the task force and the role of the CNS in facilitating research. Approximately 40 NACNS members were in attendance. The forum included a presentation of the proposed research priorities and asked for questions from the audience regarding their opinion of these identified topics as well as an open discussion regarding potential barriers anticipated for addressing identified topic areas. The audience input was compiled and included a list suggesting research agenda topics and a list of barriers NACNS members encounter when conducting research. Overall, the forum attendees agreed with the proposed NACNS agenda. Minor changes were suggested regarding the wording of agenda categories (e.g., "Palliative Care" was recommended to be changed to "Palliative Care Across the Lifespan").

Following the annual conference, the task force decided to gather information from the NACNS members via survey. The survey asked the participants to indicate if the identified areas should be included in the NACNS research agenda. In mid-2016, the survey was administered to members of NACNS and reminders were issued biweekly until it was believed that responses were adequately

TABLE 22.2 Research Agenda of the National Association of Clinical Nurse Specialists, 2017

Clinical practice application (Priority)	Patient-centered outcomes Population health management Comparative effectiveness
Health care system (Priority)	Delivery Services Costs Safety Nurse-sensitive indicators
Health care policy	Scope of practice Regulation
Health promotion	Wellness management Disease management Symptom management Quality of life Functional status
Education	Health care providers/students Patients Families Populations (vulnerable, unique) Communities
Palliative care across the life span	Neonatal Pediatric Adult Geriatric

TABLE 22.3 Strategies for the Dissemination of a Research Agenda

- Include in a strategic plan for a service line or division within an organization
- Highlight in an annual report
- Present at a conference or forum
- Announce via a press release
- Describe in an interview
- Post to the website of a relevant organization or sponsoring body
- Report in a publication with readership and impact factor that align with the agenda

collected. Approximately 10% of the NACNS members responded to the survey. During the summer of 2016, the results were analyzed. The emerging research agenda for NACNS included six board categories with two to five subcategories within each category (Table 22.2).

In early fall of 2016, a summary of the results was drafted in a memorandum for the NACNS board of directors. Endorsement of the six categories was supported by the priorities task force. The next phase will be to disseminate this research agenda. Some example strategies for dissemination of a research agenda are listed in Table 22.3.

EVALUATING RESEARCH AGENDAS

Research agendas should be flexible, relevant, updated over time, and targeted for a specific population or group. Evaluation of well-developed research agendas can be indicated by their influence on practice, policy, education, and research (Figure 22.1).

A research agenda that meets the current needs of the population it serves can be evident in a variety of practice areas. For example, research agendas can influence quality improvement projects and translation of research to practice.

Based on the steps of the legislative process, the research agenda can influence policy by informing key policy makers who can influence the outcome of proposed legislative decisions. Research agendas can be used to educate

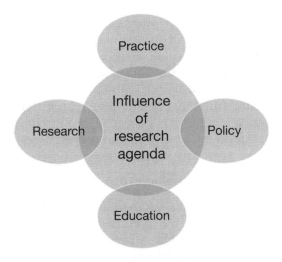

FIGURE 22.1 Areas influenced by well-developed research agendas.

legislators and those influencing policy development. The research agenda can also serve as a tool for communication with legislators. Strategic use of a research agenda can inform viewpoints of policy makers because it reflects the viewpoints of stakeholders. The ultimate impact is to increase the awareness regarding the relevance of the issues addressed in research agendas, which can have a positive impact on policy making.

Research agendas can impact education by influencing priority areas of emphasis for educators to ensure students are apprised of the more important areas for a professional group. Additionally, research agendas can be a source for idea generation for students working on master's theses or doctoral practice projects.

Lastly, research agendas can influence research by providing researchers with evidence to support directions for research studies in a specific area or health care field. They can support decisions to pursue areas of research. Depending on the detail provided in the research agenda, the researcher may be guided in understanding the state of the science in an area and directed to investigate areas that need to be further explored. Research agendas can be used in grant funding applications to support a researcher's investigational decisions.

Research Agendas and Policy Engagement

As nurses are assuming more leadership positions in health care that impact research, there is a growing need for active participation in policy develop-ment. Based on this need, students must be prepared to identify and analyze policies and regulations. The development of in-depth knowledge will increase the understanding and ultimately expertise with policy making. How CNSs can become involved in policy development depends on the will to learn and a time commitment. Some examples of strategies for increasing participation in policy making are to engage in state legislative activities; engage in board membership at the local, state, or national level; and enroll in policy internships, policy fellow-ships, or policy workshops.

For those unsure about how to engage in policy making, nurses must first identify a policy area that invokes passion and a desire to change and improve the status quo. Then, it is crucial to surround oneself with others who are passionate about the same topic (e.g., join organizations, attend meetings, join a blog, become a member of an action committee). Through networking, nurses can advocate for policy change. Fact sheets can stimulate action by guiding nurses on how to con-tact their legislators. Nurse advocacy councils within health care systems may have templates, so nurses can easily write to their lawmakers. Nurses must rec-ognize that they have the numbers or volume (e.g., registered nurses, advanced practice nurses) to have a voice that is powerful enough to effect change. Nurses must not be daunted; nurses must step up and represent (Abood, 2007).

Ethical Considerations in Policy Development

Ethical issues may arise during policy development that was influenced by a research agenda. The goal of research agenda–based policy change is to identify and evaluate the potential benefit of laws as well as the potential costs associated with them. Furthermore, when developing policies, it is important to consider

TABLE 22.4 Ethical Considerations in Pursuing Policy Based on Research Agendas

1. Are there any ethical considerations which may involve resource utilization, quality, or safety?
2. Are there scope-of-practice considerations?
3. Are there professional codes of conduct issues?
4. Is the agenda/policy consistent with regional and/or organizational values?
5. Does the agenda/policy support patients' rights and values?
6. Does the research agenda appropriately address and protect the rights of vulnerable patient populations?
7. Are there implications for ethical principles such as respecting patient autonomy (are patient choices impacted), beneficence (is there a potential for patient harm), or nonmaleficence (does the agenda/policy increase harm for anyone involved)?
8. Does the agenda/policy result in conflict among providers?
9. Does the agenda/policy incur risk from inaction by the professional?

whether a policy may make it more difficult for professionals to expand their practice. Another consideration to evaluate is whether the policy will impact the code of conduct in professional practices. These considerations may be related to the scope of nurses' practice and code of conduct. For example, a policy based on a research agenda involving nursing actions that are outside of the scope of practice will result in ethical dilemmas, which will require either policy revision or scope-of-practice revision. Inaction—or doing nothing—is also an ethical consideration or risk that can develop when policies are developed. Policies that require new nursing action may create ethical dilemmas to avoid the legal ramifications due to a lack of delivery of the "standard of care" or inaction. Questions to ask regarding ethical considerations are listed in Table 22.4.

DISCUSSION QUESTIONS

1. *Based on the information in this chapter, list at least two areas of policy change you can identify where legislation could have an impact.*
2. *Define research priorities and discuss with your classmates. Do your perceptions of research priorities differ from your peers? How? Why do you think that is?*
3. *Lastly, what methods would be ideal for the dissemination of your task force's research priorities to relevant groups? Considering the nature of the research priorities, what are some options for the frequency with which they should be reevaluated?*

ANALYSIS/SYNTHESIS

1. *If you were going to describe the importance of your issue for policy change to potential supporters, what key issues would you stress? How would you describe this to your patients?*

2. *Consider the health policy changes discussed in this chapter or those you have described in your analysis and consider the consequences if these changes are NOT enacted. In other words, what will be the impact of inaction?*
3. *What methods would be ideal for the dissemination of your task force's research priorities to relevant groups?*
4. *Considering the nature of the research priorities, what are some options for the frequency with which they should be reevaluated?*

CLINICAL APPLICATION

1. *Imagine you are selected to lead efforts to establish a research priority agenda in your health care facility/system. How would you collect data and appraise the evidence to support early formulation of a clinical research priority list?*
2. *Consider a professional society, health care system, academic setting, or government body. You have led a task force, and research priorities have been recommended by the members. List examples of expert stakeholders who would be appropriate to validate and approve the priorities.*

ETHICAL CONSIDERATIONS

1. *When thinking about research and research priorities for your clinical practice environment what kinds of ethical issues might you encounter?*

REFERENCES

Abood, S. (2007). Influencing health care in the legislative arena. *The Online Journal of Issues in Nursing, 12*(1). doi:10.3912/OJIN.Vol12No01Man02

American Association of Nurse Practitioners. (2015). Nurse practitioner research agenda. Retrieved from https://www.aanp.org/research/np-research-agenda

Melvin, C. L., Corbie-Smith, G., Kumanyika, S. K., Pratt, C. A., Nelson, C., Walker, E. R., . . . The Workshop Working Group on CVD Prevention in High-Risk Rural Communities. (2013). Developing a research agenda for cardiovascular disease prevention in high-risk rural communities. *American Journal of Public Health, 103*(6), 1011–1021. doi:10.2105/AJPH.2012.300984

Reedy, J. (2009). Creating a research agenda. Retrieved from https://www.insidehighered.com/advice/2009/05/20/creating-research-agenda

Effects of Changes in Health Policy on Nursing Organizations

The Coalition for Patients' Rights—A Coalition That Advocates for Scope-of-Practice Issues

Melinda Ray and Maureen Shekleton

Health care spending, the amount the United States spends on health care, has been an issue for decades. Health care spending hit a high of 12.7% in the 1970s. After it dropped to 5.5% in the 1990s, in the past decade we have been seeing most recently rates of health care spending in the neighborhood of 3% to 5%. The Kaiser Family Foundation reports that "Health spending in the U.S. had grown at historically low levels starting in 2008, likely due to a combination of the economic downturn and slow recovery and higher patient cost-sharing, as well as structural changes to the health system" (The Henry J. Kaiser Family Foundation, 2016).

According to the Centers for Medicare and Medicaid Services, in 2014 U.S. health care spending increased 5.3% following growth of 2.9% in 2013. This equates to $3 trillion, or $9,523 per person. This growth pattern was attributed to the implementation of the Affordable Care Act (ACA). Another way to quantify this is to look at the share of the economy devoted to health care spending. In 2014 it was 17.5%; more than 17.3% in 2013 (Centers for Medicare and Medicaid Services, 2016, p. 1). To appreciate the growth in these costs, in 1970, health spending accounted for $75 billion or $356 per resident and was 7.2% of gross domestic product (GDP; The Henry J. Kaiser Family Foundation, 2012, p. 1).

With the continued implementation of ACA health plans, it is projected that health-spending growth will continue at a higher rate than in years past. But, economists are not expecting the growth of health care spending to enter the double digits of the 1970s (The Henry J. Kaiser Family Foundation, 2016).

One mechanism to achieve cost reductions in health care services is the full utilization of a wide range of licensed, qualified health care professionals working at their full scope of practice. Although this seems like a straightforward, logical approach, its implementation is hindered by years of tradition in the provision of health care in the United States. Full utilization of a wide range of licensed health care providers creates competition between these health care professionals and traditional health care providers such as medical physicians, osteopathic physicians, and dentists. A response to this scenario has been the evolution of two coalitions—the Coalition for Patients' Rights (CPR; www.patientsrights coalition.org) and the American Medical Association's (AMA) Scope of Practice Partnership (SOPP).

One of the key strategies in moving issues forward at the federal, state, and local levels is coalition building. Coalitions are established around a common mission or purpose, and the members agree to work together to move this mission forward. Often that translates into legislation, regulation, and/or media coverage on the issue. The coalition typically elects or appoints leadership that guides the group in their work. Coalition members, typically associations, organizations and/or businesses, and other stakeholders, pool their resources and work together on the issues of concern. The CPR is an excellent example of a long-standing and effective multidisciplinary coalition.

The demands of the patient in the evolving reformed health care system are juxtaposed against the history of health care professionals in care delivery. Traditional, medically driven care is being challenged to accept the entry of qualified Advanced Practice Registered Nurses (APRNs), physician assistants (PAs), and other health care professionals who are legally qualified to provide specific health care services. This need for change has generated a strident response from organized medicine that has organized a coalition of medical physician membership organizations called the SOPP. The SOPP was formed in 2006 to challenge what physicians and osteopaths describe as "inappropriate scope of practice expansions, such as those that are not commensurate with a nonphysician provider group's education and training" (American Osteopathic Association [AOA], 2013). The stated goals of the SOPP were to protect patient safety by supporting the "team" approach to medical care. They are advocating for the physician-led, team-based medical model, which they maintain ensures that professionals with complete medical education and training are adequately involved in patient care (AOA, 2013).

Although many SOPP member organizations note that they value the contributions of nonphysician clinicians to the health care delivery system, there is a continued theme that expansion of their authority to provide services to patients should not happen without medical and osteopathic physician oversight.

The CPR was formed in response to this coalition of medical physician organizations and years of interprofessional rivalry between organized medicine/osteopathy and other health care professional groups. The CPR member organizations represent (but are not limited to) nursing, physical therapy, occupational therapy, psychology, family therapy, chiropractic physicians, naturopathic physicians, nutrition specialists, speech and hearing therapists, and foot and ankle surgeons. In the past, if one of the physician/osteopathic organizations made an effort to oppose a scope-of-practice issue for another health care provider group, that provider group would organize a targeted coalition and mount a response. The CPR has grown out of these ongoing challenges by professional medicine and optimizes the voice of a number and variety of health care provider organizations. It is rather unique to have such a large number of varied health care groups work together on scope-of-practice issues.

The CPR consists of more than 35 health care professional membership organizations. The CPR website notes there are "a variety of licensed health care professionals who provide a diverse array of safe, effective, and affordable health care services to millions of patients each year. These competent, well-prepared health care professionals complete years of education in their respective specialties, and have long been recognized at the federal and state levels as qualified and essential contributors to the U.S. health system" (CPR, 2011a).

One of the strengths of the CPR is the wide variety of health care providers that are members. This broad-based composition allows the CPR to generate a strong support from many different fronts when needed. When asked what is the most significant contribution the CPR has made to the protection and enhancement of scope of practice of health care professionals other than MDs and DOs, Maureen Shekleton, PhD, RN, FAAN, who was the Professional Relations Specialist for the American Association of Nurse Anesthetists, the organization, and until 2016 served as the co-chair of CPR, stated, "providing a unified, multidisciplinary voice for over 3 million health care professionals to support their ability to practice to the fullest extent of their preparation so that patients are allowed a choice of quality cost-effective providers through whom they can access care..." (CPR, 2011b).

CPR ACTIVITIES

The purpose of a coalition is to bring together an alliance of parties and/or groups for joint action. The CPR has worked to take a proactive approach to the issues that are of concern to its members. One important effort is in the public relations arena. Early in the formation of the coalition, members recognized the importance of having a unified communication strategy that was designed to promote the role of CPR member organizations in health care. The coalition has generated a series of press releases that articulate the added value of its members to the health care system. The CPR has also published a brochure that serves as a resource for members and the public. This brochure was developed to introduce health care professionals and consumers to the coalition. It is available as a hardcopy brochure and a downloadable one-page version that can be found on the coalition's website (CPR, 2011a).

As most scope-of-practice issues are dealt with at the state level, CPR has most recently been focused on efforts to support and assist state coalitions. The CPR members have access to a state issues-focused toolkit that they can use to support their state advocacy efforts. In addition, the CPR members have access to conference calls where members update each other on state activities. This update has the impact of allowing organizations to support each other's efforts in the states.

Dr. Shekleton identified one of the challenges the coalition faces: engaging and empowering the local affiliates of the national organizations because the actual scope battles occur at the state level. In 2011, the coalition implemented an approach they called the State-Based Coalition (SBC) Program for state/regional organizations, branches, and representatives of the national CPR organizations. The purpose of these SBCs is to enable a coordinated, proactive response by stakeholders to scope-of-practice developments at the state level, particularly attacks by the SOPP through state and local medical societies. The SBC Program works to facilitate networking and information sharing at the state level between CPR organizations and the creation of state-based CPR coalitions that reflect the national membership of the CPR. One excellent resource that is available on the coalition website (www.patientsright scoalition.org) is a virtual training session on how to build state-level coalitions that will have an impact. Some of the topics covered in this webinar include background information on the coalition: the role a coalition can play in addressing scope-of-practice issues on the state level and an overview of tools that are available to support coalition development in your state (CPR, 2011b).

THE SOPP

Between individual health care professionals of different disciplines who provide care together, there is a positive and supportive relationship between the individual medical and/or osteopathic physicians and other collegial professionals who are represented by the CPR member organizations. Unfortunately, these expert medical clinicians may not have a voice within their professional societies and associations. As a result, there is, at times, a wide gap between what many practitioners experience at the bedside and what is articulated by the medical and osteopathic association on the national policy front. Health care economics and the passage of health care reform have provided many new opportunities for all categories of health care professionals to work in new, innovative integrated health care delivery models of care. As state and federal entities have worked to find solutions to health care professional shortages and reduce medical costs, the use of all qualified health care providers has become more of a norm for best practices. Although at times this may require a modification in the state's scope of practice for a specific professional group, most often, it is a matter of regulatory and/or legislative changes at the state or federal level to allow these qualified professionals to work within their current scope of practice to provide better care to their patients.

The CPR seeks to counter efforts by professional medicine/osteopathy and specifically the efforts of the AMA's (SOPP) initiative that are designed to limit patients' choice of health practitioners. The SOPP efforts are extensive and have been artfully framed as patient protections.

According to a presentation given by Michael D. Maves, MD, MBA, chief executive officer and executive vice president, AMA, on February 18 and 19, 2010, in Geneva, Switzerland, at the World Health Professions Conference on Regulation, the membership included 49 state medical associations and the District of Columbia, 14 national medical associations, the AMA, and the AOA (and AOA's 20 state associations; Maves, 2010). Their stated interests included state and federal regulation and legislation related to the scope of practice of a variety of non-MD/DO health care providers. Some of the health care groups SOPP has specifically targeted include, but are not limited to, podiatrists, optometrists, nurse anesthetists, Nurse Practitioners, nurse midwives, psychologists, audiologists, physical therapists, chiropractors, and naturopathic physicians (Maves, 2010). Limited information is publicly available concerning the goals and planned activities of SOPP. According to the AMA website, information on the SOPP can be accessed via the AMA website's members-only site.

The presentation given by Dr. Maves identified three major initiatives to curtail the scope of practice of other members of the health care provider team. The first is strategically called the "Truth in Advertising Campaign" (AMA, 2013). This campaign highlights the SOPP's concern with the use of the title "doctor" by nonmedical providers. If an individual has an earned doctorate in a discipline such as psychology or nursing, they would require these individuals to forgo the use of their earned title and require them to identify their type of professional licensure and training. This initiative seeks to require nonmedical providers to include the full designation in their title, such as doctorate in psychology or doctorate in nursing. In an article detailing the efforts of Reps. John Sullivan (R-OK.) and David Scott's (D-GA) legislation—the Healthcare Truth and Transparency Act (H.R. 452 introduced January 21, 2011)—it was noted that the goals of these efforts are to clarify title misrepresentation and minimize patient confusion about who is providing medical care. The rhetoric used in this initiative is phrased in terms of patient protections but essentially serves to limit patient choice of health care providers. This legislation failed in the 112th Congress but variations of this legislation have been seen in a number of different states.

Two other initiatives are part of the SOPP's efforts—the AMA Scope of Practice Data Series and the AMA GeoMapping Initiative. The AMA Scope of Practice Data Series provides the AMA's analysis of the preparation and scope of practice of 10 provider groups (AMA, 2013). A number of CPR member organizations made efforts to proactively work with AMA to provide accurate information regarding their respective practitioner roles. Despite these efforts, the final products in the AMA Scope of Practice Data Series were disappointing to the CPR organizations whose members were targeted including Nurse Practitioners and nurse anesthetists as well as physical therapists, podiatrists, audiologists, naturopaths, and psychologists. In response to the AMA Scope of Practice Data Series, the coalition publicly requested that it be withdrawn. The CPR's recommendation to withdraw the Scope of Practice Data Series modules was based on many concerns, including those related to conflict of interest, inaccuracies, restricting patient access, and redundancies. The CPR maintains that there is a fundamental conflict of interest for one professional group to define the scope of practice of another (CPR, 2010). According to the CPR website, it is not reasonable for medical physicians to purport that they are seeking to protect patients when (a) there is no credible evidence to suggest that preventing patients from choosing their health care professional would, in any way, improve patient care and (b) the economic interests of MDs and DOs are intertwined with scope-of-practice issues. These efforts amount to protecting "turf," and the needs of patients are lost in the discussion (CPR, 2010). These documents are not readily available on the AMA website.

In addition to this concern, the Scope of Practice Data Series has been criticized as being "rife" with inaccuracies and misstatements about the training, education, and accreditation of health care professionals other than MDs/DOs. Despite these statements, the AMA continues to support and disseminate the Scope of Practice Data Series as advocacy documents (AMA, 2013).

The third publicly identified initiative of the SOPP is the AMA GeoMapping Initiative. This project attempts to map the practice areas of different providers on a state-by-state level. In a 2012 advocacy summary, the AMA spoke about their GeoMapping Initiative, "The AMA GeoMapping Initiative compares the practice locations of physician specialists and nonphysicians to demonstrate that, despite the claims of lack of access, health care professionals tend to practice in the same, large urban areas" (AMA, 2010, p. 5). The power of these maps lies in how they are interpreted. Many health care providers, because of restrictions in direct payment policies, must be associated with an employer in order to be reimbursed.

The CPR has spent its history anticipating and responding to these assaults to scope of practice. This is a strong coalition that is likely to continue to grow and work to represent the concerns of health care professionals. When asked, what has made CPR such a long-lasting and effective coalition, Dr. Shekleton identified that the reasons go beyond mere opposition to the SOPP efforts. He believes that the coalition members have come to the realization that the problems each discipline faces are similar to those faced by others. In other words, they see each as more alike than different. Also, the reason to counter the SOPP is not a reason to stay together. The focus has expanded to consumer education about the abilities of health care professionals other than MDs and DOs and engaging state affiliates in coalition building.

IMPLICATIONS FOR THE APRN

APRNs must actively engage in local, state, and national issues that impact their practice. There are many public policy implications to APRNs working to practice to the full extent of their scope of practice. It is critical that APRNs work to articulate and take action in concert with their colleagues on public policy issues that have an impact on patients, their family, health care providers, systems, the community, and on local, state, and federal public policy levels. In order to stay on top of these issues, APRNs should maintain memberships in their professional associations. Often, APRNs gravitate to single memberships in organizations that provide solid clinical and practice support to their members. These memberships are important, but in order to be professionally engaged in scope-of-practice issues, APRNs should also consider membership in the state nurses association and their APRN membership organizations. APRNs should seek out opportunities to be engaged on the state and local level through coalitions and state association chapters that will focus colleague efforts on key issues of importance to the APRNs in the state.

Beyond this basic level of engagement, APRNs can work on their personal policy advocacy skills. Often membership associations offer training sessions and lobby days on the state and federal levels. These sessions are excellent ways to begin to refine skills in these areas.

Coalitions form around issues of mutual interest for individuals and associations. With the advent of health care reform and the efforts to fully utilize all health care providers to the full extent of their scope of practice, the tensions with the professional medical associations are expected to continue. As with many policy issues, evaluation is not a clear-cut process. Success can, at times, be defined as passage or failure of passage of specific legislation. More often, success can be seen in more subtle results, such as legislative delay tactics, budget implications that sideline a policy discussion, and/or negotiated bill language that solves a smaller percent of the concerns a group has with specific legislation.

APRN ENGAGEMENT

Scope of practice, the core issues around which the CPR coalition is formed, requires a high level of APRN engagement for change to be realized. It is essential to see personal political activity as part of your professional role. Scope-of-practice issues are largely fought and won on the state level. Therefore, the APRN has the opportunity to invest time in building relationships with colleague APRNs and policy makers to make change over a period of time. Being engaged and active on the local and state levels allows individual APRNs to work together with each other to achieve public policy success. Although it is important that all nurses support APRNs operating under their full scope of practice, the APRN is uniquely qualified to speak to the needs of the health care system and the patients and families.

It is challenging to always measure the success of public policy issues. It is a clear success when a bill is passed or fails; but success can also be the development of a strong, well-functioning coalition, or long-term engagement of APRNs. All national competencies mention the importance of public policy awareness and engagement. An individual APRN can feel amazingly empowered when able to serve as a resource for legislators and/or to testify to the state legislature or even on the national level. Once an APRN gets involved in public policy issues, that nurse often is motivated to stay involved. The ability to represent the concerns of the profession and the needs of the patients and families the APRNs serve helps the individual APRN to achieve a new aspect of professional identity. It often motivates these individuals to stay involved and pursue other legislative and regulatory issues of concern.

DISCUSSION QUESTIONS

1. *Consider the impact of rising health care costs and the implementation of health care reform in the United States. With this in mind, discuss the advantages for payers to include a wide range of health care providers to their clients.*
2. *Identify how an APRN working at full scope of practice can contribute to decreased health care costs.*
3. *Identify and discuss the advantages of working in a coalition to represent the public policy concerns of a given issue. What could be some disadvantages to working within a coalition to advance a public policy issue and how might they be resolved? Examine the arguments presented by the AMA in their SOPP and identify how these positions would limit the scope of practice of other licensed health care providers.*

ANALYSIS, SYNTHESIS, AND CLINICAL APPLICATIONS

1. *Divide into two groups with each group selecting a position to defend. One group will represent the AMA's SOPP and the other will represent the CPR. Each group should prepare key talking points for testimony that represents their position on a scope-of-practice issue. Some scope-of-practice issues the groups might consider: expansion of prescriptive authority (Schedule III medications) for APRNs; ordering of x-rays by APRNs; ordering of home health care services for patients by Nurse Practitioners and Clinical Nurse Specialists; and use of fluoroscopy and interventional pain management by CRNAs.*
2. *Review the Truth and Transparency legislation found at www.thomas.gov/. Develop a fact sheet in opposition to this legislation from the APRN perspective.*

ETHICAL CONSIDERATIONS

1. *Consider the role that the CPR has played in recent political and policy initiatives. Contemplate the outcomes of these policies and political initiatives if the CPR did not exist. Would there be a difference in the manner in which patients would be treated? Professional disciplines?*

REFERENCES

American Medical Association. (2010). Advocacy update: AMA GeoMapping initiative provides powerful scope of practice snapshot. Retrieved from http://www.phlebology.org/20100119_Advocacy_Update.pdf

American Medical Association. (2013). Truth in advertising. Retrieved from http://www.ama-assn.org/ama/pub/advocacy/state-advocacy-arc/state-advocacy-campaigns/truth-in-advertising.page

American Osteopathic Association. (2013). Scope of practice partnership. Retrieved from http://www.osteopathic.org/inside-aoa/advocacy/state-government-affairs/scope-of-practice-partnership/Pages/default.aspx

Centers for Medicare and Medicaid Services. (2016). National health expenditures 2015 highlights. Retrieved from https://www.cms.gov/Research-Statistics-Data-and-Systems/Statistics-Trends-and-Reports/NationalHealthExpendData/Downloads/highlights.pdf

Coalition for Patients' Rights. (2010). CPR responds to AMA scope of practice modules. Retrieved from http://www.patientsrightscoalition.org/Advocacy-and-Legislation/AMA-Initiatives/Response-to-AMA-Scope-of-Practice-Modules.aspx

Coalition for Patients' Rights. (2011a). Protecting health care quality, access and choice of providers. Retrieved from http://www.patientsrightscoalition.org/default.aspx

Coalition for Patients' Rights. (2011b). State-Based Coalition (SBC) Program. Retrieved from http://www.patientsrightscoalition.org/Advocacy-and-Legislation/State-Coalition.aspx

The Henry J. Kaiser Family Foundation. (2012). *Health care costs: A primer* (pp. 2–5). Retrieved from http://kff.org/health-costs/report/health-care-costs-a-primer

The Henry J. Kaiser Family Foundation. (2016). Chart—How much is health spending expected to grow? Retrieved from http://www.healthsystemtracker.org/chart-collection/the-latest-health-spending-projections

Maves, M. (2010). Scope of practice in the United States. Proceedings from the World Health Professions Conference on Regulation, Geneva, Switzerland. Retrieved from http://www.whpa.org/whpcr2010/presentations/Michael%20Maves%20WHPCR2010.pdf

CHAPTER 24

The American Nurses Association

Lisa Summers and Andrea Brassard

With a limited number of seats at many decision-making and policy-setting tables, the American Nurses Association (ANA) is sometimes the sole voice of nursing. ANA's position has become increasingly crucial, yet sensitive, with the growth of nursing specialties and the increasing importance of varied nursing roles. As a historical convener of the larger nursing community, ANA seeks to fully and accurately represent the nursing community, including each of the four Advanced Practice Registered Nurse (APRN) roles. ANA believes strongly in the value of APRNs and their contribution to improving access to high quality, cost-effective health care services. ANA's work on "APRN issues" is wide ranging and given the nature of policy work, evolving.

This chapter briefly addresses the history and current work of ANA on behalf of APRNs and provides an overview of APRN issues: leveraging the opportunities of health system reform; addressing scope of practice barriers; gathering and disseminating workforce and payment data that will better demonstrate the economic value of nursing and achieve equitable reimbursement for APRNs; and ensuring that the role of APRNs is recognized via ANA's expansive work in the national quality enterprise.

HISTORY

ANA, founded in 1896, is the premier professional organization representing the interests of the nation's 3.6 million registered nurses. ANA advances the nursing profession by fostering high standards of nursing practice, promoting a safe and ethical work environment, bolstering the health and wellness of nurses, and advocating on health care issues that affect nurses and the public. ANA is at the forefront of improving the quality of health care for all.

ANA was first conceived by a group of 10 alumnae associations who met near New York City to discuss the feasibility of a national nursing association. In 1898, the Nurses Associated Alumnae of the United States and Canada, which was originally a part of the group, held their first convention. When the group was incorporated in the state of New York in 1901, Canada had to be dropped from the name. Individual states also started organizing at this time to begin regulating nursing, with North Carolina being the first state to do so along with New York, New Jersey, and Virginia. It was in 1911 that the Alumnae changed its name to the ANA. ANA was responsible for the first census of nursing resources in the country in 1918 and over the years has been instrumental in many other efforts that support nursing practice and welfare that nurses still benefit from today.

ANA'S Early Involvement With the APRN Movement

Clinical Nurse Specialists (CNS) and Nurse Practitioners (NPs) were the two APRN roles that were the focus of ANA's early involvement with the APRN movement. Nurse anesthetists had already organized as early as 1931 into the American Association of Nurse Anesthetists (AANA) and the nurse-midwives followed in 1955 as the American College of Nurse-Midwives (ACNM).

In the 1960s, the term "nurse practitioner" was defined by ANA's Committee on Education as "any person prepared and authorized by law to practice nursing and therefore, deemed competent to render safe nursing care" (ANA, 1965, p. 106). Following the advent of the first pediatric practitioner program at the University of Colorado, the term took on its expanded meaning.

ANA's Commission on Nursing Education developed a definition for NP for use in interpreting the federal Nurse Training Act of 1971. An NP has completed a program of study in an expanded role whose responsibility encompasses:

1. Obtaining a health history
2. Assessing health-illness status
3. Entering a person into the health care system
4. Sustaining and supporting persons who are impaired, infirm, and ill during programs of diagnosis and therapy
5. Managing a medical care regimen for acute and chronically ill patients within established standing orders
6. Aiding in restoring persons to wellness and maximum function
7. Teaching and counseling persons about health and illness
8. Supervising and managing care regimens of normal pregnant women
9. Helping parents in guidance of children with a view to their optimal, physical, and emotional development
10. Counseling and supporting persons with regard to the aging process
11. Aiding people and their survivors during the dying process
12. Supervising assistants to nurses (ANA Commission on Nursing Education, 1971)

Building on this list of NP responsibilities, ANA's Congress for Nursing Practice provided definitions for NP, nurse clinician, and CNS, stating that "Unfortunately, rather than clarifying nursing practice, all these terms and definitions have had a tendency to confuse levels of practice within the nursing professions as well as for other professions and consumers" (ANA Congress for Nursing Practice, 1974). As cited in this 1974 paper, NPs learned history taking and physical examination through continuing education or in a baccalaureate nursing programs.

ANA collaborated with other professional organizations, including the American Academy of Pediatrics and the American School Health Association, in the 1970s to issue position statements on pediatric NPs, school NPs, and geriatric NPs. ANA also accredited continuing education programs for NPs and developed certification exams for NPs and CNSs. ANA operationally defined CNSs both as expert practitioners in a specific area of clinical nursing who provide direct patient care and as change agents within the health care system (ANA Council of Family Nurse Practitioners and Clinicians, 1976, cited by Hamric & Spross, 1983)

ANA CERTIFIES CNSs AND NPs

Although specialty certification was conceived by ANA in the mid-1950s, the ANA certification program was not established until 1973 (Johnson, Dawson, & Brassard, 2010). ANA's first advanced practice certification exams were the pediatric NP in 1974; and the family NP, adult NP, and CNS in medical–surgical nursing (now known as CNS in adult health) in 1976; the adult psychiatric-mental health CNS and child/adolescent psychiatric-mental health CNS in 1977; and the gerontological NP in 1979. ANA added more certification exams for nursing administration and other nursing specialties and more NPs and CNSs. In 1990, the American Nurses Credentialing Center (ANCC) became an independent corporation. Today, ANCC offers seven APRN certifications—five NP and two CNS.

ANA'S NP COUNCILS AND THE COUNCIL OF CNSs

ANA's early involvement with APRNs included sponsoring conferences, councils, and papers. ANA held a national conference on NP education in 1974, with keynote speaker Loretta Ford, noted for founding the first NP role—the pediatric NP—and sponsored by ANA's two NP councils: the Council of Nurse Practitioners in Nursing of Children and the Council of Family Nurse Practitioners and Clinicians. These two ANA councils merged to become the Council of Primary Health Care Nurse Practitioners later in the decade. ANA released a position pamphlet "Scope of Primary Nursing Practice for Adults and Families" in 1976, which included definitions, scope, and professional responsibilities. "Family health care is a team effort. The composition of this team may include nurses, social workers, physicians, therapists, and others. It is imperative that there be mutual recognition of each profession's unique expertise." The 1976 statement foreshadows the patient-centered team idea much talked about now by including the phrase "the consumers' involvement in decisions that affect their health care is paramount."

Primary care was explored further in a 1977 monograph written by the American Academy of Nursing and published by ANA. Physical assessment skills were viewed as key to primary care services. Consumer choice of primary care provider was raised as an issue, as was direct reimbursement of nursing services. The monograph cites Barbara Bates, legendary physical assessment textbook author, who wrote "the successful nurse practitioner will integrate her new medical role with her earlier nursing role, achieving a new and balanced professional approach" (American Academy of Nursing, 1977, p. 23). The monograph also points out the distinction between nurses and physician assistants. "The PA is a physician extender who does not have an identity of his own. If the physician leaves the practice, the PA is out of a job. The nurse has her own identity, is licensed in her own right, accountable for her practice, and is in command of a separate body of knowledge" (American Academy of Nursing, 1977, p. 31). Claire Fagan's wise words regarding scope of practice continue to resonate:

> The internal professional struggles about scope are probably as serious as the external. For example, how many nurse writers have described their functions as dependent? Responsibility for one's own actions and accountability to the consumer in no way permit the notion of dependent functions for the professional in primary care. To some extent we have been willing to narrow our scope of practice by getting rid of washing floors and dishes, but we have been more tentative about expanding it. It seems to me that the scope of nursing practice is defined by what nurses are willing to be accountable for, based on their knowledge, skill, and experiential success. I believe that the scope of nursing practice is more limited by nurses' unwillingness to assume the authority that goes with responsibility (i.e., accountability) than by any other single factor. We must confront this problem, since it is clear that the scope of nursing as a professional discipline can meet most of what have been identified as primary care needs. (American Academy of Nursing, 1977, p. 41)

In addition to fear of accountability, Fagan lists four other factors that limited scope of practice in the 1970s and continue today: legal limits, educational factors, political factors, and economic factors.

ANA's Council of Clinical Nurse Specialists conducted a national survey of CNSs who were members of state nurses associations within ANA. More than 3,000 CNSs were surveyed; response rate was 74%. The vast majority of respondents, 98%, held master's degrees. The most common specialty area was psychiatric and mental health adult nursing (32%). Most of the respondents were employed by hospitals (55%); about 10% worked in private practice. The Council of Clinical Nurse Specialists published *The Role of the Clinical Nurse Specialist* in 1986.

Changing Policies on Advanced Education and Licensure

In the 1980s, ANA's positions on APRN education and practice evolved. The Council on Primary Health Care Nurse Practitioners' 1980 position statement encouraged graduate preparation of NPs and, according to the 1984 ANA house of delegates, all NPs must be prepared at the graduate level by 1990. Regarding APRN practice, ANA discouraged listing NP tasks or functions in policy or regulation "since it is inflexible and limiting to the judgment of the professional practitioner. The nurse is accountable for her practice and utilizes the breadth and depth of her educational preparation" (Waddle, 1981). ANA took a broader perspective, publishing *Scope of Practice of the Primary Health Care Nurse Practitioner* in 1986, followed by *Standards of Practice for the Primary Health Care Nurse Practitioner* in 1987.

Also in the 1980s, ANA published *Issues in Professional Nursing Practice*. Part 1 Nursing: Legal Authority for Practice described ANA policy on specialty and advanced nursing practice. Thirty years earlier, in 1954, ANA had the misguided recommendation that states insert a disclaimer at the end of the definition of nursing practice stating that "the foregoing shall not be deemed to include acts of diagnosis or prescription of therapeutic or corrective measures." This rec-ommendation (which was removed from official ANA policy in 1965) became a statutory barrier to advanced nursing practice in many states. In 1985, ANA's position was that professional organizations should establish the scope and stan-dards of advanced or specialty nursing practice. ANA advised against state reg-ulation of advanced or specialty nurse practice in the 1970s and 1980s, fearing that additional clauses in nurse practice acts that authorized state boards of nurs-ing to regulate specialty or advanced nursing practice would increase physician involvement in nursing laws and regulations. *Issues in Professional Nursing Practice* listed state examples of physician involvement including joint protocols, written agreements, and the regulation of advanced practice nursing by joint boards of medicine and nursing. ANA warned that "this kind of physician involvement relinquishes part of the legal control of nursing practice to another profession and results in a superordinate-subordinate relationship....The degree of speci-ficity of the [scope of practice] rules...is restrictive and harmful" to expansion of advanced practice

A NATIONAL ALLIANCE OF NPs

Perhaps in response to the promulgation of restrictive laws and regulations, in 1983, an NP survey conducted by *The Nurse Practitioner* journal found that NP respondents expressed the need for a strong organized voice for NPs. Fifty-five percent of the NP respondents looked "to organize forces under the auspices of the ANA" (Harper & Billingsley, 1983, p. 24). In response, ANA convened a meet-ing of six existing national NP groups: ANA's Council of Primary Health Care Nurse Practitioners, the Association of Faculties of Pediatric Nurse Practitioner and Associates Programs, the National Association of Nurse Practitioners in Family Planning, the National Association of Pediatric Nurse Associates and Practitioners, the National Organization of Nurse Practitioner Faculties, and the Nurses' Association of the American College of Obstetricians and Gynecologists. These six organizations agreed to form a national coalition of NP organizations "to promote the visibility, viability, and unity of nurse practitioners to improve the health of the nation through primary care." Coalition priorities included leg-islative and political action, marketing of the NP as a provider of health care, and communication among all participants in the coalition. The National Alliance of Nurse Practitioners was short-lived. At the 1985 national conference, ANA did not answer the call to house the National Alliance, and the formation of a new NP organization, the American Academy of Nurse Practitioners (AANP) was announced ("Nurse Practitioners," 2000). The AANP exists today as the American Association of Nurse Practitioners.

Successes and Frustration

Over the decades, there have been both successes in APRN advocacy and frus-trations. For example, in the 1980s, ANA responded decisively to an APRN mal-practice insurance crisis. ANA had sponsored malpractice insurance for nurses at the rate of $58 per year for coverage of $1,000,000 per occurrence and $3,000,000 in the aggregate per year. In 1987, Fireman's Fund, the last insurance company in the country that accepted all types of NP applicants, notified ANA that they would not continue coverage. Following discussions and pressure, they agreed to cover for one additional year those NPs who were currently covered. Fireman's Fund, however, increased the premium from $58 to $1,500 per year. ANA worked to find other insurance carriers, writing letters to Congress and testifying before the National Association of Insurance Commissioners (ANA, 1989).

Between 1992 and 1996, the Agency for Health Care Policy and Research (now the Agency for Healthcare Research and Quality) sponsored a series of clinical practice guidelines. ANA was asked to review *Clinical Practice Guideline for Depression* and expressed concern about the absence of psychiatric and mental health CNSs as providers of mental health services. Unfortunately, the final version did not mention nurses at all and ANA did not endorse the guideline (Betts, 1992).

ANA's POLICY PRIORITIES: APRNs

There are many opportunities for ANA to engage in work that will increase access to quality health care provided by APRNs. ANA focuses resources on those areas that are "cross cutting," impacting each of four APRN roles. Whether it is lobbying Congress to allow APRNs to certify patients for home health services, drafting regulatory comments to ensure that APRNs are included in new payment models, or developing resources for state nurses associations, ANA works collaboratively with other organizations representing APRNs.

Leverage the Opportunities of Health System Reform

For decades, ANA has advocated for health care reforms that would guarantee access to high-quality health care for all. ANA was the first association to endorse the creation of the Medicare program in 1965, at a time when the American Medical Association was vehemently opposing efforts to achieve national health insurance (The Kaiser Family Foundation, 2009). In 1977, ANA lobbied for the introduction of a health services bill to expand primary care services, encouraging utilization of NPs. In the 1990s, ANA collaborated with the nursing community to develop *Nursing's Agenda for Health Care Reform* (ANA, 1992; Betts, 1996).

ANA's advocacy is based on the belief that quality affordable health care is not a privilege, but a basic human right. While the Patient Protection and Affordable Care Act (PPACA, or ACA) did not go so far as to extend universal coverage, it does extend health care coverage to millions of Americans and protects many others from losing coverage. ANA has been committed to informing nurses and the public about health care reform and will continue to do so (ana.nursingworld.org/MainMenuCategories/HealthcareandPolicyIssues/HealthSystemReform.aspx).

Although *defense* of the ACA has diverted a good deal of attention from *implementation* or improvement of the law, there have been many important provisions implemented (Weston, 2015), and ANA has worked to ensure that the role of the APRN is recognized and included in regulatory language, policy documents, data collection tools, and so on. More detail on regulatory work follows.

Increased use of electronic health records and expansion of health information technology (HIT) systems has been a major component of the ACA. ANA continues to ensure that nurses are involved in the design, development, and implementation of those systems, and that APRNs are eligible for funding to enhance adoption of HIT.

Address Barriers to APRN Scope of Practice

Ensuring the ability of APRNs to practice to the full extent of their education and training has long been a policy priority for ANA. With terms like "scope of practice" and "independent" identified as a "red flag," there continues to be a need to reach a common understanding of how words like those are used in various contexts (ANA, 2016b).

Physician collaboration has always been and continues to be a hot-button issue. In 1993, ANA testified before the Physician Payment Review Commission to express its concerns about statutory requirements for collaboration:

> Advanced practice nurses are, as are all registered nurses, independently licensed and accountable for their actions. [They are]...able to deliver...services independent of their relationship with physicians or other health care providers.... Collaborating with and referring to other health providers is a matter of good professional practice...Regardless of practice setting or supervision requirements, advanced practice nurses, like most health professionals, generally maintain a network for referral to and collaboration with other professionals and maintain a means to access emergency back-up. (ANA, 1998, p. 4)

ANA leaders met with leaders of the American Medical Association in 1993–1994 to discuss collaboration issues. After much discussion and negotiation, the following definition was proposed:

> Collaboration is the process whereby physicians and nurses plan and practice together as colleagues, working interdependently within the boundaries of their scopes of practice with shared values and mutual acknowledgment and respect for each other's contribution to care for individuals, their families, and their communities. (ANA, 1998, p. 6)

This definition of collaboration was adopted by the ANA Board of Directors in 1994; the American Medical Association took no further action.

Almost 20 years later, after the release of the Institute of Medicine 2011 report *The Future of Nursing: Leading Change, Advancing Health*, 12 physicians and nurse leaders, including ANA, met to produce a document on interprofessional collaboration. This more recent effort failed following the leak of a confidential draft document and objections from organized medicine (Jablow, 2013).

ANA has worked to build partnerships beyond nursing, particularly through the Coalition for Patients' Rights (addressed in Chapter 23). The Citizen Advocacy Center has been another important ally that has brought the voice of the consumer through its Reforming Scope of Practice Initiative (Citizen Advocacy Center, 2010).

In many states, as efforts to achieve full practice authority for APRNs have advanced, analysis has revealed a disturbing trend in legislation requiring a supervised post-licensure practice or transition period, often referred to as "transition to practice." These requirements have not been based on evidence, but are the result of political compromise. As a part of ANA monitoring of state actions, and in keeping with a commitment to develop resources that serve members at the state level, ANA developed Principles for Full Practice Authority (ANA, 2016b). This document contains a table with the states that have enacted legislation with "transition to practice" barriers, and five essential principles to guide state-based advocacy on this issue.

Although legislation is often the focus of scope-of-practice efforts, ANA is attuned to many opportunities to ensure that APRNs can practice to the full extent of their education. For example, ANA sits on a number of Professional and Technical Advisory Committees (PTACs) of the Joint Commission and in that venue, seeks to facilitate the ability of APRNs to be credentialed as "licensed independent providers" in institutions.

DOCUMENT THE APRN WORKFORCE

Advocacy on behalf of APRNs requires good data on the APRN workforce. Unfortunately, those data have been difficult to gather.

For many years, the most relied on estimates of the registered nurse workforce were provided by the federal government's National Sample Survey of Registered Nurses (NSSRN) conducted by the Health Resources and Services Administration (HRSA). This survey, conducted every 4 years, profiled the demographics, educational preparation, and practice settings of RNs. In 2004, the survey was enhanced with collection of additional information about nursing specialties and APRNs. The NSSRN was last conducted in 2008, with the results published in 2010 (NSSRN, 2010).

HRSA elected to change direction for its next survey and focus on the workforce characteristics of NPs. The resultant 2012 National Sample Survey of Nurse Practitioners estimated the nursing workforce included 154,000 NPs in the United States in the 2012 survey year, although the AANP projected a much higher estimate: 205,000 NPs in 2014. HRSA leaders indicated they plan to resume implementation of the NSSRN in the Spring of 2017, and continue administering it every 4 years, as has been done in the past. HRSA plans to oversample all APRNs, but does not plan to publish role-specific surveys (as was done with the 2012 survey of NPs).

ANA's health economist tracks monthly workforce data from the Bureau of Labor Statistics (BLS) and other sources and posts regular updates on ANA's Nursing Workforce webpage. ANA also relies on data provided by the professional associations that represent the four APRN roles, and works closely with the Forum of State Nursing Workforce Centers and the National Council of State Boards of Nursing (NCSBN). The ability to gather and disseminate workforce data is critical to expanding access to APRNs.

Monitor Payment Reform and Achieve Equitable Reimbursement

In addition to workforce data, it is equally important to gather data regarding payment for services provided by APRNs. Although BLS can provide some data on nurse earnings, data on direct payments for RN services are sorely lacking. Again, ANA's health care economist has mined such available payment data as do exist, using public files of approved charges by APRN Medicare Part B providers.

APRNs' CONTINUED GROWTH AS MEDICARE PART B PROVIDERS

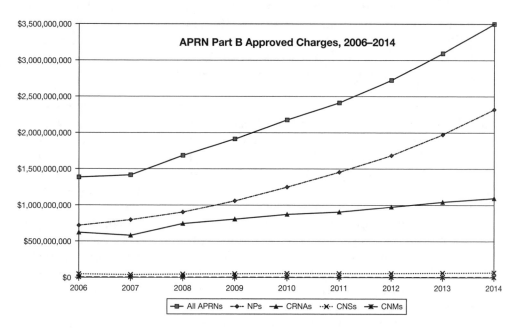

APRN, Advanced Practice Registered Nurse; CNM, Certified Nurse-Midwife; CNS, Clinical Nurse Specialists; CRNA, Certified Registered Nurse Anesthetist; NP, Nurse Practitioner.

APRNs continue to grow as an important component of the Medicare Part B provider workforce, providing care to Part B fee-for-service beneficiaries. In 2006, APRNs provided 1.25% of all Part B approved charges, at $1.38 billion. By 2014 that had increased 253% to $3.49 billion, 2.71% of total approved charges. NP approved charges more than tripled from $711 million to $2.32 billion. Certified nurse midwifes (CNMs) actually grew the fastest (although not obvious from the graph because of their much smaller shares of Part B). With the inclusion of PPACA §3114 the Affordable Care Act increased approved charges for midwives from 65% of the Medicare Physician Fee Schedule (PFS) to 100%. Approved charges for CNMs doubled from 2010 to 2011, and by 2014 total CNM approved charges had more than quadrupled relative to 2006. Total Part B approved charges increased at an annualized rate of 1.96% from 2006 to 2014. For APRNs in total the annualized increase was 12.33%. The increases, respectively, for NPs, Certified Registered Nurse Anesthetists (CRNAs), CNSs, and CNMs were 15.92%, 7.42%, 5.55%, and 19.38%.

APRN reimbursement has long been an ANA priority. In the 1980s, ANA lobbied successfully for landmark federal legislation that allowed pediatric and family NPs to be paid directly for the Medicaid services they provide. ANA lobbied effectively for direct payment to NPs, nurse midwives, and CNSs under the Federal Employees Health Benefits Plan (FEHBP). ANA currently advocates for "same payment for same service"; nurses should not be paid less for providing health care services.

The ACA has driven a number of changes seeking to shift payment from "volume to value" (U.S. Department of Health & Human Services Press Office, 2015). Purchasers and consumers (Consumer Reports, 2013) are both driving payment reform and ANA has continued to analyze reform efforts and ensure that APRNs are recognized and equitably reimbursed. ANA supports initiatives at the federal and state levels, aimed at both public and private payers, to remove barriers to direct and equitable reimbursement, including eliminating physician oversight requirements.

ANA represents the entire nursing profession on the American Medical Association Relative Value Scale Update Committee (RUC) and current procedural terminology (CPT) Committee, which influence reimbursement policy for Medicare and private payers. ANA works to ensure that APRNs are included in fee-for-service billing codes.

ANA has long taken exception to Medicare's "incident to" billing and payment policy. With respect to RNs and APRNs, "incident to" services are those provided by nurses, but billed as if they were provided by the physician and paid at PFS levels. Although Medicare has paid for "incident to" services since its inception, "Incident to was designed to reimburse physicians for the services of their employees, not to recognize the services of autonomous professionals" ("Nursing Reimbursement under Medicare and Medicaid," 1996, pp. 4–5).

Recent efforts to reform the payment system provide a window of opportunity for renewed advocacy to end incident to billing. The White Paper on an Alternative Payment Models Framework (Framework), issued by Centers for Medicare & Medicaid Services (CMS) Health Care Payment Learning & Action Network (LAN) in October 2015, enunciated several principles regarding payment and value. Principle 3 states that to the greatest extent possible, value-based incentives should reach providers who directly deliver care, a principle violated in "incident to" billing. Under the Merit-Based Incentive Payment System (MIPS), APRNs' composite scores will be biased downward because services provided to Medicare beneficiaries, but billed "incident to" a physician service, will be attributed to physicians rather than to the APRNs who actually serve those patients.

> The practice of "incident to" billing obscures the rendering provider, seriously undermining the ability of CMS to accurately calculate cost and quality performance, and hindering providers from being individually responsible and accountable for the care they render patients. A new payment system designed to incentivize high quality, value-based services must clearly and consistently identify the provider responsible for actually rendering a service, as well as ensure that Medicare claims accurately reflect the rendering provider. . . . We urge CMS to support efforts to eliminate "incident to" billing. In addition, we recommend that CMS establish modifiers to identify when a line item in a claim was provided "incident to" as well as the licensure and NPI of the actual rendering provider. Without establishing a mechanism to gather this type of clear data, CMS will be unable to accurately calculate value-based performance adjusters at a provider-specific level. (ANA, 2016a)

In today's environment, with a concerted effort to curb fraud and abuse, APRNs must be diligent in assuring that services billed "incident to" meet the requirements (ANA, 2010a). APRN graduates should ask about billing practices when applying for employment. APRN services billed "incident to" a physician constitute fraud if they involve any of these three "NP"s: **N**o **P**hysician in the office suite, **N**ew **P**atient, or existing patient with a **N**ew **P**roblem.

Quality

ANA has long played an important role in the national quality enterprise, with the development of the National Database of Nursing Quality Indicators®, and providing leadership and a strong voice for nursing in the Hospital Quality

Alliance, the National Priorities Partnership, and the National Quality Forum, among others. With new efforts to link payment and quality measures, it is imperative that APRNs be included in national performance measurement programs that were historically designed for physicians.

Of particular importance is the Medicare Access and CHIP Reauthorization Act of 2015 (MACRA). After decades of "kicking the can down the road," MACRA repealed the Medicare sustainable growth rate (SGR) methodology for updates to the PFS, often called "the doc fix." SGR was replaced with two new alternatives: the MIPS for certain eligible clinicians or groups under the PFS and Alternative Payment Models.

These new models will replace the Physician Quality Reporting System (PQRS), a system that APRNs in all four roles had participated in. In 2013, 56,006 APRNs (including 804 CNMs) were awarded $5,674,574 in PQRS incentive payments for high quality. Although ANA fully supports the use of quality measures that are transparent, actionable, evidence-based, patient-centered, and consensus-driven, ANA has warned CMS that the language in the new plans "does not fully recognize or acknowledge the essential role and expertise of clinicians other than physicians in the design and implementation of MACRA." ANA's comment letter goes on to provide specific examples.

How Does ANA Do This Substantive Work?

Nurses are the single largest group of health care professionals (3.6 million) and continue to be ranked as the most trusted professional according to the annual Gallup poll of honesty and ethics in various fields (Gallup, 2015). That is a powerful basis on which to influence policy and effectively advance a legislative agenda. Although the expertise of specialty organizations is highly valued when addressing particular health care problems or issues, policy makers (and the media) often wish to turn to one organization to learn about nursing. ANA works closely with specialty organizations through its organizational affiliates.

ORGANIZATIONAL AFFILIATES

ANA's affiliates are specialty nursing organizations that hold organizational-level membership in ANA. Working together, ANA and these organizations seek to share information and collaborate in finding solutions to issues that face the nursing profession, regardless of specialty. Although each organization maintains its own autonomy, the nursing profession and health care consumers benefit from opportunities to speak with aligned voices as a result of the collaboration that occurs with ANA and our affiliates. Four national APRN organizations are ANA organizational affiliates: the AANA, the ACNM, the National Association of Clinical Nurse Specialists, and Nurse Practitioners in Women's Health.

ANA SUPPORT FOR APRN WORK

Like many large professional associations, the ANA has several departments that work closely together to advance a series of policy and advocacy goals as determined by the board and the membership.

POLICY AND PROGRAMS

Staff with expertise in health policy, law, and economics (in addition to clinical expertise) analyze existing and proposed policies, create resources, and build strategic alliances with partners in other associations, advocacy groups, and government agencies. In the Department of Health Policy, the focus is on the nursing workforce, quality, HIT, APRN issues, and payment/reimbursement. In the Department of Nursing Practice and Work Environment, specific topics include safe staffing, safe patient handling and mobility and the Healthy Nurse, Healthy Nation™ Grand Challenge. Across departments, there is a focus on continued work to build a "culture of safety."

ADVOCACY/GOVERNMENT AFFAIRS

ANA's strength on Capitol Hill is a direct result of the collaboration and coordination of three critical components of its federal legislative program: lobbying, grassroots activities, and political action. The backbone of nursing's influence in the United States Congress is the political and grassroots activism of thousands of nurses across the country.

The lobbyists on ANA's Government Affairs (GOVA) team bring years of legislative and political experience to their work representing nurses on Capitol Hill. With the knowledge that we work better as a team (just like at the bedside), ANA's advocacy is often carried out in coalition, and there is an emphasis on building alliances with key stakeholders.

Lobbyists are most effective when paired with a strong coordinated grassroots effort, and ANA works to encourage nurses to develop and maintain relationships with their elected officials so they can more easily engage them when called to action. Joining RNAction.org, allows nurses to follow issues, including many that specifically impact APRNs, and ensure that their voice is heard.

Political action committee (PAC) is a term for committees organized for the purpose of raising and spending money in support of the campaigns of political candidates (Center for Responsive Politics, 2016). Over the past 40 years, PACs have been widely used by like-minded members of associations, labor unions, corporations, and groups of individuals to pool their resources to support candidates. The ANA–PAC is bipartisan and works directly with the national parties to recruit and support candidates who have demonstrated their belief in the legislative and regulatory agenda of the ANA.

Regulatory Work

Although working toward the passage of favorable laws is important, it is equally important to be vigilant as those laws are *implemented*. When Congress (or a state legislature) passes laws, they rarely contain enough specific language to guide their implementation completely. It is the responsibility of the federal administrative agencies to fill in the details of new or amended laws with rules and regulations. Regulations/rules are used to clarify definitions, authority, eligibility, benefits, and standards. Their development is shaped not only by the law but also with the ongoing involvement and input of professional associations like ANA, other providers, third-party payers, consumers, and other special interest groups.

The development of rules takes time and follows a defined process. The publication of the proposed rule in the Federal Register offers an opportunity for those with an interest in the particular rule to react to the draft rule before it becomes final. ANA routinely reviews the Federal Register for proposed regulations of particular interest to the nursing community, analyzing them, identifying concerns, and commenting when appropriate.

If necessary, ANA submits comments to the agency recommending changes to the proposed regulation. Earlier quotes from ANA's comment letters regarding "incident to" billing and new payment models are good examples.

Although the regulatory process often receives less attention than other policy and advocacy efforts, a recent example generated unprecedented interest. When the Department of Veterans Affairs (VA) published a proposed rule that would provide full practice authority to APRNs working in the Veterans Health Administration, the VA received an extraordinary number of comments—nearly 225,000. This example also illustrates the importance of working in coalition (in this case, Veterans Access to Quality Healthcare Alliance) and reaching out to groups outside of nursing. Prominent stakeholders, including the Federal Trade Commission, AARP, the American Hospital Association, and the Robert Wood Johnson Foundation, all joined ANA in expressing support for the rule. Further, ANA and its partners engaged in robust traditional media relations, holding a press conference at the National Press Club, as well as ongoing social media outreach to raise awareness of the issues and encourage a wide range of stakeholders to submit comments. As this text goes to press, there has not been a final ruling, but ANA will maintain resources and updates on this important issue at RNAction.org (www.rnaction.org/site/PageNavigator/nstat_take_action_VHA.html).

Communications and Social Media

A communications strategy is key to the success of any advocacy agenda. Traditional and social media can have a significant impact on the public perception of nurses, including APRNs, and on the understanding of complex policy problems. ANA fields many requests from the media and invests significant resources in communications, including social media. The "Share Your Stethoscopes" campaign, which won a media and public relations campaign award, is a recent example.

OFFICE OF GENERAL COUNSEL

Occasionally, ANA's Office of General Counsel (OGC) pursues legal action and weighs in on legal issues to protect nurses and patients and to uphold ANA's policy positions. For example, ANA, through its legal counsel, has filed and supported legal challenges to arbitrary practice restrictions in the form of laws, regulations, rules, policies, or guidelines, and has filed numerous amicus briefs in support of APRNs. In 2013, ANA and the Iowa Nurses Association, represented by attorneys in ANA's OGC, intervened in lawsuits filed by the Iowa Medical Society and Iowa Society of Anesthesiologists against the Iowa Board of Registered Nursing.[1] The physician groups challenged whether the Iowa Board of Nursing and Iowa Department of Public Health exceeded their regulatory authority by enacting rules allowing APRNs to supervise radiologic technologists using fluoroscopy machines. The case was appealed through the Supreme Court of Iowa, which ultimately found that the Department of Public Health and Board of Nursing had the power and authority to adopt the rules, and that the

In September 2015, Miss Colorado performed a monologue about her profession as a nurse during the Miss America Pageant. Hosts of *The View* mocked the performance, with one host asking why she was wearing a doctor's stethoscope. This struck a nerve and many nurses were upset at the lack of understanding and respect regarding what nurses do every day. Within hours, the ANA responded by launching a social media campaign intended to help educate the hosts as well as the public about the nursing profession. We encouraged nurses to Tweet @TheView with selfies with their stethoscopes, using the hashtag #NursesShareYourStethoscopes. Thousands of nurses shared their photos and the hashtag went viral. It put pressure on the show, resulting in over a dozen advertisers pulling ads in support of nurses. *The View* apologized and brought nurses on the show to educate viewers on the work they did and the equipment they used...including a stethoscope.

Board of Nursing rationally determined that APRN supervision of fluoroscopy was recognized by the medical and nursing professions, despite the opposition of the board of medicine and physician organizations (*Iowa Med. Soc'y v. Iowa Bd. Of Nursing*, 831 N.W.2d 826, 2013).

More recently, the ANA filed an amicus brief in a case decided by the U.S. Supreme Court, *North Carolina State Board of Dental Examiners v. Federal Trade Commission*, which stands to have significant impact on state regulatory boards, particularly in situations where the actions of a board might be seen to be anticompetitive (Summers, 2015).

CONSTITUENT AND STATE NURSES ASSOCIATIONS AND APRNs

ANA's State Government Affairs program tracks trends in nursing-related legislation in the states, but with more than 1,000 nursing and health care related bills introduced in state legislatures each session, the ANA constituent and state nurses associations (C/SNAs) are the source of information specific to state bills. Although scope of practice is the issue typically of greatest interest to APRNs, ANA and the C/SNAs also track bills and engage in advocacy related to safe staffing, mandatory overtime, safe patient handling and mobility, workplace violence, and the nurse licensure compact.

Many of the C/SNAs expend significant resources working with licensing boards, legislatures, and regulatory agencies to bring affordable and accessible quality care to the public through the full utilization of APRNs. This work has been going on for decades and continues today, evolving and responding to new political and legislative environments.

ANA is sometimes asked, "What factors are associated with legislative success at the state level?" Although many variables can impact a campaign, ANA and C/SNA experts recommend (Summers, 2012):

- Choose the right issue to move forward in the legislative arena. Not all problems need a legislative or regulatory fix. Some might be better addressed in other ways.

- Form a strong coalition. C/SNAs with favorable legal and regulatory environments tend to have a formal coalition that includes the C/SNA and the groups representing each of the four APRN roles. Strong coalitions include effective channels of communication.
- Develop a shared strategy. A strong coalition is not guaranteed to have a shared strategy, but it has a better chance at developing one.
- Extend your coalition beyond nursing. Support from other health care providers, consumer groups, and business sends a message that your issue is bigger than nursing. Partnering with physician colleagues can yield significant results.
- Create opportunity out of crisis. Successful advocacy efforts are sometimes linked to a crisis. Although we likely have no control over this factor, it may affect timing of a legislative effort if the crisis can be leveraged.
- Hire a savvy lobbyist. There is value in the regular presence of a good lobbyist who will know if an issue should be addressed legislatively and identify the best sponsors. A shared lobbyist working for the C/SNA and the APRN groups enables consistency of the message.

As noted earlier, particularly with regard to APRN scope-of-practice issues, "words matter." Language is often an issue with legislation and there is a need to replace negative language for APRNs (i.e., physician extenders) with appropriate terminology (i.e., NP and APRN). Identifying this before any enactment is crucial to ensuring inclusion of APRNs.

Sometimes advancement in one state can be the catalyst for movement in another, and ANA facilitates communication between states and sharing of "lessons learned."

Many C/SNAs have produced "white papers" or policy briefs to assist in their advocacy efforts. Not infrequently, the process of convening various organizations to collaboratively produce such a document is as beneficial as the document itself. For example, the Missouri Nurses Association (MONA) convened a task force to author a white paper entitled "A Template for Change in the State of Missouri." This document covers the state of health care in Missouri (MO), defines APRNs and their role in health care, describes barriers and recommends removal of such to support full scope of practice. It is updated regularly so it can be used to guide legislators and others who have the opportunity to make changes. In 2013, one small step forward came with the allowance of a waiver to the required physician on-site supervision in the collaborative practice agreement for rural health clinics.

The implementation of the *Consensus Model for APRN Regulation* is an area where C/SNAs have been hard at work. The West Virginia, Arizona, North Dakota, and Rhode Island nurses associations have all been successful in getting the recommendations placed into state code. In many states, a long partnership with the Board of Nursing has facilitated the process of bringing state rules and regulations into alignment with the *Consensus Model*.

Implementation of the *Consensus Model* is an example of where national- and state-based work overlap, and also an example of the role ANA plays in advocating for all four APRN roles, through continued involvement in the licensure, accreditation, certification, and education (LACE) network (see chapter 5 on *Consensus Model*).

AMERICAN NURSES CREDENTIALING CENTER (ANCC)

As credentialing became an important component of the concept of quality practice, ANA's credentialing arm, the ANCC, became a distinct and independent corporate entity in 1990. Today, ANCC provides 26 certifications of which seven are for APRN (five NP and two CNS) and 19 are specialty certifications. In addition to ANCC's credentialing programs, ANCC recognizes health care organizations that promote nursing excellence and quality patient outcomes, while providing safe, positive work environments through the Magnet Recognition Program® and Pathway to Excellence Program®. ANCC also accredits health care organizations that provide and approve continuing nursing education. ANCC also accredits nursing residency programs. ANCC's Practice Transition Accreditation Program™ establishes global standards for residency or fellowship programs that transition RNs and APRNs into new practice settings.

As implementation of the APRN *Consensus Model* progressed, ANCC updated current certifications and developed new certifications to reflect the roles and populations in the model. The new NP certifications developed were Adult-Gerontology Acute Care NP and Adult-Gerontology Primary Care NP. The Family Psychiatric-Mental Health NP certification, which covered content across the life span was renamed Psychiatric–Mental Health NP and continues to cover content across the life span. The Pediatric NP Certification was renamed Pediatric Primary Care NP to clarify the focus of this certification.

The Adult-Gerontology CNS certification was developed and the Pediatric CNS certification was updated. Both CNS certifications include content on the APRN core and wellness through acute care. Refer to the ANCC website for more details (www.nursecredentialing.org/certification.aspx#specialty and APRN Corner: Frequently Asked Questions).

DOCUMENTS ESSENTIAL FOR ALL NURSING PRACTICE

ANA, in its role as the professional organization for all nurses, continues to maintain accountability for stewardship of several professional publications considered essential resources for every nurse in every role and setting, including APRNs. These documents provide a foundation for education, credentialing, and practice: *Code of Ethics for Nurses with Interpretive Statements* (ANA, 2015a); *Nursing: Scope and Standards of Practice* (ANA, 2015b); and *Nursing's Social Policy: The Essence of the Profession* (ANA, 2010b).

CODE OF ETHICS FOR NURSES WITH INTERPRETIVE STATEMENTS

The *Code of Ethics for Nurses with Interpretive Statements* serves the following purposes:

- It is a succinct statement of the ethical values, obligations, duties, and professional ideals of nurses individually and collectively.
- It is the profession's non-negotiable ethical standard.
- It is an expression of nursing's own understanding of its commitment to society. (ANA, 2015a, p. viii)

It requires each nurse to demonstrate ethical competence in professional life. The values and obligations apply to nurses in all roles, in all forms of practice, and in all settings. The Code reflects the proud ethical heritage of nursing and is a guide for all nurses now and into the future.

NURSING: SCOPE AND STANDARDS OF PRACTICE

The ANA follows a regular cycle to review documents essential to nursing, convening workgroups to examine and, if necessary, revise the definition of nursing, scope-of-nursing-practice statement, and standards of nursing practice and accompanying competencies. Those workgroups, including APRNs, are charged to review the current practice environment, existing nursing and specialty nursing scope and standards documents, and other materials and resources to identify the best mechanism to describe contemporary nursing practice and provide a framework for practice for the next 5 to 10 years.

Nursing: Scope and Standards of Practice, Third Edition, was published in 2015 after an extended field review and public comment period, review and revision, and final approval by the ANA Board of Directors. The revised standards include additional competencies for graduate-level prepared nurses and APRNs.

Faculty members are expected to integrate this content into academic and nursing professional development curricula. Similarly nurses and other stakeholders in clinical and non-clinical practice, administration, research, and other environments should use the scope and standards and accompanying competencies for all practice activities, including such initiatives as quality improvement, development of policies and procedures, professional goal setting, and professional certification. The language of this resource can be used as a template, and is used by specialty nursing organizations to draft congruent specialty nursing scope and standards of practice. Regulatory bodies, especially state boards of nursing, are encouraged to incorporate the contemporary *Nursing: Scope and Standards of Practice* content in decision-making activities.

NURSING'S SOCIAL POLICY STATEMENT

ANA's *Nursing's Social Policy Statement* (ANA, 2015c, pp. 180–188) is a document about the relationship between the nursing profession and society. "It forms and frames both the basis for nursing's involvement with caring practices and the shape of society vis-à-vis health and health policy" (Fowler, 2015, p. 1). An example of what is called a social contract, this type of relationship, like any contract, establishes mutual and reciprocal expectations between the two parties. In the case of the contract between nursing as a profession and society as a whole, it helps frame and form such critical issues as authority for and authorization of nursing practice.

Future Focus

As ANA looks to the future, the strategic roadmap is focused on three goals: profession-wide engagement; nurse-focused innovation; and nurse-to-consumer relationships (ANA, n.d.).

ANA seeks to increase both the number and engagement of nurses with ANA, recognizing that for many APRNs, their primary affiliation is with the association that represents their role or specialty. Maintaining membership in ANA allows APRNs to help the profession speak with "one strong voice" and be a true catalyst for transforming health care and advancing the profession to improve health for all.

APRNs have demonstrated the creative thinking and persistence that have led to many innovative models of care. The American Academy of Nursing's *Raise the Voice: Edge Runners* includes several models of care led by APRNs including the 11th Street Family Health Services, the Arkansas Aging Initiative, and the Centering Health Care Institute (http://www.aannet.org/initiatives/edge -runners; http://www.aannet.org/initiatives/edge-runners/profiles).

The challenge is to foster the scale and spread of nurse-focused innovations and leverage the data and analytics that will maximize the power of nursing and add transformative value in the form of quality, cost, and safety across the care continuum.

Consumers are becoming engaged in their care as never before and nurses, particularly APRNs, are assuming new roles in a consumer-driven model. As a part of ANA's work to position nurses as integral partners in consumers' health, ANA has launched a nationwide campaign, Healthy Nurse, Health Nation: Leading the Way to Better Health, and is developing strategic partnerships to redefine the nurse-to-consumer relationship.

ANAs work will adapt to a changing environment but remain focused on the vision of all nurses as a powerful unified force in engaging consumers and transforming health and health care.

To keep abreast of ANA's policy and advocacy work on behalf of APRNs, visit the Advanced Practice Nurse webpage on *Nursing World:* nursingworld .org/EspeciallyForYou/AdvancedPracticeNurses.

DISCUSSION QUESTIONS

1. *Based on the information in this chapter, list at least two areas of policy change championed by the American Nurses Association that you can identify where legislation could have an impact.*
2. *If you were to describe the importance of ANA's work to position nurses, particularly APRNs as integral partners in consumers' health to potential supporters, what key issues would you stress? How would you describe this to your patients?*
3. *Consider ANA's policy work on behalf of APRNs discussed in this chapter and consider the impact that might occur if this work did NOT continue. In other words, what are the consequences if ANA no longer advocates for APRNs?*

ANALYSIS, SYNTHESIS, AND CLINICAL APPLICATION

1. *Describe your past or current involvement in ANA and/or your state nurses association. Were you aware of ANA's history and current work on behalf of APRNs? Is there current or future need for joint efforts of ANA and APRN organizations? Why or why not?*
2. *APRN reimbursement has long been an ANA priority. How are APRN visits billed at your clinical sites? Are your preceptor's services billed "incident to" a physician?*

3. *Are APRNs credentialed as "licensed independent providers" in the health care institution where you work or plan to work? Consider activities that you might lead to promote APRN credentialing in your workplace.*

EXERCISES/CONSIDERATIONS

1. *ANA seeks to fully and accurately represent the nursing community, including each of the four APRN roles.*
2. *With a limited number of seats at policy-making tables, ANA sometimes is the sole voice for nursing.*
3. *ANA is adapting to a changing environment but remains focused on the vision of all nurses engaging consumers and transforming health and health care.*

NOTE

1. Iowa Medical Society v. Iowa Department of Public Health and Iowa Board of Registered Nursing, Iowa District Court, Polk County, Case No. 8252 (2010) and Iowa Society of Anesthesiologists versus Iowa Department of Public Health and Iowa Board of Registered Nursing, Iowa District Court, Polk County, Case No. 8253 (2010). The two cases were eventually consolidated into a single case under case number cv 8252.

REFERENCES

American Academy of Nursing. (1977). *Primary care by nurses: Sphere of responsibility and accountability.* American Academy of Nursing monograph. Kansas City, MO: American Nurses Association.

American Nurses Association. (n.d.). 2017–2020 Strategic plan. Retrieved from http://www.nursing world.org/FunctionalMenuCategories/AboutANA/ANAStrategicPlan

American Nurses Association. (1965). First education. *American Journal of Nursing, 65*(12), 106–111.

American Nurses Association. (1989, March 2). *Press release. ANA Archives.* Kansas City, MO: Author.

American Nurses Association. (1992). *Nursing's agenda for health care reform.* Washington, DC: American Nurses Publishing.

American Nurses Association. (1998). Collaboration and independent practice ongoing issues for nursing. *Trends & Issues, 3*(5). Silver Spring, MD: Author.

American Nurses Association. (2010a). Ignorance is not a defense: Implications of heightened scruting for fraud and abuse [ANA Issue Brief]. Retrieved from http://www.nursingworld.org/MainMenuCategories/Policy-Advocacy/Positions-and-Resolutions/Issue-Briefs/Fraud-and-Abuse.pdf

American Nurses Association. (2010b). *Nursing's social policy: The essence of the profession* (3rd ed.). Silver Spring, MD: Author

American Nurses Association. (2015a). *Code of ethics for nurses with interpretive statements.* Silver Spring, MD: Author.

American Nurses Association. (2015b). *Nursing: Scope and standards of practice* (3rd ed.). Silver Spring, MD: Author.

American Nurses Association. (2016a). Letter from ANA to CMS on the merit-based incentive payment system and alternative payment model incentive under the physician fee schedule, and criteria for physician-focused payment models, dated June 27, 2016. Retrieved from http://www.nursing world.org/MIPS-APM-ANACommentLetter-062716

American Nurses Association. (2016b). ANA principles for advanced practice registered nurse (APRN) full practice authority. Retrieved from http://www.nursingworld.org/MainMenuCategories/ThePracticeofProfessionalNursing/NursingStandards/ANAPrinciples/Principles-for-APRN-Full-Practice-Authority.pdf

American Nurses Association, Commission on Nursing Education. (1971). Definition of the term "Nurse Practitioner." *ANA Archives.* New York, NY: Author.

American Nurses Association, Congress for Nursing Practice. (1974). Definition: Nurse practitioner, nurse clinician and clinical nurse specialist. *ANA Archives*. Kansas City, MO: Author.

American Nurses Association, Council of Family Nurse Practitioners and Clinicians. (1976). *Scope of primary nursing practice for adults and families*. *ANA Archives*. Kansas City, MO: Author.

American Nurses Association, Council of Primary Health Care Nurse Practitioners. (1980). *The primary health care nurse practitioner*. *ANA Archives*. Kansas City, MO: Author.

Betts, V. T. (1992, November 25). *Letter to J. Jarrett Clinton*. *ANA Archives*. Washington, DC: American Nurses Association.

Betts, V. T. (1996). Nursing's agenda for health care reform: Policy, politics and power through professional leadership. *Nursing Administration Quarterly, 20*(3), 1–8.

Center for Responsive Politics. (2016). What is a PAC? Retrieved from https://www.opensecrets.org/pacs/pacfaq.php

Citizen Advocacy Center. (2010). Scope of practice initiative. Retrieved from http://www.cacenter.org/cac/SOP

Consumer Reports. (2013). What you need to know about the Health Care Reform update. Retrieved from http://www.consumerreports.org/cro/2012/06/update-on-health-care-reform/index.htm

Fowler, M. D. M. (2015). *Guide to nursing's social policy statement: Understanding the profession from social contract to social covenant*. Silver Spring, MD: American Nurses Association.

Gallup. (2015). Americans' faith in honesty, ethics of police rebounds. Retrieved from http://www.gallup.com/poll/187874/americans-faith-honesty-ethics-police-rebounds.aspx?g_source=Social%20Issues&g_medium=newsfeed&g_campaign=tiles

Hamric, A. B., & Spross, J. (1983). *The clinical nurse specialist in theory and practice*. New York, NY: Grune & Stratton.

Harper, D. C., & Billingsley, M. C. (1983, July–August). Organizing for power. *Nurse Practitioner, 8*(7), 24–33.

Iowa Med. Soc'y v. Iowa Bd. of Nursing, 831 N.W.2d 826 (Iowa 2013).

Jablow, P. (2013, January 9). How to foster interprofessional collaboration between physicians and nurses? Retrieved from http://www.rwjf.org/en/research-publications/find-rwjf-research/2013/01/how-to-foster-interprofessional-collaboration-between-physicians.html

Johnson, J., Dawson, E., & Brassard, A. (2010). Consensus model for advanced-practice nurse regulation: A new approach. In E. M. Sullivan-Marx, D. O. McGivern, J. A. Fairman, & A. S. Greenberg (Eds.), *Nurse practitioners: The evolution and future of advanced practice* (pp. 125–142). New York, NY: Springer Publishing.

The Kaiser Family Foundation. (2009). National health insurance—A brief history of reform efforts in the U.S. Retrieved from https://kaiserfamilyfoundation.files.wordpress.com/2013/01/7871.pdf

Nurse Practitioners: Remembering the Past, Planning the Future. (2000, January 4). *Medscape*. Retrieved from http://www.medscape.com/viewarticle/408388

Nursing Reimbursement under Medicare and Medicaid. (1996, September). *Nursing Trends & Issues, 1*(3).

Summers, L. (2012). Finding the path to success in state level APRN advocacy. *The American Nurse*. Retrieved from http://www.theamericannurse.org/2012/04/02/finding-the-path-to-success-in-state-level-aprn-advocacy

Summers, L. (2015). Who's smiling now. Retrieved from http://www.theamericannurse.org/2015/07/01/whos-smiling-now

U.S. Department of Health & Human Services Press Office. (2015). Better, smarter, healthier: In historic announcement, HHS sets clear goals and timeline for shifting Medicare reimbursements from volume to value. Retrieved from http://wayback.archive-it.org/3926/20170127232849/https://www.hhs.gov/about/news/2015/01/26/better-smarter-healthier-in-historic-announcement-hhs-sets-clear-goals-and-timeline-for-shifting-medicare-reimbursements-from-volume-to-value.html

Waddle, F. I. (1981, October 6). *Letter to Jean R. H. Dickson*. Silver Spring, MD: American Nurses Association Archive.

Weston, M. J. (2015). Nurses' reaction to Supreme Court in King v Burwell. Congress Blog. *The Hill*. Retrieved from http://thehill.com/blogs/congress-blog/healthcare/246319-nurses-reaction-to-supreme-court-in-king-v-burwell

Policy and the Integration of Advanced Practice Nursing Roles in Canada: Are We Making Progress?

Denise Bryant-Lukosius, Ruth Martin-Misener, Josette Roussel,
Nancy Carter, Kelley Kilpatrick, and Linda Brousseau

In 2010, the *Canadian Journal of Nursing Leadership* published 10 papers from a decision support synthesis examining the integration of Advanced Practice Registered Nursing (APRN) roles in the Canadian health care system. The synthesis included a scoping review of the international APRN literature, 81 interviews with national and international key informants and a national roundtable with health care administrators and policy makers (DiCenso & Bryant-Lukosius, 2010). As the most comprehensive study of its kind in Canada, decision support synthesis recommendations provided a roadmap for future APRN role development. An important contribution of this study was an analysis of policy factors enabling APRN role integration, defined as the extent to which the roles are utilized to their full potential across the continuum of health care (DiCenso et al., 2010). The purpose of this chapter is to revisit policy factors to identify where progress in APRN role integration has been made. The chapter begins with a brief description of the Canadian health care system and a 2010 snapshot of factors impacting the integration of the two APRN roles recognized in Canada, the Clinical Nurse Specialist (CNS) and Nurse Practitioner (NP). Next, a framework for understanding policy factors influencing APRN role integration is described and applied to examine the current status of CNS and NP roles. Recommendations for future policy actions and the role of APRNs in implementing these actions are identified.

APRN ROLE INTEGRATION IN CANADA BY 2010

Canada has 10 provinces and three territories spread across a vast geographic area that is slightly larger than that of the United States (Wikipedia, 2016). Despite its geographic size, Canada has a small population of 35 million people, one tenth of the population in the United States (Statistics Canada, 2016). Most Canadians live in large southern urban communities bordering the United States, while 20% live in small rural, northern, and remote communities (Employment and Social Development in Canada, 2014). In the early 1890s, nurses in expanded roles were introduced to address the lack of health care services and shortages of physicians in these latter communities (Kaasalainen et al., 2010). These roles were precursors to the more formal introduction of NP and CNS roles in the 1960s and 1970s respectively.

In addition to geographic differences in resources and health needs across the country, federal and provincial/territorial health care policies have influenced the integration of APRN roles in Canada. The Canadian Constitution directs how health care services are organized and delivered (Health Canada, 2012). Provincial/territorial governments have responsibility for establishing, maintaining, and managing most health services. The federal government is responsible for health services for First Nations and Inuit people, the Canadian military, inmates in federal penitentiaries, and some refugee groups. Canada has a publicly funded health care system providing universal coverage for medically necessary hospital and physician services (Health Canada, 2012). However, other health services related to medications and rehabilitative, mental health, community, home, vision, hearing, and long-term care are not included under universal coverage, and people must pay out-of-pocket or through third-party insurance plans. The Canada Health Act ensures that provincial and territorial health care plans are administered and operated on a nonprofit basis by a public authority and meet criteria for comprehensiveness, universality, portability, and accessibility (Health Canada, 2012). Federal funding transfers to provinces/territories may be withheld if they do not adhere to Canada Health Act requirements.

The CNS is a registered nurse with a master's or doctoral degree in nursing (Canadian Nurses Association [CNA], 2009a). CNSs were introduced in acute care hospitals, in response to rising patient acuity and the growing specialization and complexity of health care. Their role was to support and improve nursing practice at the point of care (Kaasalainen et al., 2010). In 2010, the actual number of CNSs was unknown due to inconsistent or absent provincial nursing regulatory processes to identify master's prepared CNSs. There was no legal protection of the CNS title, so any nurse could self-identify as a CNS. Estimates suggested that in 2007 there were 2,354 self-reported CNSs in Canada, making up less than 1% of the nursing workforce (CNA, 2013a). About 66% of CNSs worked in hospital or outpatient settings, with some expansion into community and long-term care settings. In 2005, funding from Health Canada led to the introduction of CNSs in 600 First Nations and Inuit communities to improve health outcomes and nursing care in areas with unmet needs for maternal/child care, mental health/addictions, chronic disease management, and diabetes (Veldhorst, 2006). Stakeholders interviewed for the decision support synthesis noted variable CNS deployment within and across provinces and overall perceived there were declining numbers of CNSs (Bryant-Lukosius et al., 2010). The use of CNSs was observed to be health care administrator dependent with lack of role clarity and understanding of the CNS role as reported barriers to role introduction and sustainability. Despite international evidence about the benefits of CNS roles, especially in priority areas for health care improvement (i.e., chronic disease management, quality of care, nursing recruitment/retention), CNSs were also felt to be vulnerable to economic cutbacks due to varied involvement in direct clinical care and challenges in documenting tangible role outcomes (Bryant-Lukosius et al., 2010). Other barriers to the health systems integration of CNS roles were poor access to CNS education, lack of role funding, and lack of regulation and title protection.

NPs are registered nurses who, in 2010, had to complete an NP education program at the baccalaureate or master's level and were required to successfully write an examination to practice as an NP–Primary Health Care/All Ages, NP–Adult, or NP–Pediatric (CNA, 2009b). For two specialized areas (neonatal and anesthesia care), NPs completed a master's or post-master's diploma. In 2010, regulatory mechanisms for NPs were complete in all but one territory. They had an expanded legislated scope of practice that in most jurisdictions enabled them to autonomously diagnose, order/interpret diagnostic tests, prescribe pharmaceuticals, and perform procedures, but with some restrictions. The expansion of NP roles has been the highlight of APRN development in Canada. Between 2006 and 2010, the total number of NPs doubled from 1,129 to 2,486 and accounted for just less than 1% of the nursing workforce (Canadian Institutes of Health Information [CIHI], 2011). However, there were disproportionate numbers of NPs deployed across provinces. Primary health care reform as a policy priority and new provincial funding specifically for primary health care NPs and for team models of primary health care that included NPs contributed to increased NP deployment, especially in the province of Ontario, where 50% of all NPs worked (Donald et al., 2010). Primary health care NPs made up 80% of all NPs and were considered the backbone of rural and remote health care and the care of at-risk patient populations in urban communities (DiCenso & Bryant-Lukosius, 2010). While much progress had been made in the introduction of NP roles after 40 years, by 2010, full health systems integration had not been achieved and significant barriers to optimal role implementation remained (Donald et al., 2010; Kilpatrick et al., 2010).

FRAMEWORK FOR UNDERSTANDING POLICY FACTORS ENABLING HEALTH SYSTEMS INTEGRATION OF APRN ROLES

From the decision support synthesis study, data from the literature scoping review and key informant interviews were synthesized to identify and examine factors enabling health systems integration of APRN roles (DiCenso et al., 2010). Policy factors in two main theme areas, role development and role implementation, provided a framework for determining the required elements for optimal APRN role integration. The focus was on enabling factors, because in most cases, barriers were the mirrored absence of these factors. In addition, health care policy and decision-making responsibilities for each factor at federal, provincial/territorial, and organizational levels were identified. Related to the theme of role development, our analysis of the current state and progress in APRN role integration focuses on factors related to pan-Canadian approaches, legislation and regulation, and education as policy priorities identified by national roundtable participants (DiCenso & Bryant-Lukosius, 2010). For our second theme related to successful APRN role implementation, national leadership and funding are the focus of our analysis. Again, these factors were selected for their relevance to national roundtable recommendations (DiCenso & Bryant-Lukosius et al., 2010).

APRN ROLE DEVELOPMENT AND IMPLEMENTATION IN 2016

Pan-Canadian Approaches

Pan-Canadian approaches are those that span across provincial and territorial jurisdictions. They are important for strengthening stakeholder understanding of APRN roles, reducing variability in APRN practices and outcomes, and promoting labor mobility of the APRN workforce (DiCenso et al., 2010). Prior to 2010, two pan-Canadian initiatives made significant contributions to APRN role development. The first occurred when the CNA (2008) published and refined over time a national framework to define advanced nursing practice, outline role competencies and outcomes, and delineate requirements for educational preparation, regulation, and role support. The second was the Canadian Nurse Practitioner Initiative (CNPI), an $8.9 million investment by the federal government in 2004 to support NP role development. The policy driver for CNPI was to improve access to comprehensive primary health care. United in its determination to avoid another failed attempt to implement NPs like the one in the 1970s and 1980s (Spitzer, 1984), the nursing profession seized the opportunity to collaborate across jurisdictional boundaries and to forge national policies. Significant gains were made toward this goal with agreement on role definitions and the development of legislation and regulatory, practice, and educational frameworks for NPs. With CNPI support, the first Canadian Core Competency Framework and other supporting tools and processes were developed (CNA, 2010). For CNSs, who were becoming "invisible" in the Canadian health care landscape, building on the lessons learned from these pan-Canadian approaches was particularly important (Bryant-Lukosius et al., 2010). Since pan-Canadian approaches can be applied to a variety of areas for promoting APRN role development and implementation, they are integrated in the sections that follow related to legislation/ regulation, education, and national leadership.

Legislation and Regulation

Like the United States, Canada has a decentralized model for regulating APRN roles, where the responsibility for governance lies with provincial/territorial nursing colleges or associations. The risk of decentralized models is variability in advanced practice due to differences in scope-of-practice laws across jurisdictions, as was the case in Canada in 2010, especially for NP roles (Maier, 2015). A national roundtable recommendation was that a pan-Canadian approach be taken to standardize APRN regulatory policies, requirements, and processes across provinces/territories in order to facilitate provider mobility to respond to population health needs and improve the recruitment and retention of APRNs (DiCenso et al., 2010). For the NP role, barriers to achieving labor mobility related to jurisdictional differences in the types of NP roles eligible for licensure and registration, scope-of-practice descriptions and interpretation, and examinations accepted for licensure/certification.

The federal government exerts its power on provinces/territories to address health care issues through legal policy levers. One area that impacts on NP regulation is the federal legislation, Agreement on Internal Trade, which aims to remove mobility barriers and recognize the qualifications of all types of workers across Canada. Under this law, provincial/territorial governments must demonstrate and obtain approval through a formal process that there are differences in occupational standards or scopes of practice before they can demand additional requirements of workers. Jurisdictions violating this legislation are subject to monetary penalties.

The perception among regulators that there are differences in the scopes of practice of NPs in some provinces has been long-standing to the extent that some provinces filed a legal objection through the Agreement on Internal Trade in order to mandate additional requirements prior to licensure. To address this perception of jurisdictional difference, the Canadian Council of Registered Nurse Regulators (CCRNR), an organization formed in 2011 consisting of all 12 registered nurse regulatory colleges and associations, obtained funding to conduct a nationwide practice analysis. The purpose of the practice analysis was to describe the knowledge, skills, and abilities required of NPs practicing in three streams of regulated NP practice—adult, family/all ages, and pediatric, with the ultimate goal of informing a national approach to NP examinations, licensure, regulation, and certification (CCRNR, 2015). Conducted between 2014 and 2015, the practice analysis included subject matter experts, literature reviews, and surveys of practicing NPs and NP educators. The results indicated that NPs use the same competencies in all Canadian provinces and territories and streams of practice (CCRNR, 2015). Informed by these results, the CCRNR, in consultation with NPs in practice and education, developed a revised set of core competencies. How the practice analysis results will be used to inform countywide NP examinations for licensure/registration has not yet been reported.

The negative impact of legacy policies and the slow process for change is poignantly illustrated by legislation prohibiting NPs from prescribing controlled drugs and substances (CDS), a restriction to scope of practice that created barriers to the comprehensiveness and accessibility of services that NPs could offer Canadians. Four major legislative and policy changes, occurring over 15 years, were required to remove this barrier. The CDS Act (CDSA) is a federal legislation that formerly recognized only physicians, veterinarians, and dentists as prescribers. The first change occurred in 1996 when the definition of "practitioner" was expanded beyond these three groups to include "any other person or class of persons described as a practitioner" (Government of Canada, 2016). In 2012, the second change under the CDSA to enable NPs occurred with the passage of a new federal bill, the New Classes of Practitioners Regulation. The third change fell to the provinces/territories to determine policies and legislation for if, when, and how to proceed with NP prescribing of CDS. The fourth change was at the level of provincial/territorial nursing regulatory bodies to establish policies including standards of practice and the education and quality assurance requirements to support safe NP prescribing of CDS. As of 2017, NPs in all provinces and territories are legally able to prescribe CDS. Achieving these legislative changes is largely due to more than a decade of persistent multistakeholder lobbying by NP organizations, nurse regulators, nursing associations, and health care organizations. Federal and provincial/territorial government priorities to increase timely access to care and to address the health care needs of populations with acute, chronic, and palliative conditions, especially in communities where NPs may be the only primary care providers, created windows of opportunity to advocate for and achieve these policy changes (Forchuk & Kohr, 2009; Government of Canada, 2012).

While changes to the CDSA to support NP prescribing is a major accomplishment, the CNA continues to lobby to remove remaining legacy policy barriers at the federal level. Most of these policies relate to NP authority to complete and sign federal income tax, unemployment, and disability forms. At provincial/territorial levels, there has also been countrywide progress in reducing legislative restrictions on NP scope of practice for prescribing all drugs, referring patients to specialists and other providers, ordering of diagnostic tests, and admitting and discharging patients from the hospital. However, barriers to NP scope of practice do exist at the organizational level in terms of developing and introducing policies and institutional practices to operationalize changes to federal and provincial/territorial legislation (Bryant-Lukosius et al., 2014). Lack of administrative support, physician resistance, poor understanding of NP roles, competing changes in practice, and lack of resources may contribute to this lag in policy uptake within organizations (Sangster-Gormley, Martin-Misener, Downe-Wamboldt, & Dicenso, 2011; Tapper & Trevoy, 2014).

Regulation of the CNS role is a contentious and unresolved issue in Canada. Except for the province of Quebec, the CNS role is not regulated. In 2010, CNSs felt strongly that regulation of the role with title protection was needed to improve role clarity and role implementation and to ensure long-term role sustainability (Bryant-Lukosius et al., 2010). However, key role stakeholders including nurse regulators, health care administrators, and government policy makers did not share this view, the main reason being that CNSs did not have an expanded scope of practice beyond that of a registered nurse. Since that time, strengthening the sustainability of the health care system by optimizing skill mix and provider scopes of practice in new models of care has been a major policy priority (Nelson et al., 2014). Provincially or nationally, CNSs have yet to leverage this and other opportunities to establish a cohesive argument for role regulation that speaks to stakeholder policy priorities such as workforce mobility, public safety, quality of care, and nursing recruitment/retention.

In contrast, in Quebec, early efforts to obtain CNS regulation aligned with provincial policy priorities to move away from delegated acts to expanded scopes of practice for health care professionals in areas of high unmet health needs (Groupe de travail ministériel sur les professions de santé et des relations humaines, 2001; Ordre des infirmières et infirmiers du Québec [OIIQ], 2003a, 2003b). In 2011, title protection for specialists, including CNSs, in infection prevention and control (IPC) was obtained (OIIQ, 2011). IPC regulation is an important first step to regulate CNS roles in the province. In 2016, nursing regulators, decision makers and representatives of universities initiated the development of mechanisms to support CNS regulation and graduate-level education in Québec (Ordre des infirmières et infirmiers du Québec, 2016).

Education

The geographic size of Canada, coupled with the distribution of its relatively small population and the federal/provincial division of powers for health and education creates challenges for APRN education. The critical mass of students needed to offer specialty education in a single university is missing, as are the job opportunities for large numbers of NP specialists. Consequently, not all provinces offer adult NP programs, and those that do take a generalist perspective focusing on chronic diseases. At the other end of the life span, two neonatal NP

(NNP) programs in the country have suspended their admissions due to the costs and resources required to support a small pool of applicants. At the same time, in the province of Nova Scotia, health human resource concerns in a regional pediatric health care center have led to the reopening of an NNP program that was dormant. The need for NNP education is clear, but the sustainability of this specialty education in any one university is unrealistic. As a result, universities are beginning to talk with one another to explore how they can offer education collaboratively. For most CNSs in Canada, their only option is to enroll in a generic master's program. While such programs may prepare graduates for the non-clinical competencies expected of a CNS, they do not address specialty clinical competencies. The lack of access to education programs specifically designed to produce CNSs continues to be a serious barrier to the long-term evolution and sustainability of the role (Bryant-Lukosius et al., 2010).

Aside from the challenges with specialty education for APRN roles, there have been positive developments in NP education for family/all-ages NPs. A major challenge to the integration of NPs in Canada in 2010 was differences in the educational preparation of NPs in primary health care (Donald et al., 2010). At that time, while most programs were at the graduate level, several programs that offered NP education were at the diploma or baccalaureate level, creating role confusion among other health care providers. While there was a strong will among educators to change to graduate-level programming, educators and health care administrators faced resistance from federal and provincial/territorial governments due to their concerns about "credential creep" and funding expectations to maintain NP program admission requirements that did not disadvantage diploma-prepared nurses. Recognizing the slow pace of change and delicacy of the situation, CNPI participants set an ultimate goal of 2015 for all NP programs to be at the graduate level, a goal that was attained. The persistence of NP educators and the support of their deans and directors was a critical influence leading to this change. In those provinces with baccalaureate or diploma NP education, an argument for the need for graduate education for NPs had to be made to provincial/territorial governments. Policies contributing to the success of these arguments were the CNA (2009b) position statement on the NP role and the Advanced Nursing Practice Framework (CNA, 2008), both identifying master's education as an international standard essential to the role. The previously mentioned legislation mandating labor mobility among Canadian workers was another important influence because the mobility of NPs in provinces/territories without mandatory master's education for NPs would have been susceptible to licensing/registration refusal in provinces with master's education.

A paper in the 2010 Special Issue of the *Canadian Journal of Nursing Leadership* challenged the Canadian Association of Schools of Nursing (CASN) and NP educators to "step up to the plate" to take action to advance NP education toward achievement of the 2010 stakeholder roundtable recommendation that a pan-Canadian approach should be taken to standardize APRN educational standards, requirements, and processes (Martin-Misener et al., 2010). To that purpose, with federal funding, a task force composed of NP educators with regulator representation was struck with a mandate to work with CASN staff to develop a framework for NP education. Activities included a synthesis of relevant literature, a series of stakeholder meetings, and a national survey of NP education programs. The resulting framework consists of definitions of the terms, contextual factors influencing education based on the literature synthesis, and guiding principles and essential components (CASN, 2012).

With the removal of barriers to NP prescribing of CDS, CASN, in consultation with NP educators, identified the need for agreement on competencies for NP programs to educate students in this important new area of practice. Given the prevalence of the misuse, abuse, and diversion of CDSs in Canada, the federal government solicited proposals to address this public health challenge. CASN was successful in obtaining this funding. A pan-Canadian process similar to that for developing the national NP education framework was used to establish CDS prescribing competencies and indicators for NP education programs along with an interactive e-resource targeted for students in NP and baccalaureate education programs (CASN, 2016).

The latest development in this string of achievements is that in 2016 CASN announced approval to develop standards and procedures for a voluntary accreditation program for NP education programs. The process is being guided by an advisory committee composed of NP educators from across Canada and a CCRNR representative. While all NP programs currently undergo approval every three to five years by their provincial/territorial regulator, a pan-Canadian accreditation process offers the potential for accelerating excellence in NP education that builds on but goes beyond the requirement to ensure public safety.

National Leadership

Since 1908, the CNA has been the national professional association that now represents over 139,000 Canadian nurses in the campaign to strengthen nursing and improve Canadian health care and has, for decades, led and advocated for policies to support the health-system integration of APRN roles (CNA, 2009b). The CNA collaborates federally with the Health Human Resources policy branch of Health Canada and with intersectoral and intra- and interprofessional stakeholders across jurisdictions. Through its Canadian Network of Nursing Specialties, the CNA works closely with the Canadian Association of APNs (CAAPN) and the newly established Clinical Nurse Specialist Association of Canada (CNS–C).

One national roundtable recommendation was that the CNA should lead, in collaboration with other health professional stakeholder groups, the creation of vision statements to clearly articulate the value-added role of CNSs and NPs (DiCenso & Bryant-Lukosius, 2010). Another recommendation, while not specific to the CNA, emphasized the need for research to better understand the CNS role within the Canadian health care context. Within a year of the roundtable, both the CNA and Health Canada partnered with the Canadian Centre for APRN Research, to conduct the first national survey of CNSs (Kilpatrick et al., 2013). The study was important because it provided the first examination of CNS practice and highlighted the lack of policies, education, and organizational supports to effectively utilize the role. Study results further underscored the need to define role competencies, establish credentialing mechanisms, and develop CNS-specific graduate programs. The results of this study informed a subsequent series of CNA-led initiatives that, combined, represent the most comprehensive work focused on CNS development in Canada's history. The initiatives included a background paper (CNA, 2012), a pan-Canadian roundtable discussion to develop a national vision statement on the CNS role (CNA, 2013b), and a pan-Canadian initiative to develop core competencies for the CNS (CNA, 2014). A key to these initiatives was the use of consensus-building approaches to engage and inform stakeholders, such as APRNs, regulators, researchers, and educators, about the CNS role. Continued efforts will be required from the CNA, the CNS-C and CNSs themselves to build on, translate, and disseminate these policy documents for use in health care decision making about the role, education curricula, and day-to-day practices of CNSs.

Results of the decision support synthesis showed that stakeholders had a better understanding of the NP role compared to that of the CNS, but did not have full understanding of the benefits NPs bring to improve the health of Canadians (DiCenso & Bryant-Lukosius, 2010). To address this knowledge gap, the CNA created a campaign to promote the NP role to the general public, decision makers, and influencers, thus creating awareness, demand, and support for NPs. The three-year bilingual (French and English) campaign was implemented from 2011 to 2013 in partnership with CNA's member jurisdictions across the country. The campaign had three core strategies: (a) link NPs to meeting health-system priorities: access, patient satisfaction; (b) build demand and support for NPs among populations in proximity to communities currently served by NPs; and (c) build understanding and support for NPs among other health care professionals. Strategy 2 was adapted to focus on running the campaign in the capital cities of each participating jurisdiction, while CNA decided not to pursue Strategy 3 because of resource limitations. The impact of the campaign is difficult to assess due to changes in its evaluation methodology over the 3 years. However, recent national public polls indicate a high level of public comfort in being treated by an NP (Nanos, 2016).

As described earlier, expanding NP authority to prescribe CDS has been important to improving access to basic health care. The CNA provided national leadership, along with its jurisdictional member organizations and CAAPN, to support and promote the development of the New Classes of Practitioners Regulations under the CDSA. This ongoing work included participating in government consultations and advisory groups as well as lobbying for the process to move toward a meaningful conclusion. The successful evolution of this policy from idea to legislation is anchored by the phases in the policy cycles (Tarlov, 1999). The first phase involved CNA activities to identify, define, and raise awareness of the issue. The second phase, defined as political engagement, occurred when CNA engaged with external groups to advance the issue. CNA member organizations from provinces/territories contributed greatly to work at the federal level and also lobbied their own elected officials and government representatives.

In 2016, the Canadian federal government consulted Canadians to develop and introduce legislation on medical assistance in dying (Department of Justice, 2016). Initially, the draft legislation only addressed the physician role, leaving NPs and RNs, many of whom act as primary care providers, with unclear roles and no protection under the Criminal Code. CNA advocated extensively at the federal level to ensure the assisted dying legislation addressed the various nursing roles and acknowledged that NPs are the primary care providers for more than 3,000,000 Canadians, especially in northern, rural and remote populations and indigenous communities. It was essential that NPs be recognized among the practitioners who could assess capacity, determine eligibility, and perform the medical acts required for assisted dying (CNA, 2016). To this end, the CNA was effective in moving the discourse from physician assistance to medical assistance in dying. In June 2016, Bill C-14 to Amend the Criminal Code and to Make Related Amendments to Other Acts (Medical Assistance in Dying), now known as S.C. 2016, c. 3., became law in Canada. This law protects nurses and other health care professionals from prosecution under the Criminal Code, allows for conscientious objection, and includes NPs along with physicians as professionals who can perform medical assistance in dying.

National leadership by APRNs to promote the development and implementation of CNS roles and NPs is the responsibility of CAAPN and the CNS-C, both members of the CNA's Canadian Network of Nursing Specialties. CAAPN has been in existence for about 30 years and, as noted earlier, has worked closely with the CNA and provincial nursing and NP associations on APRN policy-related issues. With the growing expansion of NPs, much of CAAPN's focus has been on this role over the past 10 years. A stark finding from the 2010 decision support synthesis was the perceived lack of CNS leadership and voice at the national level among stakeholders (Bryant-Lukosius et al., 2010). In 2016, the CNS-C was established to provide cohesive leadership for CNSs. Revitalization of national CNS leadership will be important for addressing the barriers and risks to the long-term sustainability of this role.

Funding

Funding to introduce APRN roles was identified as a challenge in the 2010 decision support synthesis. Some progress has been made with funding for new roles in long-term care, primary care, and palliative care. Between 2010 and 2015, the number of NPs increased from 2,486 to 4,353, accounting for just more than 1% of the nursing workforce (CIHI, 2016). While significant, and welcome, the scale with which they are being introduced is insufficient to close the gap between patients' need for accessible health services and the existing lack of timely services. Funding, more than any other barrier, is proving to be a particularly difficult chasm to cross. The reasons for this are complex, rooted in the consequences of intricately interconnected policy legacies that are not easily disentangled.

Health care funding in Canada has been likened to a series of silos (Brichta & Kabilan, 2016). Funding for primary care and acute care are separate, and within each sector, physician and other health care services are separately funded. The detachment of personal remuneration and service provision creates challenges with governance and the policy levers that can be used to influence change in the quality and organization of services (Brichta & Kabilan, 2016). Within primary health care, the sector that has seen the greatest reforms in the past 15 years, there has been a movement toward alternative funding models, but most family physicians are still remunerated through fee for service. This funding is negotiated with provincial/territorial governments and protected for physician services. NPs, on the other hand, are employed by health authorities or organizations in which remuneration is almost exclusively through salary. As budgets are generally fixed, funding for NP positions comes from reallocation of funds within that overall budget. NP employers contribute to overhead costs including the salary for a receptionist who is usually employed by a health authority or organization. Overall, physicians report these overhead contributions to be inadequate. Some NPs have advocated for the right to be paid on a fee-for-service basis like physicians. Decision makers, who are attempting to move away from fee-for-service payment models where it can be difficult to control costs, have little appetite for increasing the pool of such providers. In acute care, APRN roles are funded within the organization's existing budget. With no new money for roles, administrators must choose between funding an APRN role or another type of resource. Such decisions are difficult and the evidence upon which to base decisions is often incomplete.

On a more positive note, there is a growing realization that continuing to fund the health care system using the same models will be insufficient to address Canadian population health needs (Brichta & Kabilan, 2016). The policy imperative for innovative funding models to address needed services associated with aging and the chronic disease epidemic is driving movement for change. For most provinces, health care costs consume 40% to 45% of their overall budget and continuing with the status quo will lead to escalating and unsustainable costs (Brichta & Kabilan). The reopening of federal discussions with provinces/territories on the Health Accord, in which federal transfer payments are negotiated, is an opportunity for nursing to become part of the dialogue and message the value proposition of APRN-provided care. The federal health minister has indicated that transfer payments to provinces/territories will not be increased to preserve the status quo. This policy direction is a powerful lever for innovation that could enable funding models to support expansion of APRN roles.

Leadership Support

At the organizational level, finding and sustaining funding for APRN roles is one of the most significant responsibilities of nursing leaders (Carter et al., 2010). This includes not only the funding for the role but also providing infrastructure and resources for CNSs and NPs to do their jobs effectively. Findings from 2010 suggest nursing leaders in organizations are important stakeholders who influence the successful integration of APRN roles. Through their formal and informal networks, leaders create awareness, engage other stakeholders, and enable network support and mentorship for NPs and CNSs. Nurse leaders at organizational, provincial/territorial, and national levels have been instrumental in using evidence-based tools, such as the PEPPA Framework, in policies to support successful APRN role integration (Bryant-Lukosius et al., 2013). Studies with nursing leaders have contributed to our understanding of how to promote evidence-informed decision making about the effective use of APRN roles. Delphi methodology was used with senior nursing policy advisors in all provinces/territories to understand their priority APRN issues and identify target audiences for APRN messaging (Carter et al., 2014). To address the APRN information needs of a broader range of decision and policy makers, the CNA worked in partnership with the Canadian Centre of APRN Research to create evidence briefs about the outcomes of CNS and NP roles (Kilpatrick et al., 2015). A series of rounds with national health care decision and policy makers were used to develop and refine the evidence brief.

DISCUSSION

Since 2010, pan-Canadian approaches have been effective for promoting APRN role development by influencing policy change related to legislation, regulation, and education. In addition, this approach leveraged leadership by national nursing organizations such as the CNA, CCRNR, and CASN to optimize role implementation through research, public awareness campaigns, and policies to improve role clarity including position statements and competency development. Further analysis is needed to better understand the roles and impact of provincial and territorial nursing and APRN associations on health care policies to support advanced practice at national and jurisdictional levels. Pan-Canadian approaches also focus on policy change at the federal and provincial/territorial levels, which may not translate quickly to policy changes needed at the organizational level to support advanced nursing practice. Additional strategies may be required to address APRN policy needs at organizational levels. There is limited research on APRN regulatory policies, leaving questions about what constitutes the best model for optimizing role implementation and scope of practice. Lack of regulation and outdated and restrictive regulatory policies are barriers to APRNs working to optimal scope of practice, and centralized or national models for APRN regulation may help to reduce practice variation and improve role clarity compared to decentralized models (Maier, 2015). Although Canada has a decentralized model for governing the regulation of APRN roles, pan-Canadian efforts related to NP roles over the past 6 years have led increasingly toward standardized regulations across jurisdictions and removal of federal and provincial/territorial restrictions to NP scope of practice.

International studies indicate that lack of regulation and title protection is a barrier to advanced practice, and in particular for CNS roles (Carney, 2016; Duffield et al, 2009; Heale & Rieck-Buckley, 2015). Currently, Canada has a mix of master's and nonmaster's prepared nurses working as specialists without a clear path for career development, education, or credentialing or other mechanisms to delineate which nurses are operating safely at an advanced level of practice (Kilpatrick et al., 2013). As a result, the public, health care providers, and administrators are uncertain about what CNS roles have to offer and may have unclear expectations about CNS scope of practice. The recruitment and retention of CNSs and the long-term sustainability of the CNS role, for which there is substantial international evidence about its impact on patient and health-system outcomes, are at risk due to these issues (Bryant-Lukosius et al., 2015; Kilpatrick, DiCenso, et al., 2014; Kilpatrick, Kaasalainen, et al., 2014). Moving forward, pan-Canadian processes involving CNSs and key stakeholders including nurse regulators, government policy makers and health care decision makers at national, provincial/territorial, and organizational levels should examine policy options available to them for optimizing the integration of CNS roles, including that of role regulation. Given that there is no one best practice model for APRN regulation, an open mindset should be used to examine and compare the benefits and consequences of different regulatory and nonregulatory approaches and other governance measures related to public safety, risks versus costs, evaluating performance, and role integration (Maier, 2015).

STRATEGIES TO ENGAGE IN HEALTH POLICY

The evolution of APRN roles in Canada over the past 50 plus years and the 15-year period required to legislate NP authority to prescribe CDS illustrate the complex, often painstakingly slow and incremental process of policy making in health care. The first step for APRNs to be a part of the policy-making process is to identify policy issues, be included in forums where policy agendas are being discussed, and get the attention of policy makers (Schober, Gerrish, & McDonnell, 2016). To assist APRNs to engage in these first steps, we offer a three "A" strategy to consider: *Anticipate, Align*, and *Act*. As shown with the relatively quick time it took to achieve new legislation for medically assisted dying, policy priorities and windows of opportunity to influence policy can be impacted by constantly evolving and dynamic factors such as government leadership, economics, demographics, societal needs, and public pressure. Being aware of health care trends, problems and issues is important in order to *anticipate,* prepare, and plan for future policy windows of opportunity. Preparation could include an analysis of a health care problem relevant to APRN role integration and the evidence on different policy options to address it (Brownson, Chriqui, & Stamatakis, 2009). A variety of frameworks can be used to examine policy problems and issues (Hardee et al., 2004).

Understanding policy issues is essential for identifying stakeholders APRNs can *align* with to tackle health care problems pertinent to their roles. One stakeholder group that has not seemed to play a prominent role in APRN policy initiatives to date in Canada is that of the public, including patients, families, and health care consumers. Public engagement in policy making at organizational, regional, provincial/territorial, and national health-systems levels is recognized as essential for redesign of the health system, including the optimization of APRN roles (Bryant-Lukosius, 2009; Carman et al., 2013). The public's priorities for health-system improvement such as access to care, chronic disease management, and person-centered care are highly relevant to the beneficial outcomes of APRN roles. Stronger alliances with this stakeholder group may be influential in future policy changes supportive of APRN roles.

In addition to the public, it will be important for APRNs to broaden their alignment with policy actors beyond that of stakeholder groups within nursing. For example, in keeping with their role mandate to promote quality improvement, CNSs could align with groups advocating for policies for health care system improvement. Conducting a stakeholder analysis at various stages of APRN role development and implementation is essential for optimal role integration at organization and health-systems levels, and tools exist to facilitate this analysis (Bryant-Lukosius, 2009). Proactive stakeholder analysis and engagement also permit time for APRNs to develop credibility and trusting relationships with stakeholders and to collaborate with them to inform and influence policy agendas and the policy-making process.

The term *Act* stresses the importance of APRN involvement in policy making relevant to their roles at all levels of the health system (organizational, regional, provincial/territorial, and national). APRNs must acknowledge and accept their larger role in public policy (McTeer, 2005), and everyone in an APRN role or with administrative responsibility for APRN roles needs to embrace the opportunities for change that are inherent in policy work. Doing this with confidence and savvy requires education and mentorship. Policy work is often slow and incremental and the gains made are not always tangible, in fact movement toward a desired change can be indiscernible at times. Staying optimistic, energized, and most important, persistent, can be difficult. Keeping one's gaze firmly fixed on the end goal is key, as is adjusting expectations for the timeline for change from months to years and sometimes even decades. Having knowledge of the policy cycle (Hardee et al., 2004) and knowing how to use policy levers and policy windows and build relationships with key stakeholders are critical skills. In Canada, 2-year master's programs are the entry-level preparatory education for APRN roles, and policy courses may or may not be part of the curriculum. As a result, many APRNs may assess themselves as unprepared for policy work. The accreditation program being developed by CASN offers an opportunity to position policy education more prominently in NP education curricula. Graduate and postgraduate education and practical learning experiences that facilitate exchanges with health care decision and policy makers provide opportunities for APRNs to learn the policy process through emersion and practical experiences within a policy environment (Bryant-Lukosius et al., 2013).

DISCUSSION QUESTIONS

1. *Based on the information in this chapter, list at least two areas of policy change you can identify where legislation could have an impact.*
2. *If you were going to describe the importance of your issue for policy change to potential supporters, what key issues would you stress? How would you describe this to your patients?*
3. *Consider the health policy changes discussed in this chapter or those you have described in your analysis and consider the impact that might occur if these changes are NOT enacted. In other words, what are the consequences of inaction?*
4. *What are the best ways to communicate APRN-related research to policy makers?*
5. *What are differences in health care policies between Canada and the United States and how do these policy differences impact on APRN role integration?*

ANALYSIS, SYNTHESIS, AND CLINICAL APPLICATION

1. *Discuss the ways pan approaches have or could be used in the United States to promote APRN role integration. Also, consider the barriers or challenges to such approaches.*
2. *Apply the 3 "A" strategy (Anticipate, Align, and Act) to identify ways you can become engaged in policy making relevant to the optimal integration of APRN roles.*
3. *Conduct a self-assessment and develop a learning plan to strengthen your knowledge, skills, and capacity for participating in policy making to support APRN role integration.*
4. *Conduct a stakeholder analysis and develop a plan to engage key stakeholders with varying levels of influence and support to address a health policy relevant to APRN role integration.*

EXERCISES/CONSIDERATIONS

1. *What ethical issues arise from health policies that limit full integration of APRN roles into health systems?*
2. *What responsibilities do APRNs have to address policy barriers to the effective use and integration of their roles within health systems?*

ETHICAL CONSIDERATIONS

1. *Consider the influence of another country on your health care system. Do you think that all countries should function in the same manner? How do the ethics of a health care system differ from one country to another? Does it matter?*

REFERENCES

Brichta, J., & Kabilan, S. (2016). *Funding Canadian health care in 2035: Strategic foresight scenarios*. Ottawa, Canada: Conference Board of Canada. Retrieved from http://www.conferenceboard.ca/e-library/abstract.aspx?did=7777

Brownson, R. C., Chriqui, J. F., & Stamatakis, K. A. (2009). Understanding evidence-based public health policy. *American Journal of Public Health, 99*(9), 1576–1583.

Bryant-Lukosius, D. (2009). *Designing innovative cancer services and advanced practice nursing roles: Toolkit*. Toronto, Canada: Cancer Care Ontario. Retrieved from https://www.cancercare.on.ca/cms/one.aspx?pageId=9387

Bryant-Lukosius, D., Carter, N., Donald, F., Harbman, P., Kilpatrick, K., Martin-Misener, R., ... Valaitis, R. (2014). *Report on advanced practice nursing (APN) in Canada for the Global Summit*. Philadelphia, PA: National Nurse-Led Care Consortium.

Bryant-Lukosius, D., Carter, N., Kilpatrick, K., Martin-Misener, R., Donald, F., Kaasalainen, S., ... DiCenso, A. (2010). The clinical nurse specialist role in Canada. *Nursing Leadership, 23*(Special Issue), 140–166.

Bryant-Lukosius, D., Carter, N., Reid, K., Donald, F., Martin-Misener, R., Kilpatrick, K., ... DiCenso, A. (2015). The clinical effectiveness and cost-effectiveness of clinical nurse specialist-led hospital to home transitional care: A systematic review. *Journal of Evaluation in Clinical Practice, 21*(5), 763–781.

Bryant-Lukosius, D., DiCenso, A., Israr, S., & Charbonneau-Smith, R. (2013). Resources to facilitate APN outcome research. In R. Kleinpell (Ed.), *Outcome assessment in advanced practice nursing* (3rd ed.). New York, NY: Springer Publishing.

Canadian Association of Schools of Nursing. (2012). *Nurse practitioner education in Canada: National framework of guiding principles and essential components*. Retrieved from http://www.casn.ca/2014/12/nurse-practitioner-education-canada-national-framework-guiding-principles-essential-components

Canadian Association of Schools of Nursing. (2016). Nurse practitioner education competencies for prescribing controlled drugs and substances. Retrieved from http://www.casn.ca/wp-content/uploads/2016/02/NP-Prescribing-Final-for-web.pdf

Canadian Council of Registered Nurse Regulators. (2015). Practice analysis study of nurse practitioners. Retrieved from http://www.ccrnr.ca/assets/ccrnr-practice-analysis-study-of-nurse-practitioners-report---final.pdf

Canadian Institutes for Health Information. (2011). Regulated nurses: Canadian trends 2006–2010. Retrieved from https://secure.cihi.ca/free_products/RegulatedNursesCanadianTrends2006-2010_EN.pdf

Canadian Institutes for Health Information. (2016). Regulated nurses, 2015. Retrieved from https://secure.cihi.ca/free_products/Nursing_Report_2015_en.pdf

Canadian Nurses Association. (2008). Advanced nursing practice: A national framework. Retrieved from https://www.cna-aiic.ca/~/media/cna/page-content/pdf-en/anp_national_framework_e.pdf

Canadian Nurses Association. (2009a). The clinical nurse specialist: Position statement. Retrieved from http://www.cnaaiic.ca/~/media/cna/page%20content/pdf%20en/ps104_clinical_nurse_specialist_e.pdf

Canadian Nurses Association. (2009b). The nurse practitioner: Position statement. Retrieved from http://www.cnaaiic.ca/~/media/cna/page%20content/pdf%20en/ps_nurse_practitioner_e.pdf

Canadian Nurses Association. (2010). Canadian nurse practitioner core competency framework. Retrieved from http://www.cno.org/globalassets/for/rnec/pdf/competencyframework_en.pdf

Canadian Nurses Association. (2012). Strengthening the role of the clinical nurse specialist in Canada. Retrieved from https://www.cna-aiic.ca/~/media/cna/files/en/strengthening_the_cns_role_background_paper_e.pdf?la=en

Canadian Nurses Association. (2013a). 2011 workforce profile of registered nurses in Canada. Retrieved from http://www.cnaaiic.ca/~/media/cna/files/en/2011_rn_work_ profiles_e.pdf

Canadian Nurses Association. (2013b). Strengthening the role of the clinical nurse specialist in Canada. Pan-Canadian roundtable discussion summary report. Retrieved from https://www.cna-aiic.ca/~/media/cna/files/en/clinical_nurse_specialist_role_roundtable_summary_e.pdf?la=en

Canadian Nurses Association. (2014). Pan-Canadian core competencies for the clinical nurse specialist. Retrieved from https://www.cna-aiic.ca/~/media/cna/files/en/clinical_nurse_specialists_convention_handout_e.pdf?la=en

Canadian Nurses Association. (2016). Innovative ways to provide better access to health care for all. Retrieved from https://nurseone.ca/~/media/cna/page-content/pdf-en/cna-2016-pre-budget-submission-to-standing-committee-on-finance.pdf?la=en

Carman, K. L., Dardess, P., Maurer, M., Sofaer, S., Adams, K., Bechtel, C., & Sweeney, J. (2013). Patient and family engagement: A framework for understanding the elements and developing interventions and policies. *Health Affairs, 32*(2), 223–231.

Carney, M. (2016). Regulation of advanced nurse practice: Its existence and regulatory dimensions from an international perspective. *Journal of Nursing Management, 24*(1), 105–114.

Carter, N., Lavis, J. N., & MacDonald-Rencz, S. (2014). Use of modified Delphi to plan knowledge translation for decision makers: An application in the field of advanced practice nursing. *Policy, Politics & Nursing Practice, 15*(3–4), 93–101.

Carter, N., Martin-Misener, R., Kilpatrick, K., Kaasalainen, S., Donald, F., Bryant-Lukosius, D., . . . DiCenso, A. (2010). The role of nursing leadership in integrating clinical nurse specialists and nurse practitioners in healthcare delivery in Canada. *Nursing Leadership, 23*, 167–185.

Department of Justice. (2016). *Legislative background: Medical assistance in dying (Bill C-14)*. Ottawa, Canada: Government of Canada. Retrieved from http://www.justice.gc.ca/eng/rp-pr/other-autre/ad-am/ad-am.pdf

DiCenso, A., & Bryant-Lukosius, D. (2010). *Clinical nurse specialists and nurse practitioners in Canada: A decision support synthesis*. Ottawa, Ontario, Canada: Canadian Foundation for Healthcare Innovation. Retrieved from http://www.cfhi-fcass.ca/sf-docs/default-source/commissioned-research-reports/Dicenso_EN_Final.pdf?sfvrsn=0

DiCenso, A., Bryant-Lukosius, D., Martin-Misener, R., Donald, F., Abelson, J., Bourgeault, I., . . . Harbman, P. (2010). Factors enabling advanced practice nursing role integration in Canada. *Nursing Leadership, 23*, 211–238.

Donald, F., Martin-Misener, R., Bryant-Lukosius, D., Kilpatrick, K., Kaasalainen, S., Carter, N., . . . DiCenso, A. (2010). The primary healthcare nurse practitioner role in Canada. *Nursing Leadership, 23*, 88–113.

Duffield, C., Gardner, G., Chang, A. M., & Catling-Paull, C. (2009). Advanced nursing practice: A global perspective. *Collegian, 16*(2), 55–62.

Employment and Social Development in Canada. (2014). Canadians in context. Geographic distribution. Retrieved from http://www4.hrsdc.gc.ca/.3ndic.1t.4r@-eng.jsp?iid=34

Forchuk, C., & Kohr, R. (2009). Prescriptive authority for nurses: The Canadian perspective. *Perspectives in Psychiatric Care, 45*(1), 3–8.

Government of Canada. (2012). New classes of practitioners regulations. *Canada Gazette, 146*(24). Retrieved from http://www.gazette.gc.ca/rp-pr/p1/2012/2012-05-05/html/reg1-eng.html

Government of Canada. (2016). *Controlled drugs and substances act (S.C. 1996, c. 19)*. Ottawa, Canada: Author. Retrieved from http://laws-lois.justice.gc.ca/eng/acts/c-38.8

Groupe de travail ministériel sur les professions de santé et des relations humaines. (2001). *Une vision renouvelée du système professionnel en santé et en relations humaines* (A renewed vision of the professional system in health and human relations). Rapport d'étape. Office des professions du Québec. Retrieved from https://www.opq.gouv.qc.ca/fileadmin/documents/Systeme_professionnel/01_premier%20rapport%20Bernier.pdf

Hardee, K., Feranil, I., Boezwinkle, J., & Clark, B. (2004). *The policy circle: A framework for analyzing the components of family planning, reproductive health, maternal health and HIV/Aids policies*. Policy Working Paper Series No. 11. Retrieved from http://pdf.usaid.gov/pdf_docs/Pnacy528.pdf

Heale, R., & Rieck Buckley, C. (2015). An international perspective of advanced practice nursing regulation. *International Nursing Review, 62*(3), 421–429.

Health Canada. (2012). Canada's health care system. Retrieved from http://www.hc-sc.gc.ca/hcs-sss/pubs/system-regime/2011-hcs-sss/index-eng.php#a3

Kaasalainen, S., Martin-Misener, R., Kilpatrick, K., Harbman, P., Bryant-Lukosius, D., Donald, F.,…DiCenso, A. (2010). A historical overview of the development of advanced practice nursing roles in Canada. *Nursing Leadership, 23*, 35–60.

Kilpatrick, K., Carter, N., Bryant-Lukosius, D., Charbonneau-Smith, R., & DiCenso, A. (2015). The development of evidence briefs to transfer knowledge about advanced practice nursing roles to providers, policy-makers and administrators. *Canadian Journal of Nursing Leadership, 28*(1), 11–23.

Kilpatrick, K., DiCenso, A., Bryant-Lukosius, D., Ritchie, J. A., Martin-Misener, R., & Carter, N. (2013). Practice patterns and perceived impact of clinical nurse specialist roles in Canada: Results of a national survey. *International Journal of Nursing Studies, 50*, 1524–1536. doi:10.1016/j.ijnurstu2013.03.005

Kilpatrick, K., DiCenso, A., Bryant-Lukosius, D., Ritchie, J. A., Martin-Misener, R., & Carter, N. (2014). Clinical nurse specialists in Canada: Why are some not working in the role? *Nursing Leadership, 27*(1), 62–75.

Kilpatrick, K., Harbman, P., Carter, N., Martin-Misener, R., Bryant-Lukosius, D., Donald, F.,…DiCenso, A. (2010). The acute care nurse practitioner role in Canada. *Nursing Leadership, 23*, 114–139.

Kilpatrick, K., Kaasalainen, S., Donald, F., Reid, K., Carter, N., Bryant-Lukosius, D.,…DiCenso, A. (2014). The effectiveness and cost-effectiveness of clinical nurse specialists in outpatient roles: A systematic review. *Journal of Evaluation in Clinical Practice, 20*, 1106–1123. doi:10.1111/jep.12219

Maier, C. B. (2015). The role of governance in implementing task-shifting from physicians to nurses in advanced roles in Europe, U.S., Canada, New Zealand and Australia. *Health Policy, 119*(12), 1627–1635.

Martin-Misener, R., Bryant-Lukosius, D., Harbman, P., Donald, F., Kaasalainen, S., Carter, N.,…DiCenso, A. (2010). Education of advanced practice nurses in Canada. *Nursing Leadership, 23*, 61–84.

McTeer, M. (2005). Leadership and public policy. *Policy, Politics & Nursing Practice, 6*(1), 17–19.

Nanos Research. (2016). Canadians' opinions on home healthcare and nurses. Retrieved from https://cna-aiic.ca/~/media/cna/page-content/pdf-en/canadians-opinions-on-home-healthcare-and-nurses.pdf?la=en

Nelson, S., Turnbull, J., Bainbridge, L., Caulfield, T., Hudon, G., Kendel, D.,…Sketris, I. (2014). *Optimizing scopes of practice: New models for a new health care system*. Ottawa, Ontario, Canada: Canadian Academy of Health Sciences.

Ordre des infirmières et infirmiers du Québec. (2003a). Loi 90: Loi modifiant le codes des professions et d'autres dispositions législatives dans le domaine de la santé (sanctionnée le 14 juin 2002) (Bill 90:Act to amend the Professional Code and other legislative provisions as regards the health sector [sanctioned June 14th 2002]). *Ordre des infirmières et infirmiers du Québec*, (5). Retrieved from http://www.oiiq.org/sites/default/files/uploads/pdf/l_ordre/qui_sommes_nous/gouvernance/Cahier-explicatif-PL90-5.pdf

Ordre des infirmières et infirmiers du Québec. (2003b). The scope of our profession expands. Some guidelines for understanding and taking advantage of recent changes to the Nurses Act. Retrieved from http://www.oiiq.org/sites/default/files/149A-Scope-profession-expands.pdf

Ordre des infirmières et infirmiers du Québec. (2011). A new specialty in infection prevention and control—A first in Canada. *The Journal, 5*, 1.

Ordre des infirmières et infirmiers du Québec. (2016). *Pratique infirmière avancée. Réflexion sur le rôle de l'infirmière clinicienne spécialisée* (Advanced practice nursing: Reflections on the role of the clinical nurse specialist). Publication no. 8456. Retrieved from http://www.oiiq.org/sites/default/files/8456-reflexion-role-ics.pdf

Sangster-Gormley, E., Martin-Misener, R., Downe-Wamboldt, B., & Dicenso, A. (2011). Factors affecting nurse practitioner role implementation in Canadian practice settings: An integrative review. *Journal of Advanced Nursing, 67*(6), 1178–1190.

Schober, M. M., Gerrish, K., & McDonnell, A. (2016). Development of a conceptual policy framework for advanced practice nursing: An ethnographic study. *Journal of Advanced Nursing, 72*(6), 1313–1324.

Spitzer, W. O. (1984). The nurse practitioner revisited. Slow death of a good idea. *New England Journal of Medicine, 310*(16), 1049–1051.

Statistics Canada. (2016). Canada's population estimates. First quarter 2016. Retrieved from http://www.statcan.gc.ca/daily-quotidien/160616/dq160616b-eng.htm

Tapper, L., & Trevoy, J. (2014). Key issues impacting nurse practitioner practice and integration in Alberta. Retrieved from https://albertanps.com/wp-content/uploads/2015/03/Key-Issues-for-Nurse -Practitioners-of-Alberta.pdf

Tarlov, A. R. (1999). Public policy frameworks for improving population health. *Annals of the New York Academy of Sciences, 896*, 281–293.

Veldhorst, A. J. (2006). *Practice patterns of clinical nurse specialists working with First Nations and Inuit communities* (Master's thesis). Hamilton, Ontario, Canada: McMaster University.

Wikipedia. (2016). *Geography of Canada*. Retrieved from https://en.wikipedia.org/wiki/Geography_of_ Canada

CHAPTER 26

The Future of Nursing: *Campaign for Action*

Susan Hassmiller, Susan C. Reinhard, and Andrea Brassard

BACKGROUND: THE ROBERT WOOD JOHNSON FOUNDATION

The Robert Wood Johnson Foundation (RWJF)—the nation's largest philanthropy dedicated solely to health—is working with others to build a national Culture of Health that will enable everyone in the United States to live longer, healthier lives. Since 1972, RWJF has supported research and programs targeting some of America's most pressing health issues, including expanding access to primary care. Ahead of its time in 1973, RWJF envisioned the promise of Advanced Practice Registered Nurses (APRNs) as primary care providers. Four regional demonstration projects in Alabama, California, Tennessee, and rural New England educated nurses to become Family Nurse Practitioners or Certified Nurse-Midwives. A few years later, this demonstration project transitioned to the Nurse Faculty Fellowship Program, which funded master's level nurse practitioner programs within schools of nursing between 1975 and 1982. To further increase access to primary care, RWJF created the School Health Services Program, which funded Nurse Practitioner–managed school health services between 1977 and 1984. This early RWJF funding was the impetus for federal funding for APRNs' education (Charting Nursing's Future, 2013).

In addition to funding APRN education, RWJF funded a sentinel research study on outcomes of Nurse Practitioner services provided by the Columbia University School of Nursing's Nurse Practitioner–run primary care practice. Mary Mundinger and her colleagues (Mundinger et al., 2000), in their groundbreaking article, reported that outcomes of Nurse Practitioner care—patient satisfaction, service usage, and health status—were comparable to care provided by physicians.

Strengthening the nursing profession has been an RWJF priority for many years, as evidenced by the more than $648 million in grants and contracts to support nursing education and practice programs since 1972 and more than $194 million in the past 6 years and counting (see Figure 26.1). Programs such as the RWJF Executive Nurse Fellows and Nurse Faculty Scholars, which conclude in 2017,

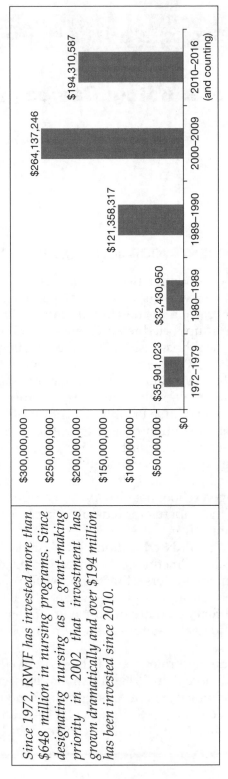

Since 1972, RWJF has invested more than $648 million in nursing programs. Since designating nursing as a grant-making priority in 2002 that investment has grown dramatically and over $194 million has been invested since 2010.

FIGURE 26.1 RWJF investments in nursing surpass $648 million.

Source: The Robert Wood Johnson Foundation.

contribute capacity-building efforts to an up-and-coming generation of nurse leaders. Other programs such as the Interdisciplinary Nurse Quality Research Initiative; the Quality, Transforming Care at the Bedside; and Safety in Nursing Education demonstrated the link between nursing care and high-quality patient outcomes. Starting in 2016, RWJF began offering four interprofessional leadership programs that represent a new four-year, multimillion dollar investment by RWJF, and one that continues a long legacy of supporting the development and diversity of leaders. These programs, which replace the single-profession programs—including RWJF nursing programs—honor the importance of teamwork and collaboration as a key ingredient for better patient outcomes.

This chapter focuses on the Future of Nursing: *Campaign for Action*, beginning with a brief description of the RWJF-funded Center to Champion Nursing in America (CCNA) and the Institute of Medicine (IOM, 2011) report *The Future of Nursing: Leading Change, Advancing Health*.

The CCNA was launched in 2007 as an initiative of RWJF, AARP, and the AARP Foundation with a mission to ensure that every American has access to a highly skilled nurse, when and where they need one (see Chapter 9 on AARP Initiatives).

In 2008, RWJF approached the IOM to propose a partnership between the two organizations to respond to the need to transform the nursing profession to become partners and leaders in improving health care. The resulting collaboration became the RWJF Initiative on the Future of Nursing at the IOM, with RWJF senior adviser for nursing Susan Hassmiller serving as the study director. The stipulation that an RWJF employee serve in this capacity was unprecedented for the IOM and served as a statement of the importance of this report for RWJF (see Chapter 4 on the IOM report by Liana Orsolini).

CAMPAIGN FOR ACTION

The Future of Nursing: Leading Change, Advancing Health was released on October 5, 2010. The *Campaign for Action* launched shortly after that at the National Summit on Advancing Health through Nursing on December 1, 2010. The *Campaign for Action* is a national initiative to guide implementation of the recommendations of the IOM report. Five pilot state action coalitions were announced at the National Summit: California, Mississippi, Michigan, New Jersey, and New York. Action coalitions are the driving force of the Campaign at the local and state levels, forming a strong, connected grassroots network of diverse stakeholders working to transform health care through nursing. Each action coalition has nurse and nonnurse ("nurse champion") leaders. Examples of the organizations that are represented by nonnurse leaders include AARP state offices, state workforce centers, state hospital associations, and large health insurers. *Campaign for Action* work on removing barriers to APRN practice and care is supported through AARP (see Chapter 9 on AARP Initiatives).

EARLY PROGRESS

By the end of the first year, action coalitions were operational in 36 states. Twelve more action coalitions joined by the end of the second year, and by 2012, all 50 states and the District of Columbia had action coalitions.

Action coalition liaisons from the CCNA provided technical assistance to assist each state with developing infrastructure, setting priorities, recruiting key stakeholders, and documenting progress. The IOM report recommendations were conceptualized as pillars to provide an infrastructure for organizing the *Campaign for Action* work: education, leadership, practice and care, interprofessional collaboration, and diversity.

At the national level, the *Campaign for Action* sparked widespread support. National organizations, such as the American Red Cross, the Healthcare Information and Management Systems Society, the National Association of Hispanic Nurses, the National Association of Public Hospitals and Health Systems, the National Medical Association, and the World Health Organization, have publicly supported the report and its key messages.

TRANSFORMING NURSING EDUCATION

To build the infrastructure for advancing education progression, the Campaign created a state- and a national-level network of nursing leaders and stakeholders to accelerate progress on goals to increase the education level of nurses. The *Campaign for Action* highlighted four promising models of nursing education progression including expanding accelerated associate degree in nursing (ADN) to master of science in nursing (MSN) programs. The accelerated ADN to MSN model can help prepare all four categories of APRNs. Regional meetings of state nursing education leaders were held to engage the action coalitions in this work. *Campaign for Action* nurse experts facilitated regional webinars to help the action coalitions develop and implement action plans to advance education progression in their states. To accelerate education progression, RWJF provided funding through the Academic Progression in Nursing (APIN) program to nine action coalitions (California, Hawaii, Massachusetts, Montana, New Mexico, New York, North Carolina, Texas, and Washington). The American Organization of Nurse Executives served as the National Program Office for this grant, as a representative of the Tri-Council of Nursing. APIN concludes in early 2017.

The *Campaign for Action's* focus on academic progression is at the core of nursing leadership and advancing nursing practice. It is built on decades of work by nursing organizations and leaders in education as well as the other pillar focus areas. For example, the APIN program recognizes the efforts of the Tri-Council for Nursing, an alliance between the American Association of Colleges of Nursing, the American Nurses Association, the American Organization of Nurse Executives, and the National League for Nursing. The Tri-Council's statement on the Educational Advancement of Registered Nurses released in May 2010 echoes many of the recommendations outlined in the IOM report.

In 2012, the American Association of Community Colleges, the Association of Community College Trustees, the American Association of Colleges of Nursing, the National League for Nursing, and the National Organization for Associate Degree Nursing issued a Joint Statement on Academic Progression for Nursing Students and Graduates. It was an unprecedented show of support for advancing opportunities for academic progression in nursing across all levels.

In 2013, RWJF convened a community college presidents' meeting. It brought community college leaders from around the country together with APIN and the

Tri-Council for Nursing. The participants called for community colleges, universities, and their clinical partners to work together to transform nursing education and prepare a highly educated nursing workforce to advance a culture of health in our country.

STATE IMPLEMENTATION PROGRAM

To further the implementation of the IOM recommendations, RWJF provided grants to 34 action coalitions through the State Implementation Program (SIP) of up to $150,000 to action coalitions to implement two priority recommendations of the IOM report. SIP required action coalitions to secure matching funds to sustain efforts over the long term. To date there are 240 additional funders that are providing resources to action coalitions, leveraging over $5 million additional dollars to the Campaign. Following four rounds of SIP funding, SIP is slated to conclude in October 2017.

The notable SIP projects include Alaska's work that culminated in successful legislation to bring Alaska's statutes in line with the APRN *Consensus Model*. Louisiana conducted a statewide survey of APRNs with content on practice environment and hospital privileges. Ohio completed the first comprehensive report on registered nurses (RN) and APRN workforce data in decades and helped develop a forecasting tool to assess future workforce needs. Tennessee's advocacy boot camp is equipping APRN students to promote legislation to remove barriers to APRN practice in

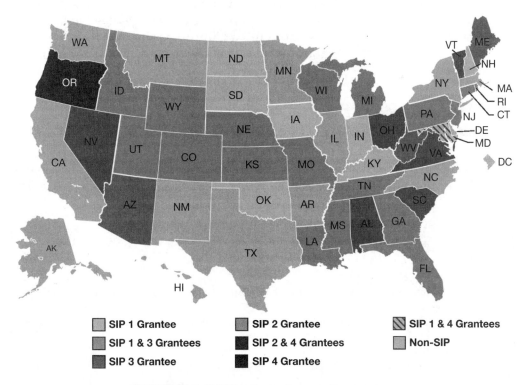

FIGURE 26.2 RWJF state implementation program.

RWJF, Robert Wood Johnson Foundation; SIP, State Implementation Program.

Source: Future of Nursing: *Campaign for Action* (n.d.).

Tennessee. Wisconsin developed the Wisconsin Diversity Assessment Tool to provide a strategic vision for increasing diversity and inclusion (see Figure 26.2).

NATIONAL SUMMITS

In 2013 and 2015, action coalitions from 50 states and the District of Columbia convened in Washington, DC, to work on transformative strategies to accelerate the on-the-ground momentum of the *Campaign for Action*. Risa Lavizzo-Mourey, MD, president, and CEO of RWJF, kicked off both summits with a conversation about the foundation's commitment to transforming health care through nursing. She called on nurses as key partners to forward the foundation's vision of a Culture of Health for all Americans. Lavizzo-Mourey noted that nurses are essential to enabling everyone to live longer and healthier lives—health is intrinsically connected to where we live, learn, work and play, and nurses are ever-present in communities. To achieve meaningful change, nurses need to partner with many others, including those outside the traditional health setting, including city and urban design, business, public transportation, and education.

Action coalition teams developed shared understandings of subsequent steps and strategy, created plans for bold action, and identified ways to attract more diverse people to work. Susan Hassmiller and Susan Reinhard, senior VP for public policy at AARP, unveiled and emphasized five Campaign Imperatives that lay the groundwork to achieve and sustain meaningful results (see Box 26.1).

Importantly, they emphasized that unless action coalitions successfully engaged stakeholders other than nurses, they would not have the requisite power, influence, and resources to make the policy and culture changes needed to implement the IOM recommendations and build a Culture of Health. Understanding that the *Campaign for Action* is about what is best for patients and communities is a core ingredient in aligning key stakeholders.

YEAR FIVE: ASSESSING PROGRESS

The 2015 Summit also marked the release of the finding of *Assessing Progress on the Institute of Medicine Report: The Future of Nursing*. This report was released by the National Academies of Sciences, Engineering, and Medicine, the new name for the IOM (National Academies of Sciences, Engineering, and Medicine, 2015). The

---

CAMPAIGN IMPERATIVES	BOX 26.1

I. Must move beyond *NURSING*
II. Must deliver short-term *RESULTS* in the coming 18 months even as you develop long-term plans
III. Must have *COURAGE* to place the right *LEADERS* at the helm or remove weak, ineffective leaders
IV. Must have *FUNDING* to sustain this work
V. Must not ignore *DIVERSE* stakeholders critical to our success

Source: Future of Nursing: *Campaign for Action* (2013) an initiative of
AARP Foundation, AARP, and the Robert Wood Johnson Foundation.
Reprinted with permission of *Campaign for Action*.

committee found that significant progress has been made toward implementing the recommendations of *The Future of Nursing* report, but more non-nursing stakeholders need to be engaged. Issue areas and recommendations are outlined next (Box 26.2).

DASHBOARD INDICATORS

The IOM report recommendations serve as a foundation to fully realize nursing's potential (see Table 26.1). Successful implementations lead to a transformed health care delivery system and improved patient care. Through extensive analysis, the *Campaign for Action*'s research team determined the best indicators to measure its progress on a national level. Moreover, just as sound evidence grounds the IOM's report recommendations, solid, reliable evidence informs its progress. Yearly, the *Campaign for Action* analyzes established data sets to evaluate where we are gaining ground and areas that require additional emphasis.

It should be noted that the second recommendation of the IOM report, to double the number of nurses with a doctorate, has been achieved, primarily through the explosive growth of Doctor of Nursing Practice (DNP) programs.

Following up on the *Assessing Progress* report, a dashboard indicator of diversity was added. Nurse program graduates by race/ethnicity and gender are compared with the U.S. population. The Campaign is also tracking the number of action coalitions with members of its' state's ethnic or racial minority nursing organization or of its' men in nursing state chapter as a voting member of its most senior executive-level policy-making body as a process measure of diversity.

The dashboard indicator on nursing leadership is now the number of nurses who report serving on boards to the Nurses on Boards Coalition. In November

---

REMOVING SCOPE-OF-PRACTICE BARRIERS	BOX 26.2

1. Build common ground around the scope of practice and other issues in policy and practice.

Achieving Higher Levels of Education

2. Continue pathways toward increasing the percentage of nurses with a baccalaureate degree.
3. Create and fund transition-to-practice residency programs.
4. Promote nurses' pursuit of doctoral degrees.
5. Promote nurses' interprofessional and lifelong learning

Promoting Diversity

6. Make diversity in the nursing workforce a priority.

Collaborating and Leading in Care Delivery and Redesign

7. Expand efforts and opportunities for interprofessional collaboration and leadership development for nurses.
8. Promote the involvement of nurses in the redesign of care delivery and payment systems.
9. Communicate with a wider and more diverse audience to gain broad support for campaign objectives.

Improve Workforce Data Infrastructure

10. Improve workforce data collection.

TABLE 26.1 Future of Nursing: *Campaign for Action* DASHBOARD Indicators and Data Sources

IOM RECOMMENDATION	INDICATOR	DATA SOURCE
Increase the proportion of nurses with a baccalaureate degree to 80% by 2020	Percentage of employed nurses with baccalaureate degree in nursing or higher degrees	American Community Survey
Double the number of nurses with a doctorate by 2020	Number of employed nurses with a doctoral degree	American Community Survey
APRNs to be able to practice to the full extent of their education and training	State progress in removing policy barriers to care by Nurse Practitioners	Center to Champion Nursing in America
Expand opportunities for nurses to lead and disseminate collaborative improvement efforts	Number of required clinical courses and/or activities at top nursing schools that include both RN students and graduate students or other health professionals	Survey of top nursing schools (as determined by U.S. News and World Report rankings) that also have graduate-level health professional schools at their academic institutions by the Philip R. Lee Institute for Health Policy Studies
Health care decision makers should ensure leadership positions are available to and filled by nurses	The number of nurses who report serving on boards to the Nurses on Boards Coalition	Nurses on Boards Coalition
Build infrastructure for collection and analysis of interprofessional health care workforce data	States that collect data on nurse education programs, supply of nurses, and demand for nurses	Forum of State Nursing Workforce Centers and the Philip R. Lee Institute for Health Policy Studies
Make diversity in the nursing workforce a priority	Pre-licensure nursing program graduates by race/ethnicity and by gender compared with the U.S. population	American Association of Colleges of Nursing, Integrated Postsecondary Education Data System (IPEDS), U.S. Census Bureau, Population Division

APRN, Advanced Practice Registered Nurse; IOM, Institute of Medicine.

Source: Future of Nursing: *Campaign for Action* (2017).

2014, RWJF, AARP, and 19 national nursing organizations came together to announce a new, nationwide effort to get 10,000 nurses onto the boards of directors by 2020. Currently, 45 action coalitions are engaged in fostering nurse leaders, and 20 action coalitions are tracking the numbers of nurses in their states serving on boards of directors. These data provide crucial information to help the Campaign monitor progress toward the 10,000 goals.

FUTURE PLANS: WHAT WILL SUCCESS LOOK LIKE?

According to former RWJF president and CEO Lavizzo-Mourey, *Campaign for Action* success would be the implementation of *The Future of Nursing* report recommendations. Success "looks like people . . . across America practicing to the full extent of their training and education. It looks like a diverse nursing workforce that is really able to start with bachelor's degree and continue to grow and provide the kind of care that we know is going to evolve over our lifetimes and beyond. It looks like, frankly, a country that . . . has a culture of health" (RWJF, 2013).

Success relies on good communication and continued evidence to support the messages that drive our action and movement toward a Culture of Health. Key messages have been developed so that action coalitions can communicate with non-nursing stakeholders such as hospital CEOs, physicians, and other audiences. Unified messages that help articulate the IOM recommendations in a way that resonates with diverse groups expand the impact of the *Campaign for Action*. Continued visibility and promotion of the importance of the IOM recommendations in addressing health care challenges are paramount to creating this culture shift within the profession, within health care, and in the community.

The Future of Nursing: Leading Change, Advancing Health continues to be the most viewed report on the National Academies of Sciences, Engineering, and Medicine website. The people viewing, buying, and printing this report are from 150 countries. With more than 1,200 mentions in major media and more than a quarter million impressions since its release, the report continues to be highly influential. It serves as an evidence base for supporting efforts toward transforming health and health care. This report has been covered or mentioned in national media such as the *New York Times*, *Wall Street Journal*, *Washington Post*, and *The Economist*.

The call from the *Campaign for Action* and the recommendations of the IOM report to transform health care through nursing have been echoed with support from several national reports. The 2012 National Governors Association report states that "to better meet the nation's current and growing need for primary care providers, states may want to consider easing their scope of practice restrictions and modifying their reimbursement policies to encourage greater nurse practitioner involvement in the provision of primary care" (National Governors Association, 2012). This recommendation was echoed in the 2014 Federal Trade Commission report (Federal Trade Commission, 2014). The American Hospital Association released a model in 2013, which calls for increased interprofessional education and practice, with APRNs responsible for diagnosing and implementing the plan of care for patients and families in healthy communities. Action coalition and national leaders have been able to use these reports as further evidence to support our messages at professional meetings and in communities (American Hospital Association, 2013).

We also measure our success through our Campaign Imperatives. Engaging key stakeholders is a *Campaign for Action* imperative. The Champion Nursing Coalition includes more than 55 diverse national organizations representing business, consumers, and health professional organizations. Health insurers such as Aetna, Cigna, and United Health Group are some of the largest employers of nurses and have historically promoted nurses to leadership positions in their organizations. Through the *Campaign for Action*, health insurers have built awareness around nurse-led health plan programs that help their members and consumers. Another Champion Nursing Coalition member, the American Hospital Association, envisions a society of healthy communities, where all individuals reach their highest potential for health. More than 30 state hospital associations have joined action coalitions to advance nursing and health care.

Sustainable funding is a campaign imperative. As noted earlier, to date 46 states report receiving external funding, which totals more than $20 million. These grants come from more than 500 institutions and 600 individuals.

The *Campaign for Action* offers an unprecedented opportunity for nurses to engage diverse health care stakeholders to improve health and health care through nursing. The nursing community is united as never before around the need to implement the IOM recommendations, and diverse stakeholders have pledged support for the Campaign. It is truly a historical time for nursing. To join this national effort, go to www.campaignforaction.org and get connected. Help shape the future of health care for all Americans.

DISCUSSION QUESTIONS

1. *Based on the information in this chapter, list at least two areas of policy change related to the Campaign for Action that you can identify where legislation could have an impact.*
2. *If you were to describe the importance of building a culture of health and well-being through nursing to potential supporters, what key issues would you stress? How would you describe this to your patients?*
3. *Consider the health policy changes discussed in this chapter or those you have described in your analysis and consider the impact that might occur if these changes are NOT enacted. In other words, what are the consequences of not implementing the recommendations of the Future of Nursing?*

ANALYSIS, SYNTHESIS, AND CLINICAL APPLICATION

1. *Describe your involvement in the* Campaign for Action. *If you are not currently involved, visit www.campaignforaction.org and join your action coalition.*
2. *Visit the Campaign Dashboard Indicators. What progress has been made nationally and in your state?*
3. *What else can the Campaign do to transform health and health care through nursing?*
4. *The* Campaign for Action *believes everyone can live their healthiest life possible, supported by a system in which nurses are essential partners. How does your current workplace consider nurses as essential partners to support a culture of health?*
5. *Consider activities at your workplace or community that you might lead to help advance the Campaign priorities.*

EXERCISES/CONSIDERATIONS

1. *APRN leadership is vital to promoting a Culture of Health.*
2. *APRN involvement in action coalitions can leverage our collective strength and influence to ensure that each of us has the opportunity to practice to the full extent of our capabilities, delivering high-quality, patient-centered care.*

REFERENCES

American Hospital Association. (2013). Workforce roles in a redesigned primary care model. Retrieved from http://www.campaignforaction.org/sites/default/files/PCwhitepaper%20FINAL%20Jan102013.pdf

Charting Nursing's Future. (2013). Celebrating a sustained commitment to improving health and health care: RWJF marks its 40th anniversary. Retrieved from http://www.rwjf.org/content/dam/files/file-queue/CNF_January%202013_Issue%2019_FINAL.pdf

Federal Trade Commission. (2014). Policy perspectives: Competition and the regulation of advanced practice nurses. Retrieved from http://www.aacn.nche.edu/government-affairs/APRN-Policy-Paper.pdf

Future of Nursing: *Campaign for Action*. (n.d.). RWJF State Implementation Program. Retrieved from https://campaignforaction.org/our-network/grantee-and-award-programs/state-implementation-program

Future of Nursing: *Campaign for Action*. (2013). Campaign imperatives. Retrieved from https://campaignforaction.org/resource/campaign-imperatives

Future of Nursing: *Campaign for Action*. (2017). Dashboard indicators. Retrieved from https://campaignforaction.org/resource/dashboard-indicators

Institute of Medicine. (2011). *The future of nursing: Leading change, advancing health.* Washington, DC: National Academies Press (prepublication copy). Retrieved from http://www.nap.edu/catalog/12956.html

Mundinger, M. O., Kane, R. L., Lenz, E. R., Totten, A. M., Tsai, W. Y., Cleary, P. D., . . . Shelanski, M. L. (2000). Primary care outcomes in patients treated by nurse practitioners or physicians: A randomized trial. *Journal of the American Medical Association, 283*(1), 59–68.

National Academies of Sciences, Engineering, and Medicine. (2015). *Assessing progress on the Institute of Medicine Report: The future of nursing.* Washington, DC: National Academies Press. Retrieved from http://www.nationalacademies.org/hmd/reports/2015/assessing-progress-on-the-iom-report-the-future-of-nursing.aspx

National Governors Association. (2012). The role of nurse practitioners in meeting increasing demand for primary care. Retrieved from http://www.nga.org/cms/home/nga-center-for-best-practices/center-publications/page-health-publications/col2-content/main-content-list/the-role-of-nurse-practitioners.html

Robert Wood Johnson Foundation. (2013). Transforming nursing to create a "culture of health." Retrieved from https://www.rwjf.org/en/about-rwjf/newsroom/newsroom-content/2013/02/transforming-nursing-to-create-a--culture-of-health-.html

UNIT VI

The Future of APRN Practice and Health Care Policy Nationally and Internationally

Health Policy for Advanced Practice Registered Nurses: An International Perspective

Madrean M. Schober

Nursing is at a crossroads worldwide, as key decision makers increasingly recognize that achieving successful health care systems for the future rests on the future of nursing. The growing presence of Advanced Practice Registered Nurses (APRNs) suggests that nurses in these roles provide leadership in achieving accessible, high-quality care, and expertise. The success of these endeavors, for the large part, depends on the development of supportive health policies, relevant policy processes, and promotional campaigns. This chapter focuses on events or policies that have impacted the development of APRN roles internationally and aims to demonstrate the complex nature of health policy and various courses of action that have influenced role development worldwide. It begins by providing an international contextual background for advanced nursing practice. Subsequent sections describe specific health policies or actions that have supported or impeded the APRN practice. Illustrations of actions in specific countries or regions of the world provide examples of the effects health policy has on role development.

BACKGROUND: THE INTERNATIONAL CONTEXT

Although the United States has defined four categories of the APRN, this title and the same delineation of advanced nursing practice are not found in other countries. The literature indicates that there is an international awareness of advanced practice role development in the United States; however, titles, role definitions, and scopes of practice are specific to the country in which the role is developing (DiCenso & Bryant-Lukosius, 2010; Gardner, Carryer, Dunn, & Gardner, 2004; Schober, 2016; Schober & Affara, 2006). To promote an understanding of these differences and enhance insight into relevant policy directives, this section provides an overview of the international milieu.

The difficulty in trying to portray advanced nursing practice from a worldwide point of view is that there is no international consensus on what this concept means. Unfortunately, confusion and lack of clarity surround attempts to define these roles from a global perspective (Donald et al., 2010; Schober, 2016). Results from a survey conducted by Pulcini, Jelic, Gul, and Loke (2010) representing 174 participants from 32 countries indicated that 13 different titles were used to refer to "advanced practice nursing." In addition, from country to country and within institutions in the same country, there are inconsistencies in role definitions, scopes of practice, educational preparation, and regulation, making it difficult to understand international development. For this chapter, the term *advanced nursing practice* (ANP) is used as an umbrella term (also used for Advanced Nurse Practitioner) and APRN refers to the individual nurse practicing at an advanced level of nursing. The author recognizes that, depending on the country, titles such as Nurse Practitioner (NP), advanced NP, Clinical Nurse Specialist, or nurse specialist among others are used. When providing specific country illustrations, the title used and/or officially approved within the country is given.

International surveys conducted from 2001 to 2014 estimated that anywhere from 30 to 60 countries were in various stages of exploring the potential for APRN roles (International Council of Nurses [ICN], 2001; Pulcini et al., 2010; Roodbol, 2004; Sastre-Fullana, De Pedro-Gomez, Bennasar-Veny, Serrano-Gallardo, & Morales-Ascencio, 2014). In June 2016, the ICN noted an increase in these numbers and announced that more than 90 countries indicated an interest in ANP through membership in the ICN NP/Advanced Practice Nursing Network. Many of these countries were noted to be in exploratory stages in distinguishing aspects of ANP.

The ICN had been following worldwide development since 1994 and noted the variations in referring to the discipline of ANP and APRN roles. To guide countries in various stages of development, in 2002 ICN suggested a definition that could be referred to and used to assist health care planners and key decision makers. The ICN defines an APRN as:

> a registered nurse who has acquired the expert knowledge base, complex decision-making skills and clinical competencies for expanded practice, the characteristics of which are shaped by the context and/or country in which s/he is credentialed to practice. A master's degree is recommended for entry level. (ICN, 2008, para. 2)

To provide further guidance for these developing nursing roles, ICN, in its ICN Regulation Series, provided *The Scope of Practice, Standards and Competencies of the Advanced Practice Nurse* (ICN, 2008), and the *ICN Framework of Competencies for the Nurse Specialist* (ICN, 2009). Both publications attempted to provide clarity to the debate over the extension of traditional nursing practice by providing frameworks for consideration.

In addition to country variations in attempts to define the APRN concept, key institutions, agencies, or individuals in pivotal positions of authority influence health policies that impact role development and the interpretation of ANP. These levels of influence differ from country to country. Pivotal individuals in positions of influence and their associated decision-making networks affect the initiation and development of APRN roles in various ways (Schober, 2016). The following sections discuss ways health policy and policy decisions have affected the launching or authorization of the APRN role.

AUTHORIZATION: LEGITIMIZING THE ROLE

In principle, as countries consider launching an APRN initiative, it would seem ideal to have a health policy in place to lend support to role development and implementation. However, multiple agencies and decision makers with various opinions and interpretations of what an APRN is or what a person in this role should do are in positions to define and shape a profile for this role (Schober, 2016). These varied ideas do not easily translate into policy-driven support for a new category of health care professionals; instead, they often can impede progress. Although the full international influence of these models in the United States is not known, representatives of countries that are seeking a successful ANP campaign often strive to emulate this country's achievements. However, from country to country, health systems vary, and policy is resulting in laws or legislation with a significantly different dynamic from what is familiar in the United States.

Who Has the Authority to Develop Health Policy Relevant to the APRN?

Patterned on the success in the United States, representatives of other countries appear to embrace this accomplishment with enthusiasm and good intentions. However, an eager approach to the APRN concept may fail to fully understand the policy processes and/or institutional structures along with the complexities of policy decisions that must be navigated to legitimize this new nursing role. In addition, the establishment of law and legislation may lag behind the actual momentum that led to the consideration of integrating APRNs into the health care workforce.

Oman

For example, since 2006 the Directorate of Nursing and Midwifery Affairs under the auspices of the Minister of Health for the Sultanate of Oman, with support from the World Health Organization—EMRO (Eastern Mediterranean Region Office), had been exploring APRN roles, especially for primary health care. Although positive sentiments continued to support this change, differences of opinion among government officials and health professionals led to a slow development in the policy system in response to this heightened interest. This dissension impeded the official launching of the APRN role for some time. A National Task Force led by the Directorate of Nursing in Oman continued to promote and lobby for the APRN concept. In June 2016, the first advanced nurse practitioner began practice in Primary Health Care and Hospital Accident and Emergency with official title protection and policies in place to authorize and legitimize the role (M. Al-Maqbali, personal communication, April 6, 2016; S. Al Zadjali, personal communication, June 12, 2016).

France

Similarly, France has been investigating the APRN role for a number of years by initially conducting pilot projects in a variety of locations throughout the country. Without any change made in the nursing act, the first education program for APRNs was launched in 2009. Two universities (École des Hautes Études en Santé Publique and the University of Marseille) set up the first master's degree program in a clinical nursing practice dedicated to preparing future advanced practice nurses. However, no policies, laws, or legislation were in place to support the advancement of nursing roles in clinical practice.

Several key institutions and agencies have the authority to influence APRN policy in France. They include:

- Ministère de la santé (Ministry of Health)
- Haute autorité de santé (HAS; High Authority of Health)
- Fédération hospitalière de France (Federation of Hospitals in France)

Two health policy documents influenced APRN development in France although there is no official authorization for the role: La coopération entre les professionnels de santé (cooperation between health professionals) and Protocole de coopération entre professionnels de santé: Mode d'emploi (Protocol of cooperation between health professionals: Directions for use. Retrieved from www.hassante.fr/portail/jcms/c_978700/protocole-de-cooperation-entre -professionnels-de-sante-mode-d-emploi and www.sante.gouv.fr/la-coope ration-entre-les-profess ionnels-de-sante.html).

The law HPST (Article 51) 2009 provided a countrywide agenda in France resulting in the beginnings of supportive legislation for APRNs, including a practice act. After years of discussion, an article introducing advanced practice in nursing and allied health professions (AHP) in France was inserted in a public health law voted by the French parliament in January 2016. This decision now needs to be implemented, but many operational aspects of this implementation process are still to be written.

As of June 2016, APRNs in France face diverse obstacles in working to integrate mainly hospital-based specialty roles into the health care workforce. Most nurses who have graduated from the early APRN program are not employed in an advanced capacity, and the original APRN program no longer exists. The lack of appropriate legislation has been the greatest difficulty encountered. The APRN roles were poorly defined in health care organizations and the added value they bring to the health care system was not rewarded with their salary. Obstacles, which hinder the implementation of APRN in France, are also observed among health care professionals, in the ranks of nurses and physicians. Fear, suspicion or rejection are the most common reactions experienced by the APRNs (C. Debout, personal communication, June 15, 2016; Schober, 2016).

Singapore

The introduction of APRNs in Singapore provides an example of the lag that can occur between the initiation of role preparation or education and the official provision of policy supportive of title protection and definition for the role. The National University of Singapore developed an APRN program following discussions among key representatives of the Ministry of Health and the university. The first group of students began their education in 2003 and completed the 18-month program in 2004. Although the policies developed through the ministry are specific in protecting the title, defining an APRN, and identifying punitive actions for persons misrepresenting themselves as an APRN without the required qualifications, these policies were not announced until 2006 following the launching of the master's program. This resulted in the initial graduates returning to their practice sites with only a vague notion of what was expected of them and no supportive health policies. Lack of role clarity among the APRNs and relevant managers, along with the lack of fundamental policies at the time, led to an environment of confusion and conflict in the early stages of role implementation (Schober, 2013, 2016).

Ireland

Health policy in Ireland provides a different perspective with the establishment of ANP and Advanced Midwife Practitioner (AMP) policies. In 2013, the National Council for the Professional Development of Nursing and Midwifery (referred to here as The National Council) released the fourth edition of the *Framework for the Establishment of Advanced Nurse Practitioner and Advanced Midwife Practitioner Posts*. The development of a career pathway by the Commission on Nursing (Government of Ireland, 1998) was created to retain expert nurses in direct patient care and served to develop clinical nursing and midwifery expertise. The establishment of the clinical pathway was a function vested in The National Council that in turn developed a definition, core concept, and competencies for the roles of the ANP and AMP. In addition, this agency determined the requirements for nurses and midwives to be accredited as an ANP or AMP, as well as giving official approval for the post (employment position) where the ANP or AMP would practice. The development of ANP/AMP roles and services was part of the strategic development of the overall health service reform in the country (Department of Health and Children, 2001, 2003). The comprehensive nature of the Irish plan provides an illustration of how ANP and AMP role development became a subset of a national health care reform and related policies.

Australia

The first NP in Australia was endorsed/authorized in the year 2000 following 20 years of exploring this option for provision of health care services in the country. Australia had six state and two territory governments with differing requirements for endorsement until July 2010, when national registration for nurses and other health professionals was implemented with the creation of the Australian Health Practitioner Regulatory Agency (AHPRA) and the Nurse and Midwifery Board of Australia (NMBA). As of September 2015, there were 1,287 endorsed NPs qualified to practice in Australia with authorization now through the Nursing and Midwifery Board (Nursing and Midwifery Board of Australia, 2017). In some ways, the original approach of health policy impacting NPs was similar to that in the United States in that authority and jurisdiction had been mainly under the separate states. With this unification, there is an effort to reevaluate and provide universal NP competency standards for the country (retrieved from www.icn-apnetwork.org; Schober, 2016).

Republic of South Africa

The state of affairs for nursing in general in a country can dictate whether health policy embraces the concept of advanced practice nursing. South Africa provides an example of how an attempt to rejuvenate the health care system and thus health policy affects all of nursing, including APRNs. The Minister of Health in South Africa introduced a number of policies to revitalize the health system in the country. This approach included the following:

- Reengineering the primary health care system
- Introducing a National Health Insurance that will be piloted at first and implemented across 14 years, each with its impact on nursing

The revised health strategy highlights the South African nurse-based health system and suggests that there is a great need for specialist nurses with advanced skills, as seen in some of the teams proposed in these policies. This highlights the need for the country for APRNs. The policy change to allow nurses to initiate antiretroviral treatment (ART) is likely the policy that brought about the largest amount of support for the APRN role in the country. From 2010 to 2012, the people who could initiate ART increased from 250 to 10,000. This has increased the life expectancy of South Africans over a period of 3 years (N. Geyer, personal communication, July 2, 2016). Refer to the subsequent section on education for discussion on how health policy influenced relevant standards for nursing education, including APRNs, in South Africa.

Saudi Arabia

Saudi Arabia provides another example of how health policy relevant to nursing in general impacts the development of APRN roles. The Kingdom of Saudi Arabia has had established nurse training programs for around 40 years, with movement away from hospital-based education to university baccalaureate and master's level programs. Although the Saudi Commission for Health Specialties (SCFHS) registers all nurses working within the kingdom, nursing as a profession still has a long way to go. The World Health Organization has recognized the need for APRNs within the Middle East including Saudi Arabia; however, there is as yet no postgraduate university education aimed at developing APRNs (Clinical Nurse Specialist or NP programs). The SCFHS has recently accredited a 12-month, full-time, hospital-based Enterostomal Therapy Education Program (wound, ostomy, and continence) aimed at developing the nursing expertise to an advanced level within this specialist field. Additionally, Saudi nurses are encouraged to avail themselves of scholarship opportunities internationally, sponsored by the Saudi government, to gain advanced clinical practice qualifications in countries such as the United Kingdom and the United States. However, to date, very few APRNs are in clinical practice within the Kingdom of Saudi Arabia (Hibbert, cited in Kleinpell et al., 2014).

Israel

Israel provides an example of how authority for APRN-like roles is granted by institutions employing these nurses while they work in this advanced capacity without national health policy or legislation supportive of the role. Like other western countries, advances in technology and the increasing aging of the population have led to increased specialization within the health care system, including the need for nurses to specialize. In addition, health services have been shown to be more limited in the peripheral regions of the country. These trends have been linked to the grassroots development of advanced practice-like roles. For example, many hospitals have positions, similar to those of the Clinical Nurse Specialist or the nurse specialist, for nurses to serve as clinical consultants or experts in roles such as pain nurse, stoma nurse, and infection control nurse. In the community, nurses who work in outpatient clinics, especially in the periphery, may practice in roles that are similar to the NP; however, their practice is very structured, and they work within very defined and prescribed medical protocols. These nurses are given the authority to perform these roles by their institutions rather than a countrywide policy. Although they have advanced clinical knowledge and function as

APRNs, these nurses do not have the legal title or authority to practice over and above any other registered nurse. They also do not have the autonomy, independence, or legal liability to practice as specialists. Most of the nurses who pioneered these roles were taught as apprentices to physicians, and some were trained by attending courses and/or conferences outside of the country.

The scope of practice for the nurse specialist in Israel continues to widen from that of the registered nurse. However, many nurse specialists practice nursing in a staff nurse role and are not implementing the role to the full extent of an expanded scope of practice. Training for the advanced role is not yet within an academic framework. That is to say, that a nurse specialist might have a master's degree in public health or nursing administration. It is not required to have a degree in advanced practice nursing. It is hoped that the nurse specialist role continues to develop and becomes incorporated into an academic framework, and that increased numbers of nurses are authorized to perform the role (retrieved October 15, 2016, from www.icn-apnetwork.org; F. DeKeyser Ganz, personal communication, May 4, 2016).

HEALTH POLICY THAT INFLUENCES APRN EDUCATION

In addition to acknowledging or authorizing the presence of APRNs in health care systems worldwide, health policies often establish education requirements for the qualified APRN before the presence of supportive health policies for the role. This section provides country-specific examples and illustrations of how governmental agencies or professional bodies have made decisions or developed policy that affects educational standards.

Republic of South Africa

In South Africa, in addition to the Ministry of Health developing new policies for health care in the country, the South African Nursing Council (SANC) has played a major role in the development of regulations for the APRN role. Given the changing health care needs of the country, there was a need to revise the scope of practice and educational preparation of nurses to fulfill these needs. This led to the development of a revised qualification framework (see Table 27.1) for nursing in the country, which for the first time established the position of APRN (in this framework, the title used is Advanced Specialist Nurse) in the hierarchy of qualifications (the breakdown of credits is 120 per academic year).

In addition, the Department of Higher Education in South Africa has had an important influence on the direction of nursing education policy. The Higher Education Act's (Act 101 of 1997) amended definition (Council on Higher Education South Africa, 1997) of *higher education programs* included nursing programs, and as such, all nursing programs from 2015 will be at a higher education level, which includes both university and nursing college programs. This also means that nursing programs will be accredited by the Council of Higher Education, not only SANC. With the newly devised qualification framework for nursing, the SANC has initiated the development of competencies and scopes of practice for specialist and advanced practice categories of nurses. Nursing professionals in the relevant fields have been participating in the exercise that would

TABLE 27.1 Revised Qualification Framework for Nursing in South Africa

NQF	QUALIFICATIONS	CREDITS	CATEGORY OF NURSE
10	Doctoral degree	360 credits at level 10	Advanced Specialist Nurse
9	Master's degree	180 credits at level 9	
8	Postgraduate diploma Bachelor's honors degree (professional degree)	120 credits at level 8 480 credits at level 8 and 96 at level 6	Specialist Nurse Registered Professional Nurse
7	Bachelor's degree Advanced diploma	360 credits at level 7 and 96 at level 5 120 credits	Registered Staff Nurse
6	Diploma	360 credits with minimum 60 at level 7 and maximum 120 at level 5	Registered Auxiliary Nurse
5	Higher certificate	120 credits	

NQF, National Quality Forum.

finally result in regulations under the Nursing Act that formalize the position of the APRN (N. Geyer, personal communication, July 2, 2016).

Ireland

ANP in Ireland as a clinical career pathway for registered nurses was formalized under a recommendation of the Commission on Nursing Report (1998). Following the release of this report, a statutory body, the National Council for the Professional Development of Nursing and Midwifery (NCNM), was established with the responsibility for setting the parameters of educational preparation and accreditation. Advanced NPs/advanced midwife practitioners (ANP/AMPs) in Ireland are expected to demonstrate "exemplary" theoretical and practical knowledge as well as "exemplary" critical thinking skills. The minimum educational requirement for an ANP/AMP in Ireland is a master's level degree relevant to the ANP/AMP practice area. Any education taken should include a major clinical component. ANP/AMPs also need to have a minimum of 7 years post-registration experience with a minimum of 5 years in their specialty practice area before they can register to practice in Ireland.

The Nursing and Midwifery Board of Ireland (NMBI) formerly, An Bord Altranais, is the independent, statutory organization which regulates the nursing and midwifery professions in the country. Registered ANPs and AMPs meet established criteria set by NMBI. In 2016 NMBI was engaged in a project to review standards and requirements for advanced practice. In advance of the change in requirements for ANP and AMP, the NMBI established a new interim revalidation process, updated application forms, updated guidelines for advanced practice portfolios and envisioned plans for matching an ANP or AMP to a position or post to become more flexible (Nursing and Midwifery Board of Ireland, 2016).

Israel

The advanced practice role exists in Israel mostly at the grassroots level; however, more recent developments and health policies have been promoting the legal authority for this role. In 2009, the first advanced practice role was approved by the Ministry of Health: the Nurse Specialist in Palliative Care. Executive order gave the legal authority for this role by the Director General of the Ministry of Health. Before this, the only formal advanced training for nurses was provided in postbasic certification courses in specific clinical areas such as critical care, oncology, geriatrics, midwifery, and dialysis. Nurses complete a theoretical and clinical program mandated by the Nursing Division within the Ministry of Health. These courses range from several months to one and a half years in length. At the end of this period, nurses take a national licensing specialization exam. The Nursing Division in the Ministry of Health determines the curriculum of the programs and administers these licensure exams. Those who receive postbasic licensure are entitled to perform certain procedures that are considered to be delegated to them from a medical practice that is beyond the scope of practice of the generalist registered nurse. These programs were often taught in schools of nursing; however, they are not within an academic framework, and no degree is offered to the graduates of these programs. However, approximately 50% of registered nurses have some post-basic certification. This high percentage is most probably because of the significant increase in salary above that of the generalist registered nurse for those who obtain post-basic certification and to the Ministry of Health requirement that certain specialty areas such as critical care units hire nurses with post-basic certification. Four universities offer master's degrees in nursing. One program focuses only on nursing research, and another on nursing education and administration with some clinical component. The third program contains theoretical courses of a clinical nature but does not include any clinical experiences. Only one university offers a master's degree in ANP where students are taught both theoretical and clinical advanced practice skills within the same program.

When countries lack policies or legislation providing specific support or governance for the APRN scope of practice, professional organizations and governmental bodies initiate nonlegislative actions to more clearly delineate this level of nursing. The following section describes this approach.

SCOPE OF PRACTICE: NATURE OF THE ROLE AND RESPONSIBILITIES

Ideally, health policies for APRNs should promote full-practice authority without placing undue restrictions on full and direct access to consultation, care coordination, and referral. Although new initiatives debate the ability of the APRN to make a diagnosis of a presenting concern or manage a full caseload, the more contentious issues emerge around prescriptive authority, reimbursement, and the establishment of autonomous practice. If health policy is absent, countries develop innovative approaches to promote and support the role.

Republic of South Africa

The challenge in South Africa remains one of designated clinical practice and prescribing by APRNs. Authorization to prescribe remains a special concession and then can only be exercised if a nurse works in the public sector. A few nurses in the private sector do have prescribing authority. This includes midwives working for themselves and nurses working in occupational health care services (occupational health is a designated service as determined by section 56 of the Nursing

Act, 2005; South African Nursing Council, 2005). Reimbursement is selectively done for self-employed nurses working in the private sector, although many medical aids (insurance schemes) do not provide any member benefit coverage for nursing/midwifery services. Self-employed wound care specialist nurses are a new group that functions as independent practitioners, and they are consulted by other practitioners, including medical practitioners (N. Geyer, personal communication, July 2, 2016).

The Netherlands

In the initial stage of development, the most important driver for the establishment of the NP (the Dutch title is " Nurse Specialist") position was the shortage of physicians. In addition, there was a desire to diminish the dominant position and power of the physicians in the political arena. In this context, the key entities influencing health policy for the APRNs are the general professional nursing organization, as well as the professional APRN organization, the national registration committee for the APRN, the Minister of Health, the universities of applied science, and insurance companies. The countrywide agenda has been in the hands of the general nursing organization, with a pivotal one-person campaign led in the early stages by Dr. Petrie Roodbol. Supported by international colleagues and under the nursing leadership, all practice acts including prescribing have been developed and implemented.

Twenty years since the introduction of the advanced nursing role in the Netherlands there are, as of 2016, 2,750 nurses educated and registered in the advanced role. They integrate medical and nursing reasoning as they fulfill the role of a clinician with a focus on human functioning, not only disease management. Provision of care includes support for patients and their families based on self-management and coping with the disease (P. Roodbol, personal communication, March 17, 2013; J. Peters, personal communication, February 17, 2016; Schober, 2016).

United Kingdom

Discussions in the UK on ANP have been long and complex because many roles have evolved in an unregulated and unplanned manner. Barton, Bevan, and Mooney (2012) indicated that the ad hoc development of advanced nursing roles, the random use of titles that imply levels of clinical expertise that cannot be verified, and varied educational development all point to the need to govern ANP at the employer level. In addition, because of the lack of health policies governing all four countries in the UK, representatives of Scotland and Wales have worked to develop guidelines, frameworks, and toolkits to support APRN roles (National Leadership and Innovation Agency for Health Care, 2010; Scottish Government, 2008; Welsh Assembly Government, 2010). As of 2016 similar guidelines have also been agreed to in England and Northern Ireland (Schober, 2016).

Barton et al. (2012) suggested that good governance regarding role development and implementation must be based on consistent expectations of the level of practice required to deliver the service and that this is best achieved through nationally agreed upon standards and processes. However, the UK has not been able to establish health policy through its Nursing and Midwifery Council that provides acceptable and universal governance; thus, individual countries have established their frameworks. Discussions in the UK on ANP have been long and complex, spanning more than 20 years since the late 1980s and early 1990s as service and strategic interest in advanced nurse roles grew (Fulbrook, 1995; Kaufman, 1996; Stilwell, 1988). Despite extensive strategic intent since then, title protection and legislation governing the profession have not been achieved. Barton et al. (2012) noted that the

> Council for Healthcare Regulatory Excellence (2008) outlined the complexity of professional regulatory issues and made it clear that, in its view, the code of professional conduct (Nursing and Midwifery Council, 2008) encompasses advanced practitioner practice, negating any need for additional formal regulation. That view led indirectly to the development of the Advanced Practice Toolkit (Scottish Government, 2008) under the auspices of Modernising Nursing Careers (Department of Health, 2006). This provided some national conformity and guidance to employers, practitioners and educators. More recently, two documents looked to governance as a mechanism of employer-led local regulation—the DH's [Department of Health] (2010) position statement on advanced practice and the Welsh framework for advanced practice. (National Leadership and Innovation Agency for Health Care, 2010, p. 2)

As of 2016, especially since devolution in the United Kingdom, it appears that there is no perceived movement to develop centrally focused health policies for APRNs. In this environment, employer-led frameworks of governance that guide the country-specific National Health Services have been proposed to fill this need.

New Zealand

A task force established by the government of New Zealand in 1998 recognized that nurses were already providing some services at an advanced level and decided to identify obstacles that might be preventing nurses from improving health care services to patients (NCNZ, 2002). This task force studied strategies to remove barriers that limited the full potential of nursing practice. The government adopted the task force recommendations. Critical to the success for the promotion of the possibility of the NP role in New Zealand was the presence of a supportive chief nursing advisor at the Ministry of Health. The presence of a person in a position of authority achieved government recognition that formal recognition and employment of NPs would improve health outcomes for the population. The Nursing Council of New Zealand (NCNZ, 2002) along with the Ministry of Health defined two clear areas of work:

- Consultation and policy development around the title, education standards and competencies
- Policy development around prescribing, including mechanisms to regulate prescribing, establish education standards, curricula and competencies (Schober & Affara, 2006, p. 57)

The action was taken by the Ministry of Health to remove barriers to NP practice, including enacting necessary legislative changes to allow prescribing. Currently, the Nursing Council of New Zealand (www.nursingcouncil.org.nz)

and the Association of Nurse Practitioners for New Zealand (www.nurse.org .nz/npnz-nurse-practitioners-nz.html) offer information about becoming an NP (now the legally protected title).

CONCLUSION

International momentum for the ANP concept and advanced practice nursing roles continues to grow. Enthusiasm for advanced nursing roles is often based on observed successes in the United States and other countries with histories of successful experiences in development. At times, eagerness to introduce these new nursing roles into health care systems is based on a limited understanding of the complexities of the development of health policy and policy processes. This chapter has sought to portray the international differences in approaching the concept of ANP and the variety of factors that influence policy that impacts role development and sustainability. The content of this chapter does not aim to provide a comprehensive view of all health policy initiatives worldwide relevant to advanced practice nurses, but rather it provides snapshots and illustrations demonstrating the variance in how health policy directives from a wide variety of government agencies, professional organizations, and other institutions influence its role and policy development. Knowledge of the complexities of how policies impact ANP and the pivotal interactions that occur among key stakeholders in the policy process provides insight into the dynamics underlying new initiatives and those in the process of maturing.

DISCUSSION QUESTIONS

1. *There is a lack of international consensus in defining ANP. Based on the information in this chapter, identify the factors that contribute to this.*
2. *If you were going to describe the importance of policy to support a new advanced practice nursing initiative in another country what key issues would you stress?*
3. *Describe the impact that might occur if policy changes supportive of ANP are not developed and enacted. Provide specific examples.*

ANALYSIS, SYNTHESIS, AND CLINICAL APPLICATION

1. *Review the international literature and generate a list of factors impacting implementation of APRN roles. Provide two to three country examples. Identify barriers and facilitators.*
2. *Convene a focus group and discuss how attention from international organizations facilitates plans for countries in the beginning stages of developing a new APRN initiative. Identify specific organizations and how they would offer support.*
3. *Based on a review of the literature and content in this chapter compare and contrast APRN development in two countries. Identify motivation for the role, implementation and whether there is a visible presence of a professional standard for practice.*
4. *Write a one page summary (include references) to present to a Minister of Health delineating why the ministry should support the inclusion of APRNs in the health care system for access to service provision.*

ETHICAL CONSIDERATIONS

1. *Ideally policy and professional regulation should support the APRN to the full extent of their educational preparation. In addition, these standards and policies offer public protection and assurance for quality of care. Discuss the ethical issues that could arise when there is no national oversight/governance or required standards guiding development for the APRN. Include consideration of an overly restrictive practice environment, the responsibility of APRNs to be proactive and interests of other decision makers to support restrictions on APRN clinical practice.*

REFERENCES

Barton, T. D., Bevan, L., & Mooney, G. (2012). Advanced nursing 2: A governance framework for advanced nursing. *Nursing Times, 108*(25), 22–24.

Council on Higher Education South Africa. (1997). Higher Education Act 101 of 1997: Higher Education and Training Law. Amendment Act 23 of 2012. Retrieved from www.che.ac.za/documents/d000004/Higher_Education_Act.pdf

Department of Health. (2006). *Modernizing nursing careers: Setting the direction.* Edinburgh, UK: Scottish Executive. Retrieved from http://www.scotland.gov.uk/Resource/Doc/146433/0038313.pdf

Department of Health. (2010). *Advanced level nursing: A position statement.* London, England: Author. Retrieved from http://www.gov.uk/government/uploads/system/uploads/attachment_data/file/215935/dh_121738.pdf

Department of Health and Children. (2001). *Quality and fairness: A health system for you.* Dublin, Ireland: Government of Ireland.

Department of Health and Children. (2003). *Business plan 2003.* Dublin, Ireland: Government of Ireland.

DiCenso, A., & Bryant-Lukosius, D. (2010). Role of clinical nurse specialists and nurse practitioners in Canada: A decision support synthesis (pp. 13–18). Ottawa, ON, Canada: Canadian Health Services Research Foundation.

Donald, F., Bryant-Lukosius, D., Martin-Misener, R., Kaasalainen, S., Kilpatrick, K., Carter, N.,… DiCenso, A. (2010). Clinical nurse specialists and nurse practitioners: Title confusion and lack of role clarity. *Canadian Journal of Nursing Leadership, 23,* 189–210.

Fulbrook, P. (1995). What is advanced practice? *Intensive and Critical Care Nursing, 11*(1), 53.

Gardner, G., Carryer, J., Dunn, S., & Gardner, A. (2004). *The nurse practitioner standards project.* Canberra, Australia: Australian Nursing and Midwifery Counsel.

Government of Ireland. (1998). *Report of the commission on nursing: A blueprint for the future.* Dublin, Ireland: Stationery Office.

International Council of Nurses. (2001). Update: International survey of nurse practitioner/advanced practice nursing roles. Retrieved from http://www.icn-apnetwork.org

International Council of Nurses. (2002). Definition and characteristics of the role. Retrieved from http://www.icn-apnetwork.org

International Council of Nurses. (2008). *The scope of practice, standards and competencies of the advanced practice nurse* (The ICN Regulation Series). Geneva, Switzerland: Author.

International Council of Nurses. (2009). *ICN framework of competencies for the nurse specialist* (The ICN Regulation Series). Geneva, Switerland: Author.

Kaufman, G. (1996). Nurse practitioners in general practice: An expanding role. *Nursing Standard, 11*(8), 44–47.

Kleinpell, R., Scanlon, A., Hibbert, D., Ganz, F., East, L., Fraser, D., … Beauchesne, M. (2014). Addressing issues impacting advanced nursing practice worldwide. *The Online Journal of Issues in Nursing, 19*(2), Manuscript 5. doi:10.3912/OJIN.Vol19No02Man05

National Council for the Professional Development of Nursing and Midwifery. (2005). *A preliminary evaluation of the role of the advanced nurse practitioner.* Dublin, Ireland: Author.

National Council for the Professional Development of Nursing and Midwifery. (2013). *Framework for the establishment of advanced nurse practitioner and advanced midwife posts* (4th ed.). Dublin, Ireland: Author.

National Leadership and Innovation Agency for Health Care. (2010). *Framework for advanced nursing, midwifery and allied health professional practice in Wales.* Lianharan, Wales: Innovation House.

Nursing Council of New Zealand. (2002). *The nurse practitioner: Responding to health needs in New Zealand* (3rd ed.). Wellington, NZ: Author.

Nursing and Midwifery Board of Australia. (2017). Regulating Australia's nurses and midwives: Registration standards (Endorsement as a nurse practitioner). Retrieved from http://www.nursingmidwiferyboard.gov.au

Nursing and Midwifery Board of Ireland. (2016). Advanced practice (nursing) & advanced practice (midwifery). Retrieved from https://www.nmbi.ie/Standards-Guidance/Current-Projects/Advanced-Practice

Nursing and Midwifery Council. (2008). *The Code: Standards of conduct, performance and ethics for nurses and midwives.* London, UK: Author.

Pulcini, J., Jelic, M., Gul, R., & Loke, A. I. (2010). An international survey on advanced practice nursing education, practice and regulation. *Journal of Nursing Scholarship, 42*(1), 31–39.

Roodbol, P. (2004). *Survey carried out prior to the 3rd ICN-International Nurse Practitioner/Advanced Practice Nursing Network Conference.* Unpublished data. Groningen, The Netherlands.

Sastre-Fullana, P., De Pedro-Gomez, J. E., Bennasar-Veny, M., Serrano-Gallardo, P., & Morales-Ascencio, J. M. (2014). Competency frameworks for advanced practice nursing: A literature review. *International Nursing Review, 61*(4) 534–542.

Schober. M. (2013). Factors influencing the development of advanced practice nursing in Singapore, Doctoral thesis, Sheffield Hallam University, Sheffield Hallam University archives. Retrieved from http://shura.shu.ac.uk/7799

Schober, M. (2016). *Introduction to advanced nursing practice: An international focus.* Cham, Switzerland: Springer.

Schober, M., & Affara, F. (2006). *Advanced nursing practice.* Oxford, UK: Blackwell.

Scottish Government. (2008*). Supporting the development of advanced nursing practice—A toolkit approach.* Retrieved from http://www.advancedpractice.scot.nhs.uk/media/1371/supporting%20the%20development%20of%20advanced%20nursing%20practice.pdf

South African Nursing Council. (2005). Nursing Act-Act No. 33 of 2005. Retrieved from http://www.sanc.co.za/publications.htm

Stilwell, B. (1988). Patients' attitudes to a highly developed extended role: The nurse practitioner. *Recent Advances in Nursing, 21,* 82–100.

Welsh Assembly Government. (2009). Post registration career framework for nurses in Wales. Retrieved from http://www.wales.nhs.uk/sites3/docmetadata.cfm?orgid=580&id=148258

Welsh Assembly Government. (2010). *Delivering a five year service, workforce and financial strategic framework for NHS Wales.* Retrieved from www.wales.nhs.uk/documents/Framework-five-year.pdf

CHAPTER 28

Credentialing Across the Globe: Approaches and Applications

Frances Hughes, Franklin A. Shaffer,
Julia Yuen-Heung To Dutka, and Catherine Coates

A combination of factors—globalization, deregulation, privatization, health care restructuring, medical tourism, and nursing shortages—have all led to an increase in focus on systems and processes, which serves to promote and validate the quality of nursing and health care globally. Credentialing is being increasingly recognized as offering an opportunity to apply formal processes to verify qualifications, experience, professional standing, and other relevant professional attributes; to assess competence, performance, and professional suitability; and to provide a safe, high-quality health care service within specific environments.

Health care has come to value accreditation in general for health care facilities and academic nursing programs as an indication of quality assurance for public protection. The industry also values recognition of excellence for individuals having met professional standards embodied in specific credentials. While credentialing for recognition of excellence has its origin mostly in English-speaking countries, it has increasingly gained importance on a global scale.

The term "credentialing" has various definitions in different contexts, depending on the nomenclature and the traditions associated with the use of the term. In some countries, credentialing refers to a process used to assign specific clinical responsibilities to health practitioners on the basis of their education. It commences on employment and continues for the period of employment. In other countries, credentialing refers to the conferring of a credential to a health professional based on the individual having met the standards specified for the credential. The credential earned is regarded as a mark of distinction and carries with it the public pronouncement that the bearer of the credential is accorded the recognition of this achievement.

THE APPLICATION OF CREDENTIALING TO NURSING

An Overview

Credentialing is a core component of clinical and professional governance or self-regulation where members of a profession set standards for practice and competence within their specialist domain beyond entry to practice. Although there is a worldwide shortage of nurses, "there is an increasing demand for nurses with enhanced skills who manage a more diverse, complex, and acutely ill patient population than ever before" (Duffield, Gardner, Chang, & Catling-Paull, 2009).

Internationally, we have guidance on the positive impact of credentialing from multiple sources. We also have opportunities to learn from both the positive and negative experiences of other countries in introducing credentialing. Evidence-based consensus, standards, and principles are important for the overarching framework for all countries. Professional nursing organizations have developed these over time but often without the accompanying ability to ensure compliance and mandate requirements. As a result, we have variability in the structure, uptake, and impact of credentialing across the globe, which may reduce its effectiveness. For example, the International Council of Nurses (ICN), through its advanced practice network, has developed policies and standards on advanced practice, which are outlined later in the text, but member countries have varying ability to mandate them.

ICN is a pillar for the global introduction of credentialing in nursing. In 2000, it established a Credentialing and Regulators Forum with the purpose of serving as a mechanism for countries with an interest in developing "dynamic regulatory processes and credentialing programs to communicate, consult, and collaborate with one another on trends, problems, solutions, etc." (ICN, 2013). This forum also provides an opportunity to promote and enable nursing's role at the forefront of health care and the development of contemporary regulatory and credentialing systems, and to advise ICN on developments and needs in regulation, credentialing, and quality assurance.

There is considerable diversity in approaches to credentialing internationally. Many countries are currently working actively on continuing education and credentialing of Nurse Practitioners (NPs) and nurses in specialty or advanced practice. It appears to be becoming increasingly common for national nursing organizations to collaborate with other associations and regulatory bodies or multidisciplinary agencies in relation to credentialing. The number and variety of agencies involved in the credentialing process appear to vary depending on the country.

Despite country variations in process and procedures, credentialing appears to be becoming increasingly accepted as a mechanism to formally recognize expertise and specific skill sets in registered nurses (Cioffi, Lichtveld, Thielen, & Miner, 2003). Countries with substantive well-established bodies are increasingly assisting others, which is important for countries with fewer resources. The international network of professional nursing bodies is crucial in maintaining professional standards and reflecting these in an overarching credentialing framework. Stronger emphasis may now be needed to galvanize this network into working on strategies for compliance to reduce variability across the globe. Professional specialty/advanced practice membership is key to achieving this compliance and reducing variability, although we must recognize that individual countries need to work within their own legislation, professional structures, and cultural and social dynamics (Newton, Pillay, & Higginbottom, 2012).

The following four case studies illustrate different credentialing approaches drawn from four different countries: New Zealand, Australia, United States, and United Kingdom.

CREDENTIALING OF REGISTERED NURSES DELIVERING MENTAL HEALTH CARE WITHIN PRIMARY HEALTH CARE SETTINGS IN NEW ZEALAND

In New Zealand, the first step toward mental health credentialing for nurses was introduced in 2011. This section describes the process used to assign specific clinical responsibilities to health practitioners on the basis of their education. A credential in mental health nursing refers to registered nurses who undertake activities in mental health but who are not specialist mental health nurses. Mental health nurses, on the other hand, are registered nurses with specific education and training in the specialty area of mental health.

Te Rau Hinegaro (Oakley-Brown, Wells, & Scott, 2006) was the first national mental health survey conducted in New Zealand and identified that people with mental health issues, including substance use, do not necessarily visit a primary health care practitioner in relation to mental health concerns. Approximately 58% of people with a serious disorder, 37% with a moderate disorder, and 19% with a mild disorder present to a health service to discuss their mental health concerns. In addition, it is well recognized that people with mental health issues are vulnerable to a wide range of other health and social problems.

Although an international evidence base demonstrating these findings was well established, this was the first study specific to New Zealand to support these international findings. At the same time, it was becoming clear that the present system was not offering nurses, employers, or consumers any certainty about the knowledge and skills required by registered nurses in order to competently and confidently provide a primary care response for people who have mental health and/or substance use issues. Clarity and consistency were required about the level of knowledge and skill needed by registered nurses working in the primary health sector in order to ensure competence and safety for people with mental health and substance use problems.

The responsibility of credentialing in New Zealand is delegated to professional bodies. In the specialty area of mental health, any registered nurse working in a primary health care service who has the knowledge, skills enhancement, and experience to apply mental health and addiction assessment, referral, and interventions in a primary care setting may apply to Te Ao Māramatanga (The New Zealand College of Mental Health Nurses) to become credentialed.

Credentialing commences on appointment and continues for the period of employment. The process is peer led and requires periodic recredentialing in order to maintain the credential. It recognizes the competence of an individual to perform agreed-upon clinical activities within a designated environment. A credential complements a nurse's existing performance review by confirming the current credentialed status of the nurse (Te Ao Māramatanga, 2013).

Applicants must complete an evidence-based record (EBR) in order to be considered for becoming credentialed in mental health nursing in primary care settings. The EBR is a record of the applicant's learning and education or training activity. Education and training are based on evidence-based New Zealand tools and guidelines (where possible) and include:

- Identifying common presenting issues
- Principles of motivating behavior change
- Screening and health promotion—for example, recognizing people who are at risk of developing moderate to severe mental illness and addiction
- Brief assessment skills
- Brief intervention skills
- Knowledge of commonly prescribed medications and their side effects
- Knowledge of community resources
- Referral and consultation pathways
- Working in shared care arrangements with specialist mental health and addiction treatment nurses/services
- Continuing management (follow-up) of people with chronic conditions, inclusive of enduring mental health illness and addictions
- Familiarity with web-based primary care packages

The EBR is then submitted to Te Ao Māramatanga's Credentialing Review Panel with the initial application and then again when recredentialing is required 3 years later. A credential awarded by Te Ao Māramatanga is valid for 3 years from the date of issue. The successful applicant receives a certificate, which is designed with space on the back to place an updated recredentialed sticker for every successful reapplication received.

The credential means that the nurse has specific skills in mental health and addiction assessment intervention in the primary health environment, but not to the level required for mental health nursing.

A credential from Te Ao Māramatanga in mental health benefits the individual nurse by ensuring that the nurse's skills in mental health and addiction meet certain standards and that the nurse will be supported to maintain and extend his or her skills. Credentialed registered nurses then become associate members of Te Ao Māramatanga. This provides access to a website with regular updates, journal articles, and other relevant information, and it provides a forum to engage with other credentialed primary care nurses.

Employers of credentialed nurses are expected to support those nurses in the development of the knowledge and skills required to main their credentialed status. This can include, for example, enabling access to relevant training and information; providing the opportunity for registered nurses to use their credentialed skills in everyday practice; and ensuring access to relevant clinical supervision and peer support, as well as review forums.

For specialist mental health nurses in New Zealand, Te Ao Māramatanga uses the term "certified," meaning they meet a set of standards in mental health nursing to hold themselves out to be recognized as mental health nurses. Te Ao Māramatanga is working on a process to introduce certification that will provide formal recognition that a registered nurse has met the professional standards for mental health nursing set by Te Ao Māramatanga, and so will then be called a certified mental health nurse. It is proposed that new graduate registered nurses will be eligible to seek certification as mental health nurses after completing a mental health new graduate program and working an additional 12 months in mental health. Existing registered nurses could follow a number of pathways, including completing the mental health entry-to-specialty-practice program, completing a postgraduate qualification or equivalent with a mental health focus, and working for 3 years or more as a registered nurse in mental health.

CREDENTIALING OF NURSES WITHIN AUSTRALIA'S HEALTH CARE SYSTEM

Unlike in New Zealand, Australia's health care system is managed at the federal level and overseen by federal governments in each of Australia's six states and two territories.

The Royal College of Nursing Australia (RCNA) has actively promoted credentialing via a range of initiatives, including establishing a national center for nurse credentialing (RCNA, 2011).

Four specialty organizations offer a credentialing service: the Australian College of Critical Care Nurses; the Australian College of Mental Health Nurses (ACMHN); PapScreen Victoria and Western Australia; and the Gastroenterological Nurses College of Australia. In order to compare and contrast the specific systems used in New Zealand and Australia, the example of credentialing mental health nurses in Australia is used as a case study.

The ACMHN is the body responsible for the credentialing of nurses in mental health. The ACMHN Credential for Practice Program (CPP) was launched nationally in October 2004, and since then over 1,100 registered nurses have been recognized as specialist mental health nurses through this program (Gendek, 2011). The ACMHN CPP is the only national credentialing program currently implemented within Australia, and it recognizes the skills, expertise, and experience of nurses who are practicing as specialist mental health nurses. The credential demonstrates to employers, professional colleagues, patients, and careers that an individual nurse has achieved the professional standard for practice in mental health nursing, as well as recognizing the contribution mental health nurses make to the mental health of the community (ACMHN, 2011).

In Australia, credentialing is a core component of clinical and professional governance, or self-regulation. Members of the profession set the standards for practice and establish a minimum requirement for entry, continuing professional development, endorsement, and recognition.

In order to apply to become a credentialed mental health nurse in Australia, applicants must demonstrate that they:

- Hold a current license to practice as a registered nurse within Australia
- Hold a recognized specialist/postgraduate mental health nursing qualification
- Have at least 12 months of experience since completing specialist/postgraduate qualification or have 3 years of experience as a registered nurse in mental health
- Have been practicing within the past 3 years

- Have acquired minimum continuing professional development points for education and practice
- Are supported by two professional referees
- Have completed a professional declaration agreeing to uphold the standards of the profession

Applicants are required to complete an EBR detailing professional activities undertaken as part of continuing professional education and continuing practice development as a mental health nurse.

CREDENTIALING OF NURSES WITHIN THE U.S. HEALTH CARE SYSTEM

The United States has well-developed credentialing and accreditation processes and systems in place in the nursing profession. While both credentialing and accreditation programs focus on quality and excellence, they are not synonymous in function and role. Credentialing is directed to the recognition of individual practitioner achievement and accreditation is the seal of approval of programs and/or organizations. For the purpose of this discussion, the focus will be on the credentialing aspects of quality recognition. Different organizations offer credentialing programs for nurses in specific specialty areas in the United States. They all have their distinct identity in the rendering of service. Three organizations are featured here for illustrative purposes.

The American Nurses Credentialing Center

The American Nurses Credentialing Center (ANCC), which is a subsidiary of the American Nurses Association, aims to promote excellence in nursing and health care globally through credentialing programs (ANCC, n.d.). It is the most significant nurse credentialing organization in the United States.

ANCC has established internationally renowned credentialing programs, which certify and recognize individual nurses in specialty areas. The organization also recognizes health care organizations for promoting safe and positive work environments and accredits continuing nursing education organizations. Under the umbrella of ANCC, the range of programs offered is:

- Accreditation program—This program recognizes the importance of high quality continuing nursing education and skills-based competency programs. ANCC accredits continuing nursing education service providers internationally. These organizations provide nurses with continuing professional development services to help them update their knowledge and skills to improve care and patient outcomes throughout their career span.
- Certification program—This program certifies and recognizes individual nurses in specialty practice areas and enables nurses to demonstrate their specialty expertise and validate their knowledge to employers and patients. Specialty exams incorporate the latest nursing practice standards, and ANCC certification empowers nurses to practice with pride and to achieve professional satisfaction.

- Pathway program—The Pathway to Excellence® Program recognizes a health care organization's commitment to creating a positive nursing practice environment. The Pathway to Excellence in Long Term Care™ program is the first to recognize this type of supportive work setting specifically in long-term care facilities. Pathway organizations focus on collaboration, career development, and accountable leadership to empower nurses.
- Magnet® recognition program—Health care organizations that achieve Magnet recognition have demonstrated nursing excellence and quality patient outcomes.

The National League for Nursing

The National League for Nursing (NLN, 2016) was the first nursing organization in the United States. It is the premier organization for nurse faculty and leaders in nursing education. Through its Commission for Nursing Education Accreditation (CNEA), it promotes excellence and integrity in nursing education at different levels of nursing education including diploma, associate's, bachelor's, master's, post-master's certificates and Doctor of Nursing Practice programs. For credentialing purposes, it offers the Certified Nurse Educator (CNE) credential.

The CNE credential establishes nursing education as a specialty area of practice and creates a means for faculty to demonstrate their expertise in this role. It communicates to students, peers, and the academic and health care communities that the highest standards of excellence are being met. A CNE credentialed nurse educator serves as a leader and a role model.

At the center of the CNE program is the CNE exam. To be deemed eligible to sit for this exam, nurse educators are required to meet both educational and experiential qualifications. In April 2016, NLN and CGFNS (Commission on Graduates of Foreign Nursing Schools) International, Inc. entered into partnership to enable qualified nurse educators across the globe to have access to the CNE credential.

Nurse educators, regardless of country of origin, must meet the criteria specified in one of the two options described below:

Option A: Must meet criteria 1 and 2
  1. Licensure
     A currently active, unencumbered, registered nurse designation in the country where currently practicing as a nurse educator.
  2. Education
     - A master's or doctoral degree in nursing with a major emphasis in nursing education or
     - A master's or doctoral degree in nursing plus a post-master's certificate in nursing education or
     - A master's or doctoral degree in nursing and nine or more credit hours of graduate-level education courses

Option B: Must meet criteria 1, 2, and 3
  1. Licensure
     A currently active, unencumbered registered nurse designation in the country where currently practicing as a nurse educator

2. Education
   A master's or doctoral degree in nursing (with a major emphasis in a role other than nursing education)
3. Experience
   Two years or more employment in a nursing program in an academic institution within the past 5 years

Pediatric Nursing Certification Board

The Pediatric Nursing Certification Board (PNCB, 2016), established in 1975, provides certification through a series of examinations for nursing professionals who care for pediatric populations. Nurses who are certified carry a body of knowledge that directly impacts patient outcomes. Qualified nurses can earn the credential designated in each of the following programs by passing the required examination:

- CPN (Certified Pediatric Nurse) certification—This certification is for registered nurses with extensive experience in pediatric practice who demonstrate knowledge and abilities related to pediatric nursing beyond basic RN licensure. Eligibility requirements include:
  a. A minimum of 1800 hours of pediatric clinical practice in the past 24 months or
  b. A minimum of 5 years as an RN in pediatric nursing *and* 3000 hours in pediatric nursing within the last 5 years with a minimum of 1,000 hours within the past 24 months
  c. A current, active, unrestricted RN license in the United States, Canada, or U.S. territory
- CPNP-PC (Certified Nurse Practitioner-Primary Care) certification—This certification is for graduates from master's degree or Doctor of Nursing Practice (DNP) degree programs or postgraduate certification programs for primary care Pediatric Nurse Practitioners (PNPs). Eligibility requirements include:
  a. Graduation from an accredited college or university that offers a ACEN (Accreditation Commission for Education in Nursing) or CCNE (Commission on Collegiate Education) accredited formal nursing master's or doctoral degree with a concentration in pediatric primary care as a NP or formal dual primary/acute care program or
  b. Graduation from a formal post-master's pediatric primary care nurse practitioner certificate program from an accredited college or university
  c. A current, active, unrestricted RN license in the United States, Canada, or U.S. territory
- CPNP-AC (Certified Pediatric Nurse Practitioner-Acute Care) certification—This certification is for graduates from master's or doctoral degree programs with a concentration in pediatric acute care as a NP. Eligibility requirements include:
  a. Graduation from an accredited college or university that offers a ACEN or CCNE accredited formal nursing master's or doctoral degree with a concentration in pediatric acute care as a NP or formal dual primary/acute care program or

   b. Graduation from a formal post-master's pediatric primary care nurse practitioner certificate program from an accredited college or university
   c. A current, active, unrestricted RN license in the United States, Canada, or U.S. territory.
 • PMHS (Psychiatric Mental Health Services) certification—This certification validates the added knowledge, skills, and expertise of Advanced Practice Registered Nurses (APRNs) in the early identification, intervention, and collaboration of care for children and adolescents with mental and behavioral health concerns. Eligibility requirements include:
   a. Graduation from an accredited college or university that offers a ACEN or CCNE accredited formal nursing master's or doctoral degree or
   b. Graduation from a formal post-master's program from an accredited college or university, with a concentration as a primary care PNP, an FNP, a family psychiatric NP, a child/adolescent psychiatric CNS, or a child/adolescent mental health CNS.
   c. A current, active, unencumbered APRN license issued by a U.S. state, U.S. territory, or Canada and current certification as an APRN in the role and population foci of primary care PNP, FNP, child/adolescent psychiatric and mental health CNS or psychiatric-mental health NP.

CREDENTIALING OF NURSES WITHIN THE UNITED KINGDOM'S HEALTH CARE SYSTEM

In the United Kingdom, the Royal College of Nursing (RCN) accredits a range of training programs and providers, while the Nursing and Midwifery Council sets the standards for nursing, midwifery, and health visiting care. The RCN follows a detailed process of accreditation, which includes systems for recruiting applicants to programs; registering and tracking applicants; and the collection and verification of evidence. The accreditation process involves peer review by expert representatives drawn from clinical, management, and educational fields of practice who have the appropriate professional background and experience (Coates, 2010). Examples of the programs accredited by the RCN include:

 • Clinical leadership program
 • Expertise and practice
 • Accredited facilitator
 • Mental health
 • Emergency nursing
 • Workplace accreditation
 • Standards for higher level practice for consultant nurses
 • Nursing and midwifery council practitioner programs

ADVANCED PRACTICE VERSUS SPECIALIZATION

Advanced practice versus specialization is increasingly emerging as an issue. As described, in New Zealand and Australia, credentialing recognizes the specialist expertise of registered nurses, but does not, however, refer to an advanced level of practice. Differentiation should occur between those registered nurses who are required to complete postgraduate programs in order to meet credential requirements. This level of educational preparation constitutes an advanced level of practice. The ICN network for advanced practice has been tackling these issues for many years through working with member countries. This process has facilitated an ongoing exchange of resources and information and helps ensure that ICN has the appropriate specialist advice.

DEFINITION

A Nurse Practitioner/Advanced Practice Nurse is a registered nurse who has acquired the expert knowledge base, complex decision-making skills and clinical competencies for expanded practice, the characteristics of which are shaped by the context and/or country in which s/he is credentialed to practice. A master's degree is recommended for entry level.

Source: ICN (approved 2002)

Characteristics

Educational Preparation

- Educational preparation at advanced level
- Formal recognition of educational programs preparing NPs/advanced nursing practice roles accredited or approved
- Formal system of licensure, registration, certification, and credentialing

Nature of Practice

- Integrates research, education, practice, and management
- High degree of professional autonomy and independent practice
- Case management/own caseload
- Advanced health assessment skills, decision-making skills, and diagnostic reasoning skills
- Recognized advanced clinical competencies
- Provision of consultant services to health providers
- Plans, implements, and evaluates programs
- Recognized first point of contact for clients

Regulatory Mechanisms—Country Specific Regulations Underpin NP/APN Practice

- Right to diagnose
- Authority to prescribe medication
- Authority to prescribe treatment
- Authority to refer clients to other professionals
- Authority to admit patients to hospital
- Legislation to confer and protect the title "Nurse Practitioner/Advanced Practice Registered Nurse"
- Legislation or some other form of regulatory mechanism specific to APRNs
- Officially recognized titles for nurses working in advanced practice roles (ICN, approved 2002)

AN OPPORTUNITY FOR GLOBAL PROCESSES AND PROCEDURES

Rising health costs and the concomitant need for high quality care have prompted the demand for APRN roles for a variety of health care services in the United States. The *Consensus Model for* APRN *Regulation: Licensure, Accreditation, Certification, and Education*—LACE (APRN Consensus Work Group & National Council of State Boards of Nursing APRN Advisory Committee, 2008) is a proposed solution to simplify and unify regulatory standards along the four major tenets of nursing education and practice with due attention to population focus specific to each role specialty. This *Consensus Model* has been endorsed by 48 organizations representing a variety of nursing professional and regulatory groups (National Council of State Boards of Nursing, 2010). This model allows for the alignment between education and practice to support the required synergy between theoretical constructs and pragmatic contexts for the preparation of APRNs. Using the consensus model as an example, harmonizing standards for preparing nurses for different roles and with different population foci could lead to a next milestone in recognizing nursing credentials on a global scale.

The feasibility of globally accepted competencies and education standards that remain locally responsive and achievable is being hotly debated. Some commentators argue that there is a need to establish transparent, standardized, and harmonized credentialing processes to ensure that migrating registered nurses can apply their skills and expertise more broadly than within their own country of education (Singh & Sochan, 2010).

Currently, there are no agreed upon standards across the globe for the awarding of nursing credentials. The ICN is in the midst of developing a new, stronger organizational structure that will lay the foundation for such standards. The comparability of the nursing credentials earned in one country to those of another country is determined using a process commonly referred to as the credential evaluation process. With the ongoing need in addressing nursing shortages and workforce sustainability, the challenge in evaluating the credentials of nurses migrating from source countries to destination countries cannot be overstated.

CGFNS International, Inc. was founded in 1977 to enable the evaluation of credentials that foreign-educated nurses earned in their respective home countries and to measure these credentials against the prevailing standards in the United States (CGFNS, 2016). Foreign-educated nurses are evaluated for eligibility to enter the United States for migration purposes. For an employment-based visa, nurses are evaluated via the VisaScreen®: Visa Credentials Assessment Services. Foreign-educated nurses whose credentials satisfy the eligibility criteria, meet English language proficiency standards, and pass the CGFNS Qualifying Exam® or the NCLEX® (National Council Licensure Examination) are issued a VisaScreen® certificate. For state licensure, nurses seeking migration can opt for the Certification Program, which is widely recognized across the jurisdictions. They can also avail themselves of the Credential Evaluation Service (CES) which provides an advisory report based on the analysis of their credentials.

Both the VisaScreen Program and the Certification Program are rooted in the tradition of certification as a method for a final determination of eligibility based on established standards (Shaffer & To Dutka, 2012, 2013). CGFNS uses the term "determinative" to signify that the adjudication of eligibility is final and that CGFNS certifies its certificate holders to have met the specified standards.

These nurses can then present their certificates to the respective authorities for processing and decision making.

The certification concept inherent in CGFNS's work for the past 40 years opens up opportunities for credentialing nurses for mobility in a fluid global environment. Thinking beyond the confines of credential evaluation as a mechanism to enable nurses to move from a source country to a destination country, credentialing as a recognition scheme through certification could be most empowering and facilitative for those who regulate as well as those who are being regulated. While jurisdictional oversight is critical to responsible and responsive care, a well-conceived and properly developed certification scheme could provide a basic credential in the form of a professional passport among countries desiring such facilitation.

Certification is about setting standards. It could conceivably serve as a platform for focusing on the core of nursing education and could provide a sound basis for conceptualizing educational standards that transcend jurisdictional boundaries. Certification as a construct may illuminate a path for building consensus around standards to provide ease in mobility of the nursing workforce.

The feasibility of applying consistent credentialing processes globally certainly needs to be examined from both a professional and a practical point of view. Education is linked to practice and the planning and delivery of care. In the case of nursing, the body of knowledge is continually growing and scopes of practice expanding. The health care system itself is complex and technology, medicines, and demands continue to change rapidly. At the core, confidence in a high-quality health care workforce that continues to be able to keep up with a fast-moving professional world, and to provide leadership within that world, is paramount.

The four case studies have illustrated that even between countries with many similarities, there are demonstrable differences, which could challenge any ability to apply consistent systems and processes with regard to credentialing. At a basic level, terminology differs among countries, and is not well understood. The terms "accreditation,"[1] "credentialing," and "certification,"[2] although connoting different shades of meaning, could end up being used interchangeably in the international scene (Coates, 2010).

In the examples of Australia and New Zealand mental health nurse credentialing, Australia's use of the term *credentialing* equates to New Zealand's term *certification*. Neither the Australian nor New Zealand example refers to an advanced level of practice; rather, they refer to the recognition of the specialist practice of experts. Confusion over terminology as well as over roles, scopes of practice, and professional boundaries of nurses in an international context has emerged in the literature (Duffield et al., 2009).

Both New Zealand and Australia have experienced changes over the last decade in their national registration processes. This has had a particular impact on mental health nurses, as up until these changes occurred, separate registrations were in situ for psychiatric nurses and they were deemed to be a nursing specialty by the fact of registration. Since 2003 in New Zealand and 2010 in Australia, these registrations have no longer been in place; thus, it became increasingly difficult to define and determine who was a mental health nurse, and confusion therefore occurred. Credentialing (Australia), and potentially, certification (New Zealand) are increasingly being seen as a way of determining who is a specialist mental health nurse.

The provision of services that are responsive to local needs is vitally important to ensuring the highest level of patient care. Providing services that ensure cultural needs and specificities are met is equally important, and it therefore becomes difficult to balance consistent processes while ensuring that services are responsive to local needs.

The application of any process or system needs also to be examined in practical terms, including legal considerations; international processes; costs; economic and political forces; marketing; minimum acceptable standards; stakeholder input; monitoring standards; and the feasibility of maintaining local, national, and global databases. An examination of international experience of credentialing enables an opportunity to establish that many of these issues exist, not only at a global level, but also within individual countries where different jurisdictions within a country have their own regional or state regulations and transferability between regions and states becomes problematic.

Under the current frameworks and rubrics, any attempts, therefore, to introduce a consistent transferrable credentialing process on an international platform could ultimately result in slowing down workforce mobility rather than enhancing it. Mutual recognition agreements that offer political solutions rather than knowledge-based solutions as the premise for mobility could be counterproductive. However, the use of certification as a methodology to ensure that an individual nurse meets a set of standards established by a duly constituted professional body could hold promise in opening up the dialogue and in reinventing the infrastructure for determining eligibility for mobility.

WHOSE ROLE TO ADMINISTER—REGULATORS OR THE PROFESSION?

A further emerging issue is the increasing debate regarding definitions and applications of "advanced practice" and "credentialing," and whether processes should be administered by regulatory organizations or by professional bodies.

> Understanding the balance between internal and external regulation is important for professionals because their regulatory systems are based on a subtle balance between these systems of control. The purpose of internal regulation (within the profession) is to ensure the advancement of nursing while serving the public interest: external regulation (outside the profession) exists chiefly to protect the public. (Joel, 2003, p. 392)

Credentialing can then play a part in internal regulation, as it is based on expert peer opinion, knowledge, and processes. In the United States, the lines do become blurred as the regulatory bodies (nursing boards) use credentialing (certification exams) as a requirement or proxy for advanced practice licensure. Thus, in the United States, advanced practice certification would be viewed as a mechanism for "public protection."

International trends show a changing emphasis in the roles of regulatory bodies. They are having an increased role in standard setting and competency assurance, but some jurisdictions are reducing their focus on advocacy and enhancement of the profession. Regulatory bodies are also experiencing a reduced role in the accreditation of nursing programs.

CONCLUSION

Credentialing is an important tool, which offers an opportunity to formally recognize that a practitioner is providing a safe, high-quality health care service within specific environments. It builds on the regulatory bodies' requirements for registration, and thus provides a more specific context of practice for specialty areas. This clarity for both employers and consumers is important, as our health care environments are more mobile and more complex, and more specialized nursing skills are being demanded on an international platform.

It is important that professional organizations in nursing be the bodies to provide the platform for credentialing. Many multinational organizations provide credentialing/accreditation/certification services, and nurses are rightly wary of being incorporated into processes that create profit for multinational groups or are equated to the same processes used in product industries. For smaller countries, we need to reach across the globe to nursing organizations that can assist and provide services to others. This then can enable nursing to provide wider, stronger networks across the globe, and nurses can become a true borderless workforce within a credentialed framework.

Today the same challenges still exist that were highlighted by Styles (Styles & Affara, 1997). Terminology and processes need to be consistent, credible, and culturally appropriate and have integrity and cultural nuances, and issues need to be addressed in any processes.

As the 21st century situates itself in the global age, the right of anyone to work anywhere, anytime, is at the forefront of consciousness of this generation across the professions. Mobility and migration will continue to increase. As individual nurses seek employment in locations that best serve their purpose, the need for certification as a credentialing mechanism will continue to grow. As human talents meet demands in the global marketplace, the sustainability of tomorrow's workforce is shaped by the credentialing processes and mandates that are in place today. The nursing profession shall rise to the challenge and apply knowledge-based solutions to recognize competence through credentialing and to balance human aspirations with meeting urgent health care needs across the globe.

DISCUSSION QUESTIONS

1. *What do you see as the benefits for practice in being credentialed?*
2. *Is credentialing just about advanced practice?*
3. *Why is there still difficultly in defining advanced practice?*
4. *What else is needed in the policy and regulatory environment to assist the development of credentialing?*
5. *What policy changes at the state and federal level in the United States could impact the credentialing process and impede or improve progress?*
6. *Compare and contrast credentialing for APRNs across the four roles and then using two or three countries from around the world.*
7. *Select two countries and use the four components of LACE to see how the components affect the advanced practice roles in those countries.*
8. *What factors impede global credentialing efforts?*

NOTES

1. Accreditation = the process for formally recognizing services and providers by establishing a set of standards.
2. Certification = the formal recognition that an individual meets set standards established by a professional body.

REFERENCES

American Nurses Credentialing Center. (n.d.). About ANCC. Retrieved from http://www.nursecreden tialing.org/About-ANCC

APRN Consensus Work Group & National Council of State Boards of Nursing APRN Advisory Committee. (2008). Consensus model for APRN regulation: Licensure, accreditation, certification, & education. Retrieved from https://www.ncsbn.org/Consensus_Model_for_APRN_Regulation_ July_2008.pdf

Australian College of Mental Health Nurses. (2011). What is credentialing? Retrieved from http://www .acmhn.org/credentialing/what-is-credentialing.html

CGFNS International, Inc. (2016). CGFNS International, Inc. Retrieved from http://www.cgfns.org

Cioffi, J. P., Lichtveld, M. Y., Thielen, L., & Miner, K. (2003). Credentialing the public health workforce: An idea whose time has come. *Journal of Public Health Management and Practice, 9*(6), 451–458.

Coates, C. (2010). *Accreditation, certification and credentialing in mental health nursing: A review of selected literature.* Report prepared for the Ministry of Health and the New Zealand College of Mental Health Nurses Te Ao Māramatanga.

Duffield, C., Gardner, G., Chang, A. M., & Catling-Paull, C. (2009). Advanced nursing practice: A global perspective. *Collegian: The Australian Journal of Nursing Practice, Scholarship and Research, 16*(2), 55–62.

Gendek, M. (2011). Recognising specialist mental health nurses—A national success. Retrieved from http://www.acmhn.org/credentialing/what-is-credentialing.html

International Council of Nurses. (n.d.). Definition and characteristics of the role. Retrieved from https:// international.aanp.org/Practice/APNRoles

International Council of Nurses. (2013). The credentialing and regulators forum. Retrieved from http://www.icn.ch/pillarsprograms/the-credentialing-forum

International Council of Nurses. (2016). Nurse practitioner and advanced practice registered nurses, defined. Retrieved from http://www.icn.ch

Joel, L. (2003). *Kelly's dimensions of professional nursing.* New York, NY: McGraw-Hill.

National Council of State Boards of Nursing. (2010). Campaign for APRN consensus. Retrieved from https://www.ncsbn.org/APRN_Consensus_Model_with Appendix_A_updated.pdf

National League for Nursing. (2016). National league for nursing. Retrieved from http://www.nln.org

Newton, S., Pillay, J., & Higginbottom, G. (2012). The migration and transitioning experiences of internationally educated nurses: A global perspective. *Journal of Nursing Management, 20*(4), 534–550.

Oakley-Brown, M. A., Wells, J. E., & Scott, K. M. (Eds.). (2006). *Te Rau Hinegaro: The New Zealand mental health survey.* Wellington, New Zealand: Ministry of Health.

Pediatric Nursing Certification Board. (2016). Pediatric nursing certification board. Retrieved from http://www.pncb.org

Royal College of Nursing Australia. (2011). International council of nurses credentialing forum 2011. Country Paper: Australia. Retrieved from https://www.acn.edu.au

Shaffer, F. A., & To Dutka, J. Y. (2012). Perspectives on credential evaluation: Future trends and regulatory implications. *Journal of Nursing Regulation, 3*(1) 26–31.

Shaffer, F. A., & To Dutka, J. Y. (2013). Global mobility for internationally educated nurses: Challenges and regulatory implications. *Journal of Nursing Regulation, 4*(3).

Singh, M. D., & Sochan, A. (2010). Voices of internationally educated nurses: Policy recommendations for credentialing. *International Nursing Review, 57*(1), 56–63.

Styles, M. M., & Affara, F. A. (1997). *ICN on regulation: Towards 21st century models.* Geneva, Switzerland: International Council of Nurses.

Te Ao Māramatanga & New Zealand College of Mental Health Nurses. (2013). Credentialing. Retrieved from http://www.nzcmhn.org.nz/Credentialing

CHAPTER 29

Advanced Practice Nursing: The Global Perspective

David Stewart, Frances Hughes,
Judith Shamian, and Moriah Ellen

The roles of Advanced Practice Registered Nurses (APRNs) have been in existence globally and under discussion in many countries for more than 50 years. The role has developed differently as a result of the different political, cultural, professional, and health environments. While developed countries like the United States, Canada, and others have made progress in introducing the roles through legislation, regulation, and education, in many countries the roles of APRNs and nurse midwives have not been formalized. The roles have not been developed to the level that the nursing community thinks will best serve global health and the citizens of the world. However an opportunity exists for the roles to be embedded and developed as a cornerstone to every health system. Under the UN Sustainable Development Goals (SDGs), all UN Member States have agreed to try to achieve universal health coverage (UHC) by 2030. This includes financial risk protection, access to quality essential health care services, and access to safe, effective, quality, and affordable essential medicines and vaccines (World Health Organization [WHO], 2016b). This level of services cannot be obtained without further development and investment in nursing roles such as APRNs.

This chapter describes some of the background work in this area by the International Council of Nurses (ICN), the WHO, and others. Furthermore this chapter discusses some of the efforts that have to be undertaken to build a universal recognition and implementation of the role for the benefit of both nursing and the public.

GLOBAL CONTEXT

What does "APRN" mean in the global community? Since 2002, the ICN (2002) has used this definition:

A nurse practitioner/advanced practice nurse is a registered nurse who has acquired the expert knowledge base, complex decision-making skills and clinical competencies for expanded practice, the characteristics of which are shaped by the context and/or country in which she or he is credentialed to practice. A master's degree is recommended for entry level.

Since this time, the definition has been debated and scrutinized. Some have suggested that the definition has led to international confusion regarding the role of APRNs. The reason for this confusion is that the APRN can take on multiple roles in the global community. It is an umbrella term in which there can be multiple roles and titles such as Nurse Specialist, Clinical Nurse Specialist (CNS), Clinical Nurse Consultant, Nurse Practitioner (NP), nurse anesthetist, nurse consultant, and nurse-midwife, and even APRN. Internationally there is no consistency among the titles in regard to the education, regulation, or practice requirements. This makes it difficult to enable comparison or transferability of practice among countries. To address this issue, the ICN is in the process of developing a guidance paper on APRN. As a result of this work, it is anticipated that there will be improved global understanding of APRN to further develop the role and improve the implementation. While the evolution of APRN roles in acute care is relatively recent, there has been a long history of the role in primary health care (PHC). While the development of the APRN concept and the evolution of the role started at a country level over the last few decades, both ICN and WHO have developed several documents that are meant to guide and support the thinking and development of the role on an international basis. The ICN has historically focused on the APRN role and its multiple facets across the entire continuum of care. This work has been highly influential on the strategies that the WHO has incorporated to meet the current and future challenges related to health and health care provision.

In 2016, the WHO released its "Global Strategic Directions for Strengthening Nursing and Midwifery: 2016–2020" (WHO, 2016a), which was informed by the ICN. A core strategy to achieve the global mandates such as UHC and the SDGs was to support the progress and implementation of APRNs. The strategy recognizes the importance of nurses to transform the way health actions are organized and how health care is delivered.

ICN AND WHO: A PERSPECTIVE ON THE APRN ROLES

The International Council of Nurses: APRN Network

Over the past few decades ICN has recognized the need to have a global nursing voice and shared agreement among the nursing community to articulate the elements associated with the APRN role. ICN has established a formal network for APRNs that can be found at the following URL: www.icn-apnetwork.org. The ICN continues to support the network and is currently engaging with the APRN community to strengthen its role and influence.

There is considerable variability across the world in regard to the APRN. For example, the nurse anesthetist APRN role is seen within Canada and the United States and several other countries globally. The role exists in other countries but not necessarily at the APRN level. For example in Africa, nurse anesthetists can be found in the Democratic Republic of Congo, in Tunisia, and more. In Asia the role is in place in Taiwan, Cambodia, and a few other countries. In the Caribbean countries the role exists in Jamaica and some other countries in the region. In 1989 the International Federation of Nurse Anaesthetists was formed and currently 41 countries are members (www.ifna-int.org).

While the concept of nurse midwives has been in existence for a long time, with or without the APRN designation, in many of the countries the concept of a community-based NP, acute care NP, CNS, and APRN in anesthesiology are virtually unknown. Furthermore while in many of the countries, nurses prescribe and do other clinical care that often is in the realm of an APRN in developed countries, there is no regulatory, educational, or infrastructure in place to recognize the role as an advanced role that builds on the role of the registered nurse (RN).

With such variability and differences, the work of the ICN's NP/APRN Network (INP/APRNN) offers the information and tools that go beyond one country's experience and help nurses, nursing organizations, policy makers, and others in each country to benefit from the richness of knowledge and information of other country-level policies and practices.

Clarifying the Role of the APRN

Among the world nations it is common that similar terms are being used for different purposes. It is important to clarify the meaning of a term. For example in some countries the reference to CNS is about an individual that has private clients can prescribe and diagnose. In other countries the very same term means a nurse with advanced preparation who provides professional support to practicing clinical nurses. Also, in other countries the two definitions above are blended so that the CNS could have private clients, prescribe, diagnose, and at the same time address nursing and system-level issues so that quality and safety are maximized. As you can see these are seemingly divergent definitions and practices.

The work that ICN has undertaken helps with understanding the role of the APRN regardless of what the person is called. This is achieved through clarifying the scope, competencies, roles, and responsibilities of an APRN on an international level.

The ICN (2005) defines the APRN scope of practice as:

> The cognitive, integrative, and technical abilities of the qualified nurse to put into practice ethical and culturally safe acts, procedures, protocols, and practice guidelines. The clinical practice of the APN is scientifically based and applicable to healthcare practice in primary, secondary, and tertiary settings in all urban and rural communities. The role also encompasses the dimensions of patient and peer education, mentorship, leadership, management and includes the responsibility to translate, utilize, and undertake meaningful research to advance and improve nursing practice. (p. 3)

Furthermore the document created by the ICN (2005) outlines what the APRN can do. The activities that an APRN can undertake include diagnosis, prescribing, initiating treatment, and more. What is essential to understand is that the APRN can do all of these within an independent scope of practice. In many of the countries that do not have a legal, regulatory, and educational framework nurses can often be found engaging in similar activities but they do it under medical delegation or without any legal and/or professional authority. Some countries do not yet have a basic "nursing act" to govern the practice and the title protection of a nurse. In those countries the practice is carried out by individuals who are considered nurses in those countries although some have had only a little academic preparation or on-the-job training.

In an effort to increase the quality and standard expectations for APRN practice, the ICN documents also clearly articulate that competencies of APRNs are built on the RN competencies and must be within a regulatory framework. Again the challenge in the majority of developing countries and some of the developed countries is that there are no regulatory frameworks in place for APRN practice and no standards or competencies defined in regulation. Furthermore, in some countries the registration as a nurse happens at the government level and often happens once in a lifetime and is not renewed on a regular basis. This brings into question the ongoing competence of the nurse. In a growing number of countries there are efforts under way to establish an independent, regulatory body whose mandate is to regulate nurses and where the licensing and regulation of APRNs should happen.

All nursing practice should be regulated (licensed and/or credentialed) (Benton & Morrison, 2009). Nursing regulatory bodies determine the requirements for license, codes of ethics and/or conduct in order to protect the public. Nursing competencies and/or standards for practice developed or recognised by regulatory bodies determine education and scope of nursing practice within defined legislative and regulatory framework. Through national (or state) nursing standards of practice, nursing demonstrates to the public, government, employers, and other stakeholders that nursing is committed to delivering quality and safe health care (Maier & Aiken, 2016). Nursing professional standards determine the level of education and describe the competencies (knowledge, skills, and judgement), professional accountabilities and responsibilities of nurses qualified to practice at different levels within a particular license. In the near future, ICN will seek to provide further clarity about the foundations on which APRN is built. ICN has commenced the development of a Professional Practice Framework for Registered Nurses. It is recognized that the context of nursing practice varies in different parts of the world. It is also acknowledged that the profession is dynamic, with changes to education, regulation, and practice as it seeks to respond to the health needs and changes to health care provision. This framework will seek to promote a common understanding of RN practice for the public, governments, health professionals, policy makers, and educators and within the profession. As such, this piece of work will provide an improved understanding of the RN, the foundation upon which the APRN sits.

The educational preparation of the APRN internationally varies significantly and can be grouped under several categories. The first category consists of those countries that have legislation in place to govern APRN practice and have a regulatory body to designate the title, to qualify individuals, and to provide clear standards that govern the educational programs that lead to APRN licensing. The second category are those countries that do not have the formal structure described and can fall into different subcategories. For example, a number of countries have "academies" and/or "specialty interest groups" with some of these countries having formal educational programs such as educational preparation to become a nurse-midwife, a community nurse, or other roles. The final category is where the functions and the advanced role that nurses assume are a result of necessity in the field and are self-taught knowledge or a result of on-the-job training. In most developed and developing countries there are an insufficient number of APRNs prepared at the graduate level to meet the standards described by ICN as the desired level of educational preparation.

Having the ICN documents that outline the competencies, standards, roles, and expectations of APRNs is extremely important and helps nurses and the governments of countries know how to move forward if there is the political and the professional will to do so. The standards and core competencies are expected to provide a foundation and broad guidelines for APRNs and contributing authorities all over the world. The expectation is that they will then develop this role within their own countries while meeting the established professional, authorized, and regulatory frameworks and requirements.

WORLD HEALTH ORGANIZATION: PRIMARY HEALTH CARE

In 2008, the WHO celebrated its 60th anniversary (soon to be its 70th) and the 30th anniversary of the Declaration of Alma-Ata on PHC (WHO, 2008). The principles underlying the declaration are still relevant today, and there is wide recognition that the principles can provide the basis for health care policy reform in many countries for the coming years. The intent and the spirit of the Alma-Ata Declaration was to have global access to primary care for ALL by the year 2000. That goal was not attained but there was significant progress in many countries. WHO and the international community reaffirmed that the essence of primary health care (PHC) services is essential in building healthy and productive societies.

Nurses and midwives embraced the Alma-Ata Declaration of 1978 and have been strong proponents of the principles that guide it as evidenced by the rapid re-orientation of professional training and transformation of nursing and midwifery practice to support PHC. With the renewed emphasis on PHC, the Office of the Nurse Scientist at WHO, together with the WHO's Global Advisory Group (GAG), have renewed their efforts to accelerate nursing's involvement and contribution to PHC. The compendium of case studies illustrating successful PHC initiatives, *"Now, more than ever; Nursing and midwifery contribute to primary health care"* (WHO, 2009), gathered by the Office of Nursing and Midwifery at the WHO, illuminates that the contribution of nurses and midwives to PHC is substantial and their experience is valuable. Examples from the compendium illustrate how nurses and midwives have contributed in all the new reform areas (case studies can be located at www.who.int/hrh/nursing_midwifery/documents/en/index.html).

WHO and many other organizations including ICN recognized that the way to global health is through PHC. The reality hit when the year 2000 came and went and the goal of "Health for ALL by 2000" was not accomplished. Several global meetings were held to review accomplishments and revitalize efforts to accelerate the attempts to build comprehensive global PHC. The 2008 WHO report dealt with the renewal of PHC and why it had not been achieved. The WHO Global Advisory Group (GAG), was established in the 1990's to make recommendations to the Director General (DG) of WHO on nursing and midwifery issues. The group also studied how nursing can accelerate its contribution to global PHC. GAG fully embraced the PHC renewal and, under the leadership of Dr. Jean Yang, the Chief Nurse Scientist of the time, undertook a tremendous amount of work to demonstrate the role and contribution that nurses generally, and NPs in particular, can make to PHC.

Examining the WHO website will provide the reader with some major documents that have been published through the past couple of decades. WHO reports worth examining further include: WHO Commission on Social Determinants of Health (SDH) *Closing the Gap in a Generation* (WHO, 2008), which describes how social factors such as poverty have an impact on the health of a population. The document identifies how new knowledge and understanding of the interrelationship of many societal variables have been observed and health is seen partly as a product of societal situations (www.who.int/social_determinants/the commission/finalreport/closethegap_how/en).

The consistent theme that emerges in evaluating the global challenges when dealing with health issues is that policy makers failed to put in place the required policies. The report urges policy makers, in health and other areas, to rise to the challenge of improving social conditions instrumental in securing health. Placing the responsibility for lack of success squarely on the shoulders of policy makers, the Commission of Social Determinants of Health champions PHC as a model that acts on the underlying social, political, and economic causes of ill health. APRNs could contribute to a lot of these issues as their proposed competencies address their abilities to do community assessment, planning, and interventions. The Millennium Development Goals (MDGs; WHO, 2011) called for the attainment of nine focused goals by 2015. Among the nine were goals to reduce infant and maternal mortality and the strengthening of health systems through renewed PHC. It was clear that PHC systems were and still are a critical component to improving health on a global scale. The MDGs did much to improve the lives of millions of people around the world. However the gap between the rich and the poor continues to grow. To address this issue, the UN has developed the SDGs. The SDGs aim to address inequalities between nations and within nations by focusing on a broader list of issues such as inequality, poverty, climate change, hunger, education, and health.

In 2017, the ICN has focused on Nurses as a Voice to lead in achieving the SDGs in its International Nurses Day (IND) publication. The publication celebrates the role nurses are playing in achieving the SDGs, but it also calls for governments and other key stakeholders to further invest in nursing, particularly APRN roles, as a means of countries meeting their agreed upon targets.

Another important document is the WHO report *Primary Health Care: Now More Than Ever* (WHO, 2008b), which revisits the 1978 Alma-Ata Declaration principles of PHC and considers the revision of the principles in light of new knowledge and 30 years of experience. In the report, new observations and learning since Alma-Ata are incorporated into the new reforms, particularly knowledge based on the social determinants of health and the MDGs.

The WHO report (2008) maintains that as societies modernize, people increasingly want to have a say in important decisions that affect their lives, including issues such as allocation of resources and organization and regulation of care.

THE ROLE OF NURSES AND MIDWIVES IN THE ALMA-ATA RENEWAL

In 1992, the World Health Assembly adopted resolution WHA45.5 on "Strengthening Nursing and Midwifery in support of strategies for Health for all"—urging the DG to establish an advisory group, which he did in 1992. The Global Advisory Group of Nursing and Midwifery (GAGNM) is thus an advisory group responsible for advising the DG on policies supporting nursing and midwifery development in WHO member states.

The DG at a meeting with GAGNM in March 2009 stated "the challenge of 'PHC/Health For All' was that key stakeholders were not involved early enough resulting in multiple definitions of the concepts, especially by professionals. For this renewal, nursing and midwifery and other health professionals should be involved."

The GAG communicated with the WHO DG that GAGNM recognizes the importance of WHO regional nursing and midwifery programs that support progress toward the achievement of health-related MDGs, particularly through improving the quality of nurse and midwife education post-qualification level. Furthermore WHO should support countries in maximizing/expanding the scope of practice of nurses and midwives. This could lead to the establishment of APRN roles using legislation, education, and regulation.

Continued international efforts and commitments being made toward improving global nursing and midwifery workforce strategies are important. The Kampala declaration and agenda for global action (2008) and the WHO Regional Office for the Western Pacific Strategic plan for strengthening health systems (2008) both call for greater government commitment to improving the health care workforce and enhancing the collection and use of reliable Human Resources for Health (HRH) data in making informed policy decisions. With continued global backing for the improvement of the health care workforce, it is hoped that international health outcomes will improve and global health targets will be met.

The 2008 Chaing Mai Declaration was made by over 700 health care professionals including nurses, doctors, midwives, and other interested stakeholders from 33 countries in the six regions of WHO. The participants were at the International Conference on New Frontiers in Primary Health Care: Role of Nursing and Other Professions. An excerpt from the declaration is provided next.

We declare that:

Nursing and midwifery is a vital component of the health workforce and are acknowledged professionals who contribute significantly to the achievements of PHC and the MDGs.
Nurses and midwives can successfully lead health teams that are essential for successful PHC to achieve MDGs.
PHC and the MDGs will not be fully achieved if the nursing and midwifery workforce continues to be neglected.
Key PHC policy decisions, at all levels, must involve nursing and midwifery leaders for effective and informed decision-making. (WHO, 2008a, p. 1)

The recommendations of this declaration call on policy makers to recognize and include nurses in decision making and planning for PHC. It also calls for legislation and educational systems to be put in place to prepare the necessary health care professionals.

UNIVERSAL HEALTH COVERAGE

In 2014, the WHO and its member states agreed to a resolution on Universal Access to Health and UHC (WHO, 2016b). This means that all people regardless of sociocultural, organizational, economic, geographical, and gender-related contexts can receive access to health care services. It also means that health systems must have in place the capacity to meet the needs of populations at any level of care, providing the infrastructure, adequate human resource capacity, and health technologies without causing financial harm. These strategies build on the basic human right that all people should be able to enjoy a healthy life.

At the sixth Global Forum for Government and Midwifery Officers in 2014 (WHO, 2014), a statement was released noting the fundamental need for continued support and evolution of the nursing role to meet the demands of UHC. It stated that nurses and midwives are critical to respond and manage the health needs of people. Nurses and midwives are the frontline professionals who use an integrated and comprehensive approach including health promotion, disease prevention, treatment, rehabilitation, and palliative care. Ten strategies around leadership and management, education and training, and collaborative partnerships were agreed upon in order to support the attainment of UHC. The progress of these strategies has not been released to date; however a real opportunity exists for APRNs to demonstrate their value in the achievement of UHC.

THE REALITY ON THE GROUND

The role and the concept of APRNs in the PHC setting is several decades old. In some of the developed countries, which will be referred to as the Organization for Economic Co-Operation and Development (OECD), countries like the United States and Canada, the role, scope, regulation, education, and practice are established but continuously evolving. The establishment of these roles came about through much research and advocacy. The same advocacy and policy push by the nursing community existed and continues to exist in several of the OECD countries to introduce and/or increase the use and availability of APRNs.

The concept of an APRN for PHC is extremely important in the low- and middle-income countries (LMC) but takes on a different meaning. In the LMC countries outside of the urban setting far too often the nurse is the primary clinician and for periods of time the only clinician. Often this person is the nurse, the midwife, the generalist, the specialist, and maker of clinical decisions. So she or he prescribes, orders tests, sutures, delivers babies, comforts those who are in need, and much more. In these circumstances the notion that there is room for a different class of practitioners on top of the nurse is great but not realistic. The key challenge for policy makers, educators, providers of fiscal resources, and the health care community, including nursing leadership, is to identify in a comprehensive manner how capacity can be built to provide the nurse with APRN knowledge and/or access to APRNs virtually.

This issue is a serious one that raises significant debates within the nursing community. Some are of the opinion that we need to advocate for the same

Western-OECD level of health care, roles, and functions because everyone should have the right to the same health care. Philosophically and ideally the ICN is in full support of these ideas. The reality is that most maternal child deaths, much of the infectious diseases, and a growing number of NCD (noncommunicable diseases, chronic diseases) can be found in much higher proportion in the LMC than in the OECD countries. Therefore we need to improve the health of the population as quickly as possible while attending to raising the scope, role, education, and research levels of health professionals and nurses in the LMC.

So What Is the Reality on the Ground?

The reality is that many RNs that work in rural communities work in the capacity of APRN without the regulatory designation and often without the desired knowledge and tools. In some countries the frontline "nurse" is not an RN but has some other designation and education level. While that is not the desired reality they still are the frontline people that deal with clinical emergencies and often they are the only one in the field. The more common reality is that there are RNs and some are RN Midwives that have gone through additional training to enhance their midwifery skills but do not have the APRN designation and level of knowledge and competencies of an APRN.

The OECD conducted a survey on APRN roles in 2009 (Delamaire & Lafrotune, 2010). The countries that participated were organized under two groups: The first group were countries with experience with APRNs, including Australia, Canada, Finland, Ireland, United Kingdom, and the United States. These countries have led the charge in building the APRN roles and getting the required infrastructure and continue to be at the forefront in pushing the boundaries and challenging the possibilities and opportunities for the roles. The second group had less experience with the APRN roles and included Belgium, Cyprus, Czech Republic, France, Japan, and Poland. These countries are distributed among three continents. The interest in the APRN role goes beyond the North American and European regions; furthermore while all these countries are members of OECD, there are different levels of country development. Countries like Poland and the Czech Republic are more recent members of OECD, versus countries like Ireland, the United States, Canada, and others who have been considered to be "developed countries" for a while. The survey results found that APRNs do two broad types of activities.

1. *Substitution:* Services formerly provided by doctors, reduce workload of doctors, improve access to care, and reduce cost.
2. *Supplementation:* New services (e.g., quality improvement), CNSs with the main aims: improve services/quality of care.

The survey findings indicate that the greatest impacts on patient care made by APRNs were in the areas of access to care, quality of care by doing some primary care as first contact for minor illnesses, and that patients were as satisfied with the APRN care or more satisfied than the care by physicians.

A study in 2016 by Maier and Aiken reviewed task shifting from physicians to nurses in primary care across 39 countries. Out of the 39 countries, 27 countries had a form of task shifting from physicians. The study recognized that globally there were reforms on policy, regulation, and education, particularly in the area of nurse prescribing. The study showed that there is an evolving trend internationally toward expanding nurse's scope of practice in primary care.

APPLICATION OF APRN PRACTICE: COUNTRY-LEVEL EXAMPLES AND DISCUSSION

Each country's experience in establishing the role of the APRN is different; often countries need to make compromises to start the role and then continue to advance the role to the optimal level of education, funding, practice, and legislation. To demonstrate this point let us explore the experience in Jamaica and the Caribbean.

The APRN role, which is called APRN, started in Jamaica in 1977 with a certificate jointly approved by the Ministry of Health and the Faculty of Medical Sciences (FMS), University of the West Indies (UWI). From the inception of the program the UWI School of Nursing, Mona (formerly Advanced Nursing Education Unit, UWI) has been responsible for curriculum development, monitoring, selection of entrants for the program, and the examination process. The dean of FMS and the permanent secretary, Ministry of Health, jointly signed the certificates for graduates.

In 2002 the program was fully transferred to the UWI with the support of the government of Jamaica. The existing certificate curriculum was upgraded and approved to a master's degree status reflecting global trends in advanced nursing practice. The master of science in nursing (MScN) for APRN is offered over five semesters. It is offered full-time and part-time.

FAMILY NP (DELIVERED AT UWI)

The credit load for the family NP is 45 credits. Applicants must be RNs and midwives and have at least 5 years current clinical practice. Applicants must have 3 years post-RN licensure/registration for Nursing Administration, Nursing Education, and CNS; and 5 years post-RN licensure/registration clinical practice as RNs in an approved recognized agency, institution, or organization where primary, secondary, tertiary, or Extended Health Care services are offered. In 2009 a new track was introduced in gerontological nursing.

CNS—GERONTOLOGY TRACK

This new track produces a cadre of nurses prepared at the advanced clinical level to provide evidence-based care to elderly persons along the wellness illness continuum at the primary, secondary, and tertiary levels of care. They will be prepared to deliver advanced nursing care in the clinical and functional areas of nursing practice. In the year 2013 only graduates from Barbados were employed as CNSs.

NPs practice in the following countries in the Caribbean Region: Antigua, Bahamas, Barbados, Dominica, Jamaica, St. Kitts, St. Lucia, Montserrat, St. Vincent, and the Grenadines. They are employed in various settings, such as government services, health centers and clinics, accident and emergency units, army, private practice, and school health (Drs. Whinney-Dehaney & Hewitt, personal communication, June 2013; Seivwright, 1982a, 1982b).

Another example that demonstrates the effectiveness of the APRN role is outlined by some comments from the government chief nurse in Zimbabwe, Mrs. Cynthia, MZ Chasokela. During a meeting hosted by WHO in Kenya in 2009 Mrs. Chasokela identified that she has been very successful in moving forward the health care and nursing agenda in her country. She described the role of nurses in PHC as community education and training in use of appropriate technology; early detection and correct diagnosis of illness and disability; effective treatment and management of conditions; routine health care work including data collection, processing, and its use for planning and decision making at the level of collection; and many more of the responsibilities often identified as part of the competencies of an APRN. She was referring to individuals with the preparation and designation of APRN as defined and recognized in some of the countries like the United States and Canada that have the education, legislation, and regulatory framework for APRNs. While many of the countries recognize the need for more advanced preparation and the need for APRNs, there is not the political climate that will allow for it to happen. These two examples clearly demonstrate the different ways that the nursing community and others advance the APRN role for the benefit of the population and the advancement of the profession.

The other area of evolution that has taken shape over the last decade and accelerated with the MDGs is the role of midwives. Historically nurses in many countries, primarily the former British colonies, as RNs went through a 12-month to 18-month specialty training to become nurse midwives. In the United States the nurse midwifery designation is considered to be at the APRN level. This is not the case in other countries. Nurses in some countries like the United Kingdom can be licensed both as nurses and midwives under two separate regulatory bodies and they do not have to keep their nursing license in order to maintain their midwifery license. The more recent trend and pressure by the International Council of Midwives (ICM) is to build direct entry programs to midwifery without having a nursing designation. This issue creates a lot of international controversy and is not supported by many in the nursing community. There is no debate about the issue that midwifery is an advanced role but whether it is a separate profession or is part of the nursing APRN role is in dispute.

To understand the issues and impact of country-specific needs for APRNs one needs to understand the country context, regulation, role of government, role of other non-nursing organizations, education system, and overall environment. The readiness of the population to consider these roles is also an essential element. This is at varying levels globally and it may be a significant amount of time before we could attest globally to a common understanding of the APRN roles.

BARRIERS TO APRN ROLES

Although the contributions APRNs make to the health of the population and the positive impact they have is clear and well documented, the existence of the role is not widespread, and even in those countries that have achieved the legislation, funding, and preparation of the APRN roles, these achievements have come only through many years of struggle and political activism. The question to be asked is why there are so many barriers to establish and implement a role that can be so useful to the health of people. The barriers mostly relate to the traditional tension between the medical and nursing profession and lack of role clarity of the different roles of APRNs and others. For example, the likelihood that the South American countries and some of the Middle East countries have a strong presence of APRNs is limited because of the high ratio of physicians per population. Until recently there were two to three doctors per nurse. Current policies are in development that are trying to even out the doctor–nurse distribution. While the APRN role is different than an MD role, the overlap is perceived to be sufficient to pose a threat to the medical profession. Politicians are reluctant to embrace an agenda that will meet stiff opposition from any major interest group. Physicians globally are considered a very strong interest group (Delamaire & Lafrotune, 2010; Pulcini, Jelic, Gul, & Loke, 2010).

Furthermore, funding is another barrier to the establishments of APRN roles. Governments, insurance companies, and other funders are hesitant to add new categories of professionals that can charge for services. National Human Resource Plans often do not include the national plan for APRNs. Lack of Educational funding and dedicated faculty to establish APRN programs are additional barriers.

The biggest barriers are often the lack of advocacy by the nursing community, and the lack of the organized nursing community to educate the public of the value and importance of the APRN role to advance the health of the nation. The health care provider community has been engaged in the discussion of the importance of teamwork, and collaboration among nurses, APRNs, doctors, and more might lead to better appreciation of the different roles and removal of some of the resistance to the APRN roles.

To resolve and/or minimize these barriers nursing groups, health care groups, the public, and government should work together. Strengthening the concept of a team education of health care professionals and team practice is one way to help the future health care professionals to gain role clarity and respect for each other's work. In the LMCs where there are too few nurses, midwives, doctors, and others, the ability to bring APRN roles to communities can make a very strong impact on the health of the community. Governments should accelerate the passing of legislative and regulatory frameworks to facilitate the APRN roles and provide the funding frameworks for both education and practice.

CONCLUSION

The need for APRNs is global. One can argue that the current reality is the inverse. In those countries where there are tremendous health care needs like in the LMC and in high-risk communities and population the need for qualified, well-prepared APRNs is tremendous, but the current reality is that those countries are most likely to require infrastructure, education, and regulation that allow and encourage the creation of APRN roles. Most often APRNs, the needed infrastructure, education, regulation, and positions can be found in the OECD countries where the burden of disease is lower.

At the same time, there are insufficient resources (both financial and human) to build an APRN system similar to those that currently exist in the OECD countries. All countries could benefit from a well-established APRN community. It is important to have a global image, plan, advocacy, agenda, and more to achieve the desired availability of APRNs. But there also needs to be a recognition that there are skills and competencies that reside in the APRN roles at some of the OECD countries that are urgently needed in the LMC. That is the challenge and the international community and the international nursing and health organizations like ICN, WHO, and International Monetary Fund must support the development of the roles and services.

DISCUSSION QUESTIONS

1. *Should APRNs practice under legislations and regulations that are unique and focused on the APRN role?*
2. *What should be the role of international nursing organizations in advancing the uptake to the APRN role?*
3. *What should be the role of global organizations like WHO and others in advancing the role of APRNs?*
4. *Compare and contrast the Social Determinants of Health report by WHO from 2008 to the health care regulations/changes of the Affordable Care Act (ACA) being faced by the United States Congress. Where does the United States excel and where does it need more focus and work? With relation to these two documents, in what areas have APRNs in the United States had influence and impact?*
5. *Why is the APRN role more formalized in the developed countries?*
6. *What can be done to remove barriers to the APRN role internationally?*
7. *What contributions can the APRN role make to the health of international communities in need?*

REFERENCES

Benton, B. C., & Morrison, A. (2009). *Regulation 2020: Exploration of the present; vision for the future* [Position statement]. Geneva, Switzerland: International Council of Nurses Clinical Nurse Specialists, Canadian Nurses Association.

Delamaire, M. L., & Lafrotune. G. (2010). Nurses in advanced roles: A description and evaluation of experiences in 12 developed countries. *OECD Health Working Paper* No. 54. doi:10.1787/5kmbrcfms5g7-en

International Council of Nurses. (2002). Definition and characteristics of the role. Retrieved from https://international.aanp.org/Practice/APNRoles

International Council of Nurses. (2005). Scope of practice, standards and competencies of the advanced practice nurses. Retrieved from http://international.aanp.org/content/docs/scopeandstandards withwatermarkrevisedwithintro1.doc

International Council of Nurses. (In Press). *Nursing care continuum framework and competencies.* Retrieved from https://siga-fsia.ch/files/user_upload/07_ICN_Nursing_Care_Continuum_Framework_and_Competencies.pdf

Maier, C. B., & Aiken, L. H. (2016). Task shifting from physicians to nurses in primary care in 39 countries: A cross-country comparative study. *European Journal of Public Health, 26*(6), 927–934. doi:10.1093/eurpub/ckw098

Pan American Health Organization. (2008, October 16–17). *Conference conclusions and recommendations.* From the International conference dedicated at the 30th anniversary of the Alma-Ata Declaration on primary health care. Almaty, Kazakhstan.

Pulcini, J., Jelic, M., Gul, R., Loke, A. Y. (2010). An international survey on advanced practice nursing education, practice, and regulation. *Journal of Nursing Scholarship, 42,* 31–39. doi:10.1111/j.1547-5069.2009.01322.x

Seivwright, M. (1982a). Nurse practitioners in primary health care, the Jamaican experience, part 1. *International Nursing Review, 29*(1), 22–24.

Seivwright, M. (1982b). Nurse practitioners in primary health care, the Jamaican experience, part 2. *International Nursing Review, 29*(2), 51–59.

World Health Organization. (2008a). The Chaing Mai Declaration: Nursing and midwifery for primary health care. Retrieved from http://www.who.int/hrh/nursing_midwifery/chiang_mai_declaration.pdf

World Health Organization. (2008b). The World Health Report 2008: Primary health care (now more than ever).

World Health Organization. (2009). *Now, more than ever: Nursing and midwifery contribute to primary health care.* Compendium of Primary Health Carestudies. Geneva, Switzerland: Author.

World Health Organization. (2011). *Global status report on noncommunicable diseases 2010.* Geneva, Switzerland: Author.

World Health Organization. (2014, May 14–15). *Nursing and midwifery workforce and universal health coverage: Forum statement.* Presented at the WHO global forum for government chief nursing and midwifery officers, Geneva, Switzerland. Retrieved from http://www.who.int/hrh/events/22May2014ForumStatement.pdf?ua=1

World Health Organization. (2016a). Global strategic directions for strengthening nursing and midwifery 2016–2020. Retrieved from http://www.who.int/hrh/nursing_midwifery/global-strategic-midwifery2016-2020.pdf?ua=1

World Health Organization. (2016b). Universal health coverage: Sustainable development goal 3. Retrieved from http://www.who.int/universal_health_coverage/en

World Health Organization, Commission on Social Determinants of Health. (2008). *Closing the gap in a generation: Health equity through action on the social determinants of health.* Geneva, Switzerland: Author.

CHAPTER 30

The Future for Nurse Practitioners

Jan Towers

Nurse Practitioners (NPs) have been around for just over 50 years. Until recently, they were the "babies" of the health professionals. They have come far and accomplished much in the short period. It has become clear that there was a need for NPs and that they have filled a significant gap in the health care world. That gap has continued to grow and so has the need for NPs.

HISTORY

In the 1960s a projected shortage of primary care providers (physicians) stimulated a search for alternative paths for providing primary care services to the citizens of the United States. That, combined with a proliferation of medics returning from the Vietnam War, stimulated an effort to expand the training of people other than physicians for the provision of primary care services. Coupled with this innovative thinking was the increasing awareness that the contribution of primary prevention, wellness programs, and a focus on patient-centered care could improve the health of the country. Examining the opportunities these conditions provided, it became clear that nurses could make a major contribution to meeting this need by expanding the scope of health care to the preventive domain. As a result, in a number of states such as North Carolina and Maryland, public health nurses began to physically assess patients coming into their well-baby and women's health clinics.

Recognizing the tremendous need and the opportunity for nurses to make a contribution in this scenario, Loretta Ford and Henry Silva, both faculty at the University of Colorado, entered into a cooperative partnership to provide primary care to children by preparing nurses to provide primary care services to pediatric patients in Colorado. The program graduated its first class of pediatric NPs in 1965 (American Academy of Nursing [AAN], 1999). The program was a success, and the role of the NP began to expand to include women's health, followed by family, adult, and geriatric care, all with great success. It was a concept whose time had come.

Initially, there were certificate programs developed through a variety of entities including continuing education programs from schools of nursing and medicine, hospitals, and other continuing education venues. As the idea of nurses providing these essential primary care services expanded, the federal government became interested in supporting the preparation of NPs and began to provide grants for the development of formal NP educational programs in the academic framework of graduate nurse education. With the provision of financial support, universities became interested in opening formal programs of study and nursing education undertook the formalization of graduate education programs to prepare NPs, first at the master's level and now at the doctoral level. This was not undertaken without controversy. The nursing community did not endorse the "expanded" role initially and worried that nurses would once again become the "handmaidens" of physicians as they took on "traditional medical activities" such as diagnosing and treating illnesses. Opposing articles were written in the major nursing journals, and NPs were often not supported by nurses in the workplace. Interestingly, the physician community was more supportive and actively participated in the early educational endeavors to prepare NPs. It was not until after the late 1990s when NPs were authorized to provide and be paid for Medicare services that organized medicine began to resist the contributions NPs could make to the provision of health care in this country.

THE CURRENT SITUATION

Now we have entered another period when a monumental shortage of health care providers is evident. With the passage of the Patient Protection and Affordable Care Act (PPACA) in 2010, one of the goals was to provide health coverage for all Americans. In 2013 there were over 41.8 million people without health insurance. This number decreased to 33 million in 2014 showing some impact (U.S. Census Bureau, 2015). Although the numbers are decreasing with the passage of the PPACA, added health care providers are necessary. NPs were and are ready to contribute to the reduction of that shortage and have been working diligently to remove barriers that prevent them from doing so.

The barriers that exist at this writing include the outdated scope-of-practice laws in some states and obsolete payment barriers at the state and federal levels. Historically, state governments control the scope of professional practice. The federal government, states, and, to a certain extent, commercial insurance carriers control payment for medical/health care services.

Scope-of-practice laws, more commonly known as practice acts, are based on state statute and regulation. They are the basis for licensure of members of the health care professions such as medicine and nursing, as well as attorneys and other service providers such as beauticians and funeral directors. Changes in scope of practice require the amending of the scope-of-practice laws within each state. As a result change in NP scope of practice has occurred state by state over the years. Efforts to build consistency from state to state, as well as to implement scope-of-practice laws that authorize NPs to practice to the full extent of their education and clinical preparation have led to the development of a stakeholder consensus document and model practice act that describes the educational preparation, national certification, and scope of practice for all APRNs, including NPs. This document has served as the basis for consistent change, recognition, and authorization of NP practice.

At this writing, 21 states and the District of Columbia have achieved plenary (full practice) authority, authorizing NPs to assess, diagnose and treat (including prescribing medication) without the supervision of another health care provider (American Association of Nurse Practitioners [AANP], 2015). (Note: This differs from "independent practice" which may or may not involve supervision or collaboration.) The remainder of the states authorize NPs to assess, diagnose and treat with some collaborative or supervisory relationship with physicians. NPs' diagnosis and treatment includes the prescription of legend drugs as well as controlled/scheduled drugs in all 50 states and the District of Columbia. Except in seven states (Arkansas, Florida, Georgia, Louisiana, Oklahoma, South Carolina, and West Virginia) NPs are authorized to independently prescribe Schedule II–V Drug Enforcement Agency controlled drugs that require federal authorization to prescribe. Arkansas and Missouri are limited to hydrocodone combination products from the Schedule II list. The remaining five states are authorized to prescribe Schedule III–V independently (Drug Enforcement Agency, n.d.). NPs are educationally prepared and able to provide the full range of primary care services to their patients.

Most recently Congress passed legislation that authorizes NPs who prescribe Schedule III–V drugs to be waivered along with physicians to provide medication assisted treatment (MAT) for opioid addiction. After completing required special education for the treatment of opioid addiction, they, like the physicians, are authorized beginning in early 2017, to treat up to 30 patients for the first year and then petition to increase the number of patients to 100 in subsequent years. (Comprehensive Addiction and Recovery Act, 2016)

Obsolete statutes and regulations in the reimbursement realm create access problems for patients. Considering certain provisions in Medicare law alone, the inability for NPs to order home health, order and supervise outpatient cardiac and pulmonary rehabilitation, admit patients to skilled nursing facilities (SNFs) and rehabilitation centers, order diabetic shoes, prosthetics and orthotics, to name a few examples, continue to create problems for safe, high quality, patient care. Although some progress has been made, such as removal of durable medical equipment (DME) barriers, expanding the ability to admit patients to hospitals and order and supervise cardiac rehabilitation in hospital settings, there is still a lot to be done. Removal of those barriers listed earlier alone would facilitate prompt care and reduction of secondary complications and stretch the dollars available for Medicare services.

Likewise obsolete statutory and regulatory language limiting a variety of services of the scope of NP practice to physician-only performance creates unnecessary barriers to the fulfillment of a variety of services as simple as required physical examinations, the ordering and coverage of services associated with chronic diseases such as chronic obstructive pulmonary disease (COPD) and diabetes, all well within the scope of practice for NPs. While NPs have been able to overcome a vast number of hurdles, lifting these additional barriers will significantly improve the profession's ability to provide needed care.

THE FUTURE

NPs have a long history of documented high quality, cost-effective care despite the barriers still to be overcome. In just a little more than 50 years, they have moved from a small group of pediatric NPs to greater than 220,000 (83% of whom are primary care providers) and growing (AANP, 2015; Goolsby, 2011).Their rate of growth is exceeding that of primary care physicians. Their acceptance among patient populations has grown by leaps and bounds (AANP, 2012a, 2012b; Newhouse et al., 2012). Increasingly, policy experts have recognized the contribution NPs can make to the health and well-being of the public, and interestingly, the media is reinforcing that worth and value.

So what should the future bring? As further steps are taken to implement new legislation, the need for health care providers expands. This applies to primary as well as specialty care. NPs have been the underpinning of primary care services to the underserved in rural and urban communities for years; their skill in providing care to the elderly and the chronically ill has been well documented. As our population grows and becomes older, the need for their services in this realm will increase significantly.

As new models of care develop, NPs have extensive opportunity to provide leadership in their development and implementation. Their nursing and primary care roots provide them with the skills that can make the new models work as they are implemented.

NEW MODELS

Medical Home

The "medical home model" is the traditional framework for NP practice. Accessible, holistic, safe, high quality personalized care, the hallmarks of the medical home, have always been the basis of NP practice. NP practices should be the cornerstone of this model, giving guidance to the health care community in its development. This model has, at the behest of the physician community, become certifiable. Entities such as National Committee for Quality Assurance (NCQA; 2016) and The Joint Commission (2016) have developed standards for the recognition of medical home practices. These standards are used to certify the eligibility of primary care practices for recognition and reimbursement in a variety of programs including Medicare and Medicaid; NP practices are eligible for recognition under these standards as medical homes (Joint Commission, 2016; NCQA, 2016; URAC, 2016). As the requirements for this model of care become the basis for inclusion and reimbursement in health care programs (public and private), it is important for NPs to be sure that their practices, wherever they are, meet these standards and are recognized as medical homes.

Accountable Care Organizations

The growth of accountable care organizations (ACOs) spurs incentives for the provision of high quality, cost-effective care. Through the practice of shared facilities, service and communication, the goals of ACOs are best met through the inclusion of NPs who have already demonstrated their worth in the realm of providing high quality, cost-effective care. Studies of Healthcare Effectiveness Data and Information Set (HEDIS) reports, use of quality indicators, and other outcome studies all demonstrate that NPs will be an asset in ACOs, whether as clinicians in a member practice or clinic, a NP practice, or a NP-owned and/or led ACO (AANP, 2012b).

Transitional and Coordinated Care

Studies have demonstrated that care coordination and follow-up care post-hospitalization reduce the number of hospital admissions. The usage of NPs in the provision of these services elevates the quality of these fundamental nursing activities with significant results. NPs should be expected to serve as clinicians as well as practice owners and managers in the provision of both transitional and coordinated care in the community. They are well prepared to provide these services with a high level of knowledge and expertise (Naylor et al., 2004).

Long-Term Skilled Nursing Care and Home Care Nursing Services

NPs are particularly well qualified to provide primary care services and medical oversight in SNFs, nursing facilities (NFs) and home nursing care programs. Their knowledge regarding the diagnosis and management of chronic illness as well as acute disease prepares them well to treat and keep patients out of hospitals, avoid complications, and maintain the quality of life for patients in these settings. The holistic approach to care provided by NPs is key to the well-being of patients under their care in both long-term NFs and home health care services (AANP, 2012a; Newhouse et al., 2011).

Quality Payment Program

With the passage of the Medicare Access and CHIP Reauthorization Act of 2015 (MACRA) the opportunity for NPs to become full and equal partners in the provision of patient-centered quality care through the Quality Payment Program (QPP) has come to fruition. With the repeal of the sustainable growth rate (SGR) billing method, NPs will be full participants in the QPP that uses various quality indicators to demonstrate their care and patient outcomes to determine their payment for services. NPs have been able to contribute to the program as it was developed and are fully capable of undertaking the requirements for participation at a high level in the program as it develops (Centers for Medicare and Medicaid Services, 2016).

It is clear that NPs are the primary care stars of the future. Their combination of nursing and medical knowledge and expertise, and their ability to integrate the two into the care they provide, as well as their expertise in the areas of health promotion and disease prevention, make them the ideal providers for the management of both acute and chronic disease and the maintenance of health in patients of all ages and walks of life.

As their numbers grow, NPs continue to provide high quality care in ever expanding settings. They have grown from a small number of clinicians providing care for children to experts in providing care to all ages and types of patients. They are the primary care providers of the future. As today's barriers are further removed, they are even better able to share their skills in the communities where they reside. Currently over 75% of NPs practice in primary care and more than 6,000 of them report that they have their practices (AANP, 2012a).

Will NPs expand their settings to include hospitals and specialty care settings? There is already evidence of the successful usage of NPs in these areas (Kleinpell & Goolsby, 2012). As models of care continue to develop, it is projected that NPs will provide increased leadership and service in these settings as well.

CONCLUSION

It is important for NPs to be at the table as new models of health care are developed, to serve as leaders in the exploration and development models that can keep the nation and the world healthier and active. It has taken a relatively short time for NPs to demonstrate their ability and their worth. If we are to have a high-level system of health care, it is important for them to take a leadership role in the development of a safe, high-level health care system for the future. The abilities are there, a bright future is waiting for NPs in both primary and acute care, but they must stay active and involved not just in the provision of care coming to them in their practices but in the development of health care policy for the future.

DISCUSSION QUESTIONS

1. *Investigate the concept of medical homes in more depth and, based on the information you find, develop an action plan for implementing the model in practice. What federal requirements need to be followed? What kind of documentation must be kept?*
2. *Which of the new models of care identified in this chapter would best fit the practice in which you are involved?*
3. *Review the components of the QPP and show how they might be applied to your area of practice or interest.*
4. *Consider the model of transitional or coordinated care and develop a practice for the care of one of the following: chronic cardiac patients, chronic diabetics patients, or chemotherapy patients.*
5. *Explore changes in NP practice should the PPACA be repealed. Which components of the PPACA have more of an impact on NP practice and reimbursement than others?*
6. *Consider the state board regulations affecting NPs in your state. What needs to change for you to be able to practice to the full extent of your education and training?*

REFERENCES

American Academy of Nursing. (1999). Living legends. Retrieved from http://www.aannet.org/about/fellows/living-legends

American Association of Nurse Practitioners. (2012a). *Position statement: Nurse practitioners in primary care.* Austin, TX: Author. Retrieved from https://www.aanp.org/images/documents/publications/primarycare.pdf

American Association of Nurse Practitioners. (2012b). *Position statement: Quality of nurse practitioner practice.* Austin, TX: Author. Retrieved from https://www.aanp.org/images/documents/publications/qualityofpractice.pdf

American Association of Nurse Practitioners. (2015). *Nurse practitioner prescriptive authority (map).* Retrieved from https://nursinglicensemap.com/advanced-practice-nursing/nurse-practitioner/nurse-practitioner-prescriptive-authority

Centers for Medicare and Medicaid Services. (n.d.). Quality Payment Program. Retrieved from http://www.qpp.CMS.gov

Comprehensive Addiction and Recovery Act of 2016, 42 USC 201 (2016).

Drug Enforcement Agency. (n.d.). Drug schedules. Retrieved from http://www.justice.gov/dea/druginfo/ds.shtml

Goolsby, M. J. (2011). 2009–2010 AANP national practitioner sample survey: An overview. *Journal of the American Academy of Nurse Practitioners, 23*(5), 266–268.

Joint Commission. (2016). Website. Retrieved from http//www.JointCommission.org/accreditation/pchi/aspx

Kleinpell, R. M., & Goolsby, M. J. (2012). American Academy of Nurse Practitioners National Nurse Practitioner Sample Survey: Focus on acute care. *Journal of the American Academy of Nurse Practitioners, 24*(12), 690–694.

Medicare Access and CHIP Reauthorization Act of 2015, 42 USC 1305 (2015).

National Committee for Quality Assurance. (2016). Website. Retrieved from http//www.ncqa.org/programs/recognition/patient centered medical home

Naylor, M., Brooten, D. A., Campbell, R. L., Maislin, G., McCauley, K. M., Schwartz, J. S. (2004). Transitional care of older adults hospitalized with heart failure. *Journal of the American Geriatrics Society, 52,* 675–684.

Newhouse, R. P., Stanik-Hutt, J., White, K. M., Johantgen, M., Bass, E. B. Zangaro, G., . . . Weiner, J. P. (2011). Advanced practice nurse outcomes 1990–2008: A systematic review. *Nursing Economic$, 29*(5), 230–250; quiz 251.

Newhouse, Weiner, J. P., Stanik-Hutt, J., White, K. M., Johantgen, M., Steinwachs, D., . . . Bass, E. B. (2012). Policy implications for optimizing advanced practice registered nurse use nationally. *Policy, Politics, & Nursing Practice, 13*(2), 81–89. Retrieved from http//ppn.sagepub.com/content/early/2012/08/29/1527154412456299

URAC. (2016). Website. Retrieved from http//www.urac.org

U.S. Census Bureau. (2015, September 16). Income, poverty and health insurance coverage in the United States: 2014. Release Number: CB15-157. Retrieved from http://www.census.gov/newsroom/press-releases/2015/cb15-157.html

CHAPTER 31

What the Future Holds for Clinical Nurse Specialist Practice and Health Policy

Sharon D. Horner

The Clinical Nurse Specialist (CNS) is an Advanced Practice Registered Nurse (APRN) prepared at the master's or doctoral level. The CNS role was originally established in the 1960s under the direction of Hildegarde Peplau at Columbia University to prepare APRNs who would provide care to persons with psychiatric and mental health problems (Spray, 1999). This new master's-level program demonstrated the high quality of care and improved patient outcomes that can be achieved by nurses with advanced practice preparation in a specialty. Taking their cue from this successful program, other colleges and universities started their own master's programs to prepare CNSs as psychiatric/mental health APRNs, and this quickly evolved to include other specialty tracks. In fact, the CNS was the first APRN role to be developed and CNS programs have always been at the graduate level—in accredited master's or doctoral programs.

The CNS is an expert clinician who works in a specialized area of nursing practice. According to the National Association of Clinical Nurse Specialists (NACNS; 2012a), "the specialty may be identified in terms of a population (e.g., pediatrics, geriatrics, women's health); a setting (e.g., critical care, emergency room); a disease or medical subspecialty (e.g., diabetes, oncology); a type of care (e.g., psychiatric, rehabilitation); and/or a type of health problem (e.g., pain, wounds, stress)" (p. 185). CNSs provide both direct and indirect care to complex and vulnerable populations in a variety of health care settings. Typically, these patients are those experiencing complex chronic or multiple chronic conditions (i.e., dual-diagnoses) and require both primary and specialty nursing care. CNSs practice in a wide variety of health care settings providing expert nursing services across the continuum of care (acute or critical inpatient care, rehabilitation, and ambulatory care). In addition, they influence the care provided to patients by consulting with nursing staffs and by implementing processes to improve health care delivery systems (Patten & Goudreau, 2012).

GOALS FOR IMPROVING PATIENT AND POPULATION HEALTH	BOX 31.1

- Work to achieve the triple aim of improving access to care, promoting preventive health care, and reducing health care costs
- Increase the effectiveness of transitioning care from hospital to home or other care settings and prevent readmissions
- Improve the quality and safety of care and reduce health care costs
- Support policies that enable CNSs to practice to the full extent of their education and training
- Appraise data to assess system progress and evaluate outcomes of care
- Maintain awareness of policy and regulatory changes that affect health care practice, health care delivery, and health care reimbursement models
- Participate as a fully contributing member of interprofessional health care teams to improve health outcomes of patients and the population

CNS, Clinical Nurse Specialist.

In recent years, there has been a convergence of initiatives aimed at improving health care delivery and health outcomes. Two key initiatives are the Institute of Medicine's (IOM) report on *The Future of Nursing: Leading Change, Advancing Health* (2011) and the Affordable Care Act (ACA). Health care policies and regulations have been developed in response to each of these key initiatives. However, there is another recurring regulatory activity the U.S. government undertakes and that is the Standard Occupational Classification (SOC) system to review the classifications of all professions. Each of these initiatives is discussed in terms of how it affects CNS practice. Box 31.1 is a summary of CNSs' goals to improve the health of patients and the health of the population.

AFFORDABLE CARE ACT

The ACA is comprised of two acts: the Patient Protection and ACA and the Healthcare and Education Affordability Reconciliation Act. Both acts were signed into law by President Barack Obama on March 23, 2010 (Cady, 2012). The triple aim of the ACA is to improve access to care, promote preventive health care, and reduce health care costs (Hynds, Hatch, & Samuels, 2014). The initiatives in the ACA focus on reducing policy-based barriers to health care access (e.g., remove insurance clauses related to preexisting conditions), establishing processes to encourage people to enroll in insurance plans that are required to provide preventive health care visits and cover screenings, and initiating processes that reward quality of care and health outcomes rather than rewarding quantity of care (Abara & Heiman, 2014; Cady, 2012). The U.S. Department of Health and Human Services (USDHHS) states the overarching goal of these policies is to assist the physicians, hospitals, health care organizations, and other health care professions by focusing on the needs of patients and aligning payments to outcomes (USDHHS, 2016).

Many ACA initiatives are designed to improve primary care services; other initiatives focus on improving patient outcomes, safety, and quality of care across the spectrum of health care delivery (Orr & Davenport, 2015). In November 2011, the Centers for Medicare and Medicaid Services (CMS) established the Shared Savings Program: accountable care organizations (ACOs) as a provision in the ACA to improve the quality of health care (CMS, 2016; DHHS, 2016). An ACO is a group of health care providers, agencies (e.g., hospitals, rehabilitation centers, outpatient clinics), and other health care–related businesses (e.g., insurers) working together to design and provide coordinated high-quality care for patients. ACOs operate on an incentive payment system based on shared savings that aligns quality performance to the payment received (CMS, 2016). When services are coordinated and not duplicated, the quality of health care delivery improves and patient outcomes improve. There are five specific domains identified that affect patient care, each with defined quality measures that are used to determine the reimbursement metrics for ACOs. In the 2016 Reporting and Performance Requirements, there were 33 quality measures listed for each of the five domains that include the patient or caregiver experience of care; care coordination; patient safety; preventative health screenings; and at-risk populations (CMS, 2016).

Currently, Medicare has several different programs to rate the quality of care provided by doctors and other clinicians. These programs include the Physician Quality Reporting System, the Value Modifier Program, and the Medicare Electronic Health Record (EHR) Incentive Program. Congress moved to streamline this process by creating the Medicare Access and CHIP Reauthorization Act of 2015 (MACRA) that was signed into law on April 16, 2015 (Haycock, Edwards, & Stanley, 2016). This legislation's purpose is twofold. It repealed the Medicare Part-B sustainable growth rate reimbursement formula and introduced a value-based reimbursement system called the Quality Payment Program (QPP). The QPP has two tracks for reimbursement: The Merit-Based Incentive Payments System (MIPS) and the Advanced Alternative Payment Models. Health care providers are assigned by the MACRA system into one of these two tracks. Most Medicare providers are assigned to the MIPS track (Clough & McClellan, 2016). Under MIPS, health care providers can choose measures and activities that fit the type of care they provide. They will be assessed on four MIPS performance categories: cost, clinical practice improvement activities, quality, and advancing care information. The MIPS score is a measure of the overall care delivered and serves as the basis for determining the Medicare quality-based payments made to health care providers (Haycock et al., 2016).

Fewer health care provider groups are assigned to the Advanced Alternative Payment Models that include projects that are CMS Innovation Center models or are part of Shared Savings Program tracks. In addition, other demonstration projects have been statutorily authorized where the health care provider group delivers well-designed high-quality and efficient care for a specified payment fee and the group accepts the risk of losing money if the delivered care costs more than the allocated payment. These demonstration projects are designed to reward high quality, efficient, and therefore cost-effective processes (Haycock et al., 2016). MACRA lays out specific criteria for determining what would qualify for the advanced Alternative Payment Model.

Implications for CNS Practice

APRNs have opportunities as the various initiatives of the ACA are implemented and health policies developed (Haycock et al., 2016). The language used to describe the health care practitioner in the ACA was "practitioners" and "providers" rather than "physician" so that APRNs can be recognized as part of the health care clinician group. The scope of practice for each APRN is determined by his or her individual state board of nursing practice (Henderson, Princell, & Martin, 2012).

Health policy is built on research, evidence-based practice, guidelines, and innovation. Health policy encourages input of the different disciplines of health care, government, and the public. The health policy landscape and structure are being laid based on the impact from many quality and patient safety initiatives. CNSs are well suited to influence health policy due to their work and focus on quality, safety, and outcomes (patient, nursing, and organizational).

Health care today is rapidly evolving and CNSs need to be involved in health policy to make their value and contribution to health care known, integrated, and supported. Support can be accomplished in many ways: through legislation that defines the scope of CNS practice in a favorable manner (e.g., to allow the CNS to practice to the full extent of the person's education [IOM, 2011]), inclusion of CNSs in reimbursement policies and inclusion in federal and state health care exchanges. CNSs historically have been involved in shaping the quality and patient safety initiatives of health care and thus are well positioned to shape health policy. One of the barriers that CNSs encounter is that at times their involvement has been too silent. Now is the time for CNSs to demonstrate their value and contributions to the health care systems and share how they positively impact delivery of care to the public.

The CNS can play a significant role in the new reimbursement models that are being developed as part of ACA initiatives. The reimbursement models are designed to incentivize health care clinician groups to undertake continuous quality improvement practices (Haycock et al., 2016). The CNS is educated in the three spheres of influence: (a) to provide care directly to patients and their families, (b) to improve health care delivery by educating staff and consulting on complex patient health care problems, and (c) to implement thoughtful and rigorous evidence-based approaches to improve health care system functioning (Delp et al., 2016; Mayo, Harris, & Burton, 2016; National CNS Competency Task Force, 2010).

The CNS has been educated in the art of systematically assessing processes, identifying barriers or challenges to be overcome, designing evidence-based solutions, guiding the health care team through the process of change, and evaluating the processes and outcomes of these changes (Mayo et al., 2016). This work is iterative and leads to continuous quality improvement. These activities can be sources of data to address the four MIPS performance categories of cost, clinical practice improvement activities, quality metrics, and advancing care information (Haycock et al., 2016). The impact CNSs have on these health care initiatives is based on the long-standing focus CNSs have always had on patient safety, quality of care, and cost-effectiveness that makes the current political, social, and economic climate the perfect time for the CNS to flourish.

TRANSITIONS IN CARE

The ACA also provided authority to section 1115A of the Social Security Act to establish the CMS Innovation Center and the Community-Based Care Transitions program (Newhouse, Barksdale, & Miller, 2015). Under the ACA, health care delivery will continue to evolve with greater emphasis on an ambulatory care delivery model (Orr & Davenport, 2015). The transition of care from hospital to outpatient setting is typically characterized by fragmentation of care. Today, hospitalized patients have higher acuities but shorter hospital stays because they are discharged to complete their recovery in other settings (Logue & Drago, 2013). In response, the ACA established the Community-Based Care Transitions Program to provide funding to support models of health care delivery across systems of care (Naylor, Aiken, Kurtzman, Olds, & Hirschmann, 2011).

The CNS plays an important role in assisting patients in their transitions in care. "Care transitions describes a continuous process in which a patient's care shifts from being provided in one setting of care to another, such as from a hospital to a patient's home or to a skilled nursing facility and sometimes back to the hospital" (Burton, 2012, p. 1). Transitions in care also include the goal of the most optimal placement of the patient based on his or her care needs. Coordination of care is integral in managing effective transitions in care, redesigning discharge from the hospital, and ultimately improved planning and communication to all care providers along the continuum of care for the patient (Laker, 2011). Effective transitions in care may help reduce health care expenditures, improve patient outcomes, increase patient satisfaction, and decrease readmissions to the hospital (Burton, 2012).

Currently, many transitions in care programs have been developed under the ACA of 2010; these were designed to help manage chronically ill patients in the safest, most cost-effective manner without compromise on quality of care (Naylor et al., 2011). CNSs have been providing transitions in care with patients with chronic diseases. When transitions in care are managed, the outcome for patients is improving quality of life and ultimately decreasing readmissions (Lovelace et al., 2016). This management of transitions of care is a perfect match for the CNS. In one way the CNS can develop a comprehensive discharge planning process based on his or her specialty (e.g., heart failure, COPD, asthma, epilepsy, diabetes); through these plans, CNSs follow patients' posthospital discharge in management of patients' symptoms, lifestyle, and other care aspects to prevent readmission to the hospital. A pilot telehealth consultation program implemented with APRNs providing assessment, diagnosis, and management of patients in rural long-term care facilities significantly reduced unnecessary hospital admissions and led to substantial cost savings estimated at $5 million over 3 years (Hofmeyer et al., 2016). Moore and McQuestion (2012) examined studies that included CNSs in the delivery of patient care to those individuals with chronic diseases. They found increased patient satisfaction, improved patient and spousal quality of life, shorter lengths of hospital stay, longer time between hospital readmission and fewer hospital readmissions, and lower costs when the CNS provided the intervention (Moore & McQuestion, 2012).

Implications for CNS Practice

Critical to the success of these initiatives are advanced nursing care practices designed to improve patient outcomes and reduce hospital readmissions (Lovelace et al., 2016). The CNS is well positioned to make critical contributions to improve the health of patients across the continuum of care by improving nursing care delivery, preventing complications, and reducing unnecessary costs (Delp et al., 2016; Hynds et al., 2014). The CNS works to ensure that the patient and family have the necessary knowledge, skills, and resources to manage care during recovery and ensures a successful transition from hospital to other care settings (Orr & Davenport, 2015).

Transition to home is a critical point in our health care system because patients and their families are feeling overwhelmed by the volume of information related to care at home, the need to perform new behaviors and at the same time deal with symptoms and fatigue of the patient's altered health state (Logue & Drago, 2013). Transitional care programs have been and continue to be developed by CNSs to provide supportive care to patients as they move between hospital and home or to extended care (Baldwin, Black, & Hammond, 2014). These CNS-led interdisciplinary transitional care programs demonstrate improved health outcomes, quality of care, and reduced hospital readmissions.

IMPROVE QUALITY AND SAFETY OF CARE AND REDUCE HEALTH CARE COSTS

Improving clinical outcomes for patients and families is, and has been, the work of the CNS. CNSs provide innovative, evidence-based, quality nursing care within their specialty. The CNS provides the leadership in assessment, development, implementation, and evaluation of programs that focus on care of a specialty population (Delp et al., 2016; National CNS Competency Task Force, 2010). In the ACO value-based payment model, patient access to care is improved, thereby improving health especially for those who are at high risk (e.g., persons who previously delayed seeking care, persons with complex and multiple chronic conditions), and better alignment of health care services with health care needs can reduce the costs of care (Vu, White, Kelley, Hopper, & Liu, 2016). Not only are cost-effectiveness, quality, and patient safety looked at as an outcome in health care, but so is patient satisfaction. This is also known as *value-based purchasing*. These are all central components of the core competencies held by the CNS. CNSs can assist through their leadership and knowledge of outcomes and patient-centered care. The leadership of the CNS is seen in leading the health care team and implementing evidence-based changes to reduce complications (Delp et al., 2016; Vu et al., 2016). CNSs can set and achieve best practices, improve patient and/ organization outcomes, and decrease health care costs. CNS practice reduces health care cost through many avenues; for example through reducing length of stay, reducing frequency of emergency room visits, increasing patient satisfaction, and reducing complications of hospitalized patients (Delp et al., 2016; Hofmeyer et al., 2016; Lovelace et al., 2016). CNSs who practice within the intensive care units have reduced the length of stays in the ICU and reduced hospital-acquired conditions (e.g., ventilator-associated pneumonia, central line infections, pressure ulcers) (Delp et al., 2016).

CNS work is also accomplished through system redesign in relation to quality and patient safety. Noting that between 44,000 and 98,000 patients die in hospitals annually due to practice-based errors, it is imperative that system redesigns are implemented to achieve patient safety (Gandhi, Berwick, & Shojania, 2016). The focus has shifted from preventing errors to reducing and preventing harm from occurring. This is truly a work of the CNS through systems leadership; consultation; coaching; collaboration; interpretation, translation, and use of evidence; and evaluation of clinical practice. CNSs have led initiatives that have significantly reduced hospital-acquired infections, injuries due to falls, central line bloodstream infections, and ventilator-associated pneumonias (Delp et al., 2016).

System redesign is accomplished through planned change, implementation of evidence-based practice, and utilization of synthesized research. CNSs are clinical expert leaders of change within organizations. They facilitate quality and safety in many ways, design and implement evidence-based programs. The programs CNSs are involved in are to prevent avoidable complications, improve the quality of care, improve the safety, prevent readmission to the hospital, reduce the length of stay, increase patient satisfaction, improve patient outcomes and reduce health care costs (Delp et al., 2016; NACNS, 2012b). CNSs need to share their innovations, tools that improve quality and patient safety with the community at large, not just within their discipline. The types of programs and initiatives that CNSs implement can help shape health policy, set standards and guidelines, and assist in meeting the needs of the patients, nursing, and organizations.

Gandhi et al. (2016) note that system change reflects three phases of knowledge development. The first phase is superficial simplicity in which a quick fix is latched onto as "the" solution. This is followed by confusing complexity in which a multitude of strategies are enacted. Finally, after testing out the many strategies, the system achieves profound simplicity in which understanding of the intersection of the many strategies is attained. Gandhi et al. (2016) indicate that in terms of patient safety, health care systems are currently in the state of confusing complexity. There are diverse safety initiatives that are focused on an array of safety targets with different approaches for each, including checklists (e.g., surgical lists, discharge lists), bundles, process standardization, barcoding, and electronic health records for prescribing and order entry. Each of these approaches has its own processes and metrics to be measured to determine the quality and effectiveness of each strategy for achieving the targeted safety goal.

Implications for the CNS

A culture of safety needs to be established and sustained in health care organizations as an integral part of how the system functions (Gandhi et al., 2016). Honesty is encouraged for effective system improvement and not as a means of identifying someone to blame. The focus is on accountability for safety, continuing review of processes, and introducing tactical strategies for protecting patients from harm. CNSs are leaders that can assist health care organizations in creating cultures that support patient safety. One way that the CNS can accomplish this is through full implementation of the core competencies of consultation, direct care, systems leadership, collaboration, coaching, research, and ethical decision making (National CNS Task Force, 2010). CNSs need to be involved in patient safety initiatives, coalitions, and centers at local, regional, state, and national levels. CNSs need to become members of patient safety initiatives and/or centers within their own health care organizations, regions, and states.

Safety briefings are a way to communicate and build awareness surrounding safety within health care organizations (Gandhi et al., 2016). These safety briefings should be done by the CNS. CNSs, for example, help create staff awareness in relation to safety issues/concerns (falls, medication errors, etc.); educate staff; integrate evidence-based information; and share unit data surrounding patient safety. CNSs can run the safety briefings and then over time assist the nursing personnel in running them by themselves. An important follow-up as a CNS would be to assist with evidence-based practice changes to the safety briefing and evaluation of clinical practice.

Patient safety and preventing harm are foundational to quality patient care and improving health outcomes. New strategies are being developed and tested, and it is imperative that the CNS remain abreast of new and innovative approaches. The CNS is a leader of patient safety initiatives that need to be disseminated to others to spread the culture of safety (Gandhi et al., 2016). In leading, it is important that CNSs know the methods, models, and tools that are available so that they can implement change and assist others in implementing change. CNSs as leaders can also provide support to staff and patients who were involved in errors and harm.

CNSs need to assist the organizations they work within or develop their own consulting companies to assist organizations in adapting to meet the rapidly moving and changing regulatory landscape, regulatory requirements, quality improvement initiatives, patient safety initiatives, and customer satisfaction and expectations. Health care organizations must be able to adapt to this rapid movement in health policy; otherwise, they may not survive, remain competitive, and fiscally responsible (Ellerbe & Regen, 2012). CNSs must assist in these efforts. CNSs should also think about how they can integrate the utilization of technology when they are transforming health care systems and environments. Ellerbe and Reagen (2012) noted that the use of technology is needed to transform nursing and improve processes that impact the delivery of safe quality care.

THE FUTURE OF NURSING

National trends, including the graying of America and anticipated shortages of nurses, physicians, and other health care providers, stimulated efforts to determine how to make the best use of the human resources currently available. In 2008, the Committee on the Robert Wood Johnson Foundation (RWJF) Initiative on the Future of Nursing was appointed by the IOM and charged to produce a report and make recommendations for the nursing profession. The Committee met for 2 years, reviewing data and reports, meeting with stakeholder groups and others. Their 2011 report, *The Future of Nursing: Leading Change, Advancing Health,* advocated for allowing nurses to practice to the full extent of their education and training. The report notes the critical role of nurses in health care delivery and has called upon nurses to provide leadership in practice and education for improved care delivery and patient outcomes. Four key messages were identified by the committee:

- Nurses at every level of nursing should practice to the full extent of their education and training.
- Nurses should achieve higher levels of education and training through improved education systems that promote seamless academic progression.
- Nurses should be full partners, with physicians and other health care professionals, in redesigning health care in the United States.
- Effective workforce planning and policy-making require improved data collection and information infrastructure. (IOM, 2011, p. 33)

In 2014, RWJF asked the IOM to convene a committee to review the progress made toward achieving the recommendations in the 2010 *Future of Nursing* report (Altman, Butler, & Shern, 2016). Much progress has been made in moving toward achieving the recommendations; however, the committee noted the increasing importance of interprofessional collaboration finds that a broader network of stakeholders need to be engaged. In 2012, the CMS issued a final rule allowing APRNs to perform all functions within their scope of practice. Nevertheless, the actual scope of APRN practice continues to be restricted based on individual state boards of nursing and legislative rules and regulations (Altman et al., 2016). The progress report identified three key themes to drive progress toward achieving *The Future of Nursing* recommendations:

- The need to build a broader coalition to increase awareness of nurses' ability to play a full role in health professions, practice, education, collaboration, and leadership
- The need to continue to make promoting diversity in the nursing workforce a priority
- The need for better data with which to assess and drive progress (Altman et al., 2016, p. 4)

Virani and colleagues (2015) compared the type, quality, and volume of services provided by physicians and APRNs to persons with cardiovascular diseases (i.e., coronary artery disease, heart failure, and atrial fibrillation) and found that the quality of care was comparable between these two provider groups and APRN care even somewhat better for the patients diagnosed with coronary artery disease. This finding supports the IOM's assertion that APRNs can provide quality health care and help fill the provider gap (2011). Investigators for the Evidence-based Synthesis Program examined the extant reports of research to develop a report for the Veterans Health Administration (VHA) on the quality of care provided by APRNs including CNSs (McCleery, Christensen, Peterson, Humphrey, & Helfand, 2014). They report that all studies found comparable outcomes for urgent care and symptom resolution within 2 weeks, hospitalizations, quality of life measures, and mortality between physicians and APRNs. The authors note that the studies' evidence is weak because there was no long-term follow-up of the patients (6 months was the longest follow-up) and generally findings should be considered inconclusive (McCleery et al., 2014).

Cox, Andersen, Santucci, Robison, and Hudson (2016) designed and tested a telephone counseling support system to improve participation in cardiomyopathy screening programs by adult survivors of childhood cancer. The program randomly assigned survivors to receive a mailed survivorship care plan only or the mailed care plan with telephone counseling provided by APRNs. The telephone counseling resulted in significantly higher participation in cardiomyopathy screening among a regionally dispersed population and was relatively low in cost to implement in comparison with reimbursement payments received for completed screenings.

Consistent with these national initiatives, in May of 2016, the VHA posted a rule in the Federal Register that would allow APRNs to function to the full scope of their education and training (Lambert-Kerzner et al., 2016). This rule is important for several reasons: In the absence of federal rules, the VHA must abide by local state laws, which are highly variable in terms of recognizing CNSs and other APRN roles, determining whether their practice is autonomous with or without physician oversight or is independent, and whether autonomous prescriptive authority is granted by a state board of nursing (National Council of State Boards of Nursing [NCSBN], 2016). This federal rule will allow for seamless and standard care practices to be implemented that allow VHA APRNs to function to the full scope of their authority regardless of the state in which the VHA hospital or clinic is located (Lambert-Kerzner et al., 2016). Granting full-practice authority to all APRNs would immediately improve access to vital health care services for veterans by reducing redundancies in services provided and delays in health care delivery. The NCSBN (2016) maintains state reference maps on APRN roles, licensure, practice authority, and implementation of the APRN Consensus Model.

Implications for CNS Practice

Central to improving health care is quality improvement initiatives, with six aims for assuring that care is safe, effective, patient-centered, timely, efficient, and equitable (IOM, 2011). CNSs need to be involved in their own professional organizations ensuring that they can practice to their full scope of education and training, per their state practice act. In addition to practicing to their full scope, CNSs must educate others about what their role is. CNSs should also take it a step beyond education and develop a template to share with others as to the work they do and outcomes of their work, and try to quantify this in relation to health care dollars saved. The organizational leadership needs to know and can speak to the benefit of having a CNS. It is the responsibility of the CNS to ensure this happens.

STANDARD OCCUPATION CLASSIFICATION

The 2010 Standard Occupational Classification (SOC) system is used by the federal government to classify workers into one of 840 detailed occupational categories. This information is used for collecting, calculating, or disseminating data. All workers are classified into one of 840 detailed occupations per their occupational definition. Detailed occupations in the SOC with similar job duties, and in some cases skills, education, and/or training, are grouped together. The Office of Management and Budget (OMB) began the multiyear process to consider revisions of the SOC in 2012 with the target of implementing the final categories in 2018. The plan is to review and revise these categories every 10 years. There is an interagency SOC Policy Committee (SOCPC) that makes recommendations for revisions based on documentation that is submitted to OMB for consideration. The public comment period for the current review closed on July 21, 2014.

In this latest round of revising the SOC system, the SOC Policy Committee of the OMB once again incorrectly categorized CNSs as general registered nurses (RNs) and not as the APRNs that they are. The NACNS is the national professional organization that represents more than 72,000 CNSs in the United States. NACNS has submitted data and documentation to demonstrate that the work performed by CNSs meets all the criteria for this role to be assigned its own distinct occupation code. This incorrect classification means that CNSs are not counted in national survey data and are not visible in workforce data. Further, the surveys that bundle CNS with RN are subject to significant error and essentially invalidate the resultant data. The committee to review progress on *The Future of Nursing* recommendations identified the need for better workforce data to determine progress and challenges (Altman et al., 2016). This decision by the SOC Policy Committee is contrary to the need for reliable and valid workforce data.

It has even more serious implications should state licensing and credentialing agencies choose to adopt the SOC classification system; then CNSs could be denied the right to function as APRNs. This decision is inconsistent with other long-standing federal decisions. Congress officially recognized CNSs as APRNs in the Balanced Budget Act of 1997, which allowed CNSs to directly bill their services through CMS. Currently, CNSs have the state-level authority to prescribe medications and other therapeutics in 39 states. Forty-three states allow the CNS to practice a range of autonomous practice. Specifically, CNSs can practice to the full extent of their education and training in 28 states and prescribe without supervision in 19 (NCSBN, 2016).

APRN *CONSENSUS MODEL*

The *Consensus Model for APRN Regulation: Licensure, Accreditation, Certification, and Education* was adopted by the nursing community in 2008. It was developed to address inconsistencies in the regulation, education, and certification of the four APRN roles—CNS, Nurse Practitioner, nurse anesthetist, and nurse midwife (APRN Consensus Work Group & the National Council of State Boards of Nursing APRN Advisory Committee, 2008). The *Consensus Model* defined six population foci for advanced practice, title protection for the APRN roles, educational requirements, and licensure as an APRN. Title protection and recognition of CNSs as APRNs is essential for improving access to care. Yet, title protection for CNSs still does not exist in all 50 states. CNSs, along with the other APRNs, need the ability to practice independently to the full extent of their education and training. The six population foci are family across the life span, neonatal, pediatrics, women/gender-related health, adult-gerontology, and psychiatric mental health.

In previous decades, CNSs were educated in a specialty (like diabetes, oncology) or a well-defined population (like pediatrics, maternity). The more recent requirement to be educated in the broad population does provide an advantage in that today many people have multiple chronic conditions (Moore & McQuestion, 2012). The diabetes CNS who was educated with the population focus on adults or adult-geriatric patients can also oversee and coordinate care for those patients with diabetes who also have heart disease or hypertension. With the growing number of people with multiple chronic conditions, this combination of broad population preparation, with specialty preparation, places the CNS in a key position to maintain high-quality care, improve the coordination of care, and facilitate transitions in care management. Most important, CNSs are functioning within their recognized scope of nursing practice.

However, given its fundamental reliance on standardized APRN examinations, the *Consensus Model* has inadvertently created more barriers to CNS practice. The lack of examinations for all of the six populations identified in the

<table>
<tr><td colspan="2">**CHALLENGES FACING CNSs DUE TO THE CONSENSUS MODEL**</td><td>**BOX 31.2**</td></tr>
</table>

- Variability in state title protection of the CNS
- Inconsistency in state adoption of the grandfathering of the CNS
- CNSs losing jobs based on misperceptions of the Consensus Model
- CNSs losing state recognition as APRN based on interpretations of the Consensus Model
- Lack of population-based CNS examinations for all six population foci

APRN, Advanced Practice Registered Nurse; CNS, Clinical Nurse Specialist.

Consensus Model and the exclusion of specialty focus in graduate preparation create undue burden on CNSs. Policy changes are needed that would address alternate mechanisms for meeting the state regulatory requirements while ensuring competence to practice as a CNS.

Implications for CNS Practice

CNSs need to be knowledgeable about regulatory implementations and policy implications that affect CNS practice. Proposed changes to federal and state laws and regulations are posted and open for public comment. The CNS must participate in this process by responding to these calls. The SOC classification has the potential to derail the efforts of CNSs to be recognized as APRNs in their states. However, other policies have been enacted that specifically include APRNs and CNSs by title that provide some protections. Inconsistencies as to how these policies are enacted can place barriers to CNS practice. The last national sample of nurse workforce that clearly defined CNSs separately from RNs was completed in 2008 by the Health Resources and Services Administration. To fill the gap in current data about CNSs, the NACNS launched the national CNS survey in 2014 to collect information about CNSs, their practice, and their level of autonomy (NACNS, 2015). NACNS has committed to collecting the national CNS census every 2 years so that trends in data can be assessed and disseminated to the nursing and health care community.

The *Consensus Model*, as the product of a national endeavor and accepted by the NCSBN and professional nursing organizations, plays an important role in recognition of the CNS as an advanced practice nursing role. More states are adopting the recommendations in the *Consensus Model*, with only nine states that do not have title protections in their regulations—at this time (NACNS, 2015). The inconsistencies in how the states implement the recommendations lead to variability in scope of practice and autonomy for CNSs. The lack of standardized examinations that lead to certification is a barrier for many CNSs. Challenges in the implementation of the *Consensus Model* are detailed in Box 31.2.

INTERPROFESSIONAL EDUCATION AND PRACTICE

The progress report on the future of nursing identified the need to work collaboratively and engage stakeholders across health care disciplines and settings to increase awareness of nurses' ability to play a full role in health care (Altman et al., 2016). The need for collaborative interprofessional health care practices is becoming increasingly apparent as the population and health care providers are aging. Health care providers are retiring, and the number of "replacement" providers is not keeping pace with the demand for health care services (Mayo et al., 2016).

While the IOM's RWJF committee on the Future of Nursing was working on this report, another group was formed in 2009 comprised of the six national associations for schools of health professions. The six professional disciplines included dentistry, nursing, medicine, osteopathic medicine, pharmacy, and public health. An expert panel with representatives from these disciplines developed the core competencies for interprofessional collaborative practice and to guide curricular development across the disciplines. The 2011 Core Competencies for Interprofessional Collaborative Practice was widely disseminated and is being implemented in health professions schools (Interprofessional Education Collaborative [IPEC], 2016). The four key competencies for successful and effective interprofessional collaboration continue to be values and ethics, roles and responsibilities, interprofessional communication, and teams and teamwork. The ultimate goal of these educational and subsequent clinical practice changes is to assist health care providers and health care organizations in achieving the ACA triple aim. Because much of the education of health care students is conducted in silos, it is critical that there be planned programs for interprofessional education if the goal of true collaboration across professions is to be attained. The Commission on Collegiate Nursing Education, one of three organizations that accredit schools of nursing, is part of the IPEC group that will begin to require IPEC competencies and learning experiences as part of the accreditation standards.

Implications for CNS Practice

The CNS has been a leader in working collaboratively in health care teams to improve system processes and health care outcomes of patients. The core competencies identified by IPEC (2016) are: (a) ethics and values to support a climate of mutual respect; (b) roles and responsibilities enacted to address health care needs of patients and promote the health of the population; (c) interprofessional communication that includes patients, families, and communities and is done in a responsive and responsible manner; and (d) teams and teamwork that develop relationships through shared values and principles of team dynamics.

CNSs can improve population health by increasing access to wellness and preventive care to populations at risk; for example, populations that are at risk for development of chronic diseases such as heart failure and diabetes. Working in ambulatory care settings, the CNS can identify patients at risk for chronic diseases through wellness and/or prevention screenings.

As life expectancy increases, people are living longer and developing chronic diseases. According to the Partnership to Fight Chronic Diseases, about 191 million people had at least one chronic disease and 75 million had two or more chronic diseases (2016). The CNS must get involved now and be a part of the teams and initiatives that are defining multiple chronic disease guidelines and outcome measures. Once guidelines and outcome measures have been developed and accepted by the health care community, these will then become part of health policy. The CNS must work with interprofessional collaborative teams to assist in developing evidence-based practice/clinical guidelines for patients with multiple chronic conditions. Policy implications need to emphasize how quality of care can be improved in the population with multiple chronic conditions due to the current lack of evidence-based standards for this population (Partnership to Fight Chronic Diseases, 2016).

Another area that has taken note of multiple chronic diseases is through the Patient-Centered Outcomes Research Institute (PCORI) with the National Priorities for Research and Research Agenda. This agenda includes multiple chronic diseases/conditions, listing the need for more research to be done. Some of the areas highlighted were in the improvement of care and outcomes; looking at other models of care, coordination of care/transitions in care for the multiple chronic condition population (Newhouse et al., 2015).

CONCLUSION

Improving access to care while maintaining quality and safety and reducing health care costs are major concerns of consumers, health care providers, federal and state governments, CMS, and other insurers. Health policy will be driving the consumer's decisions, health care dollars, research, and much more. CNSs must be part of the solution. CNSs must demonstrate their contributions in improving care, and this can be done through documentation and dissemination of their work in publications and presentations. CNSs need to be involved in research and evidence-based decisions to know what the various research agendas are in relation to health policy. Moore and McQuestion (2012) state that there is a need within research literature for CNSs to study the outcomes of the various CNS roles, initiatives that they implement, interprofessional work, impact on patients and families in all settings (e.g., community, hospital, offices, clinics, schools, correctional facilities) and throughout the health continuum through support of transitions in care, wellness and prevention, and chronic disease management (inclusive of multiple chronic disease management). Not only should this be done through research and publication, but also through the need to share successes with other health-related professionals outside of nursing.

CNSs need to become involved on many levels to make sure that CNS practice is an accepted part of health care policies. Finkelman (2013) maintains that it is critical for CNSs to get involved in policy making and to demonstrate the leadership role that CNSs take in improving patient care. CNSs need to share their work with more than our peers. Sharing can be done with employers, government officials, health care professionals outside of nursing, nurse educators, and nursing professional organizations (Finkelman, 2013). Henderson et al. (2012), discuss how nurses need to advocate for change in health policy. This can be done by participating in health policy through education of themselves, supporting the current initiatives (e.g., ACOs, patient-centered medical homes), participating in legislative activities (voting, running for office), supporting nursing organizations that are pursuing health policy changes, and educating others in health care and outside health care (Henderson et al., 2012).

CNSs must get involved in their own states with health policy and with state boards of nursing. If we do not have CNSs at the table, this may result in barriers to practice for CNSs. If barriers to practice occur, this ultimately is eliminating ability of the CNS to meet the needs of the public. CNSs need to know their resources, use them, and direct others to them. One such document for CNSs is *The Starter Kit for Impacting Change at the Government Level: How to work with your state legislators and regulators* (2012), and there are other documents provided by NACNS on their website http://www.cns.org. Barriers for APRNs still exist, with some CNSs not being able to practice to their full scope of education and training because they are not currently recognized by their state as APRNs or they lack title protection as CNSs. The future of the CNS can be changed based on individual states' implementation of legislation and language in the nurse practice act. Our future depends on it, so get involved in your state legislature to ensure that this occurs.

DISCUSSION QUESTIONS

1. *Based on the information in this chapter, list at least two areas of policy change you can identify where legislation could have an impact.*

ANALYSIS/SYNTHESIS QUESTIONS

1. *If you were going to describe the importance of your issue for policy change to potential supporters, what key issues would you stress? How would you describe these to your patients?*
2. *When thinking about CNS practice how would you describe the current state of CNS education, licensure, certification and accreditation? What health policy would you develop/create that would improve processes for CNSs?*

CLINICAL APPLICATION

1. *Think about how CNS practice impacts health care overall in acute care, critical care, public health and primary care. What would be missing if the CNS were not present in the health care systems. Would the work of the CNS be done? If so, how? If not, what impact would that have?*
2. *CNSs work within three spheres of influence. Where does health policy fit?*

ETHICAL CONSIDERATIONS

1. *Consider the health policy changes discussed in this chapter or those you have described in your analysis and consider the impact that might occur if these changes are NOT enacted. In other words, what are the consequences of inaction?*
2. *What can I do to help make these changes on a local level? Institutional level in my health care organization? State level? National level?*
3. *What changes in the health care system would occur if the CNS role were to disappear?*

REFERENCES

Abara, W., & Heiman, H. J. (2014). The Affordable Care Act and low-income people living with HIV: Looking forward in 2014 and beyond. *Journal of the Association of Nurses in AIDS Care, 25,* 476–482.

Altman, S.H., Butler, A.S., & Shern, L. (Eds.). (2016). *Assessing progress on the Institute of Medicine report: The future of nursing*. Washington, DC: National Academies Press.

APRN Consensus Work Group & the National Council of State Boards of Nursing APRN Advisory Committee. (2008). Consensus model for APRN regulation: Licensure, accreditation, certification & education. Retrieved from https://www.ncsbn.org/Consensus_Model_for_APRN_Regulation_July_2008.pdf

Baldwin, K. M., Black, D., & Hammond, S. (2014). Developing a rural transitional care community case management program using clinical nurse specialists. *Clinical Nurse Specialist, 28*, 147–155.

Burton, R. (2012, September 13). Health policy brief: Care transitions, health affairs. Retrieved from http://www.healthaffairs.org/healthpolicybriefs/brief.php?brief_id=76

Cady, R. F. (2012). Healthcare reform after the supreme court ruling: implications for nurse executives. *JONA's Healthcare Law, Ethics, and Regulation, 14*(3), 81–84.

Centers for Medicare and Medicaid Services. (2016). *Accountable care organization 2016 program quality measure narrative specifications*. Baltimore, MD: Author.

Clough, J. D., & McClellan, M. (2016). Implementing MACRA: Implications for physicians and for physician leadership. *Journal of the American Medical Association, 315*, 2397–2398.

Cox, C. L., Andersen, M. R., Santucci, A. K., Robison, L. L., & Hudson, M. M. (2016). Increasing cardiomyopathy screening in childhood cancer survivors: A cost analysis of advanced practice nurse phone counseling. *Oncology Nursing Forum, 43*, E242–E260.

Delp, S., Ward, C. W., Altice, N., Bath, J., Bond, D. C., Hall, K. D., . . . Carter, K. (2016). Spheres of influence...clinical nurse specialists: Sparking economic impact, innovative practice. *Nursing Management, 47*(6), 31–36.

Ellerbe, S., & Regen, D. (2012). Responding to Health Care Reform by Addressing the Institute of Medicine Report on the Future of Nursing. *Nursing Administration Quarterly, 36*, 210–216.

Finkelman, A. (2013). The clinical nurse specialist: Leadership in quality improvement. *Clinical Nurse Specialist, 27*, 31–35.

Gandhi, T. K., Berwick, D. M., & Shojania, K. G. (2016). Patient safety at the crossroads. *Journal of the American Medical Association, 315*, 1829–1830.

Haycock, C., Edwards, M. L., & Stanley, C. S. (2016). Unpacking MACRA: The proposed rule and its implications for payment and practice. *Nursing Administration Quarterly, 40*, 349–355.

Henderson, S., Princell, C. O., & Martin, S. D. (2012). The Patient-Centered Medical Home: This primary care model offers RNs new practice—and reimbursement—opportunities. *American Journal of Nursing, 112*(12), 54–59.

Hofmeyer, J., Leider, J. P., Satorius, J., Tanenbaum, E., Basel, D., & Knudson, A. (2016). Implementation of telemedicine consultation to assess unplanned transfers in rural long-term care facilities, 2012–2015: A pilot study. *Journal of Post-Acute and Long-term Care Medicine, 17*, 1006–1010.

Hynds, R. L., Hatch, J. L., & Samuels, J. G. (2014). The Affordable Care Act 2010. *Journal for Nurses in Professional Development, 30*, 281–286.

Institute of Medicine. (2011). *The future of nursing: Leading change, advancing health*. Washington, DC: National Academies Press.

Interprofessional Education Collaborative. (2016). *Core competencies for interprofessional collaborative practice: 2016 update*. Washington, DC: Author.

Laker, C. (2011). Decreasing 30-day readmission rates. *American Journal of Nursing, 111*(11), 65–69.

Lambert-Kerzner, A., Lucatorto, M., McCreight, M., Williams, K. M., Fehling, K. B., Peterson, J., . . . Battaglia, C. (2016). The Veterans Health Administration's proposal for APRN full-practice authority. *The Nurse Practitioner, 41*(11), 16–24.

Logue, M. D., & Drago, J. (2013). Evaluation of a modified community based care transitions model to reduce costs and improve outcomes. *BMC Geriatrics, 13*, 94. doi:10.1186/1471-2318-13-94

Lovelace, D., Hancock, D., Hughes, S. S., Wyche, P. R., Jenkins, C., & Logan, C. (2016). A patient-centered transitional care case management program: Taking case management to the streets and beyond. *Professional Case Management, 21*, 277–290.

Mayo, A. M., Harris, M., & Burton, B. (2016). Integrating geropsychiatric nursing and interprofessional collaborative practice competencies into adult-gerontology clinical nurse specialist education. *Clinical Nurse Specialist, 30*, 324–331.

McCleery, E., Christensen, V., Peterson, K., Humphrey, L., & Helfand, M. (2014). Evidence brief: The quality of care provided by advanced practice nurses. In *VA evidence-based synthesis program evidence briefs* [Internet]. Washington, DC: Department of Veterans Affairs.

Moore, J., & McQuestion, M. (2012). The clinical nurse specialist in chronic disease. *Clinical Nurse Specialist, 26*, 149–163.

National Association of Clinical Nurse Specialists. (2012a). NACNS Statement on the APRN Consensus Model Implementation. *Clinical Nurse Specialist, 26*, 185–189.

National Association of Clinical Nurse Specialists. (2012b). 2014 CNS census. Retrieved from http://nacns.org/professional-resources/practice-and-cns-role/cns-census/2014-cns-census

National Association of Clinical Nurse Specialists. (2015). Key findings from the 2014 clinical nurse specialist census. Retrieved from http://www.nacns.org/html/cns-census.php

National CNS Competency Task Force. (2010). *Clinical nurse specialist core competencies: Executive summary 2006–2008*. Philadelphia, PA: National Association of Clinical Nurse Specialists. Retrieved from http://nacns.org/html/competencies.php

National Council of State Boards of Nursing. (2016). CNS independent practice map. Retrieved from https://www.ncsbn.org/5406.htm

Naylor, M. D., Aiken, L. H., Kurtzman, E. T., Olds, D. M., & Hirshman, K. B. (2011). The importance of transitional care in achieving health reform. *Health Affairs, 30*, 746–754.

Newhouse, R., Barksdale, D. J., & Miller, J. A. (2015). The patient-centered outcomes research institute: Research done differently. *Nursing Research, 64*, 72–77.

Orr, P., & Davenport, D. (2015). Embracing change. *Nursing Clinics of North America, 50*, 1–18.

Partnership to Fight Chronic Disease. (2016). What is the impact of chronic disease on America? Retrieved from http://www.fightchronicdisease.org

Patten, S., & Goudreau, K. A. (2012). The bright future for clinical nurse specialist practice. *Nursing Clinics of North America, 47*, 193–203.

Spray, S. L. (1999). The evolution of the psychiatric clinical nurse specialist: An interview with Hildegard E. Peplau. *Perspectives in Psychiatric Care, 35*(3), 27–37.

U.S. Department of Health and Human Services. (2016). Accountable care organizations. Retrieved from https://www.medicare.gov/manage-your-health/coordinating-your-care/accountable-care-organizations.html

Virani, S. S., Maddox, T. M., Chan, P. S., Tang, F., Akeroyd, J. M., Risch, S. A., . . . Petersen, L. A. (2015). Provider type and quality of outpatient cardiovascular disease care: Insights from the NCDR PINNACLE registry. *Journal of the American College of Cardiology, 66*, 1803–1812.

Vu, M., White, A., Kelley, V. P., Hopper, J. K., & Liu, C. (2016). Hospital and health plan partnerships: The Affordable Care Act's impact on promoting health and wellness. *American Health & Drug Benefits, 9*, 269–278.

CHAPTER 32

The Certified Nurse-Midwife in Advanced Nursing Practice

Janelle Komorowski

Midwives have a long history of advocating for women and their infants. In America's early years, lay midwives often served as the only health care provider in the community. As physicians increasingly assumed dominance over the field of obstetrics in the early 20th century, demand for lay midwives dwindled. The majority of midwives who remained active were forced out of practice by legislation that made it nearly impossible to meet the qualifications for licensure. Some states went so far as to criminalize the practice of midwifery.

Although the birthplace had predominately moved from the home to the hospital setting by the early 1900s, there remained populations of women unable to access prenatal care or hospital delivery due to socioeconomic, religious, cultural, or racial disparities. In 1925, Mary Breckinridge determined to improve the condition of underserved women and children and founded what would later become the Frontier Nursing Service. Mary had served as a public health nurse during World War I and was touched by the masses of underserved women and children she encountered. She returned to England for additional training in midwifery and came back to the United States with a plan. Nurses would travel on horseback in order to reach even the most remote families, providing midwifery and public health nursing care for those who would otherwise find such services inaccessible. Mary organized a system of nurses and recruited a physician to provide consultation at a central hospital location. Within a few years, more than 1,000 families were being cared for by the nurses (Breckinridge, 1981). In 1929, Mary brought British nurse-midwives to America to work alongside her public health nurses. Around the same time in New York City, the Maternity Center Association and Lobenstein Clinic founded the first nurse-midwifery educational program in the United States, followed in 1939 by the Frontier Graduate School of Midwifery (Rooks, 1997). The profession of nurse-midwifery grew rapidly, with seven schools established by the 1950s. Nurse-midwives excelled at providing care for disadvantaged women, but their popularity also grew among the affluent as women began to recognize the benefits of the midwifery model of care.

Nurse-midwives in the United States today provide care for a disproportionately large number of women who are considered higher risk during pregnancy: adolescents, single mothers, economically disadvantaged women, the uninsured, women of color, women of low education, immigrants, and women who for various reasons seek prenatal care late in their pregnancies or not at all. Given a higher-risk population and access to fewer resources, one would expect high rates of undesirable outcomes among the women and infants for whom nurse-midwives provide care, when compared with women of means who have access to physician care. The opposite is actually the case. Nurse-midwives in the Frontier Nursing Service significantly reduced some of the highest maternal and neonatal mortality rates in the country at the time, while providing care in very remote and impoverished settings (Frontier Nursing Service, 1958).

In 1960, nurse-midwives were introduced to a hospital in Madera County, California, a medically underserved area with a high proportion of migrant workers. Half of the workers typically received either late prenatal care or none at all. Because midwifery was illegal in California at that time, a special law was passed to permit the midwives to practice in one hospital. Prematurity and neonatal death rates dropped significantly during the 3 years that the midwives cared for the indigent women. Funding for the project ended in 1963. When physicians took over the practice, prematurity and neonatal death rates returned to preproject levels (Rooks, 1997). Although many reasons for the drop and subsequent rise in prematurity and neonatal death rates were proposed, none was adequate to explain the change. Levy et al. (1971) asserted that the reason for the changes was the introduction and subsequent removal of nurse-midwives from the area. Prematurity and neonatal death rates had remained unchanged at other hospitals in the area during the time that the nurse-midwives worked, lending credence to the theory that midwifery care made the difference.

Today, Certified Nurse-Midwives (CNMs) caring for the underserved continue to achieve excellent outcomes. The Family Health and Birth Center in Washington, DC, has a 9% preterm birth rate, compared with 14.2% in the area, and a low birth weight rate that is half that of the region's (Family Health and Birth Center, 2007). The contribution of nurse-midwives to improved primary health care services for underserved women has been affirmed by the Institute of Medicine (IOM; 2011), which recommends expanding the responsibilities of nurse-midwives as primary care providers for women.

CONCEPTUAL AND THEORETICAL SUPPORT FOR NURSE-MIDWIFERY PRACTICE

The conceptual basis for nurse-midwifery practice is reflected in the Philosophy of Care outlined by the American College of Nurse-Midwives (ACNM, 2010). The Philosophy of Care emphasizes the partnership of the nurse-midwife with women, recognizes the woman as the expert in her own life and needs, and encourages the advocacy and support of the CNM for the woman's choice for her health care. Kennedy, Rousseau, and Low (2003) identified four common themes of midwifery care:

- The midwife as an instrument of care
- The woman as a partner in care

- The alliance between the woman and her midwife
- The environment of care

These themes are also identified in the ACNM's Philosophy of Care. Emphasis on the normalcy of birth resonates throughout midwifery literature. Carolan and Hodnett (2007) voiced concern that this emphasis of nurse-midwifery on the normal could lead to an exclusionary model, leaving out women with higher needs. Midwives do serve a disproportionate number of at-risk women, a number that is expected to increase as physicians leave the practice of obstetrics or limit their practices to privately insured patients. Although emphasis on the normal is a hallmark of midwifery care, CNMs have proven their ability to achieve superior outcomes even when caring for women with moderate pregnancy complications. As midwifery caseloads shift to include larger numbers of medically indigent women, the emphasis on normalcy must be extended to include those who fall into high-risk categories.

Rooks (1997) contrasts the midwifery and medical models of care, asserting that the two often overlap and are not mutually exclusive and that the optimal intertwining of the two models of care is a collaborative relationship between the nurse midwife and the physician. However, she emphasizes the unique contributions of the nurse-midwifery model in preservation of normalcy in birth, avoidance of unnecessary interventions, and acknowledgment of needs often unaddressed by the medical model. Perhaps the most significant validation of Rooks's assertions comes from Stapleton, Osborne, and Illuzzi (2013). The researchers examined records of 15,574 births that occurred in midwife-led birth centers. Outcomes show significant cost savings, a cesarean section rate of only 6% as compared with a national average of U.S. cesarean section rate for 2011 of 32.8% (Centers for Disease Control and Prevention, 2011), fewer routine interventions, and perinatal outcomes comparable with physician-attended, hospital-based births.

Although there is ample evidence to support the benefits of midwifery care, the development of a theoretical basis for midwifery knowledge is relatively recent. Credit for the beginnings of midwifery theory is given to Ernestine Wiedenbach, a nurse-midwife and nurse theorist whose work was the basis for the first written philosophy of the ACNM. Wiedenbach is credited with focusing nursing research on a patient-centered versus medical model. She theorized that nurse-midwifery should focus on meeting the patient's "need-for-help," which she defined as interventions either wanted or needed by the patient that can improve her coping abilities (Nickel, Gesse, & MacLaren, 1992).

Three middle-range theories of midwifery practice each incorporate the nurse-midwifery philosophy of care in the development of their theories. Lehrman (1981) developed the first nurse-midwifery theory to be tested. Her work focused on six constructs depicting midwifery practice and drawn from ACNM philosophy. Congruent with ACNM philosophy, Lehrman's center of focus is the patient, either the parturient or the neonate. A descriptive study by Morten, Kohl, O'Mahoney, and Pelosi (1991) validated Lehrman's prenatal care theory and suggested a correlation between the positive attitude of the nurse-midwife and desirable patient outcomes. Because she links the nurse-midwifery care processes with outcomes, Lehrman's work is a strong basis for future nurse-midwifery practice theory and research.

Thompson, Oakley, Burke, Jay, and Conklin (1989) sought to develop a middle-range theory that could explain the difference nurse-midwifery care makes in patient outcomes. Thompson identified six core principles of nurse-midwifery practice based on the ACNM philosophy. Thompson's broad theory includes specific behaviors for each concept, which will benefit future researchers in identifying correlations between nurse-midwifery care practices and patient outcomes, and may guide development of future practice guidelines.

Kennedy's theory (2000) also links superior patient outcomes to nurse-midwifery practices, but it identifies a lack of knowledge as to why such practices produce exemplary outcomes. Two assumptions underlying Kennedy's model are that exemplary practice is associated with positive outcomes for women and infants and that core philosophies and standards for the practice of nurse-midwifery are the foundation of exemplary midwifery practice. Echoing Lehrman and Thompson, a central focus of Kennedy's theory is the woman as an active participant in her care, with the nurse-midwife cast in a supporting role. Kennedy has proposed that her model be tested to confirm whether specific nurse-midwifery behaviors affect patient outcomes. She has continued to develop her theory, which is recognized by many nurse-midwives and nurse-midwifery educators as the best description of the essence of nurse-midwifery practice.

Berg (2005) proposed a theory of Genuine Caring in Caring for the Genuine and stressed the importance of balancing care for the high-risk woman in a way that meets her medical needs while still acknowledging her right to give birth in a way that honors the natural process of becoming a mother. Emphasis in Berg's model is placed on a synthesis of medical science and traditional midwifery care, which she asserts is best achieved in collaborative practice between physicians and midwives.

Fahy and Parratt (2006) proposed the concept of Birth Territory, which encompasses the birth environment, the locus of control over the birth, and the woman's physical and psychological experience of the birth. They juxtapose the concept of "midwifery guardianship" with "midwifery domination." Midwifery guardianship assumes a supportive role on the part of the midwife, whose goal is to facilitate the woman's desires and her ability to give birth normally in a physiologic manner. Midwifery domination is any action on the part of the midwife that requires the woman to submit to the midwife's directives rather than rely on her own inner knowledge. The woman may react by abandoning her intuitive ability to give birth or by responding aggressively toward the midwife in an effort to protect her intuitive abilities to give birth.

Doherty (2009) introduced the concept of the midwife–patient relationship as a "therapeutic alliance" in which the midwife and the client work together to achieve mutually agreed upon goals for client care. A therapeutic alliance is subtly differentiated from a collaborative relationship in that collaboration may be more midwife-directed; in other words, the midwife may propose to the client options from which she may choose, versus working together with the client to identify options the client would like to choose from. In the collaborative relationship, the midwife still retains the role of leader, whereas the therapeutic alliance is more a partnership of equals with differing skills.

The common thread among midwifery theories and care models is the theme of preserving the normalcy of pregnancy and birth insofar as possible, the midwife in partnership with the woman versus an authoritarian relationship, and keeping the woman as the central focus of care. As these models are tested and refined, future research will further contribute to the development of nurse-midwifery practice and philosophy.

CORE COMPETENCIES

The practice of nurse midwifery in the United States is guided by the Core Competencies of the ACNM. Although many of the competencies describe essential clinical skills for nurse-midwifery practice, significant attention is also given to recognition of parturition as a normal process and avoidance of technological interventions in the absence of clear medical need. Advocacy for the woman's right to informed choice and self-determination, health promotion, and family-centered care are also included in the Core Competencies. Although these ideals are widely espoused by nurse-midwives, Lange and Kennedy (2010) found significant discrepancies between ideal and actual practice, as identified by 245 new CNMs. In describing their final clinical practice settings before graduation, study participants reported a disconnection between the espoused core philosophy of preserving normal birth and actual clinical practices. Differences between theory and practice in the demonstration of caring behaviors were insignificant, but wide variations between theory and practice were apparent in the frequency of routine interventions and infrequent choice of nontechnological approaches when appropriate. In addition, continuous support in labor was not observed in actual practice to the degree it is emphasized in the midwifery model of care.

Vedam, Goff, and Marnin (2007) state that "there are unique competencies in perinatal management that characterize, promote, and preserve the midwifery model of care." Certainly, the ACNM Core Competencies reflect the College's belief in the uniqueness of the midwifery model; why then is there such a gap between theory and practice? The answer may lie in the barriers to practice facing today's midwives. Many of these barriers relate to health policy and can be categorized as regulatory, collegial, and financial barriers.

REGULATORY BARRIERS

As of 2012, 32 states required Nurse Practitioners (NPs) to have some degree of physician involvement in their practices. In some states, physician involvement is limited to a formal "collaborative agreement," in which the physician agrees to be available for consultation and collaboration for patients whose care falls outside the midwife's scope of practice. Other states require a supervisory relationship, with the physician signing admission and discharge orders, and cosigning all inpatient care and medication orders. Only 18 states and the District of Columbia grant primary care and prescriptive privileges to NPs without requiring any level of physician involvement. Thus, whereas certification attests that the midwife is qualified to practice independently as a primary care provider, state regulations may significantly restrict the midwife's ability to practice to the full extent of her or his training and certification.

Sonenberg (2010) attempted to assess the impact of differing state regulations on CNMs. The project was challenging due to the practice of putting the supervisory physician's name on medical records, obscuring data pertaining to midwife-attended births and outcomes. Inability to determine from records when a midwife was the care provider creates a barrier to ascertaining the effect of state regulations on midwifery practice. It also obscures data about who is providing care for disadvantaged women and the impact of CNM care on perinatal outcomes.

In addition to dealing with restrictive state regulations, the midwife who works near state borders faces additional problems. Lugo, O'Grady, Hodnicki, and Hanson (2007) stated, "Disease doesn't respect geographic boundaries, but even though patient condition, diagnosis, and management don't change, the regulations for NPs do change [between states]. When you read all 51 Nurse Practice Acts, you can't help but have an emotional reaction. There are some very strange stipulations and arbitrary limitations put on NPs, which speaks to how NP regulation is not evidence-based and needs to be cleaned up."

Safriet (2011) gives the example of an Advanced Practice Registered Nurse (APRN) licensed in two states, with differences in authority to practice between the two states. The APRN's competency does not change when crossing the state line, but reimbursement and scope of practice may be significantly different. Much of the difference can be attributed to politics, rather than sound policy. Safriet identified further problems with inconsistent state regulations as follows:

- Decision makers, even in progressive states, will often adopt the policies of the most restrictive jurisdictions. Safriet termed this as a "race to the bottom" (2011, p. 450).
- Patients living in rural or underserved areas, or those without insurance, may find themselves without adequate care due to lack of physicians who are willing and/or able to enter into a collaborative or supervisory agreement.
- Competent, well-trained APRNs may become discouraged when they are unable to practice to the full scope of their training and may relocate to more favorable practice areas leaving underserved areas even more destitute.
- Costs of care increase and creative ideas for health care delivery are stifled.
- APRNs may fear disciplinary action when even mundane activities, such as a phone consult or a birth control prescription refill, cross state lines.
- Technological advancements are restricted. For example, APRNs are increasingly utilizing telemedicine innovations, but working across state lines presents a barrier to practice and reimbursement.

Forty-one states regulate APRNs through a board of nursing, one state (Nebraska) has an advanced practice board to oversee APRN practice, and eight states have combined board of nursing and board of medicine oversight. Working to establish the board of nursing as the regulatory body for NPs in every state is a step toward increasing autonomy for APRNs. With the annual number of primary care visits expected to increase by 15.07 million to 24.26 million visits by 2019, an anticipated 4,307 and 6,940 new primary care providers will be needed to meet the demand (Hofer, Abraham, & Moscovice, 2011). Projections do not take into account changes in demand because of population growth and changes in demographics. Hauer et al. (2008) suggest projected needs for primary care providers may be grossly underreported as a result of declining numbers of medical students choosing primary care specialties. With these anticipated shortfalls, the APRN is likely to be ever more in demand, as the lower salaries, shorter educational time, and willingness of more APRNs to serve in primary care capacities can help meet the anticipated needs. It is even more critical that state regulation of APRNs become uniform, as primary care APRNs in rural areas may rely heavily on telemedicine, raising questions of licensing and scope of practice across state borders. Although physicians must also be licensed separately from state to state, they are given authority to diagnose, treat, and prescribe equally in all 50 states and the District of Columbia. In order for APRNs to step in and fill the need for primary care providers, it is imperative that they achieve uniform authority to diagnose, treat, and prescribe in all jurisdictions.

COLLEGIAL BARRIERS

As we evaluate the need for uniform scope-of-practice authority for NPs, collegial barriers must be considered. With 32 states currently requiring varying degrees of collaboration with a physician in order for the APRN to practice, physicians have a significant influence on accessibility of APRNs to the general public. Perhaps, in no specialty has this been more apparent than in that of obstetrics. Throughout the history of midwifery, physicians have been content to allow midwives to care for the patients they did not wish to manage, often because it was not financially lucrative. As the midwifery model of care became better known and the excellent outcomes achieved with midwifery care were studied and published, significant numbers of privately insured women began to seek out midwives for their primary care provider for obstetrics and gynecology. Numerous accounts exist of profitable nurse-midwifery practices abruptly shut down because of physician pressure (Hoban, 2012; Pleticha, 2004; Shaver, 2007), yet the IOM, citing the cost savings and excellent outcomes of nurse-midwifery care, urged the expanded use of nurse-midwives and utilization of Nurse Practitioners as patient-centered medical home (PCMH) leaders (IOM, 2011). Despite studies suggesting equal to better outcomes with APRN care (Newhouse et al., 2011) and nurse-midwifery care (Cragin & Kennedy, 2006; Newhouse et al., 2011), some physician groups have vehemently opposed expansion of APRNs into independent primary care and leadership of PCMHs. Citing the shorter duration of APRN education, the American Medical Association (AMA) insisted that only a physician is qualified to lead a PCMH and that the NPs should only work under the supervision or collaboration of a physician (AMA, 2010). The American Academy of Family Physicians (AAFP, 2010) agreed. Both organizations cite patient safety as their overarching concern, despite ample evidence establishing the quality outcomes of NPs in primary care roles (Newhouse et al., 2011).

The fact that many states still require some level of physician involvement in a nurse midwife's practice poses a significant practice barrier for many midwives. Even in states that grant midwives independent practice status, individual hospitals still retain the option to restrict nurse midwifery credentialing to those midwives who have a "sponsoring" physician agreement or are employees of a physician. Hospitals are not at liberty to grant midwives *more* privileges than state regulations allow but are permitted to be as restrictive as they wish in *limiting* midwifery privileges and scope of practice. Even in hospitals that only require a collaborative agreement, midwives may often feel compelled to practice in a way that violates the tenets of the ACNM philosophy. If minor complications of labor arise, which by hospital protocols mandate consultation with an obstetrician, the obstetrician may make recommendations based on the medical model of care. The nurse midwife may be compelled to comply with the obstetrician's recommendations, even when they are not evidence based, and to disregard the ACNM philosophy of care.

A further constraint to collaborative relationships is the perception of many physicians that collaboration means the APRN functions in a dependent role under a delegating physician (similar to the physician relationship with a registered nurse, but with expanded scope of practice for the APRN). In contrast, APRNs view collaboration as the consultation of one health care professional with another (Cairo, 1996), just as a family physician might consult with an obstetrician for a laboring patient in need of cesarean delivery. Shaw et al. (2005) identified the persistence of a dominant medical hierarchy, despite efforts to create team collaboration between physicians and NPs. Nurse-midwives, especially, may perceive this as a lack of respect for the differences between the midwifery and medical models of care, which can lead to job dissatisfaction and further widen the theory–practice gap.

In a literature review examining collaboration between physicians and NPs, Clarin (2007) identified several barriers to collaborative practice as follows:

- Lack of knowledge about NP scope of practice
- Lack of knowledge about NP role
- Poor physician attitude
- Lack of respect
- Poor communication
- Patient and family reluctance to receive NP care

Clarin asserts that a strategy for improving collaboration between physicians and APRNs is increased communication and education regarding the role of the APRN. Other authors disagree, suggesting that rather than focusing on increased communication and education about APRN roles, the focus should be on removing legislative barriers to completely independent APRN practice (van Soeren, Hurlock-Chorostecki, Goodwin, & Baker, 2009). When the ability of CNMs to practice independently is restricted, it limits the full potential of their benefit to vulnerable populations and underserved women. One successful APRN practice rose out of a shortage of providers for over 30,000 patients in Ontario. Eight unemployed APRNs proposed creating an APRN-led clinic. By going public with their idea, they garnered the support of the community, the media, and professional nursing organizations. The pilot project has been successful in Ontario (Heale, 2012) and could be a model for similar projects in the United States. The AARP-sponsored webinar (2012) finding seems to support Heale's findings, suggesting that a power shift involving consumers and stakeholders is the means to achieving regulatory changes.

The IOM (2011) has recommended state and federal changes that will allow NPs to exercise their full scope of practice. It is recommended that state legislatures bring their scope-of-practice regulations in line with the National Council of State Boards of Nursing Model Nursing Practice Act and Model Nursing Administrative Rules, which provide a template for the scope of advanced practice nursing. In addition, the IOM recommends that states require fee-for-service plans to cover NP services and that the Federal Trade Commission pinpoint state regulations that present barriers to practice without increasing public health and safety, and pressure states to change these regulations based on their anticompetitive effect. The IOM recommends that the Centers for Medicare and Medicaid Services (CMS) require hospitals that participate in Medicare/Medicaid programs to give NPs full medical staff eligibility and clinical/admitting privileges. Such changes would largely eliminate the collegial barriers APRNs face today.

FINANCIAL BARRIERS

NPs typically earn less than half of their closest physician counterparts, family practice physicians. Midwives have been at the forefront of fighting for equal Medicaid and Medicare reimbursement for NPs. Although the battle is not fully over, the ACNM has made great strides toward equal compensation. Nurse-midwives are now compensated equally with their physician counterparts for the same services. Even with equity in compensation, nurse-midwives still provide less costly care, because of less frequent use of expensive diagnostic tests and technological interventions during childbirth, as well as a significantly lower cesarean section rate.

Private insurers are mixed in their payment for nurse-midwife services, varying from not covering midwifery care, to excluding birth centers and home birth, to fully covering all birth options. Medicaid now covers 41% of all prenatal patients (March of Dimes, 2013), and although it grants compensation for all birth settings (where legal) and providers, the rate of compensation is so low that many practitioners cannot break even unless they have enough private-pay patients to balance out the Medicaid loss (Cowen, 2010). This can lead to rationing of Medicaid services, where clinics limit the proportion of Medicaid patients to private-pay patients in order to survive financially; in many cases, physician practices have stopped accepting Medicaid patients entirely (Hogberg, 2012; Jackson Healthcare, 2013).

Hospital budgets can present a barrier to ideal midwifery practice. Need for quick turnover of labor and delivery rooms can lead to pressure on the midwife to schedule inductions, to encourage repeat cesarean section rather than a trial of labor after cesarean (TOLAC), and to encourage patients to agree to interventions intended to hurry the normal process of labor, effecting faster delivery and consequently making more labor rooms available. Collaborating physicians, schooled in the medical model of obstetric care, may struggle to understand why the midwife objects to financially based interventions, while nursing staff may empathize with the midwife's perspective but struggle with the demands of staying within a budget while still maintaining adequate staffing for patient needs.

Additional financial barriers to midwifery practice come in the guise of safe medical care. Although midwives order fewer diagnostic tests and perform fewer technological interventions, they can still fall prey to fear of litigation, and the "I did everything I could" mentality that prompts many providers to order tests and procedures that are likely unnecessary, in an effort to protect themselves from lawsuits. Midwives especially, because of their unique practice philosophy, are likely to feel the theory–practice gap as they find themselves using tests and procedures in order to protect themselves rather than to serve in the best interests of the patient.

For some midwives, even obtaining malpractice insurance is difficult at best. Washington state is one of a few that have enacted legislation mandating that insurers take turns offering affordable coverage to NPs. In other states, insurance is mandated yet prohibitively expensive, presenting a significant economic barrier to practice. Although insurance is generally available (albeit costly) to NPs, midwives as a specialty group are often entirely excluded from coverage if they offer any intrapartum care, and even the coverage offered by the ACNM, which supports home birth as a viable choice for women, has periodically excluded home birth midwives from qualifying for professional liability insurance. This becomes an insurmountable barrier to practice if the midwife is unable to contract with insurers as a preferred provider because they mandate liability coverage for their contracted providers. To further complicate matters, some insurers have refused coverage for physicians who collaborate with midwives, citing the myth of vicarious liability (Booth, 2007). This concept suggests that the physician who collaborates with a midwife will be responsible for any actions they take before transferring care of a patient to the obstetrician, even when there is not a formal, signed collaborative agreement between the midwife and the physician. In an already litigious atmosphere, obstetricians are understandably hesitant about any collaboration they fear could increase their risk of liability.

Finally, no discussion of financial barriers would be complete without mention of the marginalized women in our society, women who do not have the financial resources to purchase health insurance, or if they qualify for Medicaid have other financial disparities that limit their access to appropriate care. These women often experience lack of resources such as transportation, lack of funds to purchase nonprescription items that Medicaid will not cover, lack of money to pay for services Medicaid either does not cover or for which they cannot find a provider who accepts Medicaid (dental care in pregnancy is a prime example), and lack of funds to provide even the most basic necessities of life for themselves: food, heat, telephone, clothing, and shelter. These are the women to whom midwives are uniquely qualified to reach out and make a difference. The PPACA purposes to make care accessible for these women, but during the time it takes to establish the system, there will continue to be women who fall through the cracks. Even after the system is in place, it is likely that new financial barriers to care will be identified; midwives need to be prepared to address these barriers. The focus of midwives on woman-centered care and serving the underserved positions them to be at the forefront of health care changes over the next decade.

OUTCOME MEASURES FOR CNM PRACTICE

The ACNM initiated a Benchmarking Project (Collins-Fulea, Moore, & Tillett, 2005) with the intended goal of practice improvement and risk reduction. In 2013, the ACNM reported on 15 outcome measures (ACNM, 2013) as follows:

- Total rate of vaginal births
- Rate of spontaneous vaginal births
- Primary C-section rate
- Total C-section rate
- VBAC success rate
- Intact perineum rate
- Episiotomy rate
- Neonatal intensive care unit admission rate

- Preterm birth rate
- Low-birth weight infant rate
- Breastfeeding initiation rate
- Breastfeeding continuation rate
- Total induction rate
- Less than 41-weeks induction rate
- Epidural use rate

Any actions that CNMs take to remove barriers to practice must always be with the goal in mind of improving quality of care. Interestingly, the benchmarking project has found that the highest proportion of practices reporting benchmark data were midwife-led and -managed practices, as opposed to those practices that are collaborative practices or physician-owned. A possible reason for this could be reflected in the numerous studies indicating better outcomes with midwifery care, considering many of the above outcome measures (Cragin & Kennedy, 2006; Johantgen et al., 2012; Newhouse et al., 2011). CNMs have a clear vision of ACNM core competencies and philosophy of care. The challenge today is to remove the barriers standing in the way of successfully implementing the midwifery model of care.

Every CNM has an ethical imperative to become involved in removing barriers that prevent midwives from practicing in accordance with the midwifery model of care. Practice constraints from collaborative agreements, financial constraints, or legislative barriers can no longer be used as a reason for providing patient care that is not in sync with one's philosophy of practice. Each CNM can become a grassroots advocate for midwifery, women, and children (ACNM, 2012a).

LOOKING AHEAD: THE IMPACT OF THE PATIENT PROTECTION AFFORDABLE CARE ACT (PPACA) ON THE FUTURE OF MIDWIFERY

Although health policy experts have offered differing opinions regarding the impact of the PPACA on health care, the state of Massachusetts serves as an example of likely outcomes of PPACA implementation. Structured similarly to the PPACA, the Massachusetts law initially resulted in an increase in emergency department visits as patients struggled to find primary care providers (PCPs). To help meet the shortfall of PCPs, Massachusetts enacted legislation facilitating the recognition and reimbursement of APRNs as primary care providers. With an anticipated increased need for PCPs as the PPACA is implemented, now is the time to press for legislative and regulatory changes recognizing APRNs as independent PCPs nationwide. The recent CMS decision to reimburse CNMs at 100% of the physician fee scale for Medicare patients opened the door for expanded nurse-midwifery services to disabled women of childbearing age, and to senior women who also benefit from midwifery's "with women for a lifetime" approach to care. Several other facets of the PPACA will also impact midwifery, as follows:

- Educational funding: Anticipating increased demand for registered nurses and APRNs, the PPACA provided for an increase in funding, not only in loans available to nursing students but also in reimbursements for graduates who are employed as nursing faculty. The increased funding helps meet the need for more nurse-midwives to provide primary care to low-risk pregnant women and Medicare/Medicaid-insured women.

- Grants for nurse-managed health clinics: The CMS is offering a number of grants and support through its Centers for Medicare and Medicaid Innovation (CMS, n.d.). In accordance with the recommendations of the IOM for an increase in the number of nurse-led clinics and PCMHs, CMS Innovation Models provide incentives for multiples types of practices, as well as proposals for innovative practice.
- Changes in how primary care is delivered: Nursing as a whole and midwives as a specialty have always emphasized preventive care and wellness. Now practices that promote wellness will be at the cutting edge of changes in the way care is delivered. Increased emphasis will be placed on cultural competency in delivery of care, with a shift to community care. Home visits for women and infants are supported by CMS, with other insurers likely to follow suit (CMS, n.d.). Midwives are the ideal leaders for care models serving vulnerable populations of women and infants. Their unique focus on pregnancy and childbirth as a normal part of a woman's life, rather than a disease, and their emphasis on keeping childbirth free of unnecessary medical interventions position midwives to make significant contributions to a holistic model of primary health care for women.
- Increased recognition of CNMs as primary care providers: APRNs are often excluded from preferred provider lists, making them less visible to the public. With the emphasis on increased utilization of APRNs as primary care providers, more options will be offered to patients as APRNs are included on preferred provider lists.

One area where the PPACA currently poses a problem for nurse-midwives is initiation of wellness exams for Medicare and Medicaid patients. Although termed an "exam," the wellness exam is not a physical examination. Rather, it is a visit that includes collection of medical and family history, medication history, list of medical providers, routine measurements such as blood pressure, weight, and body mass index (BMI), cognitive assessment, development of a screening schedule for the next 5 to 10 years, health education, and referrals for education and preventive care as indicated. Under the current language of the PPACA, nurse-midwives are not authorized to perform the initial wellness exam. CNMs may still perform the annual well-woman physical exam, which also includes collection of much of the same information comprising the wellness exam. At the time of this writing, the ACNM is in discussion with the secretary of CMS in an effort to revise the current language to be inclusive of CNMs as approved providers of the initial wellness exam (ACNM, 2012b).

In order for midwives to realize the full benefit of the PPACA to independent APRN practice, they must not only succeed in changing language that excludes midwives from recognition as providers of the initial wellness exam, but they must also work within their home states to achieve legislative and regulatory changes allowing them to practice to the full extent for which the PPACA provides. An example can be found in the recent success of the ACNM's Maryland chapter in the passage of the Maryland Birth Options Preservation Act. The Act removed supervisory language and replaced it with the ACNM guideline that calls for midwives to have a written plan for collaboration, consultation, and referral (ACNM, 2008). Other state chapters have achieved similar successes. For midwifery to remain a viable and growing profession in the coming years, every midwife must give serious consideration to becoming personally involved in working to remove barriers to practice.

REMOVING BARRIERS TO PRACTICE

Clarin (2007) proposed six strategies for removing barriers to APRN practice:

- Educate physicians to understand the APRN role and scope of practice
- Train medical students with graduate nursing students
- Work toward uniformity of education and certification requirements for APRNs
- Apply integrated collaboration models when developing new APRN positions
- Require all team members to be responsible for improvement of communication
- Practice interdisciplinary rounds with APRNs and physicians to demonstrate the APRN's ability and involvement in medical management

Quinn (in AARP, 2012) asserts that change will require an advocacy approach. In order to remove practice barriers, CNMs will need to make a power shift. This can be performed by creating a coalition of multiple stakeholders: nurses, APRNs, consumers, payers, and businesses affected by the practice barriers. In most states that have outdated practice laws, the power lies with those who have the most money. Policy makers will vote according to who is supporting them financially and who is voting for them. Although nurses do not have as strong an economic base as physicians, they have the numbers to significantly influence a vote for or against a politician. Consumers can also significantly impact a vote by sheer numbers. As demonstrated in the Ontario NP clinic project (van Soeren et al., 2009), concerned consumers were able to effect a change in outdated practice laws simply by their vote.

Restrepo (2012) suggested ways that the individual APRN can become involved in removing barriers to practice:

- Discontinue use of the term "mid-level practitioner" as it implies a lesser quality care provider
- Emphasize our professional standing and our unique contributions to health care, especially in the areas of health promotion, coordination of care, disease prevention, and palliative care
- Become actively involved in your specialty professional organization, whether by contributing financially, politically, or both
- Contribute to research contributions submitted not only to nursing journals but also to other non-nursing publications in order to reach a larger professional audience

Whether by educating physician colleagues, becoming active in grassroots advocacy campaigns, contributing financially to professional organizations, providing information to legislators, or sharing information on the professional capabilities of APRNs on a one-to-one basis with consumers, each CNM has the ability—and the obligation—to fight for the future of midwifery and advanced practice nursing.

DISCUSSION QUESTIONS

1. *Based on the information in this chapter, identify two issues you consider to be most urgently in need of policy change in your practice area, state, or nationwide.*
2. *If you were going to describe the importance of these two issues for policy change to potential supporters, what key issues would you stress? How would you describe this to your patients in a way that would motivate them to contact the appropriate legislators?*
3. *Consider the health policy changes discussed in this chapter or those you have described in your analysis and consider the impact that might occur if these changes are NOT enacted. In other words, what are the consequences of inaction?*

ANALYSIS, SYNTHESIS, AND CLINICAL APPLICATION

1. *Ellen is a nurse midwife caring for a 22-year-old G1P0 in early labor. Two hours ago, the patient's exam was 4 cm/70%/–3/posterior with 30-second contractions every 7 minutes. The patient was smiling and talking through contractions. Ellen's exam now shows the patient to be 4 cm/100% effaced/0 station/anterior, with 45-second contractions every 3 minutes. The patient is breathing hard with each contraction and expressing doubt that she can handle natural labor. The charge nurse of the labor and delivery unit informs Ellen that they need the bed for this patient, and urges her to either augment labor to expedite delivery or discharge the patient to home because "she is not progressing." The patient does not want to go home, does not want augmentation, and is relying on Ellen's support to help her have a natural birth. Ellen knows that augmentation will make it more difficult for her patient to have a natural birth.*
   - *Which aspects of the ACNM philosophy of care are important to consider in Ellen's situation?*
   - *Which core competencies apply in this situation?*
   - *How can Ellen advocate for her patient in this situation?*
   - *Can Ellen be an advocate for her patient while still being supportive of the charge nurse's concerns? Why or why not?*
2. *Mary Beth has been one of four midwives in an all-midwifery practice at a busy city hospital for the last 8 years. The midwives in her group deliver about 35% of the babies born in the hospital each year and collaborate with two private groups of obstetricians. The midwives' practice is the only one in the city that accepts Medicaid. The obstetricians will take Medicaid referrals of women who are too high-risk for midwifery care, but otherwise will not see Medicaid patients due to low reimbursement. Mary Beth's friend in the hospital credentialing department tells her the physicians are discussing rescinding their collaborative agreement for "sponsorship" of hospital privileges for midwives. They want the midwives to perform all the prenatal and postpartum care for the Medicaid patients, while the obstetricians will manage intrapartum care, allowing them to collect the majority of the Medicaid fee. The midwives do not want to stop attending births, but need their collaborative agreement with the obstetricians in order to continue to practice in their state.*
   - *Which aspects of the ACNM philosophy of care are important to consider?*
   - *Which core competencies apply in this situation?*

- *What strategies can Mary Beth and her group use in approaching the obstetricians?*
- *Imagine Mary Beth practices in a state that authorizes independent practice of nurse-midwives. Would the obstetricians' proposal present a regulatory barrier or a collegial barrier, or both? Why?*
- *What strategies might Mary Beth and her group use to approach hospital administrators about a bylaw revision that would allow the midwives to practice independently, without a physician "sponsor"?*

EXERCISES/CONSIDERATIONS

1. *Review the information at the Grassroots Advocacy page of the ACNM website at www.midwife.org/Grassroots-Advocacy. Choose one of the suggested actions and discuss the steps necessary to implement it.*
2. *Discuss collaborative practice with CNMs in your area.*
   - *Is their collaborative relationship formal (as in a written agreement) or informal?*
   - *Have the CNMs you talk with ever felt compelled, due to the hierarchical nature of their collaborative relationship, to practice in a way that conflicts with the ACNM philosophy of care?*
   - *What do the CNMs feel would improve collaboration in their practice setting?*
3. *Imagine your ideal practice setting a decade from now. How will it be different from your practice today? What steps can you take now to achieve that ideal practice?*

ETHICAL CONSIDERATIONS

1. *Certified nurse-midwives who do not have collegial collaborative agreements may face ethical dilemmas if they are compelled to engage in practices they know are not evidence-based or that conflict with the ACNM philosophy of care. Which is the greater ethical responsibility in this case: to provide the midwifery model of evidence-based care to one patient, or to cooperate with collaborating physicians' preferred practices in order to maintain collaborative agreements? Are there other possible solutions?*
2. *Judith has just started a new job as a certified nurse midwife on a busy labor unit. The hospital bylaws require her to consult with an obstetrician in the event a patient has a baby suspected to be larger than 4,000 g. Her patient's baby is estimated at 4,200 g by a 39-week ultrasound performed today. The patient has otherwise been healthy, negative for gestational diabetes, and had a 22-pound weight gain with a starting BMI of 24. This is the woman's first baby and her Bishop's score is 2. The woman does not want to be induced. The consulting obstetrician instructs Judith to admit her patient and begin an induction for suspected macrosomia. Judith knows that the evidence does not support the benefit of induction of labor for suspected macrosomia in the absence of gestational diabetes, and that an induction may increase her patient's risk of needing a cesarean birth.*
   - *What ethical principles apply to this situation?*
   - *Which aspects of the ACNM philosophy of care are most important to consider?*
- *If the obstetrician insists that Judith needs to induce the patient, regardless of evidence presented, how should Judith respond?*

REFERENCES

American Academy of Family Physicians. (2010). AAFP takes issue with IOM report calling for greater nursing role. Retrieved from http://www.aafp.org/online/en/home/publications/news/news -now/professional-issues/20101006iomnursingreport.html

American Association of Retired Persons. (2012, October 17). Removing barriers to APRN practice and care: The consumer perspective. Future of Nursing: *Campaign for Action*, at the Center to Champion Nursing in America. Retrieved from http://www.campaignforaction.org/webinar/ removing-barriers-aprn-practice-and-care-consumer-perspective

American College of Nurse Midwives. (2008). Supplement to ACNM annual report 2008. Retrieved from http://www.midwife.org/ACNM/files/ccLibraryFiles/Filename/000000000522/annual report2008_supplement.pdf

American College of Nurse Midwives. (2010). Our philosophy of care. Retrieved from http://www .midwife.org/Child-Page-3

American College of Nurse Midwives. (2012a). Grassroots advocacy. Retrieved from http://www .midwife.org/Grassroots-Advocacy

American College of Nurse Midwives. (2012b). Midwives and Medicare after health care reform. Retrieved from http://www.midwife.org/Midwives-and-Medicare-after-Health-Care-Reform

American College of Nurse Midwives. (2013). 2013 ACNM benchmarking project: Summary data. Retrieved from http://www.midwife.org/acnm/files/ccLibraryFiles/Filename/000000004435/ General-Summary-2013.pdf

American Medical Association. (2010). AMA responds to the IOM report on future of nursing. Retrieved from http://www.oalib.com/references/14154284

Berg, M. (2005). A midwifery model of care for childbearing women at high risk: Genuine caring in caring for the genuine. *Journal of Perinatal Education, 14*(1), 9–21.

Booth, J. W. (2007). An update on vicarious liability for certified nurse midwives/certified midwives. *Journal of Midwifery and Women's Health, 52*(2), 153–157.

Breckinridge, M. (1981). *Wide neighborhoods* (2nd ed.). Lexington: University Press of Kentucky.

Cairo, M. J. (1996). Emergency physicians' attitudes toward the emerging NP role: Validation versus rejection. *Journal of the American Academy of Nurse Practitioners, 8*(9), 411–417.

Carolan, M., & Hodnett, E. (2007). 'With woman' philosophy: Examining the evidence, answering the questions. *Nursing Inquiry, 14*(2), 140–152.

Centers for Disease Control and Prevention. (2011). Births: Method of delivery. Retrieved from http:// www.cdc.gov/nchs/fastats/delivery.htm

Centers for Medicare and Medicaid Services. (n.d.). Innovation models. Retrieved from http://www .innovation.cms.gov/initiatives/index.html#_Expand

Clarin, O. A. (2007). Strategies to overcome barriers to effective nurse practitioner and physician collaboration. *Journal for Nurse Practitioners, 3*(8), 538–548.

Collins-Fulea, C., Moore, J. J., & Tillett, J. (2005). Improving midwifery practice: The American College of Nurse-Midwives' benchmarking project. *Journal of Midwifery and Women's Health, 50*(6), 461–471. Retrieved from http://www.midwife.org/ACNM/files/ccLibraryFiles/Filename/ 000000000189/PIIS1526952305003302.pdf

Cowen, T. (2010, December 11). Following the money, doctors ration care. *New York Times*. Retrieved from http://www.nytimes.com/2010/12/12/business/12view.html?_r=0

Cragin, L., & Kennedy, H. P. (2006). Linking obstetric and midwifery practice with optimal outcomes. *Journal of Obstetric, Gynecologic, and Neonatal Nursing, 35*(6), 779–785.

Doherty, M. E. (2009). Therapeutic alliance: A concept for the childbearing season. *Journal of Perinatal Education, 18*(3), 39–47.

Fahy, K. M., & Parratt, J. A. (2006). Birth territory: A theory for midwifery practice. *Women Birth, 19*(2), 45–50.

Family Health and Birth Center. (2007). Briefing Statement to the Committee on Health of the Council of the District of Columbia, 2/22/07. As cited in ACNM (2007). Issue brief: Reducing health disparities. Retrieved from http://www.midwife.org/ACNM/files/ACNMLibraryData/ UPLOADFILENAME/000000000112/Health_Care_Disparities_Issue_Brief_10_07.pdf

Frontier Nursing Service. (1958). Summary of the first 10,000 confinement records of the Frontier Nursing Service. *QBull Frontier Nursing Service, 33,* 45–55.

Hauer, K. E., Durning, S. J., Kernan, W. N., Fagan, M. J., Mintz, M., O'Sullivan, P. S., & Schwartz, M. D. (2008). Factors associated with medical students' career choices regarding internal medicine. *Journal of the American Medical Association, 300*(10), 1154–1164.

Heale, R. (2012). Overcoming barriers to practice: A nurse practitioner-led model. *Journal of the American Academy of Nurse Practitioners, 24*(6), 358–363.

Hoban, R. (2012). Midwives and doctors tussle over home births, but it's pregnant women who are affected. Retrieved from https://www.northcarolinahealthnews.org/2012/08/17/midwives -doctors-tussle-over-home-births-but-its-pregnant-women-who-are-affected

Hofer, A. N., Abraham, J. M., & Moscovice, I. (2011). Expansion of coverage under the Patient Protection and Affordable Care Act and primary care utilization. *Milbank Quarterly, 89*(1), 69–89.

Hogberg, D. (2012, August). The next exodus: Primary-care physicians and Medicare. National Policy Analysis. Retrieved from http://www.nationalcenter.org/NPA640.html

Institute of Medicine. (2011). *The future of nursing: Leading change, advancing health.* Retrieved from https:// www.nap.edu/read/12956/chapter/1

Jackson Healthcare. (2013). Physician practice trends survey 2012. Retrieved from http://www.jackson healthcare.com/media-room/surveys/physician-practice-trends-survey-2012.aspx

Johantgen, M., Fountain, L., Zangaro, G., Newhouse, R., Stanik-Hutt, J., & White, K. (2012). Comparison of labor and delivery care provided by certified nurse-midwives and physicians: A systematic review, 1990 to 2008. *Women's Health Issues, 22*(1), 73–81.

Kennedy, H. P. (2000). A model of exemplary midwifery practice: Results of a Delphi study. *Journal of Midwifery & Women's Health, 45*(1), 4–19.

Kennedy, H. P., Rousseau, A. L., & Low, L. K. (2003, September). An exploratory metasynthesis of midwifery practice in the United States. *Midwifery, 19*(3), 203–214.

Lange, G., & Kennedy, H. P. (2010). Student perceptions of ideal and actual midwifery practice. *Journal of Midwifery & Women's Health, 51*(2), 71–77.

Lehrman, E. J. (1981). Nurse-midwifery practice: A descriptive study of prenatal care. *Journal of Nurse Midwifery, 26*, 27–41.

Levy, B. S., Wilkinson, F. S., & Marine, W. M. (1971). Reducing neonatal mortality rates with nurse-midwives. *American Journal of Obstetrics and Gynecology, 109*, 50–58.

Lugo, N. R., O'Grady, E. T., Hodnicki, D. R., & Hanson, C. M. (2007). Ranking NP state regulation: Practice environment and consumer healthcare choice. *American Journal for Nurse Practitioners, 11*(4), 8–24.

March of Dimes. (2013). Medicaid coverage of births: U.S. 2001–2003. PeriStats. Retrieved from http:// www.marchofdimes.com/peristats/level1.aspx?reg=99&top=11&stop=154&lev=1&slev=1&obj =1&dv=cr

Morten, A., Kohl, M., O'Mahoney, P., & Pelosi, K. (1991). Certified nurse-midwifery care of the postpartum client: A descriptive study. *Journal of Nurse-Midwifery, 36*(5), 276–288.

Newhouse, R. P., Stanik-Hutt, J., White, K. M., Johantgen, M., Bass, E. B., Zangaro, G., & Weiner, J. P. (2011). Advanced practice nurse outcomes 1990–2008: A systematic review. *Nursing Economic$, 29*(5), 1–22.

Nickel, S., Gesse, T., & MacLaren, A. (1992). Ernestine Wiedenbach: Her professional legacy. *Journal of Nurse-Midwifery, 37*(3), 161–167.

Patient Protection and Affordable Care Act. (2010). One Hundred Eleventh Congress of the United States of America at the Second Session. Retrieved from http://www.gpo.gov/fdsys/pkg/ BILLS-111hr3590enr/pdf/BILLS-111hr3590enr.pdf

Pleticha, K. (2004). The birth battle: Doctors, midwives, and the politics of pregnancy. *Parent: Wise, 1*(1). Retrieved from: http://www.parentwiseaustin.com/Archive/2004-04/ Birth-Battle-Doctors-Midwives-and-Politics-Pregnancy

Restrepo, G. (2012, October 25). Advanced practice nursing: The future is now. *The Clinical Advisor.* Retrieved from http://www.clinicaladvisor.com/advanced-practice-nursing-the-future-is-now/ article/265419/#

Rooks, J. (1997). *Midwifery and childbirth in America.* Philadelphia, PA: Temple University Press.

Safriet, B. (2011). Appendix H: Federal options for maximizing the value of advanced practice nurses in providing quality, cost-effective health care. In Committee on the Robert Wood Johnson Foundation Initiative on the Future of Nursing (Ed.), *The future of nursing: Leading change, advancing health.* Washington, DC: National Academies Press.

Shaver, K. (2007, May 18). Birth centers' closures limit delivery options. *The Washington Post*, pp. B1–B5.

Shaw, A., deLusignan, S., & Rowlands, G. (2005). Do primary care professionals work as a team: A qualitative study. *Journal of Interprofessional Care, 19*(4), 396–405.

Sonenberg, A. (2010). Medicaid and state regulation of nurse-midwives: The challenge of data retrieval. *Policy, Politics, and Nursing Practice, 11*(4), 253–259.

Stapleton, S. R., Osborne, C., & Illuzzi, J. (2013). Outcomes of care in birth centers: Demonstration of a durable model. *Journal of Midwifery & Women's Health, 58*(1), 3–14.

Thompson, J. E., Oakley, D., Burke, M., Jay, S., & Conklin, M. (1989). Theory building in nurse-midwifery. *Journal of Midwifery & Women's Health, 4*(3), 120–130.

van Soeren, M., Hurlock-Chorostecki, C., Goodwin, S., & Baker, E. (2009). The primary healthcare nurse practitioner in Ontario: A workforce study. *Nursing Leadership, 22*(2), 58–72.

Vedam, S., Goff, M., & Marnin, V. N. (2007). Closing the theory–practice gap: Intrapartum midwifery management of planned home births. *Journal of Midwifery & Women's Health, 52*(3), 291–300.

CHAPTER 33

Health Care Policy and Certified Registered Nurse Anesthetists: Past, Present, and Future

Christine S. Zambricki

Certified Registered Nurse Anesthetists (CRNAs) are Advanced Practice Registered Nurses (APRNs) who, as anesthesia professionals, safely administer *approximately 43 million anesthetics* to patients each year in the United States according to the American Association of Nurse Anesthetists (AANA) 2016 Practice Profile Survey (AANA, 2016b). CRNAs have a proud history of integrating nursing care with specialized knowledge and skill in administering anesthesia and treating pain. The success of the nurse anesthesia profession in the public policy arena over time has not been a matter of chance; it has been a matter of choice. The early leaders of this profession were amazing women who taught so many lessons that resonate today. Nurse anesthetists such as Alice Magaw and Agatha Hodgins had ideas of consequence that predicted and ensured the centrality of CRNAs in contemporary health care delivery.

For a student of the history of nurse anesthesia in America, the most astonishing fact about current challenges is that contemporary health policy issues have roots deeply embedded in the past. Turf wars are not new, nor are battles for reimbursement or attempts to restrict the scope of practice. Examining the oldest nursing specialty's saga from its 19th-century beginnings to the present not only brings to light many compelling characters, but it also lays to rest numerous myths and allows us to come to grips with the most pressing national health issues of our time. What follows are lessons that we need to learn—but have not—from the history of this storied profession.

BRIEF HISTORICAL BACKGROUND/RELEVANT LITERATURE

Surgery in the early 1800s was a barbaric enterprise, requiring physical force to immobilize the patient only to have many patients die from postoperative surgical infections in the following days. Nurses in the late 19th century were essential contributors to the two significant advances that paved the way for the "Golden Age of Surgery." Without the ability to prevent surgical infections and the capacity to render a patient insensible to pain, surgery could not progress.

Although the relationship between germs and disease was not completely understood at that time, Florence Nightingale's emphasis on cleanliness, hygiene, and ventilation proved dramatically successful, reducing the death rate in British army hospitals in the 1850s from 40% to 2% (Porter, 2001, p. 226). The world took notice when Nightingale began her *Notes on Hospitals* (1863) with the prescient admonition: "It may seem a strange principle to enunciate as the very first requirement in a Hospital that it should do the sick no harm" (Nightingale, 1863, Preface). Florence Nightingale's words still hold true today. If she could see APRNs now, how proud she would be of their leadership and steadfast commitment to patient care.

With the opening of the first formal school of nursing in New York in 1873, nursing began to achieve recognition in the United States as a respectable profession rooted in the science of Nightingale's work. At about the same time, sterile gowns, gloves, and instruments were replacing street clothes, bare hands, and water-rinsed instruments and sponges in the operating room. With the emergence of nursing as a legitimate career choice and the acceptance of asepsis, the foundation for safe surgery was falling into place.

The only barrier remaining to achieve Nightingale's obligation to "do the sick no harm" in surgery was the need for a qualified provider to deliver anesthesia safely and efficiently. Once again, professional nursing fulfilled the need and made possible the advancement of contemporary surgery.

Modern anesthesia began in the 1840s with the introduction of diethyl ether for use as a general anesthetic. It would be decades before the administration of anesthesia became safe and predictable. In the years following the demonstration of the anesthetizing properties of diethyl ether, there were no nurse anesthetists, no anesthesiologists, and it was well recognized that "the life of the patient, no less than the success of the operation, is jeopardized by the careless and ignorant manner in which this important part of the procedure is carried out by a novice just out of medical school" ("The Professional Anaesthetizer," 1897). Initially, anesthesia duties were assigned to the least experienced medical school graduates. These younger interns were more interested in observing the surgery than in monitoring the patient, and the lack of vigilance during the administration of anesthesia resulted in significant mortality.

During the Civil War, there were reports of nurse anesthetists using chloroform to anesthetize soldiers in battlefield hospitals, and the demand began to grow for nurse anesthesia services (Sudlow, 2000, p. 9; Thatcher, 1953, pp. 33, 54). After the war, to meet the need for dedicated and focused anesthesia providers, surgeons recruited Catholic nursing nuns to train them as nurse anesthetists. The earliest existing records documenting the anesthetic care of patients by nurses were those of Sister Mary Bernard in 1887 at St. Vincent's Hospital in Erie, Pennsylvania (Thatcher, 1953).

In the late 1800s, working with the Mayo brothers in Rochester, Minnesota, nurse anesthetist Alice Magaw, known as the "Mother of Anesthesia," greatly contributed to the fund of knowledge in anesthesia. Magaw perfected techniques for administration of open-drop ether and chloroform, documenting the personal administration of 14,000 surgical anesthetics without a single mortality in 1906

(Koch, 1999). Based on the observations of her work, medical leaders turned to nursing as a solution to the need for professional, dedicated anesthetists. Looking at the roots of nurse anesthesia practice, what distinguished nurse anesthetists from the beginning were the "touch" component of the care, coupled with technical excellence, and quality patient outcomes. The need for specific training in anesthesia was pressing, and doctors and nurses came from across the globe to learn anesthesia techniques from Magaw and Mayo. Dr. J. M. Baldy, president of the American Gynecologic Society, summed up the current state of affairs in his presidential address in 1908 when he said: "The general administration of anesthetics as it is performed today is the shame of modern surgery, is a disgrace to a learned profession, and if the full unvarnished truth concerning it were known it would be but a short while before it were interfered with by legislative means—and properly so. . . . Many brainy women, fully capable of being trained to this responsible position, have entered the nursing profession and it is from this source that we may look for a solution to our difficulties" (Baldy, 1908).

By World War I, there were four formalized, postgraduate educational programs training nurse anesthetists. In 1915, nurse anesthetists Agatha Hodgins and Dr. George Crile (cofounder of the Cleveland Clinic), having perfected the administration of nitrous oxide/oxygen anesthesia, opened Lakeside (Hospital) School of Anesthesia in Cleveland, Ohio. Through Hodgins's leadership and vision, the alumni association of this program was the nucleus for the formation of the AANA.

With the increasing professional recognition of nurse anesthetists, physicians became attracted to the field. A number of legal challenges ensued, the most famous being *Frank v. South* (1917) in the state of Kentucky. In this case, the Jefferson County Medical Society claimed that Margaret Hatfield, a nurse anesthetist, was illegally practicing medicine. The Supreme Court of Kentucky ruled that using discretion and making independent judgments in the process of giving anesthesia was legitimate nursing practice. Approximately 20 years later, *Chalmers-Francis v. Nelson* (1936) was decided in a manner similar to *Frank v. South,* and anesthesia was determined to be both the practice of medicine and the practice of nursing. Thus, the foundation for nurse anesthesia practice was firmly established in U.S. law.

Today, CRNAs are APRNs, prepared at the master's or doctoral level, with specialized education in anesthesia and pain management. More than 50,000 CRNAs administer over 32 million anesthetics in the United States each year (AANA, 2016b).

CRNAs administer anesthesia for all types of surgical cases, from the simplest to the most complex. CRNAs are the predominant anesthesia professionals in rural America; in some states, CRNAs are the sole providers in nearly 100% of the rural hospitals. CRNAs work in all settings in which anesthesia and pain care are delivered: traditional hospital surgical suites and obstetrical delivery rooms; ambulatory surgical centers; in the offices of dentists, podiatrists, and plastic surgeons; and in pain clinics. In 24% of all U.S. counties, CRNAs are the sole anesthesia professionals. Nurse anesthesia predominates in veterans' hospitals and the U.S. Armed Forces. More than 900 full-time CRNAs are employed by the Department of Veterans Health Administration (U.S. Department of Veterans Affairs, 2016).

According to the U.S. Department of Labor, all four types of APRNs, including nurse anesthetists, will be in high demand through the 2014 to 2024 decade, particularly in medically underserved areas such as inner cities and rural areas (U.S. Bureau of Labor Statistics, U.S. Department of Labor, 2016). Employment projections for nurse anesthetists predict a 19% growth rate for the decade, primarily because of an increase in the number of individuals who have access to health insurance and the continuing aging of the baby boomer generation, who require more surgical procedures as they live longer and seek more active lives than previous generations. For a multitude of reasons, 21st-century surgical volume continues to increase year after year without any sign of abatement. CRNAs continue to command significantly higher salaries than other APRNs, regardless of educational level or practice setting (Yox, Stokowski, McBride, & Berry, 2016).

Ninety percent of America's CRNAs are members of the 50,000-member AANA. This is a high percentage of membership by any measure. Men make up more than 40% of nurse anesthetists while making up less than 10% of nurses in general. Since its founding by Agatha Hodgins in 1931, the AANA has placed its responsibilities to the public above or equal to its responsibilities to its membership. The education of nurse anesthetists has been a priority throughout the history of the AANA. The AANA's certification exam was first administered in 1945, nurse anesthesia educational programs were nationally accredited in 1952, a voluntary continuing education program was approved in 1969, and a mandatory continuing education became effective in 1978. In 1986, a bachelor's degree in nursing or a related degree was required for admission to nurse anesthesia programs, and by 1998 all programs were required to be at the graduate level, awarding at least a master's degree. Doctoral education for entry into nurse anesthesia practice will be required by 2025.

The Council on Accreditation of Nurse Anesthesia Educational Programs (COA) is the accrediting agency for the 119 nurse anesthesia programs in the United States, its territories, and protectorates (COA, 2017a), as well as for three nurse anesthesia fellowship programs (COA, 2017b). The COA's mission is to grant public recognition to nurse anesthesia programs and institutions that award post-master's certificates, master's, and doctoral degrees that meet nationally established standards of academic quality and to assist programs and institutions in improving the educational quality (COA, 2016a).

The National Board of Certification and Recertification for Nurse Anesthetists (NBCRNA) is a not-for-profit corporation comprising the Council on Recertification and the Council on Certification of Nurse Anesthetists. The mission of the NBCRNA is to promote patient safety through credentialing programs that support lifelong learning (NBCRNA, 2016a).

NBCRNA credentialing provides assurances to the public that certified individuals have met objective, predetermined qualifications for providing nurse anesthesia services. Although state licensure provides the legal credential for the practice of professional nursing, private voluntary certification indicates compliance with the professional standards for practice in nurse anesthesia. The certification credential for nurse anesthetists has been institutionalized in health care facilities, and it has been recognized through malpractice litigation, state nurse practice acts, and state rules and regulations.

To become a CRNA, a licensed registered nurse must graduate from a nationally accredited nurse anesthesia educational program and pass the national certifying examination administered by the Council on Certification of Nurse

Anesthetists. CRNAs are recertified via the Continued Professional Certification (CPC) Program which is based on 8-year periods comprised of two 4-year cycles. In addition to practice and state licensure requirements, the CPC requires continuing education credits, completion of prescribed learning modules, and a pass/fail examination (NBCRNA, 2016b).

CONCEPTUAL AND THEORETICAL SUPPORT

CRNAs are anesthesia professionals who have been providing anesthesia care and managing pain in the United States for nearly 150 years. The conceptual framework for CRNA practice originates with the scope, standards, guidelines, and position statements set forth by the AANA. As with APRNs, the practice of nurse anesthesia is also grounded in the theoretical framework contained within *The Consensus Model for APRN Regulation: Licensure, Accreditation, Certification, and Education*, approved in 2008 by the National Council of State Boards of Nursing (NCSBN) along with 44 other nursing organizations including the AANA (NCSBN, 2008). This model is currently being implemented on a state-by-state basis with the goal of uniformity of state regulations throughout the country (NCSBN, 2016).

The AANA Scope of Nurse Anesthesia Practice offers guidance for CRNAs and health care institutions regarding the scope of nurse anesthesia practice, recognizing that scope is continuously evolving based on patient and community needs, as well as the development of new science and technology. Contemporary CRNA practice encompasses the responsibilities associated with anesthesia practice, as well as pain management. CRNAs, like all health care providers, work as members of interprofessional teams. Every CRNA is individually responsible for the quality of services he or she renders (AANA, 2013c). Recognizing the inevitability of overlapping scope of practice with physicians and others, CRNAs' scope of practice is grounded in benefits to the public regarding quality and access to care within a competency framework.

The practice of anesthesia is a specialty in both nursing and medicine. Anesthesia practice is defined as the art and science of rendering a patient insensible to pain by the administration of anesthetic agents and related drugs and procedures. CRNA scope of practice also includes, but is not limited to, the management of pain associated with obstetrical labor and delivery, management of acute and chronic ventilatory problems, and the management of acute and chronic pain. Education, practice, and research in the specialty are to promote competent anesthesia care encompassing the diversity of patient populations, age, ethnicity, and gender (AANA, n.d.-a, n.d.-b, n.d.-c, 2016b).

The AANA has adopted a *Code of Ethics* to guide nurse anesthetists in fulfilling their obligations as professionals. CRNAs practice nursing by providing anesthesia and related services such as advanced monitoring and pain management. They accept the responsibility conferred on them by the state, the profession, and the society. Each CRNA has a personal responsibility to uphold and adhere to these ethical standards (AANA, 2013a). The observance includes responsibility to patients, competence, responsibilities as a professional, responsibilities to society, and ethical behavior regarding research, business practices, and endorsement of products and services.

The Consensus Model for APRN Regulation: Licensure, Accreditation, Certification, and Education (2008) defines APRN practice, describes the APRN regulatory model, identifies the titles to be used, defines each specialty, and describes the emergence of new roles and population foci. APRNs, including CRNAs, are defined as licensed independent practitioners who are expected to practice within standards established or recognized by a licensing body. As such, the CRNA is accountable to patients, the nursing profession, and the licensing board to comply with the requirements of the state nurse practice act, and for the quality of advanced nursing care rendered; for recognizing limits of knowledge and experience, and planning for the management of situations beyond the APRN's expertise; and for consulting with or referring patients to other health care providers as appropriate (The Joint Dialogue Group, 2008).

APPLICATION TO APRN PRACTICE

Throughout nurse anesthesia history, key turning points have been marked by nurse anesthetist leaders who were political entrepreneurs. They had visionary ideas, noticed weaknesses in the status quo, and prevailed on decision makers to act to achieve political change.

The major health policy challenges for nurse anesthetists fall into one of the two general categories: scope of practice and reimbursement. In general, the scope of practice is determined at the state level, and decisions drive reimbursement at the federal level. The reality is that these two policy issues are inextricably connected because access to reimbursement is essentially a form of economic credentialing. Thus, payment impacts scope. Similarly, the scope of practice drives reimbursement with a direct link between what services a professional is authorized to provide and payment under the current fee-for-service system.

The Patient Protection and Affordable Care Act (PPACA; United States Public Law 111-148, March 23, 2010) implemented significant changes to how health care is paid for in the United States. Alternative delivery and payment models such as accountable care organizations and health insurance exchanges were created as innovations to pay for more covered lives. It is incumbent on every nurse anesthetist to understand the value of his or her services as health care policy evolves. Medicare reimbursement methodology is important to CRNAs because the federal government is the largest health insurance program in the country and also because federal programs are used as a template for private insurers in the states. CRNAs must understand the nuances of anesthesia reimbursement policy beginning with the current system.

Medicare payment policy is outlined in statutes, regulations, and Medicare manuals. Examples of key importance to CRNAs include

- Omnibus Budget Reconciliation Act of 1986
- 42 CFR §410.69, 42 CFR §414.60
- Medicare Claims Processing Manual
- Chapter 12—Physician/Non-physician Practitioners
- Section 50, Payment for Anesthesiology Services
- Section 140, CRNA Services

There are four components of Medicare payment. Of these four, Part A and Part B are of special significance for nurse anesthetist health care policy initiatives.

Part A—Hospital Coverage includes the Conditions of Participation, Conditions for Coverage, and Interpretive Guidelines. Part A also includes the provisions for a reasonable-cost pass-through payment for CRNA services in critical access hospitals. The Conditions of Participation and the Conditions for Coverage outline requirements for hospitals, ambulatory surgery centers, critical access hospitals, and other facilities to participate in the Medicare program. Surveyors use the Interpretive Guidelines to ascertain compliance with the Conditions of Participation and the Conditions for Coverage.

For a health care organization to participate in and receive payment from the Medicare or Medicaid programs through Part A, it must be certified as complying with the Conditions of Participation and the Conditions for Coverage. State agencies conduct surveys on behalf of the Centers for Medicare and Medicaid Services (CMS) to determine compliance. National accrediting organizations must adopt, at a minimum, these standards that meet the federal requirements if they wish to be recognized by CMS. CMS grants these accrediting organizations "deeming" authority to "deem" a health care organization as meeting the Medicare and Medicaid requirements. If the health care organization has "deemed status" from a national accrediting organization, it is not required to undergo a Medicare survey and certification process. However, Medicare is always free to survey in addition to the national accrediting organization if the CMS wishes. Examples of national accrediting organizations that have deeming status from CMS include The Joint Commission (TJC), the Healthcare Facilities Accreditation Program (HFAP) and Det Norske Veritas (DNV) or "The Nordic Truth."

Part B—Physician Services describes conditions of payment for anesthesia services when provided by CRNAs, anesthesiologists, and anesthesia assistants. Part B also authorizes payment for related services that are medical and surgical in nature rather than anesthesia services. These include such things as pain management, Swan–Ganz catheter insertion, and emergency intubation. In addition, Part B sets forth conditions of payment for medical direction and medical supervision, as well as teaching rules.

The remaining two Medicare components are less relevant to nurse anesthesia health care policy. Part C refers to Medicare Advantage HMO, and Part D describes coverage for the Medicare Drug Benefit.

Policy issues rarely occur in a vacuum. The core competencies of CRNA practice exist in a political context of special interests, cost containment, and partisan politics. The following case examples are illustrative of the intersection among access, quality, and cost in a market framed by politics and timing. More than any other APRN specialty, CRNAs have historically experienced the most vigorous and organized resistance from their counterpart anesthesiology physician specialists, particularly as it relates to the scope of practice.

The following real-life examples provide an overview of the strategies and tactics employed which resulted in both public policy success and disappointments directly linked to the professional practice of CRNAs in the United States.

The first case study involves the construct of "physician supervision" as it relates to health care payment policy and state scope of practice. The second example details issues related to the delivery of chronic pain management services by CRNAs and the reimbursement for those services. The third situation revolves around APRN full scope of practice in the Veterans Health Administration (VHA) hospitals. In these cases, strategy and interventions are effectively linked with core competencies and outcomes to impact health care policy.

Elimination of Part A Medicare Requirements for Physician Supervision

The concept of "physician supervision" has been misinterpreted, misused, and misunderstood since its inception. In our complex health care world, the reality is that no one, neither the physician nor the nurse, practices independently. Particularly in the surgical environment, there must be and will always be an interprofessional collaboration and cooperation among members of the operating room team. The concept of supervision for highly trained professionals does not fit the reality of contemporary practice in which each brings his or her expertise to the team to provide the very best care for the patient.

The Medicare Part A Conditions of Participation requires physician supervision of nurse anesthetists unless an individual state opts out of that requirement. References regarding physician supervision requirements are contained in facility-specific sections within the Conditions of Participation and Conditions for Coverage. This supervision of CRNAs may be by the operating physician or by an anesthesiologist. At the time of writing (Table 33.1), 17 states have opted out of the Medicare physician supervision requirement for CRNAs (Figure 33.1). There is no opt-out mechanism for anesthesiology assistants (AAs), who must always be supervised, not just by a physician, but by an anesthesiologist too. How did health care policy arrive at this juncture, with physician supervision required and a governor allowed to opt out of the law or opt back in without any requirement for public comment or state legislative oversight?

Organized medicine has long held the belief that the delivery of anesthesia is solely the practice of medicine, despite court decisions to the contrary. After a long hiatus following the *Chalmers-Franci v. Nelson* decision in 1936, the issue of physician supervision became prominent once again in the late 20th century (Blumenreich, 2000). Congress had provided additional financial support for physician education in an attempt to reduce health care costs by increasing the number of doctors. As a result, the number of physicians surged in the last quarter of the century, and the number of anesthesiologists tripled. At the same time, the Captain of the Ship doctrine, in which the surgeon is responsible for all damages caused by hospitals and hospital employees, was on the wane. Some anesthesiologists at this time sought to persuade hospitals and surgeons that they were at a greater risk when working with nurse anesthetists as compared to anesthesiologists. However, fears in this regard were unwarranted, as "the same legal principles that governed the liability of a surgeon for the negligence of a nurse anesthetist also governed the liability of a surgeon for the negligence of an anesthesiologist and had nothing to do with supervision. The issue was whether the surgeon controlled the procedure that gave rise to the injury" (Blumenreich, 2000, p. 407), regardless of whether the procedure was performed by a CRNA or an anesthesiologist.

The CMS Part A reimbursement rules for hospital reimbursement historically required that nurse anesthetists be supervised by either an anesthesiologist or by the procedural physician such as a surgeon or an obstetrician. In December 1997, CMS published a proposed rule that would allow state law to determine

TABLE 33.1 Physician Supervision Language in CMS Conditions of Participation

HEALTH CARE FACILITY	CMS CONDITIONS OF PARTICIPATION
Hospitals	42 CFR §482.52(a)(4)
Ambulatory surgery centers	42 CFR §416.42(b)(2)
Critical access hospitals	42 CFR §485.639(c)(2)

CMS, Centers for Medicare and Medicaid Services.

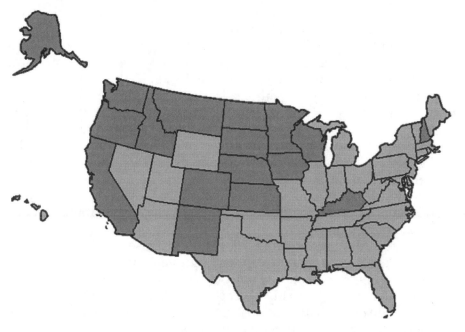

FIGURE 33.1 Opt-out states as of January 2016 (dark gray states).

Source: American Association of Nurse Anesthetists (2016b).

which professionals would be permitted to administer anesthetics and the level of supervision required. This proposed change was based on the "lack of evidence to support maintaining a special federal requirement for physician supervision of CRNAs" (62 Fed. Reg. 56762, 2001, p. 56762).

The final rule to eliminate federal physician supervision requirements for CRNAs furnishing anesthesia services in hospitals, ambulatory surgical centers (ASCs), and critical access hospitals (CAHs) was published on January 18, 2001 to be effective March 19, 2001. In promulgating the final rule, CMS stated "We have found no compelling scientific evidence that an across-the-board federal physician supervision requirement for CRNAs leads to better outcomes" (62 Fed. Reg. 4674, 2001, p. 4674).

Anesthesiologists and organized medicine had vehemently opposed the elimination of physician supervision during the rulemaking period, although there was no evidence to support the position that supervision adds value regarding cost or quality. During the comment period, thousands of letters were written, both for and against, and ultimately the agency issued a final rule eliminating the federal requirement for physician supervision of nurse anesthetists.

Some say that making policy is like making sausage: It is not a pretty sight. What happened subsequently is a practical example of the impact of politics and timing. During the interval between publication of the final rule and the effective date of the rule, a new president of the United States took office and immediately pulled back all proposed and final rules of the previous administration that had not yet been implemented. The result was that the final rule eliminating physician supervision was essentially dead. The new administration delayed implementation in March, postponed implementation again in May, and after much negotiation and advocacy, the baby was split and the compromise that resulted left both sides unhappy. In November 2001, CMS implemented a final rule maintaining physician supervision with the proviso that states may opt out of this federal government requirement (62 Fed. Reg. 56762, 2001).

The process for opt out is simple. The governor of the state must send a letter to CMS informing Medicare that the state will opt out, that this decision is consistent with state law, and that the governor has consulted with the State Boards of Medicine and Nursing. The governor does not need to obtain the permission of the boards but merely consult with them. The governor does not need to get approval from CMS to opt out but only provide notification. When CMS receives the written communication signed by the governor, the opt out is in effect, and the physician supervision requirement for Part A reimbursement no longer applies in that state.

In retrospect, despite the bitter pill of compromise, the benefit of the final rule was that it created a unique opportunity to conduct a retrospective study comparing the difference in patient outcomes between states that had opted out and states that had not. This study was executed, and the results of this research demonstrated conclusively that there is no harm found when nurse anesthetists work without supervision by physicians (Dulisse & Cromwell, 2010).

Repealing the federal Medicare requirement for physician supervision remains a strategic goal for the nurse anesthesia profession. This rule is an example of unnecessary government regulation that is not evidence-based. The scope of practice and supervision requirements are best determined at the state level, and in today's challenging environment, health care facilities need the flexibility to innovate in determining the best anesthesia care delivery model. Contemporary anesthesia practice is extremely safe (Li, Warner, & Lang, 2009) and of the highest quality; therefore, communities may look at factors such as cost and access when seeking to meet the unique needs of their patient population.

As mentioned, physician supervision is a requirement for Medicare Part A payment to hospitals outlined in the Conditions of Participation. It is important to recognize the distinction between physician supervision as a condition of health care facility reimbursement in Part A and the payment methodology for medical direction and physician supervision in Medicare Part B payment to providers. This distinction is critical, as recent findings relative to provider payment practices raise questions about the federal requirement for supervision in Part A. Physician supervision is a Part A requirement for hospital reimbursement, and it refers to general supervision by either an anesthesiologist or by the procedural physician such as a surgeon. Part B provider reimbursement includes the construct of medical direction and also a different construct of medical supervision.

These refer only to anesthesiologists and describe two different ways that anesthesiologists get paid when they work with CRNAs.

There are three options for CRNA practice relative to the Medicare Part A supervision requirement. CRNAs may personally provide anesthesia care without physician supervision if a state has opted out of the federal supervision requirement. Where states have not opted out of the supervision requirement, the operating physician may supervise the CRNA or the CRNA may be supervised by an anesthesiologist. In contrast, federal law requires that anesthesiology assistants must always be supervised by an anesthesiologist.

Professional reimbursement for anesthesia providers is governed by Part B of Medicare. In 1987, through the strong legislative advocacy of the AANA and others, CRNAs became the first nursing group to be paid directly by Medicare reimbursement when the Omnibus Reconciliation Act became law (AANA, 2013c). Part B describes the payment methodology for two types of services—anesthesia services and related services (medical and surgical)—when provided by CRNAs, anesthesiologists, and anesthesia assistants. Part B also defines teaching rules for situations where anesthesiologists or CRNAs are being paid for supervising residents or nurse anesthesia students.

There are three options for Medicare CRNA reimbursement in Medicare Part B. CRNAs are paid 100% of the allowable physician Medicare fee when providing anesthesia services, if there is no anesthesiologist billing medical direction or medical supervision for the same patient. In this case, the CRNA may also be paid 100% for each of the two patients if the CRNA is supervising two students. Alternatively, a nurse anesthetist receives only 50% of the payment when an anesthesiologist is billing either medical direction or medical supervision for that same case.

Payment for an anesthesia service performed by a CRNA may be made to the CRNA or the individual or entity that the CRNA has an employment or contractual relationship with if the CRNA signs over his or her billing rights. This is commonly applied to a CRNA group, an anesthesiologist group, or a health care facility. The conditions for a CRNA to be paid require that the CRNA accept assignment; that is, the CRNA must accept the Medicare payment as payment-in-full for the service and not bill the balance to the patient. CRNAs must personally provide the service, or they may supervise nurse anesthesia students.

In contrast, there are four options by which Medicare pays an anesthesiologist for anesthesia services through Part B reimbursement. They may be paid for personally providing anesthesia services (100% payment), for medically directing CRNAs (50% payment) for each of up to four cases, for medically supervising CRNAs (three base units plus one additional base unit if present for induction) for each case, and for supervising residents (100% payment for each of two residents).

An anesthesiologist may meet the requirement for Part A supervision of the CRNA and yet not bill medical supervision or medical direction in Part B. By law, the operating physician is never eligible to be paid for anesthesia services in Part B, even if he or she is serving as the supervising physician for Part A requirements for facility reimbursement. In other words, either an operating physician or an anesthesiologist may be designated the supervising physician of the CRNA to meet Part A supervision requirements, but only the anesthesiologist may bill for medical direction or medical supervision for Part B professional billing. If an anesthesiologist provides Part A physician supervision but does not bill for medical direction or medical supervision for a given patient, then the CRNA may bill for 100% of the fee for having personally provided the anesthesia care. Whenever the anesthesiologist bills Part B for medical direction or medical supervision, then the CRNA must revert to the option of 50% billing.

Anesthesiologists are permitted to bill for medical direction of up to four concurrent cases. To be compliant with Medicare requirements, when billing Part B medical direction, the anesthesiologist is required to fulfill seven steps (Table 33.2) for each case. At the time of enactment, the Medicare agency emphasized that these seven steps were payment requirements and not the quality-of-care standards (U.S. Department of Health and Human Services [USDHHS], Health Care Financing Administration, 1998).

Anesthesiologists are also allowed to bill for Part B medical supervision for more than four procedures concurrently. This is called Part B medical supervision. When billing medical supervision, the anesthesiologist is paid three base units per case. If the anesthesiologist documents presence at induction, one additional unit is allowed per case for a maximum of four base units for unlimited cases.

The current reimbursement system allowing anesthesiologists to be paid for "medically directing" or "supervising" CRNAs has been widely criticized as an additional cost with no evidence of an increase in safety. The alternative—to pay a single payment to the provider giving the anesthetic to a single patient, whether CRNA or anesthesiologist—would cut costs dramatically for facilities and taxpayers. Such a payment scheme would also promote proper usage of each of two independent, fully-trained, full-service anesthesia providers, thus dramatically reducing any current or future anesthesia provider shortages. With a single payment for a single patient, current fraudulent billing practices would also be eliminated (Horowitz, 2016).

Regardless of whether or not a state has opted out of Part A physician supervision requirements, CRNAs in all states can bill for personally provided anesthesia care in Medicare in Part B. In order to properly bill for services, anesthesiologists and CRNAs must use "modifiers" or codes that describe how the providers are involved in the patient's care (Table 33.3).

TABLE 33.2 Tax Equity and Financial Responsibility Act (TEFRA). Seven Required Steps for Anesthesiologists to Legally Bill for Medical Direction of up to Four Cases

ANESTHESIOLOGISTS BILLING MEDICAL DIRECTION ARE REQUIRED TO MEET SEVEN STEPS
Perform a preanesthetic examination and evaluation
Prescribe the anesthesia plan
Personally participate in the most demanding aspects of the anesthesia plan including, if applicable, induction and emergence
Ensure that any procedures in the anesthesia plan that he or she does not perform are performed by a qualified individual as defined in operating instructions
Monitor the course of anesthesia administration at frequent intervals
Remain physically present and available for immediate diagnosis and treatment of emergencies
Provide indicated postanesthesia care

Source: Conditions for Payment (2001).

TABLE 33.3 CMS Modifiers for CRNAs and Anesthesiologists

ANESTHESIA PROVIDER	ANESTHESIA SERVICE	MODIFIER	PAYMENT
CRNA	Personally performed	QZ	100%
	CRNA providing service when anesthesiologist bills for medical direction	QX	50%
	CRNA providing service when anesthesiologist bills for medical supervision	QX	50%
	CRNA personally performed service with two students	QZ	100% for each of up to two cases
	CRNA providing supervision of two students when anesthesiologist bills for medical direction	QX	50% base units + discontinuous time units
Anesthesiologist	Personally performed	AA	100%
	Medical supervision of >4 concurrent cases	AD	Three base units per case plus 1 unit if documented presence at induction
	Medical direction of one CRNA	QY	50%
	Medical direction of two, three, or four concurrent procedures while meeting the seven steps for all cases	QK	50% for each case
	Supervision of a resident	GC	100% for each of up to two cases
	Medical direction of two CRNAs supervising two students each	QK	50% for each case

CMS, Centers for Medicare and Medicaid Services; CRNA, Certified Registered Nurse Anesthetists.
Source: USDHHS, CMS (2013).

To make things even more complex, the anesthesia payment calculation is based on a formula that includes base units, known as relative value units, a taxonomy adopted by Medicare that is related to the complexity of the case and time units that are calculated by dividing actual time by 15-minute intervals. For example, an appendectomy is 6 base units and coronary bypass surgery is 20 base units. The total units are multiplied by a Medicare conversion factor set annually that varies with state and often with location in the state to arrive at a total charge. Generally, Medicare pays 80% of this total charge, and either the patient's Medicare gap insurance policy or the patient is responsible for the remaining 20%. The formula for calculating payment is

Total units (Base units + Time units) × conversion factor =
Total anesthesia professional Part B charge

The following is an example of how Medicare pays for anesthesia services in the case of a 90-minute appendectomy when a CRNA and/or anesthesiologist is involved in the case. There are 6 relative value units for an appendectomy. It is also important to note that anesthesia time is paid in increments of 15 minutes. Medicare determines an amount paid per billing unit annually. This amount varies with state and with a region in a state and is known as the conversion factor. After computing the fee for the case, Medicare pays 80% of the total. Reimbursement for the appendectomy is

6 (base units) +6 (15-minute time units) = 12 (total units) 12 (total units) × $21.00 (sample conversion factor) = $ 252.00 × 0.8 (Medicare pays 80%) = $201.60

The anesthesiologist is deemed to have met the Medicare requirement to be reimbursed for medical direction if he or she has performed and documented all seven criteria for each concurrent case.

See *Medicare Claims Processing Manual*, Chapter 12, Section 50 for other modifiers; available at www.cms.gov/Regulations-and-Guidance/Guidance/Manuals/downloads/clm104c12.pdf.

An anesthesiologist may medically direct up to four rooms. To be paid for medical direction, the anesthesiologist must comply with the seven steps described in the Tax Equity and Financial Responsibility Act (TEFRA). If the anesthesiologist bills for Part B medical direction, then the anesthesiologist and the CRNA each receive 50% of the payment for the case. The anesthesiologist receives $100.80, and the CRNA receive $100.80. If the anesthesiologist is medically directing four concurrent cases, then he or she receives a total compensation that is the sum of 50% of the payment for each of the four concurrent cases. Although it is more likely that a medically directing anesthesiologist in the real world would be medically directing four different types of cases, for the sake of this example, if the anesthesiologist were to medically direct four concurrent appendectomies, he or she would receive $403.20. At the same time, each CRNA would receive 50% of the total amount paid for each individual case.

An anesthesiologist may medically supervise five or more rooms, according to Part B payment rules. In the case of Part B medical supervision, the anesthesiologist does not need to comply with the seven TEFRA steps to be paid. The anesthesiologist who is medically supervising is paid three base units for each case. If the anesthesiologist documents being present on induction, he or she is paid one additional base unit for that case. When an anesthesiologist bills Part B medical supervision, each CRNA receives 50% of the payment for that case. In the appendectomy example, the CRNA receive $100.80. The anesthesiologist is paid 3 (base units) × $21.00 (conversion factor) = $63.00 per case. For concurrent medically supervised cases where the anesthesiologist documents presence at induction, the anesthesiologist receive $84.00 (an additional base unit of $21).

Of the anesthetics you administer, how often is an anesthesiologist involved in the following activities?

An anesthesiologist or a CRNA may personally provide the anesthetic care without the involvement of medical direction or medical supervision. In this case, the CRNA or the anesthesiologist who is personally providing the appendectomy anesthetic will receive the full Medicare payment of $201.60.

Of the anesthetics you personally administer, how often is an anesthesiologist involved in the following activities?

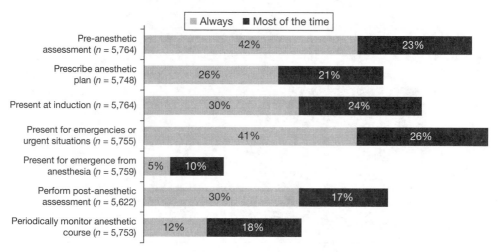

FIGURE 33.2 AANA membership data on compliance with the seven steps.
Source: American Association of Nurse Anesthetists (2011).

For years, nurse anesthesia annual survey responses reported that anesthesiologists do not comply with the seven steps for medical direction in the majority of cases (Figure 33.2). The concept of medical direction as a measure of anesthesiologist work effort was further undermined when *Anesthesiology*, the official publication of the American Society of Anesthesiologists, published a review of one year of data from a tertiary hospital showing that lapses in compliance commonly occurred during first-case-of-the-day starts even with a 1:2 medical direction ratio (Epstein & Dexter, 2012). According to the study, anesthesiologists' failure to comply with the steps required to qualify for payment is substantial (Figure 33.3).

Medical direction adds unnecessary cost to the health care system. Without evidence to support the value proposition of medical direction for every case, having two anesthesia providers when one is sufficient is not consistent with the best use of the resources, particularly in light of health workforce shortages. The "one size fits all" approach does not take into account the individual needs of a patient based on health status, anesthetic plan, or type of procedure. Whether the cases are cataract procedures or open heart surgery, one anesthesiologist may be paid for medically directing up to four cases.

Compliance with the seven steps required for reimbursement results in operating room delays while patients, surgeons, and staff in the operating room waiting for the anesthesiologist to finish in one room. Many hospitals stagger starts by 15 minutes to accommodate this revolving anesthesiologist model but do not stagger employee start times, with shifts beginning at the top of the hour. The cost of this staffing inefficiency is multiplied by the number of operating room team members impacted: at a minimum, a CRNA, an operating room nurse, and a surgical tech for each operating room. At an estimated cost of $20 per minute, the operating room is considered the most expensive real estate in the hospital (Marshall, Steele, & Associates, 2013). Recognizing that the cost of operating

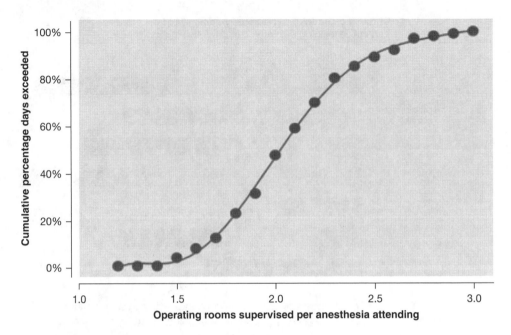

FIGURE 33.3 Lapses in anesthesiologist compliance with requirements for
medical direction payment.

Source: Epstein and Dexter (2012).

room time is variable based on many factors (Macario, 2010), all organizations, including hospitals, have compelling reasons to reduce costs.

Administrative costs associated with an anesthesia team care model are greater than with personally provided anesthesia. Medical direction incurs a greater administrative burden because two anesthesia bills must be generated rather than one. Unfortunately, in too many cases this results in denials, two appeals, and two appeal decisions, multiplying the administrative burden of providing care.

In addition, hospital administrators are often incorrectly led to believe that they must have an anesthesiologist to supervise the CRNAs. It is not uncommon for anesthesiologist groups to require the hospital to pay a subsidy to make up for the income shortfall that the anesthesiologist group perceives will result from direct reimbursement for the case volume that is available. Subsidies to anesthesiologist groups represent a significant cost to health care facilities. The 2012 Subsidy Study by HealthCare Performance Strategies reports that subsidies have risen substantially since the past 5 years to approximately $160,090 per anesthetizing location. Extrapolating based on the previous 2008 study, it is estimated that U.S. hospitals with more than 25 beds pay well over $158 billion in anesthesiology subsidies annually (Health Performance Strategies, 2012).

From the 20,000 foot view, scrutiny of the cost of various anesthesia delivery models suggests that CRNA-only anesthesia is the most economically viable under the widest range of conditions and case volumes. Analysis of claims data to compare the cost of providing anesthesia by provider type and by delivery model demonstrates that CRNAs deliver quality care most cost-effectively when compared with medically directed or anesthesiologist-only services. CRNAs are also the most cost-effective providers regarding the cost to educate. The total estimated expense of preanesthetic and anesthetic graduate education for a CRNA is $161,809, whereas for an anesthesiologist it is $1,063,795 (Hogan, Seifer, & Moore, 2010).

Complete transparency of anesthesia workforce practices and billing is necessary to capture the anesthesia care experience at a granular level. Often what happens in the operating room stays behind closed doors, and policy makers do not realize the reality of how the operating room functions. Systematic monitoring of the safety and quality of care, measured against prices, costs, and work effort of various providers, reduces waste and rewards high-value care while eliminating duplication of services.

Chronic Pain Management

Contemporary challenges to CRNA practice are neither new nor unexpected. For nearly a decade, organized medicine has attempted to restrict CRNA scope of practice, control the anesthesia market through supervision and other requirements, and limit the reimbursement for CRNA services. Facing health policy problems head-on has profound effects, with long-lasting impact beyond present-day concerns. Surgery and pain management are inflection points where patients can emerge healthier than before, and CRNAs are facilitators of that process. For the greatest good of the public, it is critical to ensure that patients continue to have access to CRNA pain care that is known to be of high quality, to cost less than alternatives, and to be offered in their home community. This second case study speaks to strategies and interventions in health care policy advocacy relative to CRNAs' role in chronic pain management.

Chronic pain management is an evolving field that deals with the treatment of intractable pain, generally of duration beyond what is expected based on the patient's condition. On January 1, 2013, Medicare implemented a final rule that reinforced, and in some cases restored, the long-standing policy of directly reimbursing CRNAs for chronic pain management services. The story of this recent challenge to CRNA scope of practice and reimbursement, including the historical context, policy foundation, and political strategy, provides a captivating example of the effective use of timing, data, and coalition building to accomplish health policy goals. In this case, the goal of nurse anesthesia is the goal of APRNs as articulated by the Institute of Medicine (IOM): nurses should practice to the full extent of their education/training (IOM, 2010).

On March 17, 2011, Noridian Administrative Services (Noridian) issued a bulletin entitled "CRNA Practice and Chronic Pain Management" notifying providers and the public that as a Medicare Administrative Contractor (MAC), Noridian would cease the practice of reimbursing CRNAs for chronic pain management services. Noridian's policy would have the effect of reducing or eliminating access to treatment for unrelenting chronic pain experienced by many Medicare beneficiaries, particularly in rural areas and in frontier states. Under the direction of a new Noridian Medical Director for Part B reimbursement, the bulletin took the position that CRNAs were not adequately trained to provide chronic pain management services, thus making an unfounded distinction between other related services such as acute pain management and the delivery of chronic pain care. Within months, a second MAC, Wisconsin Physician

Services, Inc. (WPS), issued a similar bulletin borrowing heavily from the language used in the Noridian statement.

A local coverage determination (LCD) is a decision about whether a contractor cover a particular service; it delineates the circumstances under which the service is considered reasonable and necessary (USDHHS, CMS, 2012b, Ch. 13, §13.1.3). From a policy perspective, the Noridian notices had the same impact as an LCD, yet there was no opportunity for comment as is required when an LCD is released. CMS directs that LCDs "shall be based on the strongest evidence available" (USDHHS, CMS, 2012b, Ch. 12, §13.7.1), yet Noridian and WPS issued denials of payment without any evidence base for these decisions in terms of quality, outcomes, access, or cost.

For more than 2 decades, Medicare law had supported reimbursement of chronic pain management services administered by CRNAs as permitted by the state law. The Social Security Act recognizes CRNAs, Nurse Practitioners, and Clinical Nurse Specialists as providers of "medical and other health services" (42 U.S.C. § 1395x[s], 2011). The Omnibus Reconciliation Act of 1986 (Public Law 99-509) called for direct payment for the services of a CRNA under Medicare Part B, beginning in 1989. The Medicare regulation implementing the law states, "Medicare Part B pays for anesthesia services and related care furnished by a CRNA who is legally authorized to perform the services by the State in which the services are furnished" (42 CFR § 410.69[a]).

The *Medicare Claims Processing Manual* provides further guidance on what is meant by "related care," stating that "[p]ayment can be made for medical or surgical services furnished by non-medically directed CRNAs if they are allowed to furnish those services under State law. These services may include . . . pain management. . . . Payment is determined under the physician fee schedule" (USDHHS, CMS, 2012a, Ch. 12, 140.4.3). Medicare does not make a distinction between "chronic pain management" and "acute pain management" when referring to "related services" or "medical and surgical services" that CRNAs are authorized to provide and be paid for. "Pain management" is an intentionally broad term, encompassing all pain management services that CRNAs are permitted to furnish under state law. The term "pain management" is not defined anywhere in statutes, regulations, or regulatory guidance.

Through these citations, it is clear that Medicare policy provided for the coverage of pain management services provided by CRNAs without physician supervision.

> Anesthesia service furnished by CRNAs can be medically directed or non-medically directed, but related care services are medical or surgical services, not anesthesia procedures, and are therefore not subject to the general medical direction rules." "Payment for related care services furnished by CRNAs on or after January 1, 1992 will be consistent with payment for physicians." "We will recognize separate payment for the same related care services furnished by anesthesiologists or CRNAs. (Part B and Other Services Payment, 1992)

At various points, Medicare states that payment for related care services furnished by a CRNA is consistent with payment for a physician and that separate payment is recognized for the same related care services whether furnished by anesthesiologists or CRNAs. As previously mentioned, the hospital Conditions of Participation for anesthesia services under Part A require physician supervision of CRNAs for "anesthesia services" (unless a state has opted out). There is no Part A or Part B requirement for physician supervision of CRNAs providing "medical or surgical" services such as pain management, insertion of Swan–Ganz catheters, central venous pressure lines, emergency intubation, or the preanesthetic examination and evaluation of a nonsurgical patient.

When Noridian and WPS ceased payment for CRNA pain services, they questioned aspects of pain care relative to the scope of practice of CRNAs. The question of scope is rightfully within the authority of each state, not the authority of an insurance company or Medicare. The federal statute is clear on the role of state law in determining CRNA scope of practice. "The term 'services of a certified registered nurse anesthetist' means anesthesia and related care furnished by a certified nurse anesthetist . . . which the nurse anesthetist is authorized to perform as such by the State in which the services are furnished" (42 U.S.C. § 1395x[bb][1], 2011). States define the scope of practice in general terms to allow for the evolution of patient needs, health care technology, and professional education over time. The states in these jurisdictions permitted and in some cases required a CRNA to perform a thorough diagnostic assessment and develop a treatment plan—the very things that the MAC said CRNAs were not qualified to do. Medicare law makes clear that CRNAs may be reimbursed for pain management services if they are allowed to furnish those services under the state law.

The linkage between pain practice and core competencies is delineated in the national standards set forth by the AANA, the COA, and the NBCRNA. CRNAs' specialized training in pain management is recognized in nurse anesthesia program accreditation standards (COA, 2016b), the scope of practice (AANA, 2013b), position statements (AANA, n.d.-a, n.d.-b, n.d.-c, 2016a), and guidelines for core clinical privileges (AANA, 2013b).

To be certified, a CRNA must have graduated from a nationally accredited program whose curriculum includes training to develop pain-management skills. This rigorous graduate-level curriculum includes content in pain management, anatomy, pharmacology, chemistry, biochemistry, physics, patient assessment, and advanced principles of anesthesia practice. Student nurse anesthetists complete a minimum of 550 clinical cases, including the full scope of procedures, techniques, and specialty practice caring for patients with all comorbidities and levels of risk. The average student graduates with over 100 clinical cases in regional anesthesia (NBCRNA, 2014).

The NCSBN considers CRNAs, Nurse Practitioners, and Clinical Nurse Specialists all to be APRNs, "licensed independent practitioners who are expected to practice within standards established or recognized by a licensing body," recognizing the CRNA for pain management and anesthesia-related skills (NCSBN, 2008). The American Nurses Association supports CRNA pain practice, stating that "through extensive approved continuing education programs, CRNAs further advance and refine their skills in all areas of practice including pain management. CRNAs' authority to make independent professional judgments and utilize multiple anesthetic techniques including all forms of regional techniques…is critical to meeting a vast array of chronic pain management and surgical needs at a reasonable cost" (*Spine Diagnostic Center of Baton Rouge v. Louisiana State Board of Nursing*, 2008).

Pain medicine is an evolving field with rapid advances in technology, pharmacology, and imaging propelling the specialty forward at lightning speed. The education and skills required to administer many chronic pain management procedures are based on the same foundation as those that CRNAs use every day as they perform various blocks for surgical and labor analgesia. With the advent of high-tech imaging and new approaches, advances in the pain specialty are happening at an increasing speed. Contemporary pain practice was unknown as recently as 20 years ago, a reality that requires every pain practitioner to keep up with workshops, fellowships, hands-on coursework, and wet-lab experiences. CRNAs who specialize in pain management are held to the same standard of professional accountability as any CRNA; that is, to maintain competency relative to their practice specialization.

ACCESS, COST, AND QUALITY IMPERATIVES

There are compelling policy considerations in favor of CRNA-provided chronic pain care and elimination of physician supervision in all practice settings, both public and private. Chief among these are access to care in rural and frontier communities and reducing health care cost while maintaining or improving the quality of care. Pain care in the United States provides an exemplary for examining the access, cost and quality imperatives for CRNAs as APRNs.

These issues were addressed in the 2011 IOM report to Congress, which the PPACA required, in recognition of chronic pain's growing impact on the Americans and on the economy. This report estimates that 100 million American adults suffer from chronic pain at the cost of more than $650 billion per year. The report notes that "a number of barriers . . . including regulatory, legal, institutional, financial and geographic . . . limit the availability of pain care" (IOM, 2011). According to survey data, 3,360 CRNAs indicated that they specialize in pain management and the same year, the American Board of Anesthesiology (ABA) recognized 3,900 physicians as pain subspecialists. The number of pain management specialists is inadequate to meet this public health challenge.

In many rural and frontier areas, Medicare beneficiaries must travel hundreds of miles to access alternative care, and CRNAs often are the only health care professionals trained in pain management in these communities. In these cases, referring practitioners choose to refer their patients to CRNAs for high-quality pain care, and patients choose to receive their care from a CRNA in their local community rather than travel long distances. This practice is the essence of patient-centered care: providing services where and by whom the patient selects. Without the CRNAs to administer chronic pain management services, Medicare beneficiaries in vast rural and frontier areas would lose access to vital treatment, which could result in poor health care outcomes, lower quality of life, and unnecessary costs to patients, Medicare, and the health care system. According to a case study analysis by the Lewin Group (2012), using real-life situations of four individuals living in rural communities representing different geographic locations throughout the United States, the direct medical costs of alternatives such as surgery or nursing home care range from 2.3 times to more than 150 times the cost of a CRNA providing these services in the community. By choosing not to reimburse CRNAs for pain care, Noridian and WPS were limiting or eliminating access to legitimate pain specialists and requiring beneficiaries to seek other more costly, more inconvenient, and in some cases, more dangerous alternatives.

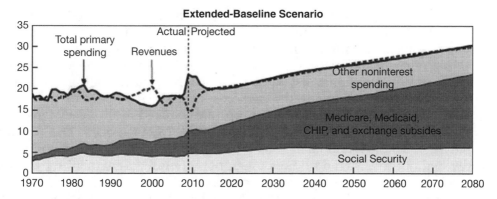

FIGURE 33.4 Federal health care spending impact on federal budget projections.

CHIP, Children's Health Insurance Program.

Another important health care policy consideration is the economics of chronic pain management provided by CRNAs. At a time when there is national concern about the cost of federal health care spending (Figure 33.4), the economics of reimbursement for CRNA-provided services versus more expensive physician-provided services cannot be overlooked. It is more economical for a facility to employ a CRNA than a physician when both possess the requisite training and skills. CRNAs typically provide anesthesia services at the lowest economic cost and do not require subsidization from the health care facility (Hogan et al., 2010).

This case study is an excellent example of why APRNs such as CRNAs must become involved in policy development. The rationale for such sponsorship lies beyond protecting reimbursement and scope of practice. Advanced practice nursing advocacy is essential to ensuring access to quality care for patients and reducing health disparities.

What accounts for the fact that nurse anesthetists are recognized as leaders in health care advocacy and influence? Much of the explanation can be found in the growing power of public opinion, brought about by the spread of education, communication technology, mass media, and professional organizations—all of which have heightened recognition of the benefits of CRNA care regarding cost, quality, and access. For APRNs, outcomes and core competencies are linked to professional practice at a level that is significantly distinguishable from registered nurse practice even at the expert level. As a result, APRNs must invest heavily in health policy development at a personal and a professional association level.

The AANA adopted a two-pronged approach to support access to CRNA pain care. Coined Protect My Pain Care, this initiative was built on a foundation of a tactical team and a strategic group. The strategic group met monthly to provide the 30,000-foot view, evaluating results of efforts to date, changing direction or cadence when needed, and staying focused on progress toward meeting goals and objectives. The tactical team met weekly to update operational activities, including grassroots action, grass tops activity (large organizations), public relations and communication, state support, research, legislative impact, and regulatory influence.

Through essential work of the tactical team, Protect My Pain Care employed devices such as the establishment of an online micro-site for patients and providers. The group enlisted the support of the community of interest such as AARP, the National Rural Health Association, and many state boards of nursing and state hospital associations. The tactical team oversaw a grassroots campaign of CRNAs, referring physicians, patients, and their families who wrote more than 4,000 letters in support of CRNA-provided pain care. The Lewin Group published case studies showing the high cost of alternative pain care without CRNAs. Democratic and Republican groups participated in focus sessions that provided insights into the importance of having the right to choose one's health care provider. Through the tactical team advocacy work, legislators and their staff reached out to CMS and others to support continued payment for CRNA pain services to protect their home state citizens.

At the request of this network of stakeholders, including professional organizations, patients, hospitals, and physicians, access to pain care by CRNAs was protected. The Medicare agency published a final rule on November 1, 2012, stating that "Anesthesia and related care means those services that a certified registered nurse anesthetist is legally authorized to perform in the state in which the services are furnished." The agency noted in its descriptive preamble, "we agree with commenters that the primary responsibility for establishing the scope of services CRNAs are sufficiently trained and thus should be authorized to furnish, resides with the states."

In doing so, the Medicare agency maintained a consistent national policy authorizing direct reimbursement of chronic pain management services provided by CRNAs, as well as adjunct imaging, and Evaluation and Management Services that nurse anesthetists are allowed to furnish under state law. CMS removed regulatory barriers to access for CRNA pain care and deferred to states for the scope-of-practice decisions. Noridian's and WPS's decision to withhold payment for CRNA chronic pain management services was overturned.

EVALUATION

Although health care costs continue to grow at an unsustainable rate, Congress and health care policy makers continue to seek ways to make health care work better, cost less, be more accessible to patients, and be of higher quality. Landmark research and advisory papers published over time underscore the value of CRNAs in promoting crucial societal goals. This scientific evidence base has been a powerful foundation for actions, interventions, and strategies aimed at developing robust health care policy. Key studies and papers are summarized in the following paragraphs.

Numerous research studies have found no significant differences among nurse anesthetists in mortality or anesthesia complications (Hoffman, Thompson, Burke, & Derkay, 2002; Needleman & Minnick, 2008; Pine, Holt, & Lou, 2003; Simonson, Ahern, & Hendryx, 2007). The quality of care by all anesthesia providers is excellent, resulting in a very low incidence of anesthesia-related morbidity or mortality. Although these previous studies have demonstrated the high quality of nurse anesthesia care, the results of a 2010 study published in *Health Affairs* (Dulisse & Cromwell, 2010) led researchers to recommend that costly and duplicative supervision requirements for CRNAs should be eliminated. The study analyzed outcome by type of professional and found that there are no differences in patient outcomes based on whether a CRNA delivered the anesthesia without physician supervision, an anesthesiologist delivered it, or a CRNA supervised by an anesthesiologist did. The study compared anesthesia patient outcomes (mortality and complications) in 14 states that opted out of the Medicare physician supervision requirement for CRNAs from 2001 to 2005 with those that did not opt out. As of 2013, 17 states have opted out. From a population-health perspective, the researchers found that anesthesia has continued to grow safer in opt-out and non-opt-out states alike. There was no difference in outcomes in the states that had opted out when compared to the states that had not. Based on the evidence contained in this study, the authors concluded that "we recommend that CMS allow certified registered nurse anesthetists in every state to work without the supervision of a surgeon or anesthesiologist" (Dulisse & Cromwell, 2010, p. 1469). Reviewing the study, the *New York Times* stated, "In the long run, there could also be savings to the health care system if nurses delivered more of the care" ("Who Should Provide Anesthesia Care?," 2010).

Among all anesthesia delivery models, nurse anesthesia care is 25% more cost-effective than the subsequent least costly model, according to a Lewin Group study published in *Nursing Economic$* (Hogan et al., 2010). Based on claims data, researchers determined that CRNAs practicing independently were the lowest cost to the private payer. As CRNAs safely provide the full range of anesthesia services, the use of additional duplicative supervision represents additional health care cost that can be saved or allocated elsewhere in the health system, while maintaining a high standard of quality and patient safety. The authors also compared the marginal cost of preanesthesia and anesthesia graduate education between nurse anesthetists and anesthesiologists. The total estimated direct costs of education and clinical experience before anesthesia education and during anesthesia graduate education were found to be $161,809 for a CRNA and $1,083,795 for an anesthesiologist (Hogan et al., 2010, p. 168). As both CRNAs and anesthesiologists provide high-quality care using the same skill set and techniques for all types of surgical procedures and all categories of patients, the contrasting cost to society of training these two categories of anesthetists gives pause during times of fiscal uncertainty.

To ensure patient access to high-quality care, a 2010 IOM report, *The Future of Nursing,* recommended that APRNs should be able to practice to the full extent of their education and training (IOM, 2010). By eliminating regulatory and other policy barriers to the use of APRNs, including CRNAs, the health care system makes the most efficient use of the available workforce of health care professionals. This ensures patient access to high-quality care and promotes local control of health care delivery.

ETHICAL CONSIDERATIONS

At this point, it is helpful to explore the relationship between the economics of health care and ethical practices in the health care system. Why do policies continue over time although they are wasteful and there are better alternatives? A practical recommendation to reduce the unsustainable rising health care costs is to incorporate evidence-based decision making when creating health care policy. A case in point includes requirements for physician supervision that have no evidence base or the promulgation of regulations that make it more difficult for lower-cost providers to give needed pain care.

The standard response to health care needs in the United States is more: more highly trained physician specialists and more access to top technology. After more than a century of progress in education, pharmaceuticals, and technology, resulting in huge gains in patient safety, as a country, we have failed to articulate a health care delivery system that is efficient and cost-effective.

Health care coverage must be affordable and sustainable for society. Health care policy should promote access to high-quality care that is effective, efficient, safe, timely, patient-centered, and equitable (IOM Committee on Consequences of Uninsurance, 2004). These societal needs support the premise that all health care providers should practice at the top of their education, training, and license.

In the conceptual framework of bioethics, questions concerning access to health care are directly related to principles of justice. Justice in this context relates to whether people who require services receive them. Concepts of fairness, health care services as a "right," and availability of these resources to those who need them come into play. Case in point: pain in America is a compelling health care challenge. Disparities in access to care, the severity of suffering, and the cost to society are just a few of the contributing factors. There are substantial differences in pain prevalence and rates of undertreatment in vulnerable populations. Access to pain care is far from equitable. Race and ethnicity, geographic variation, and education and income impact availability of pain care. Attempts to prevent qualified pain care providers, such as nurse anesthetists, from delivering needed care to vulnerable populations legitimately raise the question of justice.

Do nurse anesthetists have any obligation to improve the health care system? The Code of Ethics for the CRNA requires that nurse anesthetists fulfill an individual, professional responsibility to society in "promoting community and national efforts to meet the health needs of the public" (AANA, 2013a). CRNAs have an obligation to try to change the system as a part of their duty to patients. Despite the explosion in knowledge, innovation, and capacity to manage catastrophic conditions, the U.S. health care system "falls short on such fundamentals as quality, outcomes, cost, and equity" (IOM, 2012).

FUTURE OF NURSE ANESTHESIA

Despite the many accomplishments of the profession of nurse anesthesia to date, there is much more to be done in the future. The need still exists in the profession to transform practice. CRNAs should practice to the full extent of their education and training. Obstacles to accomplishing this goal remain at the federal and state levels in the form of outdated statutes, rules, and regulations that are based on historical politics rather than a base of evidence. Despite the armed services usage of CRNAs in their full practice roles, the VA's failure to eliminate physician supervision for CRNAs must still be addressed. On the reimbursement front, barriers still exist to CRNA practice, particularly at the state and local health care plan levels. In 2013, the AANA began a program of state reimbursement advocacy with the establishment of the State Reimbursement Specialist (SRS) program. The SRS serves as a coordinator of contacts with state reimbursement decision makers and is the clearinghouse for all information regarding state health plan reimbursement, including private plans, federal and state exchanges, Medicaid plans, and the MACs. In the coming years, this program will develop to be a powerful strategic tool as more reimbursement battles shift from the federal to the state level.

In the future, the nurse anesthesia profession must continue to evolve in transforming the education of the CRNAs. Nurse anesthetists must achieve high levels of education and training, evolving to the minimal standard of a doctoral degree by the year 2025. There has been a strong movement in this direction, and efforts must not get sidetracked along the way. To accomplish this goal, current faculty must return to obtain their doctoral degrees in large numbers, and educational programs must design flexible curricula that accommodate the needs of working professionals using advanced technology and innovative teaching approaches. Lifelong learning is moving to a continuing competency model that includes competency-based modular offerings as well as interval testing. The area of pain management holds tremendous promise for the nurse anesthesia profession to take a leading role in designing comprehensive pain care education that follows the holistic model put forth by the IOM in the 2012 report *Pain in America* (IOM, 2012). Through these efforts and others, the profession of nurse anesthetist can remain at the forefront of advancing nursing education for the future.

There is a great opportunity for nurse anesthetists to become full partners with physicians and other health professionals in redesigning health care and the health care system. With their advanced education and expert clinical knowledge, nurse anesthetists are prime candidates to assume leadership roles in health care systems and the university setting. The profession needs to accelerate efforts to advance the placement of CRNAs on decision-making boards and regulatory bodies to contribute the special expertise of nurse anesthetists to the advancement of an imaginative and successful future for our country's health care system.

To accomplish this future vision, the profession of nurse anesthesia, in collaboration with the accrediting body and the certification/recertification board, must seek to strengthen data integrity relative to the CRNA workforce, anesthesia and pain care quality outcomes, and the best educational approaches. Effective workforce planning and policy making require an improved information infrastructure. Although there is strong evidence demonstrating the quality of nurse anesthesia practice, the cost advantage of nurse anesthesia care, and the reach of nurse anesthetists in providing access to disparate populations, it is not enough. There are many questions that remain to be answered, and the profession must step up to the plate in a leadership role to contribute to this essential body of knowledge.

There are still many opportunities for nurse anesthesia leadership in addressing these pressing challenges and contributing to the betterment of society. CRNAs, working through the professional association, can facilitate the use of evidence-based clinical practice guidelines in anesthesia and pain management practice. Nurse anesthetists must engage in lifelong learning, accessing, managing, and applying new evidence to deliver safe care. CRNAs must find ways to fully involve patients for a truly patient- and family-centered approach to anesthesia and pain care. As payment models shift to reward desired care outcomes, payment models will change, and CRNAs must be ready for plan designs that support high quality, team-based care. The profession of nurse anesthetist must increase the availability of information about the quality, cost, and outcomes of their care, with full transparency for payers and decision makers. Nurse anesthetists have always been leaders in nursing and the health professions as a whole. Concepts of continuous learning and quality improvement must be incorporated into professional education, certification, and accreditation requirements. The imperatives are clear, but the roadmap has yet to be drawn.

CONCLUSION

CRNAs, and all APRNs, have a key role to play in the development of our nation's health care policy. CRNA's superior knowledge and skill in anesthesia and pain care makes them uniquely qualified to improve the health care system for their patients and society. With greater education comes greater responsibility, and nurse anesthetists are well positioned to use their significant talents for the greater good of society's health care delivery system.

As clinical experts, as educators, as administrators, and as researchers, CRNAs must use their experience at the leading edge of patient care to drive change that is needed. Throughout their history to the present, nurse anesthetists have been defined by providing access to excellent quality care at less cost than alternative providers. The success of the nurse anesthetist profession during times of crisis is well-documented, and the contributions during times of war well recognized.

Every nurse anesthetist must become involved, at some level, in influencing health care reform. Advocacy may involve writing a letter or sending an e-mail to a member of Congress, making an appointment in the district to meet with a legislator, or attending a town hall meeting in the community. CRNAs may become involved in lobbying days in their state or Washington, DC. Nurse anesthetists must build strong relationships on both sides of the aisle as an investment in the future. Attend conferences to stay current on key issues for the profession or make a contribution to the political candidate of their choice is a form of personal advocacy. State nurse anesthesia associations welcome volunteers with interest in government relations. At the national level, the AANA offers many opportunities for leadership, including becoming a Federal Political Director or a State Reimbursement Director or joining the CRNA-PAC Committee. With 90% of nurse anesthetists belonging to the professional association, CRNAs have a high level of engagement and a high level of responsibility. Beneficial change to the anesthesia delivery system requires attention by CRNAs through focused advocacy, education, and research. Nurse anesthetists must be willing to challenge the system when it is in patients' best interests to do so while understanding that health care spending competes with other important needs of society, and efforts to reduce costs mean better access to care for all. The future is bright for this storied profession as health policy incentives align to reward the value that CRNAs bring to the patient experience.

DISCUSSION QUESTIONS

1. *Three examples are provided in this chapter that describes major policy changes related to nurse anesthesia practice. Compare these three initiatives regarding the end result being a success, a compromise, or a failed initiative? Analyze the*

context for each example to provide a hypothesis for the reason that the outcome was achieved. What gaps were present in the advocacy strategy for each example? What is the impact of the outcome on cost, quality, and access to anesthesia services?

2. *Anesthesia care is safer than ever in the history of the specialty. In the advent of new anesthesia techniques, drugs, and enhanced training, anesthesia mortality risk has declined 100-fold to less than one in 100,000, according to recent studies. What are the implications of this improvement in outcomes for health care policy relative to nurse anesthetists? How does the increase in safety relate to advocacy efforts?*

ANALYSIS, SYNTHESIS, AND CLINICAL APPLICATION

1. *Synthesize the lessons learned from the regulatory experience with physician supervision to analyze the issue of nondiscrimination as it relates to scope of practice. The Affordable Care Act (Sec. 1206) contains a "nondiscrimination" provision that prohibits health plans from discriminating against qualified health care providers by licensure. Where are the likely sources of opposition to the language? What arguments could be made against the nondiscrimination provision? What bullet points would you make if asked to provide a written comment during the notice-and-comment rule-making process by CMS?*

EXERCISES/CONSIDERATIONS

1. *Challenges to advanced nursing practice will continue as economic pressure increases and changes in health care policy advance. Compare and contrast the advantages and disadvantages using advanced practice nurses from (a) the physician perspective, (b) societal perspective, (c) the health care institution perspective, and (d) the patient perspective.*

ETHICAL CONSIDERATIONS

1. *A bill has been introduced that allows payment for telemedicine supervision of nurse anesthetists in rural hospitals. Discuss this proposal regarding the ethical considerations for health care sustainability. Develop a strategy for advocacy to address this proposal and describe the following: a community of interest, opponents and supporters, key talking points, and elements of a media plan.*

REFERENCES

American Association of Nurse Anesthetists. (n.d.-a). About us. Retrieved from http://www.aana.com/aboutus/Pages/default.aspx

American Association of Nurse Anesthetists. (n.d.-b). Certified registered nurse anesthetists at a glance. Retrieved from http://www.future-of-anesthesia-care-today.com/pdfs/CRNAs_At_A_Glance.pdf

American Association of Nurse Anesthetists. (n.d.-c). Qualifications and capabilities of the certified registered nurse anesthetist. Retrieved from http://www.aana.com/ceandeducation/becomeacrna/Pages/Qualifications-and-Capabilities-of-the-Certified-Registered-Nurse-Anesthetist-.aspx

American Association of Nurse Anesthetists. (2011). Member profile survey 2011. Unpublished data.

American Association of Nurse Anesthetists. (2013a). Code of ethics for the certified registered nurse anesthetist. Retrieved from http://www.aana.com/resources2/professionalpractice/Documents/PPM%20Code%20of%20Ethics.pdf

American Association of Nurse Anesthetists. (2013b). Guidelines for core clinical privileges for certified registered nurse anesthetists. Retrieved from http://www.aana.com/resources2/professional practice/Pages/Guidelines-for-Core-Clinical-Privileges.aspx

American Association of Nurse Anesthetists. (2013c). Scope of nurse anesthesia practice. Retrieved from http://www.aana.com/resources2/professionalpractice/Documents/PPM%20Scope%20 and%20Standards.pdf

American Association of Nurse Anesthetists. (2016a). A holistic approach to pain management: Integrated, multimodal, and interdisciplinary treatment [Position statement]. Retrieved from http://www .aana.com/resources2/professionalpractice/Pages/A-Holistic-Approach-to-Pain-Management .aspx

American Association of Nurse Anesthetists. (2016b). Certified registered nurse anesthetists fact sheet. Retrieved from http://www.aana.com/ceandeducation/becomeacrna/Pages/Nurse-Anesthetists-at-a-Glance.aspx

Baldy, J. M. (1908). The nurse as an anesthetist. *American Journal of Nursing, 8,* 979–982.

Blumenreich, G. A. (2000). Supervision. *AANA Journal, 68*(3), 404–408.

Chalmers-Francis v. Nelson, 6 Cal. 2d 402 (1936).

Conditions for Payment: Medically Directed Anesthesia Services, 42 C.F.R. § 415.110 (2001).

Council on Accreditation of Nurse Anesthesia Educational Programs. (2016a). About COA. Retrieved from http://home.coa.us.com/about/Pages/default.aspx

Council on Accreditation of Nurse Anesthesia Educational Programs. (2016b). Standards for accreditation of nurse anesthesia educational programs. Retrieved from http://home.coa.us.com/ accreditation/Documents/2004%20Standards%20for%20Accreditation%20of%20Nurse%20 Anesthesia%20Educational%20Programs,%20revised%20June%202016.pdf

Council on Accreditation of Nurse Anesthesia Educational Programs. (2017a). List of accredited educational programs. Retrieved from http://home.coa.us.com/accredited-programs/Documents/ LOAP%20June%202017.pdf

Council on Accreditation of Nurse Anesthesia Educational Programs. (2017b). List of accredited fellowships. Retrieved from http://home.coa.us.com/accredited-programs/Documents/LOAF%20 August%202017.pdf

Dulisse, B., & Cromwell, J. (2010). No harm found when nurse anesthetists work without supervision by physicians. *Health Affairs, 29*(8), 1469–1475.

Epstein, R., & Dexter, F. (2012). Influence of supervision ratios by anesthesiologists on first-case starts and critical portions of anesthetics. *Anesthesiology, 116,* 683–691. Retrieved from http://anesthesiology. pubs.asahq.org/article.aspx?articleid=2443431

Frank v. South, 175 Ky. 416, 194 S.W. 375 (1917).

Health Performance Strategies. (2012). *Anesthesia subsidy surveys* (pp. 1–8). Ft. Lauderdale, FL: Author.

Hoffman, K., Thompson, G., Burke, B., & Derkay, C. (2002). Anesthetic complications of tympanostomy tube placement in children. *Archives of Otolaryngology Head & Neck Surgery, 128*(9), 1040–1043.

Hogan, P., Seifer, R., & Moore, C. (2010). Cost effectiveness analysis of anesthesia providers. *Nursing Economic$, 28*(3), 159–169.

Horowitz, J. (2016) Want to save a quick 20 billion in healthcare? *The Hill.* Retrieved from http://thehill .com/blogs/pundits-blog/healthcare/306639-want-to-save-a-quick-20-billion-in-healthcare

H.R.5985—The Department of Veterans Affairs Expiring Authorities Act of 2016. (2016). Retrieved from https://www.congress.gov/bill/114th-congress/house-bill/5985

Institute of Medicine. (2010). *The future of nursing: Leading change, advancing health.* Washington, DC: National Academies Press.

Institute of Medicine. (2011). *Relieving pain in America: A blueprint for transforming prevention, care, education, and research.* Washington, DC: National Academies Press.

Institute of Medicine. (2012). *Best care at lower cost: The path to continuously learning health care in America.* Washington, DC: National Academies Press.

Institute of Medicine, Committee on Consequences of Uninsurance. (2004). *Insuring America's health: Principles and recommendations.* Retrieved from http://nationalacademies.org/hmd/ reports/2004/insuring-americas-health-principles-and-recommendations.aspx

Joint Dialogue Group. (2008). The consensus model for APRN regulation: Licensure, accreditation, certification, and education. Retrieved from https://www.ncsbn.org/aprn.htm

Koch, E. (1999). Alice Magaw and the great secret of open drop anesthesia. *AANA Journal, 67*(1), 33–38. [Includes a reprint of Magaw's article "A review of over fourteen thousand surgical anesthesias."]

The Lewin Group. (2012). Cases: Costs of alternative pain management paths. Retrieved from http://www.lewin.com/s~/media/Lewin/Site_Sections/Publications/CRNAPainMgt CaseStudies.pdf

Li, G., Warner, B., & Lang, B., (2009). Epidemiology of anesthesia-related mortality in the United States, 1999–2005. *Anesthesiology, 110*(4), 759–765.

Macario, A. (2010). What does one minute of operating room time cost? *Journal of Clinical Anesthesia, 22*(4), 233–236.

Marshall, Steele, & Associates. (2013). Operating room efficiency program. Retrieved from http://www .marshallsteele.com/OREfficiencyProgramOverview.pdf

National Board of Certification and Recertification of Nurse Anesthetists. (2014). Summary of NCE and SEE performance and clinical experience September 1, 2013 through August 31, 2014. Retrieved from https://www.nbcrna.com/certification/SiteAssets/Pages/Program-Administration/ NCESEE_AnnualSummary2015_0115.pdf

National Board of Certification and Recertification of Nurse Anesthetists. (2015). *Annual report.*

National Board of Certification and Recertification of Nurse Anesthetists. (2016a). Mission and vision. Retrieved from http://www.nbcrna.com/about-us/Pages/Mission_Vision_ValueStatements .aspx

National Board of Certification and Recertification of Nurse Anesthetists. (2016b). CPC program/ recertification. Retrieved from http://www.nbcrna.com/cpc/Pages/default.aspx

National Council of State Boards of Nursing. (2008). The consensus report. Retrieved from https://www .ncsbn.org/FINAL_Consensus_Report_070708_w._Ends_013009.pf

National Council of State Boards of Nursing. (2016). Consensus model implementation status. Retrieved from https://www.ncsbn.org/5397.htm

Needleman, J., & Minnick, A. (2008). Anesthesia provider model, hospital resources, and maternal outcomes. *Health Services Research, 44,* 464–482.

Nightingale, F. (1863). *Notes on hospitals: Preface.* London, UK: Longman, Green, Longman, Roberts and Green.

Omnibus Budget Reconciliation Act of 1986, Pub. L. No. 99–509.

Part B and Other Services Payment (57 Fed. Reg. 33878 et seq., July 31, 1992).

Patient Protection and Affordable Care Act. (2010). Pub. L. No. 111–148, §2702, 124 Stat. 119, 318–319. Retrieved from http://www.gpo.gov/fdsys/pkg/BILLS-111hr3590enr/pdf/BILLS-111hr3590enr.pdf

Pine, M., Holt, K., & Lou, Y. (2003). Surgical mortality and type of anesthesia provider. *AANA Journal, 71*(2), 109–116.

Porter, R. (2001). *The Cambridge illustrated history of medicine* (p. 206). New York, NY: Cambridge University Press.

Services of a certified registered nurse anesthetist or an anesthesiologist's assistant: Basic rule and definitions, 42 C.F.R. § 410.69 (2011).

Simonson, D., Ahern, M., & Hendryx, M. (2007). Anesthesia staffing and anesthetic complications during cesarean delivery: A retrospective analysis. *Nursing Research, 56*(1), 9–17.

62 Fed. Reg. 4674 (January 18, 2001) (to be codified at 42 CFR Parts 416, 482, and 485).

62 Fed. Reg. 56762 (November 13, 2001) (to be codified at 42 CFR Parts 416, 482, and 485).

Spine Diagnostic Center of Baton Rouge v. Louisiana State Board of Nursing. (2008). Docket No. 09 C 1444, Supreme Court of Louisiana, Brief of Amici Curiae by the American Nurses Association, Louisiana State Nurses Association, Louisiana Alliance of Nursing Organizations in Support of the Application for Writ of Certiorari Filed by the Louisiana State Board of Nursing through the Louisiana Department of Health and Hospitals and the Louisiana Association of Nurse Anesthetists.

Sudlow, L. L. (2000). *A vast army of women: Maine's unaccounted forces in the American Civil War.* Gettysburg, PA: Thomas Publications.

The professional anaesthetizer. (Editorial). (1897). *Medical Record (NYC), 51,* 522. 18.

Thatcher, V. S. (1953). *History of anesthesia with emphasis on the nurse specialist.* Philadelphia, PA: J. B. Lippincott.

42 U.S.C § 1395x(s)(11) (2011).

42 U.S.C. § 1395x(bb)(1) (2011).

U.S. Department of Labor, Bureau of Labor Statistics. (2016). Nurse Anesthetists, Nurse Midwives, and Nurse Practitioners. *Occupational Outlook Handbook, 2016–17 Edition.*, Retrieved from https://www.bls.gov/ooh/healthcare/nurse-anesthetists-nurse-midwives-and-nurse-practitioners.htm

U.S. Department of Health and Human Services, Centers for Medicare and Medicaid Services. (2012a). *Medicare claims processing manual* [Pub. 100-04]. Retrieved from https://www.cms.gov/Regulations-and-Guidance/Guidance/Manuals/Internet-Only-Manuals-IOMs-Items/CMS018912.html

U.S. Department of Health and Human Services, Centers for Medicare and Medicaid Services. (2012b). *Medicare program integrity manual* [Pub. 100-08]. Retrieved from https://www.cms.gov/Regulations-and-Guidance/Guidance/Manuals/Internet-Only-Manuals-IOMs-Items/CMS019033.html

U.S. Department of Health and Human Services, Centers for Medicare and Medicaid Services. (2013). CMS Manual System Pub 100-04 Medicare Claims Processing Centers Transmittal 2716. Retrieved from https://www.cms.gov/Regulations-and-Guidance/Guidance/Transmittals/Downloads/R2716CP.pdf

U.S. Department of Health and Human Services, Health Care Financing Administration. (1998). Medicare program: Revisions to payment policies and adjustments to the relative value units under the physician fee schedule for calendar year 1999. *63 Fed. Reg. 58843*, Nov. 2, 1998.

U.S. Department of Veterans Affairs. (2016). Advanced practice registered nurses. Retrieved from https://www.federalregister.gov/documents/2016/12/14/2016-29950/advanced-practice-registered-nurses

Who should provide anesthesia care? (2010, September 6, Opinion Section). *New York Times*. Retrieved from http://www.nytimes.com/2010/09/07/opinion/07tue3.html?_r=0

Yox, S. B., Stokowski, L. A., McBride, M., & Berry, E. (2016). *Medscape ARPN salary report 2016*. Retrieved from http://www.medscape.com/features/slideshow/aprn-salary-report?src=WNL_specrep_nursesalary_161213_MSCPEDIT_aprn&uac=142362HX&impID=1252731&faf=1#page=1

CHAPTER 34

Advocacy, Policy, and Politics in Action: A Case in Point—Full Scope of Practice Within the VA Health System

Christine S. Zambricki

Building on the previous chapter's overview of health care policy and nurse anesthesia, this chapter presents a final case study, describing the efforts to incorporate full practice authority for all Advanced Practice Registered Nurses (APRNs) within the Veterans Health Administration (VHA) Handbook. In contrast to the examples of success outlined in the prior chapter, this VA story provides a concrete example of how an advocacy initiative may be decided on politics rather than policy merits.

Despite months of coordinated efforts in the legislative, regulatory, research, grassroots, and grasstops arenas, in the end, the politics of physician opposition proved formidable and the final rule did not include CRNAs for full scope-of-practice authority within the VA hospital system. Certified Registered Nurse Anesthetists (CRNAs) were excluded from the rule. CRNAs were the only group of APRNs excluded from the rule. A historical perspective of the context and the activities of various stakeholders involved in this rocky multiyear journey will prove informative.

In 2012, the VA Office of Nursing Services (ONS) highlighted the goal that APRNs will function as independent licensed professionals regardless of the state in which they were licensed (ONS, 2012), a recommendation of the Advanced Practice Nursing Advisors (APNA) structure within the VA health system. The APNA's role within the VA structure is to establish, implement, and evaluate the strategic plan for APRNs in the VA serving in an advisory capacity for strategic planning, issues, and activities such as privileging, role utilization, scope of practice, recruitment and retention, and prescriptive authority.

Subsequently, the American Association of Nurse Anesthetists (AANA) met with Chief Nursing Officer Cathy Rick, RN, PhD, NEA-BC, FACHE, FAAN, to learn more about the proposed change and how nurse anesthetists could support this mutual goal. While the intent was to reduce variability in practice across the entire VA health care system and to increase Veteran patients' access to care, an overarching goal for both the U.S. Department of Veterans Affairs, Office of Nursing Services and the AANA was to achieve alignment with key recommendations from the Institute of Medicine (IOM) relative to the future of nursing (IOM, 2010). The ONS was updating the VHA Nursing Handbook in early 2013. Dr. Rick was confident that these changes would be incorporated into the revisions because support was building within the VA system to do so. APRN practice had been advancing in all of the armed services and the VA was next in line.

Shortly before the changes to the handbook were to be finalized, the American Society of Anesthesiologists (ASA) became aware of the proposed revisions and actively lobbied to pull it back from the brink. The ASA began amassing congressional friends in opposition, AANA did the same, and "Dear Colleague" letters from both sides were sent to the Secretary, ultimately canceling each other out. As the year progressed, organized medicine became aware of the proposed changes and the ASA joined the American Medical Association and a host of other national physician organizations, as well as 43 state medical societies and associations in asking the Veterans Health Administration (VHA) to put the changes on hold before finalizing the draft version of the Nursing Handbook. By fall of 2013, physician opposition had coalesced, resulting in 66 medical organizations penning a letter on October 28, 2013, to Robert Petzel, MD, VA Undersecretary for Health, urging that the handbook ensure support of physician-led health care teams and state-based licensure.

In 2014, the VHA scandal broke. The press was awash with reports of a pattern of negligence in the treatment of United States military veterans. The public consciousness was raised, and policy makers were suspicious of any policy that might appear to compromise the care of veterans. The Nursing Handbook revisions were put on hold.

VA leadership changed. In June 2014, the department announced several changes aimed at accelerating veterans' access to quality health care and rebuilding their trust in the system. Dr. Carolyn Clancy was named Interim Undersecretary for Health to help get the VHA back on track. She would serve in this capacity until a new undersecretary was named. Carolyn Clancy, MD, would replace Robert Jesse, MD, PhD, as acting Undersecretary for Health. Dr. Jesse had assumed the position following the resignation of Robert Petzel, MD. In the midst of heated controversy over the proposal designating APRNs as independent practitioners, Dr. Clancy, with 23 years of distinguished service at the federal Agency for Healthcare Research Quality, supported the changes and had signed off on the revisions to the Nursing Handbook.

Meanwhile, the fight migrated to the congressional halls. Committees of jurisdiction held hearings. Grassroots campaigns raged. The ASA was very effective in engaging highly vocal and passionate supporters on the Hill. With 17 physicians in Congress and huge political action committee (PAC) coffers, every time that Dr. Shulkin testified before a congressional committee he was attacked with vehement diatribe regarding the proposed changes to the Nursing Handbook as it related to CRNAs. Ultimately, everyone just wanted it to be over; the issue became a hot-button that wore down staff in offices that supported the change. The message was that the VA had done bad things to veterans, and now they wanted to have anesthesia provided by nurses.

In March 2015, leadership changed again at the VA. Robert A. MacDonald was confirmed as Secretary of Veterans Affairs and Dr. David J. Shulkin was appointed VHA Undersecretary for Health. Dr. Clancy returned to her position as VA Assistant Deputy Undersecretary for Health for Quality, Safety and Value.

With new leadership at the VA, the message and the approach took a new direction. The issue of APRN full scope of practice was removed from the Nursing Handbook revision process and would be considered on its own within the administrative rulemaking process. At the same time, the terminology changed from Licensed Independent Practitioner (LIP) to full practice providers.

On September 1, 2015, RAND Corporation issued a report to the U.S. Department of Veterans Affairs titled Independent Assessment of the Health Care Delivery System and Management Processes of the Department of Veterans Affairs (RAND, 2015). With accessibility and timeliness of care as long-standing areas of concern within the VA, the Veterans Access, Choice and Accountability Act of 2014 Section 201 had called for this independent assessment. RAND cited a shortage of specialty providers within the VA, including those in anesthesiology. The report identified 14 comments discussing the lack of anesthesia service/support as a barrier to providing care, including for urgent cases such as cardiovascular surgery as well as nonurgent procedures such as endoscopy and colonoscopy. While the researchers sparingly mentioned the use of nurse anesthetists, they did refer to a 2010 study in which no harm was found when nurse anesthetists worked without supervision by a physician that analyzed 7 years of Medicare data (Dulisse & Cromwell, 2010). In the final recommendation of this study, Dulisse wrote, "Based on our findings, we recommend that (Centers for Medicare and Medicaid services) allow certified registered nurse anesthetists in every state to work without the supervision of a surgeon or anesthesiologist."

On May 25, 2016, the VA issued a proposed rule to amend the VA medical regulations to permit full practice authority of four roles of VA APRNs including CRNAs (Federal Register, 2016) when they were acting within the scope of their VA employment. The VA provided a 60-day comment period. On May 29, 2016, in a very unusual next step, the VA Office of Public and Intergovernmental Affairs issued a press release in which Dr. Shulkin stated that the VA did not seek to change the VA policy on the role of CRNAs (Office of Public and Intergovernmental Affairs, 2016). During the ensuing comment period from May through July 2016, the VA received 223,296 comments on the proposed rule. Over 104,000 of those comments were opposed to giving CRNAs full practice authority and 46,000 comments expressed support of CRNAs being allowed to work autonomously.

The Federal Trade Commission (FTC) commented in support of the proposed rule. The FTC has historically been in favor of APRNs working to the full extent of their education and training and believed that the impact of the regulation on competition in the private sector would ultimately benefit consumers. The FTC's main interest was the extent to which the VA action would yield information about new models of care delivery and broaden the availability of health care services nationwide.

Meanwhile the grassroots, grasstops, and legislative advocacy raged on. The comment period was marked by intensive lobbying, more letters and phone calls to Members of Congress, and more letters and phone calls to the VA from members of Congress. Hearings were held by the Committees of Jurisdiction. Both the AANA and the ASA were able to get bills introduced to show that there was congressional support for their position. Both sides launched huge campaigns that were successful in getting veterans and their families, as well as veterans' organizations, to weigh in with support for their respective positions.

Within the AANA, every bit of focus was on this issue. The AANA grassroots effort was in full swing, with over 100 local veterans groups supporting full practice rights as well as local American Legions and Gold Star Mothers. The AANA launched a huge media campaign in DC and ran ads on veterans' sites all over the country, resulting in thousands of veterans writing in support. CRNAs who are veterans contacted the organizations that they were part of and got their support. The grassroots campaign included all aspects of social media incorporating campaign hashtags, tele town halls for AANA members, and digital ads. The AANA developed a microsite.

Specific veterans' communities were targeted by zip code around military bases and hospitals. When all was said and done, the AANA achieved 50% to 60% participation of its 50,000 members in this effort.

The ASA opted to go through the appropriations process, pushing for language in the final report that provided full scope for Nurse Practitioners (NPs), Clinical Nurse Specialists (CNSs), and nurse midwives and excluding CRNAs. The AANA found themselves in a very hard battle, as some of the nurse anesthetists' congressional friends signed on to the bill thinking they were being supportive. The physicians were able to engage Members of Congress emotionally to a greater extent than the CRNAs, resulting in very negative comments in committee, angry and emotional exchanges, and even boos on the house floor. At the final moment, the anti-CRNA language was removed from the Appropriations Report, and the resulting neutral language was claimed as a victory by both sides. On Memorial Day and July 4, the ASA was on the national mall obtaining signatures on petitions that were later submitted as public comments to the proposed rule. The ASA put conducted surveys and published survey results with little traction. Accurate cost and access data were difficult to obtain by either side. The ASA also set up a microsite "Protect SafeVACare."

Throughout this process, the nursing coalition remained strong and refused to fragment. The AANA and other nursing organizations established a microsite called Veteransaccesstocare.org. The NPs kicked in a really effective TV campaign. The American Nurses Association had close ties with the White House. Despite pressure to break away from the CRNAs, the nursing community did not support any legislative language unless it contained all four APRN groups. The nursing coalition held weekly calls and the AANA held daily meetings with their internal government affairs team and weekly calls with strategy teams including state government affairs and the practice division. The AANA Federal Political Directors in every state achieved goals for numbers of letters and calls, and developed a phone tree that was used to contact every AANA member in every state.

On June 30, 2016, the Commission on Care published its Final Report. Congress had created a Commission on Care in response to the scandal over VHA employees' manipulation of the data systems to cover up long appointment scheduling delays. The Commission on Care was charged with reviewing the congressionally mandated comprehensive independent assessment of VHA care delivery and management systems, to examine access to care and to evaluate how veterans' care should be organized and delivered over the next 2 decades.

In the midst of the comment period on the proposed rule, the Commission on Care recommended that clinical operations be enhanced through more effective use of health professionals—particularly optimizing the use of APRNs. With less than 2 weeks to go before the comment period closed, the Commission's recommendation supported the proposed rule to grant direct access to VA APRNs. The Commission deliberations were informed by the Independent Assessment Report, 26 days of public meetings, testimony from a broad range of experts and stakeholders, site visits, and their recommendations submitted to the President in accordance with the Veterans Access, Choice, and Accountability Act of 2014 (Commission on Care, 2016).

Following the end of the comment period, the VHA APRN Full Practice Authority proposed a final rule that was moved to the White House Office of Management and Budget (OMB), Office of Information and Regulatory Affairs for final review. This action must take place prior to the final publication of rules in the Federal Register. The VA's proposal to provide veterans direct access to care provided by NPs and other APRNs in VA facilities had taken another critical step forward. The OMB had up to 90 days to review the proposed final rule, after which they must either publish a final rule in the Federal Register or return it to the VA for revision. During this time, opponents in the physician community continued to take steps to derail the implementation. New legislation to prohibit the implementation of the proposed VA rule relating to practice authority of APRNs was introduced in the House of Representatives and ultimately failed to move forward. With the new administration coming in mid-January, there was also concern that delaying publication of the final rule might allow the new administration to put a hold on or cancel the APRN provision prior to its publication as a final rule.

On September 29, 2015, language contained in early versions of H.R.5985—the Department of Veterans Affairs Expiring Authorities Act of 2016, which is mainly a funding bill extending the VA's authority to collect co-payments for nursing home care, and extending authority for several pilot programs—prevented the VA from assigning any independent anesthetist duties to CRNAs. However, due to strong lobbying by the nursing organizations during the legislative process, that provision was removed from the final version of the law, which passed Congress and was presented to the White House.

The final rule was published on December 13, 2016. The VA will allow three types of NPs—Certified Nurse Practitioner (CNP), CNS, and Certified Nurse-Midwife (CNM)—"to practice to the full extent of their education, training and certification, without the clinical supervision or mandatory collaboration of physicians," according to the new rule slated to take effect from January 13. CRNAs were the only group of APRNs excluded from the rule (U.S. Department of Veterans Affairs, 2016).

The VA stated that their position to not include CRNAs in the final rule did not stem from CRNAs' inability to practice to the full extent of their professional competence, but rather from VA's lack of access problems in the area of anesthesiology. The VA requested further comment on whether there are access issues or other unconsidered circumstances that might warrant their inclusion in a future rulemaking. In the final rule, the VA acknowledged that there are difficulties hiring and retaining anesthesia providers, but described the situation as improving. The final rule cites the fact that in fiscal years 2011 through 2015, CRNAs were in the top 10 VHA Occupations of Critical Need, and they are in 12th place in fiscal year 2015. Despite projection forecasts cited in the RAND study of a 19% increase in demand for VA health care services nationwide from FY2014 to FY2019, the VA still concluded that allowing CRNAs to practice to the full extent of their training would not improve access to care.

The issue of full practice authority for CRNAs within the VA system remains for future rulemaking. The addition of nurse anesthetists to this regulation would have wide-ranging benefits to the VA health system. First and foremost, eliminating supervision of CRNAs would establish a model of care in which one anesthesia provider cares for one patient, eliminating the cost of expensive anesthesia providers whose only job is "supervising" other qualified anesthesia providers and who do not give anesthesia themselves. This model would result in significant cost savings and preempt any future workforce shortages. Continued supervision causes delays in operating room function and pays two people for one job. The removal of supervision requirements for nurse anesthetists will give veterans better access to more health care professionals for anesthesia services and critical pain management services. One of many areas in which they could provide help is the opioid epidemic—the overuse of morphine-like drugs that produce euphoric side effects for those in chronic pain, which some veterans are afflicted by.

When the rule was finalized on December 13, 2016, it drew more than 5,000 comments on both sides of the issue. It remains to be seen whether the VA will do the right thing for veterans anesthesia care in future rulemaking. In retrospect and despite a yeoman's collective effort of multi-modal advocacy, it is clear that organized nursing could have done more. The issue became much bigger than the VA rule and thus required many years of building high-level relationships with the majority party in order to achieve success. In the end, all of the arguments made for and against did not decide the issue.

This last advocacy example is a perfect exemplar of a resolution that is purely political for an issue that no one wanted to touch due to the intense passion and partisan nature of the participants. At one point in the midst of heated arguments, the VA Undersecretary for Health testified that he did not want to pass this issue along to the next undersecretary. In the end that is exactly what happened with the proviso that if access problems arise, they can change it in the future.

Postmortem. Fast forward to November 2016 and the newly elected president appoints this same Dr. David Shulkin, Undersecretary for Health, as the secretary of VA and a member of the new president's cabinet. This denouement provides yet one more kernel of truth to the age-worn admonition "Don't burn bridges—you'll be surprised how many times you'll have to cross the same water."

DISCUSSION QUESTIONS

1. *How has increased interprofessional practice among APRNs and other practitioners resulted in improved health outcomes for patients, families, and communities?*
2. *How can health coaches and community workers affect the practice of APRNs?*
3. *Is a transition to practice residency really necessary for APRNs, especially since research shows good health outcomes of APRNs who never had such a residency?*
4. *Are there any practice barriers in your state and if so what are they and what does this mean for your practice?*
5. *What reason(s) might an APRN choose to earn a PhD over a DNP?*

ANALYSIS, SYNTHESIS, AND CLINICAL APPLICATION

1. *Interview leaders in your state or district's Action Coalition and analyze the extent to which your state has implemented any or all of the eight recommendations of* The Future of Nursing *report.*
2. *Interview an APRN who works in a NHMC about his/ her practice in relation to the eight recommendations of* The Future of Nursing *report. Ask them their concerns about the health of the community in which they serve and what their ideas are to promote the health of their community.*
3. *Find an APRN who is racially/ethnic neither white nor a female and ask them what (if any) the barriers were for them to become an APRN. Ask them how their diversity enhances their nursing practice.*
4. *What are several ways you can enhance your cultural competencies? Why does this matter?*

EXERCISES/CONSIDERATIONS

1. *APRNs will have to learn ways of increasing interprofessional practice, especially if their state allows independent practice.*
2. *APRNs will increasingly be asked to extend their practices by engaging in trans disciplinary teams such as including community health workers.*
3. *APRNs will increasingly work with registered nurses in increasingly complex care environments in the ambulatory setting.*
4. *APRNs will increasingly use telehealth to manage patients with chronic illness, engage in "hospital at home" programs, provide consultation, determine if patients are appropriate for transfer, and improve access to palliative care consultations and services.*
5. *APRNs will increase their engagement in population/preventive health measures.*

REFERENCES

Commission on Care. (2016). Final report: A missed opportunity. Retrieved from https://cv4a.org/commission-care-final-report-missed-opportunity

Dulisse, B., & Cromwell, J. (2010). No harm found when nurse anesthetists work without supervision by physicians. *Health Affairs, 29*(8), 1469–1475.

Federal Register. (2016). Advanced practice nurses. A proposed rule by the Veterans Affairs Department. Retrieved from https://www.federalregister.gov/documents/2016/05/25/2016-12338/advanced-practice-registered-nurses

Institute of Medicine. (2010). *The future of nursing: Leading change, advancing health.* Washington, DC: National Academies Press.

Office of Nursing Services, Veterans Administration Health Care. (2012). *Annual report 2012: VA Nursing: Shaping healthcare from the veteran patient's perspective.* Retrieved from https://www.va.gov/nursing/docs/2012onsannualrptweb.pdf

Office of Public and Intergovernmental Affairs, Veterans Administration. (2016). Press release. Retrieved from https://www.va.gov/opa/pressrel/pressrelease.cfm?id=2793

RAND. (2015). Independent assessment of the health care delivery systems and management processes of the Department of Veterans Affairs. Retrieved from http://www.va.gov/opa/choiceact/documents/assessments/Assessment_B_Health_Care_Capabilities.pdf

U.S. Department of Veterans Affairs. (2016). *Advanced practice nurses. Final rule.* Retrieved from https://www.gpo.gov/fdsys/pkg/FR-2016-12-14/pdf/2016-29950.pdf

Health Policy Acronyms

ACA	Affordable Care Act
ACP	advance care planning
ACI	advancing care information, also see meaningful use
ACO	accountable care organization, also see MSSP
AENT	Advanced Education Nursing Traineeships
AHRQ	Agency for Healthcare Research and Quality
ANET	Advanced Nursing Education Traineeship
APM	Alternative Payment Model;
Advanced APM	Advanced Alternative Payment Model
APTC	advanced premium tax credit
ASC	ambulatory surgery center
ASPE	[Office of the] Assistant Secretary for Planning and Evaluation
AUC	Appropriate Use Criteria B
AV	actuarial value
BHP	Bureau of Health Professions
BPCI	Bundled Payments for Care Improvement Initiative
CAC	Certified Application Counselor
CAH	critical access hospital
CAHPS	Consumer Assessment of Healthcare Providers and Systems
CAMH	CMS Alliance to Modernize Healthcare
CAP	Consumer Assistance Program
CCIIO	Center for Consumer Information and Insurance Oversight
CCM	chronic care management
CCNA	Center to Champion Nursing in America
CDC	Centers for Disease Control and Prevention
CEHRT	Certified Electronic Health Record Technology
CFR	Code of Federal Regulations
CHC	community health center
CHIP	Children's Health Insurance Program
CIN	clinically integrated network
CJR	Comprehensive Care for Joint Replacement Model
CME	continuing medical education
CMMI	Centers for Medicare and Medicaid Innovation (Innovation Center)

CMS	Centers for Medicare and Medicaid Services
COB	coordination of benefits
COBRA	Consolidated Omnibus Budget Reconciliation Act
CO-OP	Consumer Operated and Oriented Plan
CoP	conditions of participation
CPC+	Comprehensive Primary Care Plus
CPCI	Comprehensive Primary Care Initiative
CPI	consumer price index
CPR	Coalition for Patients' Rights
CPIA	clinical practice improvement activities
CPS	composite performance score
CPT	current procedural terminology
CSR	cost-sharing reduction
CQM	clinical quality measure
CY	calendar year
DEA	Drug Enforcement Agency
DME	durable medical equipment
DOJ	Department of Justice
DRG	diagnosis-related group
DSH	disproportionate share hospital
eCQM	electronically specified clinical quality measure
ECP	essential community provider
EHB	essential health benefits
EHR	electronic health record
E&M	Evaluation and Management Services
EMR	electronic medical record
EOB	explanation of benefits
EPs	eligible professionals
EPO	exclusive provider organization
EPSDT	early periodic screening, diagnostic & treatment services
ERISA	Employee Retirement Income Security Act
ESI	employer-sponsored insurance
eRx	electronic prescribing
FDA	Food and Drug Administration
FEHBP	Federal Employees Health Benefits Program
FFM/FFE	Federally Facilitated Marketplace/ Federally Facilitated Exchange
FFS	fee-for-service
FPL	federal poverty level
FQHC	Federally Qualified Health Center
FQHC-APCP	Federally Qualified Health Center, Advanced Primary Care Practice
FSA	flexible spending account
FTC	Federal Trade Commission
FY	fiscal year
GAO	Government Accountability Office
GINA	Genetic Information Nondiscrimination Act
GME	graduate medical education
GNE	graduate nursing education
GPCI	geographic practice cost index

GPRO	Group Practice Reporting Option
HAC	hospital-acquired condition
HAI	hospital-associated infection
HCBS	home and community-based services
HCC	hierarchical condition categories
HCFA	Health Care Financing Administration
HCFAC	Health Care Fraud and Abuse Control
HCPCS	Healthcare Common Procedure Coding System
HCPLAN	Health Care Payment Learning and Action Network
HCR	health care reform
HDHP	high-deductible health plan
HEDIS	Healthcare Effectiveness Data and Information Set
HIE	Health Information Exchange
HIPAA	Health Insurance Portability and Accountability Act of 1996
HIM/HIX	health insurance marketplace/health insurance exchange
HIT	health information technology
HITECH	Health Information Technology for Economic and Clinical Health Act
HPHS	high-performing health system
HPSA	health professional shortage area
HHS	Department of Health and Human Services
HMO	health maintenance organization
HOPD	hospital outpatient department
HPSA	health professional shortage area
HRP	high-risk pool
HRSA	Health Resources and Services Administration
HSA	health savings account
IAH	Independence at Home (demonstration project)
ICD-10-CM	International Classification of Diseases, 10th Revision, Clinical Modification
ICU	intensive care unit
IDS	integrated delivery system
IHI	Institute for Healthcare Improvement
IMPACT	Improving Medicare Post-Acute Care Transformation Act of 2014
IOASE	in-office ancillary services exception
IOM	Institute of Medicine (now called NAM)
IPAB	Independent Payment Advisory Board
IPPS	Medicare Hospital-Inpatient Prospective Payment System
IT	information technology
JNC	Joint National Committee on Prevention, Detection, Evaluation, and Treatment of High Blood Pressure (now in its eighth publication)
LCD	local coverage determination
LTC	long-term care
LTCH	long-term care hospital
LTSS	long-term social services
MA	Medicare Advantage
MAC	Medicare Administrative Contractor
MACPAC	Medicaid and CHIP Payment and Access Commission

MACRA	Medicare Access and CHIP Reauthorization Act of 2015
MAGI	modified adjusted gross income
MCO	managed care organization
MDH	Medicare-dependent hospitals
MDP	measure development plan
MedPAC	Medicare Payment Advisory Commission
MEI	Medicare Economic Index
MHI	mental health integration
MIPPA	Medicare Improvements for Patients and Providers Act of 2008
MIPS	Merit-Based Incentive Payment System
MLR	minimum loss rate
MMA	"Medicare Modernization Act" or the Medicare Prescription Drug, Improvement, and Modernization Act of 2003
MPAPC	Multi-Payer Advanced Primary Care Practice Model
MPFS	Medicare Physician Fee Schedule
MSMG	multi-specialty medical group
MSPB	Medicare Spending per Beneficiary
MSSP	Medicare Shared Savings Program, also known as the ACO program
MTM	Medication Therapy Management
MU	meaningful use of certified EHR technology
MUA	medically underserved area
NAM	National Academy of Medicine (former IOM)
NAT	nurse anesthesia traineeships
NCQA	National Committee for Quality Assessment
NHLBI	National Heart, Lung and Blood Institute
NHSC	National Health Service Corps
NIH	National Institutes of Health
NMHC	nurse-managed health clinics
NNCC	National Nursing Centers Consortium
NPI	National Provider Identifier
NPP	National Priorities Partnership
NPRM	notice of proposed rule making
NQF	National Quality Forum
NQS	National Quality Strategy
NTA	Nurse Training Act
OAA	Older Americans Act (1965-reauthorized in 2016)
OCM	Oncology Care Model
OCR	Office for Civil Rights
OECD	Organization for Economic Co-Operation and Development
OEP	open enrollment period
OIG	Office of the Inspector General
OMB	Office of Management and Budget
ONC	Office of the National Coordinator for Health Information Technology
OON	out of network
OOP	out of pocket
OPPS	[Medicare Hospital] Outpatient Prospective Payment System
PBM	pharmacy benefit manager
PCMH	patient-centered medical home

PCORI	Patient-Centered Outcomes Research Institute
PCHH	Primary Care Health Home
PDP	Prescription Drug Plan under Medicare Part D
PECOS	Medicare Provider Enrollment, Chain and Ownership System
P4P	pay for performance
PFPMs	physician-focused payment models
PFS	Physician Fee Schedule
PGP	Physician Group Practice (demonstration project)
PHS	Public Health Service
PMPM	per-member/per-month
POS	Point-of-Service Plan
PPACA	Patient Protection and Affordable Care Act
PPI	Public Policy Institute (within AARP)
PPO	preferred provider organization
PQRS	Physician Quality Reporting System (CMS)
PTAC	Professional and Technical Advisory Committee
QA	quality assurance
QCDR	Qualified Clinical Data Registry
QE	qualified entity
QHP	Qualified Health Plan
QI	quality improvement
QIO	Quality Improvement Organization
QPP	Quality Payment Program
QRUR	Quality and Resource Use Reports
QSEN	Quality and Safety Education for Nurses
RAC	recovery audit contractor
RBRVS	resource-based relative value scale
RUC	AMA/Specialty Society, Relative Value Update Committee
RVU	relative value unit
SAMHSA	Substance Abuse and Mental Health Services Administration
SBC	summary of benefits and coverage
SBM/SBE	state-based marketplace/state-based exchange
SCHIP	State Children's Health Insurance Program (see CHIP)
SEP	special enrollment period
SGR	sustainable growth rate
SHIPS	State Health Insurance Programs
SHOP	Small Business Health Options Program
SNF	skilled nursing facility
SNP	Special Needs Plan
SPM/SPE	State Partnership Marketplace/ State Partnership Exchange
SPP	specialty pharmacy provider
SSA	Social Security Administration
SSDI	Social Security Disability Income
SSI	supplemental security income
TANF	Temporary Assistance for Needy Families
TCPI	transforming clinical practice initiative
TERFA	Tax Equity and Fiscal Responsibility Act (of 1982)
TIN	tax identification number

TMA	transitional medical assistance
TPA	third-party administrator
UCR	usual, customary and reasonable charges
UHC	universal health coverage
URAC	an accreditation and benchmarking agency (like NCQA)
USDHHS	U.S. Department of Health and Human Services
VBP	hospital value-based purchasing
VM	value-based payment modifier

Index